TENTH EDITION

ZOLLINGER'S ATLAS OF SURGICAL OPERATIONS

E. Christopher Ellison, MD, FACS

Interim Dean and Robert M. Zollinger Professor of Surgery and Distinguished Professor
The Ohio State University College of Medicine and Wexner Medical Center
Columbus, Ohio

Robert M. Zollinger, Jr., MD, FACS

Professor Emeritus, Department of Surgery, Case Western Reserve
University School of Medicine and University Hospitals
Clinical Professor of Surgery, University of Arizona College of Medicine
Formerly, Instructor in Surgery, Harvard Medical School and the Peter Bent Brigham Hospital
Tuscon, Arizona

ILLUSTRATIONS FOR TENTH EDITION BY
Marita Bitans

ILLUSTRATIONS FOR PREVIOUS EDITIONS BY
**Marita Bitans, Jennifer Smith, Carol Donner,
Mildred Codding, Paul Fairchild, and William Ollila**

Mc
Graw
Hill
Education

New York   Chicago   San Francisco   Lisbon   London   Madrid   Mexico City
Milan   New Delhi   San Juan   Seoul   Singapore   Sydney   Toronto

Zollinger's Atlas of Surgical Operations, Tenth Edition

1 2 3 4 5 6 7 8 9 0 DSS/DSS 20 19 18 17 16

ISBN: 978-0-07-179755-9
MHID: 0-07-179755-6

NOTICE

Medicine is an ever-changing science. As new research and clinical experience broaden our knowledge, changes in treatment and drug therapy are required. The authors and the publisher of this work have checked with sources believed to be reliable in their efforts to provide information that is complete and generally in accord with the standards accepted at the time of publication. However, in view of the possibility of human error or changes in medical sciences, neither the authors nor the publisher nor any other party who has been involved in the preparation or publication of this work warrants that the information contained herein is in every respect accurate or complete, and they disclaim all responsibility for any errors or omissions or for the results obtained from use of the information contained in this work. Readers are encouraged to confirm the information contained herein with other sources. For example and in particular, readers are advised to check the product information sheet included in the package of each drug they plan to administer to be certain that the information contained in this work is accurate and that changes have not been made in the recommended dose or in the contraindications for administration. This recommendation is of particular importance in connection with new or infrequently used drugs.

This book was set in Minion Pro by Aptara, Inc.
The editors were Brian Belval and Christie Naglieri.
The production supervisor was Richard Ruzycka.
Project management was provided by Nomeeta Devi, Aptara, Inc.
The cover designer was Dreamit, Inc.
RR Donnelley/Shenzhen was printer and binder.

Library of Congress Cataloging-in-Publication Data

Ellison, E. Christopher, author.
  Zollinger's atlas of surgical operations / E. Christopher Ellison, Robert
M. Zollinger, Jr. ; illustrations for tenth edition by Marita Bitans ;
illustrations for previous editions by Marita Bitans, Jennifer Smith, Carol
Donner, Mildred Codding, Paul Fairchild, and William Ollila. – Tenth
edition.
      p. ; cm.
  Atlas of surgical operations
  Includes bibliographical references and index.
  ISBN 978-0-07-179755-9 (hardcover) – ISBN 0-07-179755-6 (hardcover)
  I. Zollinger, Robert Milton, Jr., 1934- , author. II. Title. III. Title:
Atlas of surgical operations.
  [DNLM: 1. Surgical Procedures, Operative–Atlases. WO 517]
  RD41
  617.9'1–dc23
                                                    2015034896

McGraw-Hill books are available at special quantity discounts to use as premiums and sales promotions, or for use in corporate training programs. To contact a representative, please e-mail us at bulksales@mcgraw-hill.com.

CONTENTS

PREFACE

Some 75 years ago, this ATLAS was created to document proven and safe operative techniques in common use by general surgeons. Many improvements and changes have occurred in the previous nine editions including use of stapled techniques for gastrointestinal anastomoses and minimally invasive surgery. These two techniques were joined in full flower in the ninth edition wherein what was once considered advanced laparoscopic techniques in the 1990s is now in common use and taught as essential elements in most surgical residency training programs.

In this new 10th edition several important improvements have been made. We have engaged Associate Editors as content experts who have helped identify new procedures that should be included and who have made significant improvements to existing content. Nineteen new surgical operations have been added. These include eight procedures that we think are essential to the practice of general surgery including axillary lymphadenectomy, insertion of a CAPD catheter, fasciotomy, escharotomy, insertion of an inferior vena caval filter, ventral hernia repair using the technique of open component parts separation, ureter repair, and basic thoracoscopy. In addition we have included four additional complex gastrointestinal procedures namely laparoscopic esophageal myotomy, sleeve gastrectomy for morbid obesity, transhiatal esophagectomy and transthoracic esophagectomy. The vascular surgery section now contains new variations on femoral thrombectomy, femorofemoral bypass, saphenous vein laser ablation, and thrombectomy of the superior mesenteric artery. Finally we added laparoscopic hand-assisted donor nephrectomy and kidney transplantation.

A major editorial reorganization has also occurred with the addition of 18 Associate Editors whose special expertise has been channeled into discrete body system–oriented chapters. This reorganization should make it easier to find operations whose titles no longer use roman numerals. The authors and the associate editors have critically reviewed and updated this entire 10th edition. The scientific content of all operative procedures from indications through postoperative care have been made current with significant improvements in about 50 chapters of text and art.

During the preparation of the 10th edition we received valuable input from Brian Belval at McGraw Hill and Donna Sampsill in the Department of Surgery at The Ohio State University. In the ninth edition, color processing and printing technology had advanced such that our medical illustrators, could add color to both old and new plates for improved anatomic clarity in more lifelike or realistic settings. For this 10th edition our medical illustrator, Marita Bitans, has prepared new artwork plates in high definition color with computer-generated graphics that now replace the original pen and ink sketches using white chalk scratch board.

We have also created an online Historical Supplement available at **www.ZollingersAtlas.com** to provide open access to many now historical operations that over the last 70 years have been deleted from succeeding editions of the ATLAS. Many were replaced by newer procedures often involving modern technologies such as stapling, laparoscopy, or minimally invasive image-guided procedures. Others were rarely performed and a few were eliminated because of evolving indications. Additionally, in the past the authors and artists had page limitations imposed by the mechanical construction of the folio-sized ATLAS and the capacity of its binding. That is to say, heavily coated paper stock was needed for quality art reproduction and for the prevention of "strike through" of printed material on the backside of each page. The result was a restriction to about 500 pages—a size reached by the mid-1980s. At that point, the addition of any new or modern procedures such as stapling or laparoscopy required the pruning out of operations that (1) were rarely done—for example, portal/systemic shunts, or (2) were done by the increasing numbers of surgical specialists—for example, thoracic/pulmonary operations.

Furthermore, the authors and the publisher feel that many once popular operations should not be lost, but rather archived in this electronic Historical Supplement of the ATLAS where there are no page limitations. Many of these archived operations are still performed in specialized or complex situations because general surgeons by the nature of their practice, not infrequently encounter one of a kind events that are not in the text books. In these circumstances the surgeon must create an operative solution in real time. These solutions often rely upon general principles and experience, perhaps aided by one of these "old" operations. This may be particularly true in regions where expensive operative equipment such as staplers or disposable laparoscopic instruments are not available.

Today many medical libraries cannot afford to purchase and store all published texts, or even all the major printed medical journals. However, the internet is truly worldwide and accessible to almost all medical/surgical facilities and physicians. We trust this electronic Historical Supplement will help fill in some of the historical surgical technique reference gaps.

As Dr. Cutler graciously allowed his original coauthor to continue on after him, so my father did with me. Now it is my turn. Dr. E. Christopher Ellison has become the new lead principle author who will continue the ATLAS. Dr. Ellison is the other son of the Z-E syndrome. He is the Robert M. Zollinger Professor in the Department of Surgery at the Ohio State University Medical Center. He has accepted the primary responsibility for the ATLAS and its migration back to Columbus and the OSU Department of Surgery, where Dr. Zollinger Senior nurtured the ATLAS for over 40 years. Finally, of additional historic note, all of Dr. Zollinger's papers plus the text and artwork from all earlier editions are now archived in the Medical Heritage Center within the OSU Prior Health Sciences Library where these materials are catalogued and available online.

E. Christopher Ellison, MD
Robert M. Zollinger, Jr., MD

ASSOCIATE EDITORS

Doreen M. Agnese, MD, FACS
Skin, Soft Tissue, and Breast
Associate Professor of Clinical Surgery
The Ohio State University
College of Medicine and Wexner Medical Center
Columbus, OH

P. Mark Bloomston, MD, FACS
Gall Bladder, Bile Ducts, Liver, and Pancreas
Ft. Myers, FL

James H. Boehmler, IV, MD
Extremities
Georgetown, TX

William B. Farrar, MD, FACS
Skin, Soft Tissue, and Breast
Professor of Surgery
Dr. Arthur G. & Mildred C. James-Richard J.
Solove Chair in Surgical Oncology
The James Cancer Center Chair in Surgical Oncology
Director, The Stefanie Spielman Comprehensive Breast Center
The Ohio State University College of Medicine and Wexner Medical Center
Columbus, OH

Jeffrey M. Fowler, MD, FACS
Genitourinary
Gynecologic Procedures
Vice Chair and Professor
John G. Boutselis M.D. Chair in Gynecology
The Ohio State University College of Medicine and Wexner Medical Center
Hilliard, OH

Alan E. Harzman, MD, FACS
Small Intestine, Colon, and Rectal
Assistant Professor of Clinical Surgery
Director, General Surgery Residency Program
The Ohio State University College of Medicine and Wexner Medical Center
Columbus, OH

Jeffrey W. Hazey, MD, FACS
Hernia
Associate Professor of Surgery
Director, Division of General and Gastrointestinal Surgery
The Ohio State University College of Medicine and Wexner Medical Center
Columbus, OH

Robert S. D. Higgins, MD, MSHA, FACS
Thoracic Surgery
Transplantation
The William Stewart Halsted Professor
Chair and Surgeon-in-Chief
Johns Hopkins University School of Medicine Department of Surgery
Baltimore, MD

Larry M. Jones, MD, FACS
Skin and Soft Tissue
Professor of Clinical Surgery
The American Electric Power Foundation Chair in Burn Care
The Ohio State University College of Medicine and Wexner Medical Center
Columbus, OH

Gregory J. Lowe, MD
Genitourinary
Ureter Repair
Columbus, OH

W. Scott Melvin, MD, FACS
Esophagus and Stomach
Professor of Surgery
Vice Chairman for Clinical Surgery
Division Chief, General Surgery
Director, Advanced GI Surgery
Montefiore Medical Center/Albert Einstein College of Medicine
Bronx, NY

Susan Moffatt-Bruce, MD, PhD, FACS
General Abdomen and Thorax
Associate Professor of Surgery
Chief Quality and Patient Safety Officer
Associate Dean, Clinical Affairs for Quality and Patient Safety
The Ohio State University College of Medicine and Wexner Medical Center
Columbus, OH

Peter Muscarella, II, MD, FACS
Pancreas
Esophagus and Stomach
Associate Professor of Surgery
Montefiore Medical Center/Albert Einstein College of Medicine
Bronx, NY

Bradley J. Needleman, MD, FACS
Esophagus and Stomach
Associate Professor of Clinical Surgery
Medical Director, Comprehensive Weight Management and Bariatric
Surgery Center
Director, Center for Minimally Invasive Surgery
The Ohio State University College of Medicine and the Wexner Medical Center
Columbus, OH

Ronald P. Pelletier, MD, FACS
Genitourinary
Transplantation
Associate Professor of Surgery
Director, Kidney Transplantation
The Ohio State University College of Medicine and Wexner Medical Center
Columbus, OH

Kyle A. Perry, MD, FACS
Esophagus and Stomach
Associate Professor of Surgery
The Ohio State University College of Medicine and Wexner Medical Center
Columbus, OH

John E. Phay, MD, FACS
Endocrine
Head and Neck
Associate Professor of Clinical Surgery
The Ohio State University College of Medicine and Wexner Medical Center
Columbus, OH

Jean E. Starr, MD, FACS
Vascular Procedures
Associate Professor of Clinical Surgery
The Ohio State University College of Medicine and Wexner Medical Center
Columbus, OH

Patrick S. Vaccaro, MD, FACS
Vascular Procedures
Luther M. Keith Professor of Surgery
Division Director, Vascular Diseases & Surgery
The Ohio State University College of Medicine and Wexner Medical Center
Columbus, OH

COORDINATING EDITOR

Dennis E. Mathias
Publications Editor
Department of Surgery
The Ohio State University College of Medicine and Wexner Medical Center
Columbus, OH

SECTION I
BASICS

CHAPTER 1

SURGICAL TECHNIQUE

Asepsis, hemostasis, and gentleness to tissues are the bases of the surgeon's art. Nevertheless, recent decades have shown a shift in emphasis from the attainment of technical skill to the search for new procedures. The advances in minimally invasive techniques have allowed the surgeon great flexibility in the choice of operative techniques. Nearly all operations may be performed by an open or a minimally invasive laparoscopic technique. The surgeon must decide which approach is in the best interest of the individual patient. In addition, application of robotic surgery has added a new dimension to the surgical armamentarium. Throughout the evolution of surgery it has been recognized that faulty technique rather than the procedure itself was the cause of failure. Consequently it is essential for the the young, as well as the experienced surgeon, to appreciate the important relationship between the art of performing an operation and its subsequent success. The growing recognition of this relationship should reemphasize the value of precise technique.

The technique described in this book emanates from the school of surgery inspired by William Stewart Halsted. This school, properly characterized as a "school for safety in surgery," arose before surgeons in general recognized the great advantage of anesthesia. Before Halsted's teaching, speed in operating was not only justified as necessary for the patient's safety but also extolled as a mark of ability. Despite the fact that anesthesia afforded an opportunity for the development of a precise surgical technique that would ensure a minimum of injury to the patient, spectacular surgeons continued to emphasize speedy procedures that disregarded the patient's welfare. Halsted first demonstrated that, with careful hemostasis and gentleness to tissues, an operative procedure lasting as long as 4 or 5 hours left the patient in better condition than a similar procedure performed in 30 minutes with the loss of blood and injury to tissues attendant on speed. The protection of each tissue with the exquisite care typical of Halsted is a difficult lesson for the young surgeon to learn. The preoperative preparation of the skin, the draping of the patient, the selection of instruments, and even the choice of suture material are not so essential as the manner in which details are executed. Gentleness is essential in the performance of any surgical procedure.

Young surgeons have difficulty in acquiring this point of view because they are usually taught anatomy, histology, and pathology by teachers using dead, chemically fixed tissues. Hence, students regard tissues as inanimate material that may be handled without concern. They must learn that living cells may be injured by unnecessary handling or dehydration. A review of anatomy, pathology, and associated basic sciences is essential in the daily preparation of young surgeons before they assume the responsibility of performing a major surgical procedure on a living person. The young surgeon is often impressed by the speed of the operator who is interested more in accomplishing a day's work than in teaching the art of surgery. Under such conditions, there is little time for review of technique, discussion of wound healing, consideration of related basic scientific aspects of the surgical procedure, or the criticism of results. Wound complications become a distinct problem associated with the operative procedure. If the wound heals, that is enough. A little redness and swelling in and about wounds are taken as a natural course and not as a criticism of what took place in the operating room 3 to 5 days previously. Should a wound disrupt, it is a calamity; but how often is the suture material blamed, or the patient's condition, and how seldom does the surgeon inquire into just where the operative technique went wrong?

The following detailed consideration of a common surgical procedure, appendectomy, will serve to illustrate the care necessary to ensure successful results. Prior to the procedure, the verified site of the incision is marked with the surgeon's initials by the operating surgeon. Then the patient is transferred to the operating room and is anesthetized. The operating table must be placed where there is maximum illumination and adjusted to present the abdomen and right groin. The light must be focused with due regard for the position of the surgeon and assistants as well as for the type and depth of the wound. These details must be planned and directed before the skin is disinfected. A prophylactic antibiotic is administered within 1 hour of the skin incision and, in uncomplicated cases, is discontinued within 24 hours of the procedure.

The ever-present threat of sepsis requires constant vigilance on the part of the surgeon. Young surgeons must acquire an aseptic conscience and discipline themselves to carry out a meticulous hand-scrubbing technique. A knowledge of bacterial flora of the skin and of the proper method of preparing one's hands before entering the operating room, along with a sustained adherence to a methodical scrub routine, are as much a part of the art of surgery as the many other facets that ensure proper wound healing. A cut, burn, or folliculitis on the surgeon's hand is as hazardous as the infected scratch on the operative site.

The preoperative preparation of the skin is concerned chiefly with mechanical cleansing. It is important that the hair on the patient's skin is removed with clippers immediately before operation; preferably in the operating suite after anesthetization. This eliminates discomfort to the patient, affords relaxation of the operative site, and is a bacteriologically sound technique. There should be as short a time-lapse as possible between hair removal and incision, thus preventing contamination of the site by a regrowth of organisms or the possibility of a nick or scratch presenting a source of infection. The skin is held taut to present an even, smooth surface, as the hair is removed with power-driven disposable clippers. The use of sharp razors to remove hair is discouraged.

Obviously, it is a useless gesture to scrub the skin the night before operation, and to send the patient to the operating room with the site of incision covered with a sterile towel. However, some surgeons prefer to carry out a preliminary preparation in elective operations on the joints, hands, feet, and abdominal wall. Historically, this would involve scrubbing the skin with a cleansing agent several times a day for 2 or 3 days before the surgery. Today the patient may be instructed to shower using a specialized cleansing agent, preferably chlorhexidine gluconate, the evening before and the day of the surgery. Intravenous antibiotics are ordered to be administered within 1 hour of the planned incision.

In the operating room, after the patient has been properly positioned, the lights adjusted, and the proper plane of anesthesia reached, the final preparation of the operative site is begun. An assistant, puts on sterile gloves, and completes the mechanical cleansing of the operative site with sponges saturated in the desired solution. Chlorhexidine gluconate is the ideal cleansing agent. The contemplated site of incision is treated first; the remainder of the field is cleansed with concentric strokes until all of the exposed area has been covered. As with all tinctures and alcohols used in skin preparation, caution must be observed to prevent skin blisters caused by puddling of solutions at the patient's side or about skin creases. It is important to allow the prep solution to dry completely before draping in order to minimize a fire hazard. This usually requires 3 minutes with chlorhexidine gluconate. Similarly, electrocardiographic (ECG) and cautery pads should not be wetted. Some surgeons prefer to paint the skin with an iodine-containing solution or a similar preparation.

A transparent sterile plastic drape may be substituted for the skin towels in covering the skin, avoiding the necessity for towel clips at the corners of the field. This draping is especially useful to cover and wall off an ostomy. The plastic is made directly adherent to the skin by a bacteriostatic adhesive. After application of the drape, the incision is made directly through the material, and the plastic remains in place until the procedure is completed. When, for cosmetic reasons, the incision must accurately follow the lines of skin cleavage, the surgeon gently outlines the incision with a sterile inked pen before the adhesive plastic drape is applied. The addition of the plastic to the drape ensures a wide field, that is, surgically, completely sterile, instead of surgically clean as the prepared skin is considered. At the same time, the plastic layer prevents contamination should the large drape sheet become soaked or torn.

Superficial malignancies, as in the case of cancer of the skin, lip, or neck, present a problem in that a routine vigorous mechanical scrub is too traumatic causing irritation or bleeding. Gentle preparation with painting is preferred. Following hair removal with clippers, a germicidal solution should be applied carefully. Similarly, the burned patient must have special skin preparation. In addition to the extreme tissue sensitivity, many times gross soil, grease, and other contaminants are present. Copious flushing of the burned areas with isotonic solutions is important as mechanical cleansing is carried out with a nonirritating detergent.

Injuries such as the crushed hand or the open fracture require extreme care, and meticulous attention to skin preparation must be observed. The hasty, inadequate preparation of such emergency surgery can have disastrous consequences. A nylon bristle brush and a detergent are used to scrub the area thoroughly for several minutes. Hair is removed by an electric clipper for a wide area around the wound edges. Copious irrigation is essential after the skin is prepared, followed by a single application of a germicide. An antibacterial sudsing cleanser may be useful for cleansing the contaminated greasy skin of the hands or about traumatic wounds.

When the skin has been prepped and the patient has been positioned and draped, then a *TIME OUT* is done. During this time, all physicians and staff must stop what they are doing and listen and verify the information presented, including the patient's name, scheduled procedure including the correct site, allergies, and whether preoperative antibiotics were administered and when as shown in TABLE 1 of Chapter 3.

The skin incision is made with a scalpel. The deeper tissues may be incised with electrocautery using a blended current. Some surgeons prefer electrocautery rather than ligatures to control smaller bleeders. If the energy level is too high, this will produce tissue necrosis potentially devitalizing a larger zone of tissues on either side of its incision.

Some surgeons prefer electrocautery rather than ligatures to control smaller bleeders. Heavy suture materials, regardless of type, are not desirable. Fine silk, synthetics, or absorbable sutures should be used routinely. Every surgeon has his or her own preference for suture material, and new types are constantly being developed. Fine silk is most suitable for sutures and ligatures because it creates a minimum of tissue reaction and stays securely knotted. If a surgeon's knot is laid down and tightened, the ligature will not slip when the tension on the silk is released. A square knot then can be laid down to secure the ligature, which is cut close to the knot. The knots are set by applying tension on the ligature between a finger held beyond the knot in such a plane that the finger, the knot, and the hand are in a straight line. However, it takes long practice to set the first knot and run down the setting, or final knot, without holding the threads taut. This detail of technique is of great importance, for it is impossible to ligate under tension when handling delicate tissue or when working in the depths of a wound. When tying vessels caught in a hemostat, it is important that the side of the jaws of the hemostat away from the vessel be presented so that as little tissue as possible is included in the tie. Moreover, the hemostat should be released just as the first knot is tightened, the tie sliding down on tissue not already devitalized by the clamp. One-handed knots and rapidly thrown knots are unreliable. Each knot is of vital importance in the success of an operation that threatens the patient's life.

As the wound is deepened, exposure is obtained by retraction. If the procedure is to be prolonged, the use of a self-retaining retractor is advantageous, since it ensures constant exposure without fatiguing the assistants. Moreover, unless the anesthesia is deep, the constant shifting of a retractor held by an assistant not only disturbs the surgeon but also stimulates the sensory nerves. Whenever a self-retaining retractor is adjusted, the amount of tissue compression must be judged carefully because excessive compression may cause necrosis. Difficulty in obtaining adequate exposure is not always a matter of retraction. Unsatisfactory anesthesia, faulty position of the patient, improper illumination, an inadequate and improperly placed incision, and failure to use instruments instead of hands are factors to be considered when visibility is poor.

Handling tissues with fingers cannot be as manageable, gentle, or safe as handling with properly designed, delicate instruments. Instruments can be sterilized, whereas rubber gloves offer the danger that a needle prick or break may pass unnoticed and contamination may occur. Moreover, the use of instruments keeps hands out of the wound, thus allowing a full view of the field and affording perspective, which is an aid to safety.

After gentle retraction of the skin and subcutaneous tissue to avoid stripping, the fascia is sharply incised with a scalpel in line with its own fibers; jagged edges must be avoided to permit accurate reapproximation. The underlying muscle fibers may be separated longitudinally with the handle of the knife or electrocautery depending on the type of incision. Blood vessels may be divided between hemostats and ligated. After hemostasis is achieved, the muscle is protected from trauma and contamination by moist gauze pads. Retractors may now be placed to bring the peritoneum into view.

With toothed forceps or hemostat, the operator seizes and lifts the peritoneum. The assistant grasps the peritoneum near the apex of the tent, while the surgeon releases hold on it. This maneuver is repeated until the surgeon is certain that only peritoneum free of intra-abdominal tissue is included in the bite of the forceps. A small incision is made between the forceps with a scalpel. This opening is enlarged with scissors by inserting the lower tip of the scissors beneath the peritoneum for 1 cm and by tenting the peritoneum over the blade before cutting it. If the omentum does not fall away from the peritoneum, the corner of a moist sponge may be placed over it as a guard for the scissors. The incision should be made only as long

as that in the muscle since peritoneum stretches easily with retraction, and closure is greatly facilitated if the entire peritoneal opening is easily visualized. When the incision of the peritoneum is completed, retractors can then be placed to give the optimum view of the abdominal contents. The subcutaneous fat should be protected from possible contamination by sterile pads or a plastic wound protector. If the appendix or cecum is not apparent immediately, the wound may be shifted about with the retractors until these structures are located.

Although some consider it is customary to pack off the intestines from the cecal region with several moist sponges, we are convinced that the less material introduced into the peritoneal cavity the better. Even moist gauze injures the delicate superficial cells, which thereafter present a point of possible adhesion to another area as well as less of a barrier to bacteria. The appendix is then delivered into the wound and its blood supply investigated, with the strategic attack in surgery always being directed toward control of the blood supply. The blood vessels lying in the mesentery are more elastic than their supporting tissue and tend to retract; therefore, in ligating such vessels, it is best to transfix the mesentery with a curved needle, avoiding injury to the vessels. The vessel may be safely divided between securely tied ligatures, and the danger of its slipping out of a hemostat while being ligated is eliminated. The appendix is removed by the technique depicted in Chapter 48, and the cecum is replaced in the abdominal cavity. Closure begins with a search for sponges, needles, and instruments, until a correct count is obtained. In reapproximating the peritoneum, a continuous absorbable suture is used.

With the peritoneum closed, the muscles fall together naturally unless they were widely separated. The fascia overlying the muscles is carefully reapproximated with interrupted sutures and the muscles will naturally realign their positions. Alternatively, some surgeons prefer to approximate the peritoneum, muscle, and fascia in a one-layer closure with interrupted sutures.

Coaptation of the subcutaneous tissues is essential for a satisfactory cosmetic result. Well-approximated subcutaneous tissues permit the early removal of skin sutures and thus prevent the formation of a wide scar. Subcutaneous sutures are placed with a curved needle, large bites being taken through Scarpa's fascia, so that the wound is mounded upward and the skin edges are almost reapproximated. The sutures must be located so that both longitudinal and cross-sectional reapproximation is accurate. Overlapping or gaping of the skin at the ends of the wound may be avoided readily by care in suturing the subcutaneous layer.

The skin edges are brought together by interrupted sutures, subcuticular sutures, or metal skin staples. If the subcutaneous tissues have been sutured properly, the skin sutures or staples may be removed on the fifth postoperative day or so. Thereafter, additional support for minimizing skin separation may be provided by multiple adhesive paper strips. The result is a fine white line as the ultimate scar with less of a "railroad track" appearance, which may occur when skin sutures or staples remain for a prolonged time. To minimize this unsightly scar and lessen apprehension over suture removal, many surgeons approximate the incision with a few subcutaneous absorbable sutures that are reinforced with strips of adhesive paper tape.

Finally, there must be proper dressing and support for the wound. If the wound is closed per primam and the procedure itself has been "clean," the wound should be sealed off for at least 48 hours so it will not be contaminated from without. This may be done with a dry sponge dressing.

The time and method of removing skin sutures are important.

Lack of tension on skin sutures and their early removal, by the third to fifth day, eliminate unsightly cross-hatching. In other parts of the body, such as the face and neck, the sutures may be removed in 48 hours if the approximation has been satisfactory. When retention sutures are used, the length of time the sutures remain depends entirely on the cause for their use; when the patients are elderly or cachectic or suffer from chronic cough or the effects of radiation therapy, such sutures may be necessary for as long as 10 to 12 days. A variety of protective devices (bumpers) may be used over which these tension sutures can be tied so as to prevent the sutures from cutting into the skin.

The method of removing sutures is important and is designed to avoid contaminating a clean wound with skin bacteria. After cleansing with alcohol, the surgeon grasps the loose end of the suture, lifts the knot away from the skin by pulling out a little of the suture from beneath the epidermis, cuts the suture at a point that was beneath the skin, and pulls the suture free. Thus, no part of a suture that was on the outside of the skin will be drawn into the subcutaneous tissues to cause an infection in the wound. The importance of using aseptic technique in removing sutures and subsequent dressing under proper conditions cannot be overemphasized. Adhesive paper strips, colloids, or glue, when properly applied, can make skin sutures unnecessary in many areas.

The example of the characteristics of a technique that permits the tissues to heal with the greatest rapidity and strength and that conserves all the normal cells demonstrates that the surgeon's craftsmanship is of major importance to the patient's safety. It emphasizes the fact that technical surgery is an art, which is properly expressed only when the surgeon is aware of its inherent dangers. The same principles underlie the simplest as well as the most serious and extensive operative procedure. The young surgeon who learns the basic precepts of asepsis, hemostasis, adequate exposure, and gentleness to tissues has mastered his or her most difficult lessons.

Moreover, once surgeons have acquired this attitude, their progress will continue, for they will be led to a histologic study of wounds, where the real lessons of wound healing are strikingly visualized. They will also be led to a constant search for better instruments until they emerge finally as artists, not artisans.

The surgeon unaccustomed to this form of surgery will be annoyed by the constant emphasis on gentleness and the time-consuming technique of innumerable interrupted sutures. However, if the surgeon is entirely honest and if he or she wishes to close all clean wounds per primam, thus contributing to the patient's comfort and safety, all the principles that have been outlined must be employed. Fine suture material must be utilized—so fine that it breaks when such strain is put on it as will cut through living tissue. Each vessel must be tied securely so that the critically important vessel will always be controlled. Strict asepsis must be practiced. All this is largely a matter of conscience. To those who risk the lives of others daily, it is a chief concern.

CHAPTER 2 ANESTHESIA

Anesthesiology as a special field of endeavor has made clear the many physiologic changes occurring in the patient during anesthesia. The pharmacologic effects of anesthetic agents and techniques on the central nervous system and the cardiovascular and respiratory systems are now better understood. New drugs have been introduced for inhalation, intravenous, spinal, and regional anesthesia. In addition, drugs, such as muscle relaxants and hypotensive or hypertensive agents, are used for their specific pharmacologic effect. Older anesthetic techniques, such as spinal and caudal anesthesia, have been improved by the refinement of the continuous technique and more accurate methods of controlling the distribution of the administered drug. Marked advances in anesthesia have taken place in pulmonary, cardiac, pediatric, and geriatric surgery. Improved management of airway and pulmonary ventilation is reflected in the techniques and equipment available to prevent the deleterious effects of hypoxia and hypercarbia. An increased understanding of the altered hemodynamics produced by anesthesia in the ill patient has resulted in better fluid, electrolyte, and blood replacement preoperatively in patients with a decreased blood volume and electrolyte imbalance, thus allowing many patients once thought to be too ill for surgery, the opportunity for safe operative care.

Although the number of anesthesiologists has increased within recent years, it still is not enough to meet the increased surgical load. Surgeons, therefore, may find that they will be assigned certified registered nurse anesthetists (CRNAs) to administer anesthesia. Although CRNAs have excellent training they must be supervised by a physician. Hence the surgeon must bear in mind that in the absence of a trained anesthesiologist, it is the surgeon who is legally accountable should catastrophe from any cause, compromise the outcome of the surgical procedure. Under these circumstances, the surgeon should be knowledgeable about the choice of anesthetic agents and techniques, and their indications and complications. Further, he or she should be familiar with the condition of the patient under anesthesia by observing the color of blood or viscera, the rapidity and strength of the arterial pulsation, and the effort and rhythm of the chest wall or diaphragmatic respirations. Knowing the character of these conditions under a well-conducted anesthesia, the surgeon will be able readily to detect a patient who is doing poorly.

It is this point of view that has caused us to present in this practical volume the following short outline of modern anesthetic principles. This outline makes no pretense of covering fully the physiologic, pharmacologic, and technical details of anesthesiology, but it offers to the surgeon some basic important information.

GENERAL CONSIDERATIONS The intraoperative role of the anesthesiologist as a member of the surgical team is severalfold, including the assurance of adequate pulmonary ventilation, maintenance of a near-normal cardiovascular system, and conduction of the anesthetic procedure itself. One cannot be isolated from the other.

VENTILATION Preventing the subtle effects of hypoxia is of prime importance to the anesthesiologist. It is well known that severe hypoxia may cause sudden disaster, and that hypoxia of a moderate degree may result in slower but equally disastrous consequences. Hypoxia during anesthesia is related directly to some interference with the patient's ability to exchange oxygen. This commonly is caused by allowing the patient's tongue partially or completely to obstruct the upper airway. Foreign bodies, emesis, profuse secretions, or laryngeal spasm may also cause obstruction of the upper airway. Of these, aspiration of emesis, although rare, represents the greatest hazard to the patient. General anesthesia should not be administered in those patients likely to have a full stomach unless adequate protection of the airway is assured. A common guideline in adults with normal gastrointestinal motility is a 6- to 8-hour interval between the ingestion of solid food and induction of anesthesia. In addition, members of the surgical team should be capable of performing endotracheal intubation. This will reduce the possibility of the patient's asphyxiating, as the endotracheal tube is not always a guarantee of a perfect airway. Other conditions known to produce a severe state of hypoxia are congestive heart failure, pulmonary edema, asthma, or masses in the neck and mediastinum compressing the trachea. As these conditions may not be directly under the anesthesiologist's control, preoperative evaluation should be made by the surgeon, the anesthesiologist, and appropriate consultants. In complex airway cases, the patient may be intubated using topical anesthetics and a flexible fiberoptic bronchoscope that serves as an internal guide for the overlying endotracheal tube.

Before any general anesthetic technique is commenced, facilities must be available to perform positive-pressure oxygen breathing, and suction must be available to remove secretions and vomitus from the airway before, during, and after the surgical procedure. Every effort should be expended to perform an adequate tracheobronchial and oropharyngeal cleansing after the surgical procedure, and the airway should be kept free of secretions and vomitus until the protective reflexes return. With the patient properly positioned and observed, all these procedures will help to reduce the incidence of postoperative pulmonary complications.

CARDIOVASCULAR SUPPORT Fluid therapy during the operative procedure is a joint responsibility of the surgeon and the anesthesiologist. Except in unusual circumstances, anemia, hemorrhage, and shock should be treated preoperatively. During the operation transfusions should be used with caution as there can be significant risks associated with transfusions. Most patients can withstand up to 500 mL of blood loss without difficulty. However, in operative procedures known to require several units of blood, the blood should be replaced as lost as estimated from the quantity of blood within the operative field, the operative drapes, and the measured sponges and suction bottles. The intravascular volume can be expanded by cross-matched packed red blood cells, specifically indicated for their oxygen-carrying capacity, when the hematocrit (Hct) is ≤23% to 25% or the hemoglobin (Hb) is ≤7 g/dL. In emergency situations when blood is not available, synthetic colloids (dextran or hydroxyethyl starch solutions), albumin, or plasma may be administered to maintain an adequate expansion of blood volume. All blood products are used with caution because of the possibility of transmitting homologous viral diseases. Infusions of Ringer's lactate (a balanced electrolyte solution), via a secure and accessible intravenous catheter, should be used during all operative procedures, including those in pediatrics. Such an arrangement allows the anesthesiologist to have ready access to the cardiovascular system, and thereby a means of administering drugs or treating hypotension promptly. In addition, large, centrally placed catheters may be used to monitor central venous pressure or even cardiac performance if a pulmonary artery catheter is placed into the pulmonary vasculature. As many modern anesthetic agents may produce vasodilation or depression of myocardial contractility, anesthesiologists may volume load patients with crystalloid solutions. This maintains normal hemodynamic parameters and a good urine output. However, this fluid loading may have serious after effects in some patients; thus the anesthesiologist must monitor the type and volume of fluids given to the patient during the operation and communicate this to the surgeon.

The patient's body position is an important factor both during and after the operation. The patient should be placed in a position that allows gravity to aid in obtaining optimum exposure. The most effective position for any procedure is the one that causes the viscera to gravitate away from the operative field. Proper position on the table allows adequate anatomic exposure with less traumatic retraction. With good muscle relaxation and an unobstructed airway, exaggerated positions and prolonged elevations become unnecessary. The surgeon should bear in mind that extreme positions result in embarrassed respiration, in harmful circulatory responses, and in nerve palsies. When the surgical procedure is concluded, the patient should be returned gradually to the horizontal supine position, and sufficient time should be allowed for the circulatory system to become stabilized. When an extreme position is used, extremity wrappings should be applied and the patient should be returned to the normal position in several stages, with a rest period between each one. Abrupt changes in position or rough handling of the patient may result in unexpected circulatory collapse. After being returned to bed, the patient should be positioned for safe respiration. The patient is observed for unobstructed breathing and stable hemodynamic parameters until he or she is sufficiently alert.

Anesthesia in the aged patient is associated with an increased morbidity and mortality. Degenerative diseases of the pulmonary and cardiovascular systems are prominent, with the individual being less likely to withstand minor insults to either system. Sedatives and narcotics should be used sparingly in both the preoperative and postoperative periods. Regional or local anesthesia should be employed in this age group whenever feasible. This form of anesthesia decreases the possibility of serious pulmonary and cardiovascular system complications and at the same time decreases the possibility of serious mental disturbance that can occur following general anesthesia. Induction and maintenance of anesthesia can be made smoother by good preoperative preparation of the respiratory tract. This begins with cessation of smoking prior to admission and continues with vigorous pulmonary care that may involve positive-pressure aerosol therapy and bronchodilators. A detailed cardiac history in preoperative workup will uncover patients with borderline cardiac failure, coronary insufficiency, or valvular disease, who require specialized drug treatment and monitoring.

ANESTHETICS As most patients are anxious in the preoperative period, premedication with an anxiolytic agent is often given in the preoperative holding area. Once upon the operating table, the patient is preoxygenated before being induced rapidly and smoothly with an intravenous hypnotic and narcotic.

Induction of a full general anesthesia requires airway control with either a laryngeal mask airway (LMA) or an endotracheal tube, whose placement may require transient muscle paralysis.

Muscle relaxants such as succinylcholine or nondepolarizing neuromuscular blocking agents should be used for those operations requiring muscular looseness if it is not provided by the anesthetic agent. By the use of these drugs, adequate muscular relaxation can be obtained in a lighter plane of anesthesia, thereby reducing the myocardial and peripheral circulatory depression observed in the deeper planes of anesthesia. In addition, the protective reflexes, such as coughing, return more quickly if light planes of anesthesia are maintained. Finally, however, it is important to note that the mycin-derivative antibiotics may interact with curare-like drugs so as to prolong their effect with inadequate spontaneous respiration in the recovery area and may lead to extended respiratory support.

When the maximum safe dosages of local anesthetic agents are exceeded, the incidence of toxic reactions increases. These reactions, which are related to the concentration of the local anesthetic agent in the blood, may be classified as either central nervous system stimulation (i.e., nervousness, sweating, and convulsions) or central nervous system depression (i.e., drowsiness and coma). Either type of reaction may lead to circulatory collapse and respiratory failure. Resuscitative equipment consisting of positive-pressure oxygen, intravenous fluids, vasopressors, and an intravenous barbiturate should be readily available during all major operative procedures using large quantities of local anesthesia. The intensity of anesthesia produced by the local anesthetic agents depends on the concentration of the agent and on the size of the nerve. As the size of the nerve to be anesthetized increases, a higher concentration of anesthetic agent is utilized. Since the maximum safe dose of lidocaine (Xylocaine) is 300 mg, it is wise to use 0.5% lidocaine when large volumes are needed.

The duration of anesthesia can be prolonged by the addition of epinephrine to the local anesthetic solution. Although this prolongs the anesthetic effect and reduces the incidence of toxic reactions, the use of epinephrine is not without danger. Its concentration should not exceed 1:100,000; that is, 1 mL of 1:1,000 solution in 100 mL of local anesthetic agent. After the operative procedure has been completed and the vasoconstrictive effect of the epinephrine has worn off, bleeding may occur in the wound if meticulous attention to hemostasis has not been given. If the anesthetic is to be injected into the digits, epinephrine should not be added because of the possibility of producing gangrene by occlusive spasm of these end arteries, which do not have collaterals. Epinephrine is also contraindicated if the patient has hypertension, arteriosclerosis, and coronary or myocardial disease.

In any surgical practice, occasions arise when the anesthesiologist should refuse or postpone the administration of anesthesia. Serious thought should be given before anesthesia is commenced in cases of severe pulmonary insufficiency; with elective surgery in the patient with myocardial infarction less than 6 months prior; severe unexplained anemia; with inadequately treated shock; in patients who recently have been or are still on certain drugs such as monoamine oxidase (MAO) inhibitors and certain tricyclic antidepressants that may compromise safe anesthesia; and, finally, in any case in which the anesthesiologist feels he or she will be unable to manage the patient's airway, such as Ludwig's angina, or when there are large masses in the throat, neck, or mediastinum that compress the trachea.

CARDIAC MORBIDITY AND MORTALITY Cessation of effective cardiac activity may occur at any time during an anesthetic or operative procedure performed under local or general anesthesia. Many etiologic factors have been cited as producing cardiac dysfunction; however, acute or prolonged hypoxia is undoubtedly the most common cause. In a few instances, undiagnosed cardiovascular disease such as severe aortic stenosis or myocardial infarction has been the cause of cardiac standstill. Many sudden cardiac complications relate to anesthetic technique and they are often preceded by warning signs long before the catastrophe actually occurs. Common anesthetic factors include overdosage of anesthetic agents, either in total amount of drug or in speed of administration; prolonged and unrecognized partial respiratory obstruction; inadequate blood replacement with delay in treating hypotension; aspiration of stomach contents; and failure to maintain constant vigilance over the anesthetized patient's cardiovascular system. The last factor is minimized by the use of the precordial or intra-esophageal stethoscope, a continuous electrocardiogram, end-tidal CO_2, and oxygen saturation monitoring.

Mortality and morbidity from cardiac events can be minimized further by having all members of the surgical team trained in the immediate treatment of sudden cardiac collapse. Successful treatment of sudden cardiac collapse depends upon immediate diagnosis and the institution of therapy without hesitation. Diagnosis is established tentatively by the absence of the pulse and blood pressure as recognized by the anesthesiologist and confirmed by the surgeon's palpation of the arteries or observation of the absence of bleeding in the operative field. The Advanced Cardiac Life Support protocols developed by the American College of Cardiology provide a reasonable guide to resuscitation. It is imperative that external cardiac compression and the establishment of a clear and unobstructed airway be instituted immediately. Intravenous administration of epinephrine is appropriate. If adequate circulation is being produced, a pulse should be palpable in the carotid and brachial arteries. Many times, oxygenated blood being circulated through the coronary arteries by external compression will be sufficient to start a heart in asystole. If the heart is fibrillating, it should be defibrillated. Defibrillation may be accomplished by electrical direct current, which is the preferred method. If all of these resuscitative measures are unsuccessful, then thoracotomy with direct cardiac compression or defibrillation may be considered in an equipped and staffed operating room setting.

The treatment of a patient revived after a cardiopulmonary arrest is directed toward maintaining adequate cardiopulmonary ventilation and perfusion, and preventing specific organ injuries such as acute renal tubular necrosis or cerebral edema. This may involve vasoactive drugs, steroids, diuretics, or hypothermia.

CHOICE OF ANESTHESIA The anesthesiologist's skill is the most important factor in the choice of anesthesia. The anesthesiologist should select the drugs and methods with which he or she has had the greatest experience. The effects of the drugs are modified by the speed of administration, total dose, the interaction of various drugs used, and the technique of the individual anesthesiologist. These factors are far more important than the theoretical effects of the drugs based on responses elicited in animals. With anesthetic agents reported to have produced hepatocellular damage, certain precautions should be observed. This is particularly important in patients who have been administered halogenated anesthetic agents in the recent past, or who give a history suggestive of hepatic dysfunction following a previous anesthetic exposure. Further, the halogenated anesthetic agents should be used cautiously in patients whose occupations expose them to hepatocellular toxins or who are having biliary tract surgery.

The following factors about the proposed operation must be considered: its site, magnitude, and duration; the amount of blood loss to be expected; and the position of the patient on the operating table. The patient should then be studied to ascertain his or her ability to tolerate the surgical procedure and the anesthetic. Important factors are the patient's age, weight, and general condition as well as the presence of acute infection, toxemia, dehydration, and hypovolemia. Hence, there is a dual evaluation: first, of the overall state of the patients' vital organ systems and, second, of the superimposed hazards of the disease.

The patient's previous experience and prejudices regarding anesthesia should be considered. Some patients dread losing consciousness, fearing loss of control; others wish for oblivion. Some patients, or their friends, have had unfortunate experiences with spinal anesthesia and are violently opposed to it. An occasional individual may be sensitive to local anesthetics or may have had a prolonged bout of vomiting following inhalation anesthesia. Whenever possible, the patient's preference regarding the choice of anesthesia should be followed. If that choice is contraindicated, the reason should be explained carefully and the preferred procedure should be outlined in such a way as to remove the patient's fears. If local or spinal anesthesia is selected, psychic disturbance will be minimized and the anesthetic made more effective if it is preceded by adequate premedication.

PRELIMINARY MEDICATION   If possible, the patient should be visited by the anesthesiologist prior to the operation. The anesthesiologist should have become acquainted with the patient's condition and the proposed operation. He or she must evaluate personally the patient's physical and psychic state and, at this time, should inquire about the patient's previous anesthetic experience and about drug sensitivity. The anesthesiologist should question the patient about drugs taken at home and be sure that medicines requiring continued administration, such as beta-blockers or insulin, are continued. Further inquiry should be made concerning drugs (such as corticosteroid drugs, antihypertensive drugs, MAO inhibitors, and tranquilizers) that may have an interaction with the planned anesthesia. If the patient is taking any of these drugs, proper precautions should be taken to prevent an unsatisfactory anesthetic and surgical procedure.

Preoperative medication is frequently a part of the anesthetic procedure. The choice of premedication depends on the anesthetic to be used. Dosage should vary with the patient's age, physical state, and psychic condition. Premedication should remove apprehension, reduce the metabolic rate, and raise the threshold to pain. Upon arriving in the operating suite, the patient should be unconcerned and placid.

CHAPTER 3

PREOPERATIVE PREPARATION AND POSTOPERATIVE CARE

For centuries the surgeon's chief training was in anatomy, almost to the exclusion of other aspects of the art. Only in the 20th century did the increasing scope of surgery and unremitting efforts to reduce the number of deaths and complications to a minimum lead inevitably to the realization that a sound understanding of physiology is as important as a thorough grounding in anatomic relationships. In the 21st century, there is increasing interest in evidence-based preoperative and postoperative care and the application of scientific knowledge and compassion to restore the patient to a normal physiologic state and equilibrium as readily as possible after minor or major surgery. The discipline of surgical critical care represents the ultimate merging of the art of surgery with the science of physiology.

PREOPERATIVE PREPARATION The surgeon of the 21st century is concerned not only with the proper preoperative preparation of the patient and technical conduct of an operative procedure but also with the preparation of the operating room and an understanding of the problems created by illness in the patient as a whole. Because of the complexities of a patient population with many medical comorbid conditions, preoperative preparation may require a team approach. It is important for the surgeon to understand potential complications and their prevention and recognition. In the ideal situation, the preoperative preparation of the patient begins the ambulatory setting prior to admission. The surgeon assesses the patient and determines the need for surgery for the specific diagnosis. The surgeon advises the patient on the benefits and risks of the procedure in general as well as those that are specific to the operation being recommended. Informed consent is more than a signature on a piece of paper: it is a process of discussion and a dialogue between the surgeon and patient in which the patient has the opportunity to ask questions. The surgeon should also include a discussion of the possible use of blood products, and if deemed appropriate, advise the patient about autologous blood donation. In assessing the patient's condition it is important to identify major health issues. Pulmonary pathology including chronic obstructive pulmonary disease and asthma should be identified. Any departure from the norm disclosed by the history, physical examination, or the various procedures enumerated below may call for further specialty referral and treatment in concert with the patient's primary physician. Likewise, history of a myocardial infarction, valvular heart disease, or a previous coronary intervention may suggest the need for cardiac clearance and assessment by a cardiologist. Finally most patients undergoing major procedures are seen prior to surgery by an anesthesiologist. This is especially important if they are class III or IV according to the American Society of Anesthesiologist (ASA). Written or verbal communication with the referring physician and primary care physician is important in order to facilitate continuity of care.

In many situations, the primary care physician may be engaged to help ready the patient for surgery. The primary physician may then set in motion diagnostic and therapeutic maneuvers that improve control of the patient's diseases, thus optimizing his or her status for anesthesia and surgery. Even simple "oral and respiratory prophylaxis," for example, the ordering of dental care and treatment of chronic sinusitis or chronic bronchitis, can be beneficial. Restriction of smoking combined with expectorants for a few days may alleviate the chronic productive cough that is so likely to lead to serious pulmonary complications. The surgeon should supervise any special diets that may be required, apprise the family and patient of the special requirements, and instill in the patient that peace of mind and confidence which constitutes the so-called psychologic preparation. The patient should inform the surgeon of any food or drug idiosyncrasies, thus corroborating and supplementing the surgeon's own observations concerning the patient as an operative risk.

It is helpful to require the patient to cough to determine whether his or her cough is dry or productive. In the presence of the latter, consultation with pulmonary medicine may be helpful and surgery may be delayed for the improvement that will follow discontinuance of smoking and the institution of repeated daily pulmonary physical therapy and incentive spirometry in addition to expectorants and bronchodilating drugs as indicated. In the more serious cases, the patient's progress should be documented with formal pulmonary function tests, including arterial blood gases. Patients with other chronic lung problems should be evaluated in a similar manner.

In general, electrocardiograms are routinely obtained, especially after the age of 50. A stress test, radionuclide imaging scan, or ultrasound echo test may be useful for screening, while coronary angiogram, carotid Doppler ultrasounds, or abdominal vascular scans may be performed if significant vascular disease is present or requires correction before an elective general surgery operation.

Standard preoperative considerations include antibiotic prophylaxis and preventive measures for venous thromboembolism. In addition, some surgeons have the patient bathe with antiseptic soap the day prior to the operation. If any special diet or bowel preparation is necessary, the patient is so advised and given the necessary instructions or prescriptions. Intravenous antibiotics should be ordered to be administered within 1 hour prior to the incision. Some antibiotics have specific administration requirements. The surgeon may consult with the hospital pharmacy concerning the optimal timing of antibiotic administration for vancomycin, gentamicin, or other less commonly employed antibiotic preparations.

Hospitalized patients are frequently more ill than those seen in an ambulatory setting. In this setting, the surgical team works with the medical team to bring the patient into physiologic balance prior to surgery. Recommendations of pulmonary and cardiac consultants should be followed to improve the patient's risk for surgery. The hospitalized patient may be separated from his or her family and may be depressed or have anxiety. The surgeon's reassurance and confident manner can help the patient overcome some of the psychologic stress of illness.

Particularly for the hospitalized patient, assessment of nutritional status with measurement of albumin and prealbumin or other markers, pulmonary and cardiac function is necessary. If the patient is malnourished, then this should optimally be corrected prior to surgical intervention if the condition permits. Enteral feedings are preferred. In some cases with oropharyngeal obstruction, a percutaneous endoscopic gastrostomy may be performed to provide access. Feeding with prepared formulas may be necessary. If gastrointestinal access cannot be obtained, total parenteral nutrition (TPN) may be necessary. Although about 1 g of protein per kilogram of body weight is the average daily requirement of the healthy adult, it is frequently necessary to double this figure to achieve a positive nitrogen balance and protect the tissues from the strain of a surgical procedure and long anesthesia. The administered protein may not be assimilated as such unless the total caloric intake is maintained well above basal requirements. If calories are not supplied from sugars and fat, the ingested protein will be consumed by the body like sugar for its energy value.

If for any reason the patient cannot be fed via the gastrointestinal tract, parenteral feedings must be utilized. On occasion, a deficient oral intake should be supplemented by parenteral feedings to ensure a daily desirable minimal level of 1,500 calories. Water, glucose, salt, vitamins, amino acids, trace minerals, and intravenous fats are the elements of these feedings. Accurate records of intake and output are indispensable. Frequent checks on the liver, renal, and marrow functions along with blood levels of protein, albumin, blood urea nitrogen, prothrombin, and hemoglobin are essential to gauge the effectiveness of the treatment. One must be careful to avoid giving too much salt. The average adult will require no more than 500 mL of normal saline each day unless there is an abnormal loss of chlorides by gastrointestinal suction or fistula. Body weight should be determined daily in patients receiving intravenous fluids. Since each liter of water weighs approximately 1 kg, marked fluctuations in weight can give warning of either edema or dehydration. A stable body weight indicates good water and calorie replacement.

In catabolic states of negative nitrogen balance and inadequate calorie intake, usually due to the inability to eat enough or to a disrupted gastrointestinal tract, intravenous TPN using a central venous catheter can be lifesaving. Ordinarily, a subclavian or jugular catheter site is used. At present, these solutions contain a mixture of amino acids as a protein source and carbohydrates for calories. Fat emulsions provide more calories (9 calories per gram versus 4 for carbohydrates or protein) and lessen the problems of hyperglycemia. In general, the TPN solutions contain 20% to 25% carbohydrate as glucose plus 50 g of protein source per liter. To this are added the usual electrolytes plus calcium, magnesium, phosphates, trace elements, and multiple vitamins, especially vitamins C and K. Such a solution offers 1,000 calories per liter and the usual adult receives 3 L per day. This provides 3,000 calories, 150 g of protein, and a mild surplus of water for urinary, insensible, and other water losses. Any component of the TPN solution can be given in insufficient or excessive quantities, thus requiring careful monitoring. This should include daily weights, intake and output balances, urinalysis for sugar spillage, serum electrolytes, blood sugar and phosphate, hematocrit, and liver function tests with prothrombin levels in specific instances. Other than catheter-related problems, major complications include hyperglycemia with glucosuria (solute diuresis) and hyperglycemic nonketotic acidosis from overly rapid infusion. Reactive hypoglycemia or hypophosphatemia (refeeding syndrome) may occur after sudden discontinuance of the infusion (catheter accident).

Another major complication involves infection, and strict precautions are needed in preparing the solutions and handling the infusion bottles, lines, and catheters in order to prevent related blood stream infections. Guidelines from the CDC for the prevention of catheter-related blood stream infections should be followed. Prior to insertion standard hand hygiene procedures are followed. During insertion maximal sterile barrier precautions are employed. The skin is prepared with a >0.5% chlorhexidine preparation. If there is a contraindication to chlorhexidine then tincture of iodine, an iodophor or 70% alcohol can be used as alternatives prior to catheter insertion or with dressing changes. The dressing used to cover the central venous catheter is with sterile gauze, or sterile transparent, semipermeable dressing. Topical antibiotic ointment is avoided, except for dialysis catheters, because the potential to promote fungal infection and antimicrobial resistance. The catheter is replaced if the dressing becomes damp, loosened, or visibly soiled. In the adult, for short-term use central venous catheters gauze dressings are replaced every 2 days and for transparent dressings every 7 days. The same guidelines apply to children unless there is risk of catheter dislodgement which may be considered. There is evidence that central venous lines should be routinely replaced in order to avoid related bold stream infections. If the patient is not receiving blood products or fat emulsions, administration sets that are used continuously, including secondary sets and add-on devices should be changed no more frequently than at 96-hour intervals, but at least every 7 days. Fungemia or gram-negative septicemia should be guarded against, and ideally the catheter system should not be violated for drawing blood samples or for infusion of other solutions. Sepsis does not contraindicate the use of intravenous nutrition, but chronic septicemia without obvious etiology is the indication for removal and culturing of these catheters.

Vitamins are not routinely required by patients who have been on a good diet and who enter the hospital for an elective surgical procedure. Vitamin C is the one vitamin usually requiring early replacement, since only a limited supply can be stored in the body at any one time. In some instances (severe burns are one example), massive doses of 1 g daily may be needed. Vitamin B complex is advantageously given daily. Vitamin K is indicated if the prothrombin time is elevated. This should be suspected whenever the normal formation of vitamin K in the bowel is interfered with by gastric suction, jaundice, the oral administration of broad-spectrum antibiotics, starvation, or prolonged intravenous alimentation. Objective evidence of improved nutrition may be documented with rising serum protein concentrations, especially albumin, prealbumin, and transferrin, or with the return of a positive skin test for immunocompetence. Certainly if the patient's condition requires urgent treatment, surgery should not be delayed to correct preoperative malnutrition, and the surgeon should plan methods of postoperative nutrition including the possible placement of a feeding jejunostomy or planning on TPN.

Blood transfusions may be needed to correct severe anemia or to replace deficits in circulating blood volume. Properly spaced preoperative transfusions can do more to improve the tolerance for major surgery in poor-risk patients than any other measure in preparation. Blood should be given if the patient is anemic. Such deficits have often been found even when the hemoglobin and hematocrit are normal, as they will be when both plasma volume and red cell volume are contracted concurrently. This situation has been dramatically termed "chronic shock," since all the normal defenses against shock are hard at work to maintain the appearance of physiologic equilibrium in the preoperative period. If the unsuspecting surgeon fails to uncover the recent weight loss and, trusting the hemoglobin, permits the patient to be anesthetized with a depleted blood volume, vasoconstriction is lost and vascular collapse may promptly ensue. The hemoglobin level should be brought to approximately 10 g/dL or the hematocrit to 30% before elective surgery in which a significant blood loss is anticipated or if the patient has limited cardiopulmonary reserve.

Time for the restoration of blood volume and caution are both necessary, especially in older people. If the initial hemoglobin is very low, the plasma volume must be overexpanded. Packed red cells are specifically needed rather than whole blood. Each 500 mL of blood contains 1 g of salt in its anticoagulant. As a result, cardiac patients may have some difficulty with multiple transfusions from the salt or plasma loading, and diuretics can be very helpful. There has also been some concern about the potassium in blood stored a week or more. This should never prevent a needed transfusion, but it is a consideration in massive transfusions in emergency situations.

Patients requiring treatment for acute disturbances of the blood, plasma, or electrolyte equilibrium present a somewhat different problem. Immediate replacement is in order, preferably with a solution that approximates the substances being lost. In shock from hemorrhage, replacement should be made with electrolyte solutions plus blood, although plasma substitutes, such as dextran or hydroxyethyl starch solutions, can provide emergency aid in limited amounts (up to 1,000 mL) until blood or plasma is available. In severe burns, plasma, blood, and normal saline or lactated Ringer's solution are in order. In vomiting, diarrhea, and dehydration, water and electrolytes will often suffice. In many of these patients, however, there is a loss of plasma that is easy to overlook. For instance, in peritonitis, intestinal obstruction, acute pancreatitis, and other states in which large internal surfaces become inflamed, much plasma-rich exudate may be lost, with no external sign to warn the surgeon until the pulse or blood pressure becomes seriously disturbed. Such internal shifts of fluid have been called "third space" losses. These losses may require albumin plus electrolyte solutions for proper replacement. It is because of these internal losses that many cases of peritonitis or bowel obstruction may require colloid replacement during their preoperative preparation.

In all such acute imbalances, a minimum of laboratory determinations will include serum or plasma sodium, potassium, chloride, bicarbonate, glucose, and urea nitrogen. Calcium, magnesium, and liver function tests may be useful, while arterial blood gases with pH, bicarbonate concentration Po_2 and Pco_2 enable accurate and repeated evaluation of the respiratory and metabolic components involved in an acidosis or alkalosis. Systemic causes of metabolic acidosis or alkalosis must be corrected. In either case, potassium may be needed. It should be given in sufficient quantity to maintain a normal serum level but only after the urine output is adequate to excrete any excess. Although the laboratory data are useful, the key to adequate replacement therapy is found in the patient's clinical course and in his or her intake–output record. Evidence of restoration is found in a clearing mentation, a stable blood pressure, a falling pulse rate and temperature curve, improved skin turgor, and an increase in urine output.

Antibiotic agents have proved their usefulness in preparing the patient whose condition is complicated by infection or who faces an operation where infection is an unavoidable risk. For procedures on the large bowel, preparation with certain oral preparations combining nonabsorbable antibiotics, purgatives, and zero-residue high-nitrogen diets will reduce the presence of formed stool and diminish the bacterial counts of the colon and theoretically result in safer resections of the lower bowel. In jaundiced patients and in others seriously ill with liver disease, cleansing and minimizing bacterial metabolism within the bowel may provide the necessary support through a major operative intervention. Decompression of an obstructed, septic biliary tree from above by percutaneous transhepatic catheterization or from below by endoscopic retrograde cholangiopancreatography (ERCP) provides bile for culture and antibiotic sensitivity studies. These maneuvers may also buy time for further preoperative resuscitation that lessens the risk of an urgent operation. The beneficial action of the antibiotics must not give the surgeon a false sense of security, however, for in no sense are they substitutes for good surgical technique and the practice of sound surgical principles.

The many patients now receiving endocrine therapy require special consideration. If therapeutic corticosteroid or adrenocorticotropic hormone (ACTH) has been administered within the preceding few months, the same drug must be continued before, during, and after surgery. The dose required to meet the unusual stress on the day of operation is often double or triple the ordinary dose. Hypotension, inadequately explained by obvious causes, may be the only manifestation of a need for more corticosteroids. Some later difficulties in wound healing may be anticipated in patients receiving these drugs.

Preoperative management of diabetes requires special consideration. Guidelines change periodically so the surgeon should consult the institution's practice guideline reference or the endocrinologist or primary care physician for assistance. Some general considerations as recommended at the Ohio State University Medical Center are outlined below. First morning procedures are preferred. The HbA1c should be reviewed (i.e., for intermediate/high risk). If poor glycemic control is identified (HbA1c >9%), the patient should be referred to the primary physician or endocrinologist for medication adjustment. The surgeon may consider postponing nonemergent surgery or procedures until medication adjustments are made. The patient should be instructed to hold all metformin-containing products 1 day prior to surgery. If the patient has inadvertently taken metformin and will undergo any procedure that will compromise renal function, the surgeon may consider **canceling** the case. If the patient will **not** undergo a procedure that may impair renal function, it is **not necessary to cancel** the case. If the patient uses other oral or noninsulin injectable diabetes medications (Symlin, Byetta) the morning of the procedure, withholding of these medications should be discussed with the primary care physician, endocrinologist, and anesthesiologist if possible. Likewise, short-acting insulin (lispro, aspart, glulisine) may be held the morning of the procedure unless the patient uses correction dosing in the fasting state. Adjustments in basal insulin (NPH, glargine, and detemir) should be made by the primary physician or endocrinologist. For morning surgery the evening dose of NPH or lente insulin may be reduced by 20% and the morning dose by 50%. For once a day basal insulin (glargine, detemir), the dose of the evening before or the morning of may be reduced by 20%. For split-mixed insulin (70/30, 75/25, 50/50), the prior evening dose may be reduced by 20% and the morning of dose by 50%. During continuous infusion of insulin with a pump, one may consider a 20% reduction in basal rates to begin at midnight prior to the scheduled surgery. For procedures lasting 3 hours or less, the infusion may be continued. For procedures lasting more than 3 hours, the continuous infusion should be discontinued and intravenous insulin infusion started according to the institutional protocol and/or according to the recommendations of the endocrinologist.

The patient's normal blood pressure should be reliably established by multiple preoperative determinations as a guide to the anesthesiologist. An accurate preoperative weight can be a great help in managing the postoperative fluid balance.

Well-prepared surgeons will assure themselves of a more than adequate supply of properly cross-matched blood and blood products if a coagulopathy is anticipated. In all upper abdominal procedures, the stomach should be decompressed and kept out of the way. It has a tendency to fill with air during the induction of anesthesia, but this may be minimized by inserting a nasogastric tube prior to operation or after endotracheal intubation. In cases of pyloric obstruction, emptying the stomach will not be easy; nightly lavages with a very large Ewalt tube may be required. A Foley catheter may be used to keep the bladder out of the way during pelvic procedures. Postoperatively, this can be a great help in obtaining accurate measurements of urine volume at hourly intervals, particularly when there has been excessive blood loss or other reason to expect renal complications. In general, a good hourly urine output of 40 to 50 mL per hour indicates satisfactory hydration and an adequate effective blood volume for perfusion of vital organs. Finally, the surgeon should forewarn the nursing staff of the expected condition of the patient after operation. This will assist them in having necessary oxygen, aspirating apparatus, special equipment or monitors, and so forth at the patient's bedside upon his or her return from the recovery room.

The anesthesiologist should interview each patient prior to operation. In those with serious pulmonary or constitutional diseases in need of extensive surgery, the choice of anesthesia is an exacting problem with serious consequences. Hence, the surgeon, the anesthesiologist, the primary physician, and appropriate consulting specialists may want to confer in advance of surgery in these complicated cases.

In scheduling the procedure, the surgeon will consider the specific equipment needed. This may include but not be limited to electrocautery or other energy sources, special scopes such as a choledochoscope, intraoperative ultrasound, grafts or prosthetics, and the need for fluoroscopy. In addition, one might consider the method of postoperative pain control. Is an epidural appropriate for postoperative pain management, or will a patient-controlled analgesic pump suffice? If the former is considered, the anesthesia team should be made aware as additional time would need to be factored for placement so as not to delay the procedure. In addition, the decision for invasive monitoring should be made in collaboration with anesthesia. Finally, if any consultants are anticipated to be needed at surgery, such as a urologist for placement of a ureteral stent, these arrangements should be established prior to the day of the operation.

OPERATIVE MANAGEMENT The surgical and anesthesia teams and nursing have the responsibility of ensuring the safety of the patient during the operative procedure. On the day of surgery prior to the operation, the key responsibility of the surgeon is to mark the site or side of the surgery. The use of surgical checklists may be helpful in improving patient safety. The outline shown in TABLE 1 is based on the World Health Organization (WHO) Guidelines for Safe Surgery (2009).

Before induction of anesthesia, the nurse and an anesthesia team member confirm that: (1) the patient has verified his or her identity, the surgical site, procedure, and has signed an informed consent; (2) the surgical site has been marked; (3) the patient's allergies are identified, accurate, and

TABLE 1 CHECKLIST FOR SAFE SURGERY

1. **Sign In (Before Induction)**—Performed Together by Surgeon, Nursing and Anesthesia
   - Team Members Introduce Themselves by Name and Role
   - Patient Identification
     Procedure
     Site and Side
     Confirmed Consent
     Blood Band
     Allergies
   - Confirmation of Site Marking, when applicable
   - Anesthesia Assessment
     Anesthesia Machine Check
     Monitors functional?
     Difficult Airway?
     Suction Available?
     Patient's ASA status
   - Blood Available
     Anticipated Blood Loss Risk
     Equipment Available
2. **Time Out (Before Skin Incision)**—Initiated/Led by Surgeon
   - Confirm Team Members/Introduce Themselves
   - Operation To Be Performed
   - Anticipated Operative Course
   - Site of Procedure
   - Patient Positioning
   - Allergies
   - Antibiotics Given—Time
   - Imaging Displayed
3. **Sign Out (Procedure Completed)**—Performed by OR Team
   - Performed Procedure Recorded
   - Body Cavity Search Performed
   - Uninterrupted Count
     Sponges
     Sharps
     Instruments
   - Counts Correct
     Sponges
     Sharps
     Instruments
   - Specimens Labeled
   - Team Debriefing

communicated to the team members; (4) the patient's airway and risk of aspiration have been assessed and, if needed, special equipment for intubation procured; (5) blood is available if the anticipated blood loss is greater than 500 mL; and (6) a functional pulse oximeter is placed on the patient. Best safety practices in the operating room include taking a timeout. Before the skin incision is made, the entire team takes a timeout. This means they stop what they are doing and focus on the safety of the patient. During this timeout the team orally confirms: (1) all team members by name; (2) the patient's identity, surgical site, and procedure; (3) that prophylactic antibiotics have been administered ≤60 minutes before the operation; (4) special equipment is available; (5) imaging results for the correct patient are displayed; and (6) review of anticipated surgical and anesthesia critical events including sterility of the equipment and availability and whether there is an anticipated fire safety hazard. At the completion of the procedure and prior to the patient leaving the operating room, the team orally confirms: (1) the procedure as recorded; (2) correct sponge, needle, and instrument counts if applicable; (3) the specimen is correctly labeled, including the patient's name; (4) any issues with equipment that need to be addressed; and (5) key concerns for the postoperative management of the patient. A debriefing with the team is helpful in reinforcing safe practices and correcting any process issues in future cases. If the patient is being admitted to an intensive care unit (ICU) bed, then there needs to be written and oral communication with the receiving team concerning the above.

POSTOPERATIVE CARE Postoperative care begins in the operating room with the completion of the operative procedure. The objective, like that of preoperative care, is to maintain the patient in a normal state. Ideally, complications are anticipated and prevented. This requires a thorough understanding of those complications that may follow surgical procedures in general and those most likely to follow specific diseases or procedures.

The unconscious patient or the patient still helpless from a spinal anesthesia requires special consideration, having to be lifted carefully from table to bed without unnecessary buckling of the spine or dragging of flaccid limbs. The optimum position in bed will vary with the individual case.

Patients who have had operations about the nose and mouth should be on their sides with the face dependent to protect against aspiration of mucus, blood, or vomitus. Major shifts in position after long operations are to be avoided until the patient has regained consciousness; experience has shown that such changes are badly tolerated. In some instances, the patient is transferred from the operating table directly to a permanent bed which may be transported to the patient's room. After the recovery of consciousness, most patients who have had abdominal operations will be more comfortable with the head slightly elevated and the thighs and knees slightly flexed. The usual hospital bed may be raised under the knees to accomplish the desired amount of flexion. If this is done, the heels must also be raised at least as high as the knees, so that stasis of blood in the calves is not encouraged. Patients who have had spinal anesthesia ordinarily are kept in bed for several hours to minimize postanesthetic headache and orthostatic hypotension.

Postoperative pain is controlled by the judicious use of narcotics. New techniques include the continued infusion of preservative-free morphine (Duramorph) into an epidural catheter which is left in place for several days or the use of a patient-controlled analgesia (PCA) intravenous infusion system containing morphine or meperidine. It is a serious error to administer too much morphine. This will lower both the rate and amplitude of the respiratory excursions and thus encourage pulmonary atelectasis. Antiemetic drugs minimize postoperative nausea and potentiate the pain relief afforded by narcotics. Some newer antihistamines also sedate effectively without depressing respirations. On the other hand, patients should be instructed to make their pain known to the nurses and to request relief. Otherwise, many stoic individuals, unaccustomed to hospital practice, might prefer to lie rigidly quiet rather than disturb the busy staff. Such voluntary splinting can lead to atelectasis just as readily as does the sleep of morphia.

Although postoperative care is a highly individual matter, certain groups of patients will have characteristics in common. The extremes of life are an example. Infants and children are characterized by the rapidity of their reactions; they are more easily and quickly thrown out of equilibrium with restriction of food or water intake; they are more susceptible to contagious diseases that may be contracted during a long hospitalization. Conversely, the healing processes are swifter, and there is a quicker restoration to normal health. The accuracy of their fluid replacement is a critical matter, since

their needs are large and their little bodies contain a very small reserve. Infants require 100 to 120 mL of water for each kilogram of body weight each day; in dehydration, twice this amount may be allowed.

The calculation of fluid needs in infants and children has been related to body surface area. Pocket-sized tables are available for the quick determination of surface area from age, height, and weight. In this system, from 1,200 to 1,500 mL of fluid per square meter are provided for daily maintenance. Parenteral fluids should contain the principal ions from all the body compartments (sodium, chloride, potassium, calcium) but not in high or "normal" concentrations. Solutions containing electrolytes at about half isotonic strength and balanced for all the ions are now available. Those containing only dextrose in water are best avoided. Colloids, such as blood or albumin, are indicated in severely depleted infants and whenever acute losses occur, just as in adults. Ten to 15 mL per kilogram of body weight may be given slowly each day.

The body weight should be followed closely. Very small infants should be weighed every 8 hours, and their orders for fluid therapy reevaluated as often. Infants and children have a very low tolerance for overhydration. Since accidents can happen everywhere, the flask for intravenous infusion hanging above an infant should never contain more water than the child could safely receive if it all ran in at once—about 20 mL per kilogram of body weight.

Elderly patients likewise demand special considerations. The elderly population is rapidly expanding in numbers; and with age, their medical diseases and treatments become more complex. The aging process leaves its mark on heart, kidneys, liver, lungs, and mind. Response to disease may be slower and less vigorous; the tolerance for drugs is usually diminished; and serious depletions in the body stores may require laboratory tests for detection. Awareness of pain may be much decreased or masked in the aged. A single symptom may be the only clue to a major complication. For this reason, it is often wise to listen carefully to the elderly patient's own appraisal of his or her progress, cater to any idiosyncrasies, and vary the postoperative regimen accordingly. Elderly patients know better than their physicians how to live with the infirmities of age. For them, the routines that have crept into postoperative care can become deadly. Thoracotomy and gastric tubes should be removed as soon as possible. Immobilizing drains, prolonged intravenous infusions, and binders should be held to a minimum. Early ambulation is to be encouraged. Conversely, if an elderly patient is not doing well, the surgeon should have a low threshold to place such an at-risk senior in an ICU after a complicated operation. In this setting, the patient will be monitored more frequently than on the floor; also, critical pulmonary, hemodynamic, and metabolic treatments may be pursued more aggressively.

As long as a postoperative patient requires parenteral fluids, accurate recordings of the intake and output and daily body weight are essential for scientific regulation of water and electrolytes. Then the amount and type of fluid to be given each day should be prescribed individually for each patient. Intake should just equal output for each of the important elements: water, sodium, chloride, and potassium. For each of these, a certain loss is expected each day in the physiology of a normal person. In TABLE 2, these physiologic losses are listed in part A. There are two major sources of loss requiring replacement in every patient receiving intravenous fluids:

TABLE 2 INTRAVENOUS FLUID REPLACEMENT FOR SOME COMMON EXTERNAL LOSSES

	mEq per Liter			IV Replacement with			
	Na⁺	Cl⁻	K⁺	Volume of Water	Saline or L/R	Dex/W	Add K⁺
A. Physiologic							
Skin, lungs	0	0	0	800 mL	—	800 mL	—
Good urine flow	40	50	30	1,200 mL	500 mL	700 mL	Optional
B. Pathologic							
Heavy sweating	50	60	5	350 mL/°C fever	½ either	½	—
Gastric suction	60	90	10	mL for mL output	½ saline	½	Add 30 mEq/L
Bile	145	100	41	mL for mL output	1 either	—	—
Pancreatic juice	140	75	4	mL for mL output	1 either	—	—
Bowel (long tube)	120	100	10	mL for mL output	1 either	—	Add 30 mEq/L
Diarrhea	140	100	30	mL for mL output	1 either	—	Add 30 mEq/L

(1) vaporization from skin and lungs, altered modestly by fever, but with a net average of about 800 mL per day in an adult; and (2) urine flow, which should lie between 1,000 and 1,500 mL daily. (In the normal stool, the loss of water and electrolytes is insignificant.) About 2,000 mL of water per day satisfy the normal physiologic requirements. It is a common error to administer too much salt in the form of normal saline in the immediate postoperative period. Normal losses are more than satisfied by the 4.5 g available in 500 mL of normal saline or a balanced electrolyte solution such as lactated Ringer's (L/R) solution. Many patients do well on less unless there is pathologic fluid loss from suction or drainage. The remainder of the normal parenteral intake should be glucose in water, as the nutritional requirements of the patient dictate.

To the physiologic output must be added, for replacement purposes, any other loss of body fluids that may result from disease. Some common sources for pathologic external losses are listed in part B of TABLE 2. In any of these losses, appropriate replacement depends upon an accurate intake–output record. If perspiration or fistulae are seeping large quantities of fluid on dressings or sheets, these may be collected and weighed. These fluids should be replaced volume for volume. All of these losses are rich in electrolyte content, and their replacement requires generous quantities of saline and electrolytes, in contrast to the very small amounts needed for normal physiologic replacement. Selection of the appropriate intravenous solutions may be made from a knowledge of the average electrolyte content in the source of the loss. TABLE 2 provides some of these data and suggests formulae by which intravenous restitution may be made. Thus, 1,000 mL of nasogastric suction output may be effectively replaced by 500 mL of saline plus 500 mL of dextrose and water with extra potassium chloride (KCl) added. Approximations of the formulae to the closest 500 mL are usually satisfactory in the adult. However, when losses arise from the gastrointestinal system below the pylorus, some alkaline lactate or bicarbonate solutions will eventually be necessary. When large volumes are being replaced, the adequacy of the therapy should be checked by daily weighing and by frequent measurement of serum electrolyte concentrations. When 3 to 6 L or more of intravenous fluids are required daily, the precise selection of electrolytes in this fluid becomes very important. The day should be broken into 8- or 12-hour shifts, with new orders for the fluid volume and electrolyte mixture at the start of each time interval. These new estimates are based upon repeated and updated measurements of body weight, input and output data, serum electrolytes, hematocrit, and the electrolyte composition of abnormal fluid losses and urine. The old principle of dividing the problem into smaller segments will improve the ability to conquer it.

The administration of potassium requires special consideration. Although this is an intracellular ion, its concentration in the plasma must not be raised above 6 mEq/L during any infusion, or serious cardiac arrhythmias may result. Ordinarily, when the kidneys are functioning properly, any excess potassium is quickly excreted and dangerous plasma levels are never reached. Small quantities of potassium should be added to the intravenous infusion only after good postoperative urine flow has been established. There are huge intracellular stores of this ion, so that there need be no rush about giving it. On the other hand, pathologic fluid losses from the main intestinal stream—the stomach or bowel—are rich in potassium. After a few days of such losses, sufficient depletion can occur to produce paralytic ileus and other disturbances. Therefore, it is best to give potassium generously, once the urine output is clearly adequate, and to monitor its level with plasma electrolyte tests or the height of the T wave in the electrocardiogram in urgent situations.

Surgeons should interest themselves in the details of the patient's diet after surgery. Prolonged starvation is to be avoided. On the first day, the diet may need to be restricted to clear liquids, such as tea. Fruit juices may increase abdominal distention and are best omitted until the third postoperative day. In a convalescence proceeding normally, a 2,500-calorie diet with 100 g of protein may often be started on the second or third postoperative day. Weighing should continue at twice-weekly intervals after diet is resumed. Weight portrays the nutritional trend and may stimulate more efficient feeding or a search for hidden edema in the case of too rapid a gain.

Ordinarily, constant gastrointestinal suction will be employed after operations upon the esophagus or resections of the gastrointestinal tract and in the presence of peritonitis, ileus, or intestinal obstruction. If ileus or intestinal obstruction appears postoperatively, a nasogastric tube may be used for decompression of the stomach and indirectly the small bowel.

The long Cantor tube is rarely used for distal decompression, as it cannot be easily passed into the small bowel. The tube is usually kept in place for 2 to 5 days and removed as normal bowel function returns. This will be evidenced by resumption of peristalsis, the passage of flatus, and the return of appetite. When it is anticipated that gastrointestinal suction will be needed for a more prolonged time, a gastrostomy placed at operation may provide gratifying comfort to the patient. It has proved efficient in maintaining suction and keeping distention to a minimum, particularly in the elderly patient with chronic lung disease, whose nasopharyngeal space must be kept as clear of contamination as possible. Feeding by way of a jejunostomy catheter or a gastrostomy tube may also be of value, particularly in the patient who is unable to swallow or who has difficulty in maintaining an adequate caloric intake.

No set rule can be laid down for the particular time at which a patient is permitted out of bed. The tendency at present is to have the patient ambulatory at the earliest possible moment, and most patients may be allowed out of bed on the first day after the operation. A longer period of rest may be essential to patients who have recently been in shock or who suffer from severe infection, cardiac insufficiency, cachexia, severe anemia, or thrombophlebitis. The principle of early ambulation has unquestionably speeded up the recovery period, accelerated the desire and tolerance for food, and probably decreased the incidence and severity of respiratory complications.

The surgeon should distinguish between ambulation and sitting in a chair; the latter actually may favor deep venous thrombosis. Every surgeon should establish a method of assisting patients out of bed and should teach these principles to those responsible for the bedside care. On the evening of the operation, the patient is encouraged to sit on the edge of the bed, kick his or her legs, and cough. Such patients are urged to change their position in bed frequently and move their legs and feet. The following day, the patient is turned on the side (wound side down) with the hips and knees flexed. This brings the knees to the edge of the bed, and an assistant then helps raise the patient sideways to a sitting position as the feet and lower legs fall over the side of the bed. The patient then swings the legs and moves feet to the floor, stands erect, breaths deeply, and coughs several times. Following this, the patient takes 8 or 10 steps and sits in a chair for 10 minutes, then returns to bed by a reversal of the foregoing steps. Once the patient has been up, he or she is encouraged at first to get up twice daily and later on to be up and walking as much as health and strength condition permit.

A sudden decrease in vital capacity may signal an impending pulmonary complication or an inflammatory process (abscess) adjacent to the diaphragm. Likewise, electrolyte imbalance, abdominal distention, or tenderness may decrease the vital capacity. Incentive spirometry is a helpful adjunct, particularly for those patients who will not or cannot breathe well for themselves. Frequent deep breathing and coughing in the postoperative period assist in clearing the bronchial tree of fluid collection, whereas ultrasonic or nebulized mists may be needed to loosen dried secretions. In such patients, pulmonary physical therapy with clapping, positive-pressure inhalation with bronchodilators, and postural drainage may be required. Daily examination with palpation of the calves and popliteal and adductor regions should be performed by the surgical team. Increase in calf circumference may be due to the edema of an otherwise unsuspected deep venous thrombosis (DVT). The onset of phlebitis has been clearly related to slowed venous return from the lower extremities during operation and postoperative immobility. Venous stasis can be reduced by wearing elastic stockings, elastic wrappings, or sequential compression stockings to the calves. In high-risk patients, including those with a history of DVT, perioperative anticoagulation should be considered.

With the occurrence of a DVT, anticoagulant therapy should be instituted at once, so that disabling or fatal pulmonary embolism may be avoided. Thrombosis is to be considered always as a potential complication; it appears to be more common in elderly and obese individuals, in infective states, and in malignant disease. Early ambulation has not eradicated this dreaded complication, and a sudden cardiopulmonary collapse several uneventful days after surgery may signal a pulmonary embolus from silent DVT.

Disruption of abdominal wounds is fortunately infrequent. It is more common in patients who have extensive surgery for carcinoma or obstructive jaundice. Contributing factors may be vitamin C deficiency, hypoproteinemia, steroid use, vomiting, abdominal distention, wound infection, or a need to cough excessively if preoperative tracheobronchial toilet was not well accomplished. The disruption is rarely recognized before the 7th day and is exceedingly rare after the 17th and 18th days. A sudden discharge from the wound of a large amount of orange serum is pathognomonic of dehiscence. Investigation may disclose an evisceration with a protruding loop of bowel or merely lack of healing of the walls of the wound. The proper treatment consists of replacing the viscera under sterile conditions in the operating room and closing the wound by through-and-through interrupted inert sutures of heavy size (as described in Chapter 10).

The surgeon must assume the responsibility for all untoward events occurring in the postoperative period. This attitude is necessary for progress. Too often surgeons are content to explain a complication on the basis of extraneous influences. Although the surgeon may feel blameless in the occurrence of a cerebral thrombosis or a coronary occlusion, it is inescapable that the complication did not arise until the operation was performed. Only as surgeons recognize that most sequelae of surgery, good and bad, are the direct results of preoperative preparation, of performance of the operative procedure, or of postoperative care will they improve his or her care of the patient and while attempting to prevent all avoidable complications.

CHAPTER 4

AMBULATORY SURGERY

Ambulatory or outpatient surgery is applicable to relatively few chapters in this *Atlas*. However, the repair of inguinal, femoral, and small umbilical hernias, breast biopsies, excision of skin tumors, and many plastic procedures are commonly performed in an ambulatory setting. In addition, many gynecologic procedures as well as certain orthopedic, otolaryngologic, and other procedures are performed in this area. The decision for or against ambulatory surgery may depend on the facilities available, as well as on the presence of an in-house anesthesiologist, recovery room, and observational unit. If all of these are available, some surgeons will also perform minimally invasive or laparoscopic procedures. Many patients tend to feel reassured by plans for ambulatory surgery, which in the majority of instances does not involve hospital admission. Obviously, the guidelines for this approach may well be altered by the patient's age and any changes in physical status.

The surgeon is responsible for making the specific decision for or against ambulatory surgery provided that the patient finds it acceptable. The attitude of the patient, the nature of the surgical problem, the depth of family support that will be available postoperatively, and the type of facility in which the procedure is to be performed must all be taken into consideration. Hospital guidelines usually indicate the procedures found to be appropriate and acceptable to that particular institution as defined in their credentialing of operative privileges and procedures. The surgeon may perform very minor surgical excisions in a properly equipped office and more extensive procedures in a freestanding facility or one associated with a hospital that provides anesthesiologists, equipment, and personnel competent to handle unexpected emergencies.

Since the general surgeon will depend upon the use of local anesthesia for many patients undergoing ambulatory surgery, it is important to be familiar with the limitations on the amount of each local anesthetic that can be safely injected. A review of the nerve supply to the area involved is advisable. Although reactions to local anesthetics are relatively uncommon, the signs and symptoms, which may include convulsive seizures, should be recognized, and preparation should be made for the early administration of some type of anticonvulsant.

Anesthesiologists tend to triage patients into several categories as defined by the American Society of Anesthesiologists (ASA). In ASA category I are patients who have no organic, physiologic, biochemical, or psychiatric disorders. The pathologic process being operated upon is localized and not systemic. In ASA category II, patients have a mild to moderate systemic disturbance caused either by the condition to be treated or by other pathophysiologic processes. Examples are mild diabetes or treated hypertension. Some would add all neonates under 1 month of age and all octogenarians. ASA category III includes patients with severe disturbances or disorders from whatever cause. Examples include those with diabetes requiring insulin or patients with angina pectoris. The presence of an anesthesiologist is essential in the majority of patients in ASA categories II and III.

Ambulatory surgery requires that the final physical evaluation of the patient by the surgeon be performed as near the date of the procedure as practical. Many ambulatory surgery centers start this process by having the patient fill out a checklist like those shown in FIGURES 1 and 2. This information is reviewed by the surgeon, the admitting nurse, and the anesthesiologist. The patient is assigned to the proper category. ASA categories I and II patients are generally excellent candidates for ambulatory surgery, whereas ASA category III patients should be carefully selected in consultation with the anesthesiologist.

The period between the examination and the performance of a procedure may be as long as 2 to 4 weeks, but in the winter months, a shorter period may be desirable because of the frequency of upper respiratory disorders. Patients should be informed that the development of even suggestive symptoms of an upper respiratory infection is a possible indication for postponing the elective procedure.

Patients may also be required to have blood studies, which often vary with age or organ system impairment. A sickle cell screen is done if clinically indicated, and a hematocrit is usually sufficient for ASA category I patients under the age of 40. Thereafter, renal function tests (BUN or creatinine) and blood glucose tests are added followed by an electrocardiogram (especially in males) and a chest radiograph. ASA category III patients who have cardiovascular disease, insulin-dependent diabetes, and specific organ system diseases such as those involving kidneys, liver, or lung require thorough medical and surgical evaluation before being scheduled for an ambulatory operation. Medical control of the diseases must be optimized, and a preprocedure consultation with the anesthesiologist may be appropriate.

PREANESTHETIC EVALUATION

NAME _____ PHONE # _____

PROPOSED OPERATION _____ SURGEON _____

DATE OF PROPOSED OPERATION _____ AGE _____ HT _____ WT _____

PLEASE CHECK (✓) EACH QUESTION YES OR NO. IF YOU DO NOT UNDERSTAND ANY QUESTION, PLEASE PLACE A QUESTION MARK (?) IN THE "YES" OR "NO" COLUMN.

RECENT OR PRESENT ILLNESS	YES	NO	REMARKS
A COLD IN PAST 2 WEEKS			
BRONCHITIS OR CHRONIC COUGH			
ASTHMA, HAY FEVER			
CROUP			
PNEUMONIA. TUBERCULOSIS OTHER LUNG INFECTION			
PULMONARY EMBOLUS			
EMPHYSEMA			
SHORTNESS OF BREATH			
ANY OTHER LUNG TROUBLE			
DO YOU SMOKE?			
HOW MUCH?			
DATE OF LAST CHEST X-RAY			
HEART FAILURE			
HEART MURMUR			
HIGH BLOOD PRESSURE			
LOW BLOOD PRESSURE			
CHEST PAIN, ANGINA			
HEART ATTACK(S)			
PALPITATIONS: IRREGULAR OR FAST HEARTBEAT			
DATE OF LAST EKG			
BACK OR NECK PAIN OR INJURY			
SLIPPED DISC, SCIATICA			
CONVULSIONS, EPILEPSY			
STROKE OR DIZZINESS			
NERVE OR MUSCLE WEAKNESS			
THYROID TROUBLE			
DIABETES			
LOW BLOOD SUGAR			
ANEMIA			
SICKLE CELL ILLNESS, BLEEDING OR CLOTTING PROBLEMS			
BLOOD TRANSFUSIONS?			
INFANT DEVELOPMENT PROBLEMS, DOWN'S SYNDROME, PREMATURITY, SLOW GROWTH AND DEVELOPMENT			

Figure 1 Preanesthetic evaluation.

The presence of an anesthesiologist provides guidance for the control of anxiety in children and adults alike by appropriate preoperative medication. Sedation with midazolam (Versed) can provide a short interval of pleasant forgetfulness while the local anesthetic is being injected. Analgesia may be needed; standard narcotics (like meperidine) and short-acting synthetic ones (like fentanyl) are effective. Should the patient require a limited general anesthesia, thiopental plus nitrous oxide or continuous infusion of propofol (Diprivan) offers the advantage of rapid emergence. Among the conduction anesthesia techniques, a short-duration spinal is possible, but epidural infusions are preferred as the patients need not await return of motor function to their legs and urinary bladder.

The rigid routines of a major operating room in a busy hospital are adhered to in the ambulatory surgical setting. A careful, detailed record of the procedure, the anesthesia, and the recovery period is made.

In many instances, the resulting scar is quite important. Distortion of the skin and subcutaneous tissues by the injection of the local anesthetic agent must be recalled because the incision adheres to the direction of the lines of skin cleavage. The avoidance of administering epinephrine along with the anesthetic agent decreases the incidence of postoperative bleeding or discoloration of the wound from delayed oozing. The skin incision should be of sufficient length to ensure adequate exposure. While electrocoagulation can be used, individual ligation of active bleeding vessels is better. The type of suture material, as well as the type of suturing, need not vary from the traditional technique of the surgeon.

All specimens removed must be submitted for microscopic evaluation by the pathologist. Patients should be informed of any abnormal findings, unless it seems more judicious to inform the next of kin, with a full written statement of the reasons for doing this on the patient's record.

Closure of the skin should be done very carefully, whether the procedure is for cosmetic purposes or for the local excision of a benign tumor. Some believe subcutaneous closure is less painful than clips or sutures that penetrate the skin. Others prefer to use adhesive strips that tend to take the

RECENT OR PRESENT ILLNESS		YES	NO	REMARKS
LIVER TROUBLE: HEPATITIS, JAUNDICE, CIRRHOSIS				
STOMACH TROUBLE, ULCERS, HIATAL HERNIA, GALL BLADDER				
KIDNEY TROUBLE, STONES, INFECTION, DIALYSIS				
MENTAL OR EMOTIONAL ILLNESS				
OTHER ILLNESS NOT MENTIONED				
FEMALES: ARE YOU PREGNANT?				
DO YOU DRINK ALCOHOL?				
USE OTHER RECREATIONAL DRUGS?				
LIST PREVIOUS SURGERIES:	DATE			
DATE OF MOST RECENT ANESTHETIC TYPE				
HAVE YOU HAD ANY UNUSUAL REACTION TO ANESTHESIA?				
HAS ANY BLOOD RELATIVE HAD AN UNUSUAL REACTION TO ANESTHESIA?				
DO YOU HAVE DENTURES OR LOOSE TEETH, CAPS, CROWNS OR BRIDGES?				
DO YOU WEAR CONTACT LENSES, HEARING AID, OR A PHYSICAL PROSTHESIS?				
ARE YOU ALLERGIC TO ANY MEDICATIONS? (LIST)				
ARE YOU TAKING (OR HAVE YOU RECENTLY TAKEN) MEDICATIONS?				
FOR BLOOD PRESSURE				
DIURETICS (WATER PILLS)				
DIGITALIS, DIGOXIN, LANOXIN (OTHER HEART MEDICINE)				
CANCER CHEMOTHERAPY				
TRANQUILIZERS, SLEEPING TABS, SEDATIVES, ANTIDEPRESSANTS				
BLOOD THINNERS, ANTICOAGULANT				
EYE DROPS				
PAIN PILLS OR SHOTS				
STEROIDS, CORTISOL, MEDROL, PREDNISONE				
INSULIN (WHAT KIND?)				
OTHER				
I HAVE ANSWERED THE QUESTIONS CONCERNING MY HEALTH TO THE BEST OF MY KNOWLEDGE.				

SIGNED _____ DATE _____

_____
RELATIONSHIP (IF OTHER THAN PATIENT)

Figure 2 Patient checklist.

GENERAL HOMEGOING POSTOPERATIVE INSTRUCTIONS

TO: _____ FOLLOWING: _____

DOCTOR'S NAME: _____ PHONE NUMBER: _____

PLEASE OBSERVE THE FOLLOWING INSTRUCTIONS TO INSURE A SAFE RECOVERY FROM YOUR SURGERY.

DIET:
1. Drink water, apple juice or carbonated beverages as tolerated.
2. Eat small amounts of foods such as Jell-O, soup, crackers, as tolerated. Progress to normal diet if you are not nauseated.
3. Avoid alcoholic beverages for 24 hours.

MEDICATIONS:
1. Take as directed.
2. If pain is not relieved by your medication, call your physician.
3. Dizziness is not unusual.
4. Avoid drugs for allergies, nerves or sleep for 24 hours.

ACTIVITIES:
1. Rest at home; limit activity; do not engage in sports or heavy work until your doctor gives you permission.
2. ALLOW 24 HOURS BEFORE:
   — driving or operating hazardous machinery (sewing machine, drills, etc.).
   — signing important papers.
   — making significant decisions.
3. Children having had surgery should not be left unattended.

WOUND/DRESSING:
1. Observe area for bleeding; if dressing becomes soaked or fresh bright red bleeding occurs, apply pressure and call your doctor at once.
2. Do not change dressing until instructed by your doctor.
3. Keep incisional area clean and dry.

If you are concerned and are unable to reach your doctor, go to the hospital's emergency room.

Call your doctor's office for follow-up appointment.

These instructions have been explained to the patient, family or friend and a copy has been given to same.

Patient Signature: _____

Date: _____   Nurse Signature: _____

Figure 3 General homegoing postoperative instructions.

tension off the line of closure. The dressing should be as simple as possible, unless a compression dressing is desired. Most dressings can be removed in 2 or 3 days and bathing resumed.

It should be suggested that upon their return home, patients will find a few hours in bed desirable while the effects of the drugs administered are diminished. They should be instructed to find the position most likely to give postoperative comfort. For example, the patient undergoing repair of an inguinal hernia should have less discomfort if the knee on the operated side is moderately flexed over a pillow. Some will be more comfortable with support for the scrotum with an ice cap placed intermittently over the area of the incision.

The patient undergoing ambulatory surgery should take plenty of fluids for several days. A mild cathartic is helpful in counteracting the effect of any preoperative narcotics, as well as reducing tension on the wound from straining at stool. Stool softeners (like mineral oil) may prove to be useful if prolonged inactivity or narcotic use is anticipated.

Written instructions like those shown in FIGURE 3 should be reviewed with the patient and particularly with the responsible family member who is taking the patient home. An informed caregiver at home is an essential part of the ambulatory surgery experience. If a relative or a caregiver is not available, then consideration should be given to overnight observation of the patient. These instructions should cover the areas of medications, diet, activities, and wound care. The feeling of relief that "it is over" does not permit the patient to test the strength of the surgical closure or the stability of recovery from the anesthetic or any drugs that may have been given. Most patients are cautioned to refrain from driving, operating hazardous machinery, or making important decisions for 24 hours. They should be instructed how to reach the surgeon and be given the telephone number of the hospital emergency department in case of an urgent emergency. A follow-up telephone call by the ambulatory surgery center or the surgeon on the day after operation serves to verify that recovery is proceeding satisfactorily. Most patients greatly appreciate this evidence of concern. A written appointment time for return evaluation and checkup is given.

Patients having ambulatory surgery do surprisingly well, and most seem to prefer this approach to the long-established tradition of hospitalization. It must be admitted that this approach places more preoperative responsibility on the patient, as well as on the surgeon, to meet all the requirements for the performance of a procedure. The patient must take the time not only to be evaluated by the surgeon but to have all the laboratory and radiographic examinations taken care of in advance. Since the tests and the physician's final evaluation may precede the day of operation by several weeks, the patient must take responsibility to inform the surgeon of any special developments, such as a change in condition or the occurrence of an upper respiratory infection.

The period of recovery before the patient can return to work depends on the extent and type of surgical procedure. It is hoped that ambulatory surgery will shorten the period of disability and ensure more prompt correction of the indications for operation.

SECTION II
SURGICAL ANATOMY

ARTERIAL BLOOD SUPPLY TO THE UPPER ABDOMINAL VISCERA

The stomach has a very rich anastomotic blood supply. The largest blood supply comes from the celiac axis (1) by way of the left gastric artery (2). The blood supply to the uppermost portion, including the lower esophagus, is from a branch of the left inferior phrenic artery (3). The left gastric artery divides as it reaches the lesser curvature just below the esophagogastric junction. One branch descends anteriorly (2a) and the other branch posteriorly along the lesser curvature. There is a bare area of stomach wall, approximately 1 to 2 cm wide, between these two vessels which is not covered by peritoneum. It is necessary to ligate the left gastric artery near its point of origin above the superior surface of the pancreas in the performance of a total gastrectomy. This also applies when 70% or more of the stomach is to be removed. Ligation of the artery in this area is commonly done in the performance of gastric resection for malignancy so that complete removal of all lymph nodes high on the lesser curvature may be accomplished.

A lesser blood supply to the uppermost portion of the stomach arises from the short gastric vessels (4) in the gastrosplenic ligament. Several small arteries arising from the branches of the splenic artery course upward toward the posterior wall of the fundus. These vessels are adequate to ensure viability of the gastric pouch following ligation of the left gastric artery as well as of the left inferior phrenic artery. If one of these vessels predominates, it is called the *posterior gastric artery;* its presence becomes significant in radical gastric resection. Mobilization of the spleen, following division of the splenorenal and gastrophrenic ligaments, retains the blood supply to the fundus and permits extensive mobilization at the same time. The blood supply of the remaining gastric pouch may be compromised if splenectomy becomes necessary. The body of the stomach can be mobilized toward the right and its blood supply maintained by dividing the thickened portion of the splenocolic ligament up to the region of the left gastroepiploic artery (5). Further mobilization results if the splenic flexure of the colon, as well as the transverse colon, is freed from the greater omentum. The greater curvature is ordinarily divided at a point between branches coming from the gastroepiploic vessels (5, 6) directly into the gastric wall.

The blood supply to the region of the pylorus and lesser curvature arises from the right gastric artery (7), which is a branch of the hepatic artery (8). The right gastric artery is so small that it can hardly be identified when it is ligated with the surrounding tissues in this area.

One of the larger vessels requiring ligation during gastric resection is the right gastroepiploic artery (6) as it courses to the left from beneath the pylorus. It parallels the greater curvature. The blood supply to the greater curvature also arises from the splenic artery (9) by way of the left gastroepiploic artery (5).

Relatively few key arteries need to be ligated to control the major blood supply to the pancreas. When the duodenum and head of the pancreas are to be resected, it is necessary to ligate the right gastric artery (7) and the gastroduodenal artery (10) above the superior surface of the duodenum. The possibility of damaging the middle colic vessels (11), which arise from the superior mesenteric artery and course over the head of the pancreas, must always be considered. This vessel may be adherent to the posterior wall of the antrum of the stomach, and it may course over the second part of the duodenum, especially if the hepatic flexure of the colon is anchored high in the right upper quadrant. The anterior and posterior branches of the inferior pancreaticoduodenal artery (12) are ligated close to their points of origin from the superior mesenteric artery (13). Additional branches directly to the third portion of the duodenum and upper jejunum also require ligation.

The body and tail of the pancreas can be extensively mobilized with the spleen. The splenic artery located beneath the peritoneum over the superior surface of the pancreas should be ligated near its point of origin (9). The dorsal pancreatic artery (14) arises from the splenic artery near its point of origin and courses directly into the body of the pancreas. Following the removal of the spleen, the inferior surface of the body and tail of the pancreas can be easily mobilized without division of major arteries. When the body of the pancreas is divided, several arteries will require ligation. These include the inferior (transverse) pancreatic artery (15) arising from the splenic artery and the greater pancreatic artery (16).

The blood supply to the spleen is largely from the splenic artery arising from the celiac axis. Following ligation of the splenic artery, there is a rich anastomotic blood supply through the short gastric vessels (4), as well as the left gastroepiploic artery (5). The splenic artery is usually serpentine in contour, as it courses along the superior surface of the pancreas just beneath the peritoneum. Following division of the gastrosplenic vessels, it is advantageous to ligate the splenic artery some distance from the hilus of the spleen. The gastric wall should not be injured during the division of the short gastric vessels high in the region of the fundus. Small blood vessels entering the tail of the pancreas require individual ligation, especially in the presence of a large spleen and accompanying induration in the region of the tail of the pancreas.

The colon has been displaced inferiorly as indicated by the arrow to allow visualization of the Gastric, Hepatic, Pancreatic and Duodenal vessels. The blood supply to the gallbladder is through the cystic artery (17), which usually arises from the right hepatic artery (18). In the triangular zone bounded by the cystic duct joining the common hepatic duct and the cystic artery, Calot's triangle, there are more anatomic variations than are found in any other location. The most common variations in this zone, which is no larger than 3 cm in diameter, are related to the origin of the cystic artery. It most commonly arises from the right hepatic artery (18) after the latter vessel has passed beneath the common hepatic duct. The cystic artery may arise from the right hepatic artery more proximally and lie anterior to the common hepatic duct. Other common variations include origin of the cystic artery from the left hepatic artery (19), the common hepatic artery (8), or the gastroduodenal artery (10); additionally, these cystic arteries may have uncommon relationships to the biliary ductal system. The variations in the hepatoduodenal ligament are so numerous that nothing should be ligated or incised in this area until definite identification has been made. ■

1 Celiac axis
2 Lt. gastric - 2a anterior branch
3 Lt. inf. phrenic

4 Short gastrics
5 Lt. gastroepiploic
6 Rt. gastroepiploic
7 Rt. gastric
8 Com. hepatic
9 Splenic
10 Gastroduodenal
11 Middle colic
12 Post. and ant. (sup. and inf.)
   pancreaticoduodenals
13 Sup. mesenteric
14 Sup. (dorsal)
   pancreatic
15 Inf. (transv.)
   pancreatic
16 Greater pancreatic

17 Cystic
18 Rt. hepatic
19 Lt. hepatic

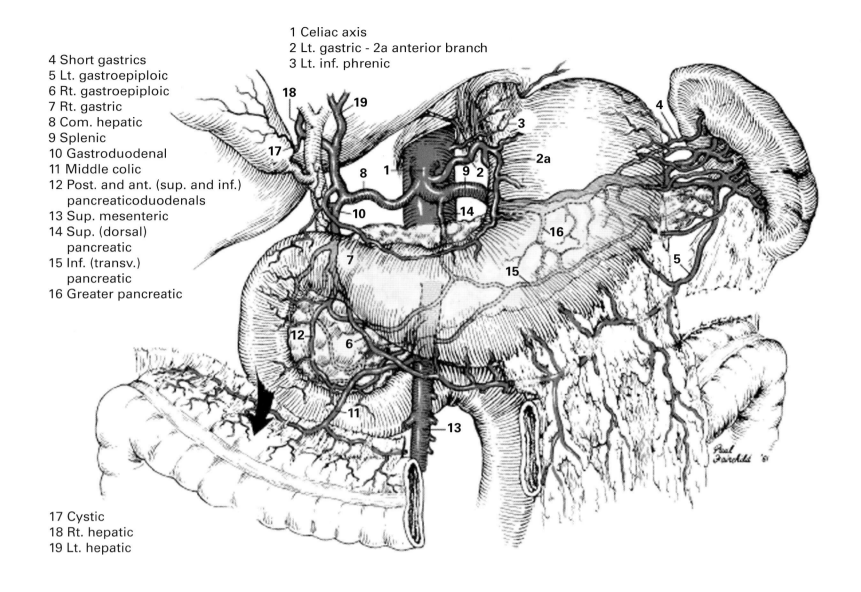

CHAPTER 6

VENOUS AND LYMPHATIC SUPPLY TO THE UPPER ABDOMINAL VISCERA

The venous blood supply of the upper abdomen parallels the arterial blood supply. The portal vein (1) is the major vessel that has the unique function of receiving venous blood from all intraperitoneal viscera with the exception of the liver. It is formed behind the head of the pancreas by the union of the superior mesenteric (2) and splenic (3) veins. It ascends posterior to the gastrohepatic ligament to enter the liver at the porta hepatis. It lies in a plane posterior to and between the hepatic artery on the left and the common bile duct on the right. This vein has surgical significance in cases of portal hypertension. When portacaval anastomosis is performed, exposure is obtained by means of an extensive Kocher maneuver. Several small veins (4) from the posterior aspect of the pancreas enter the sides of the superior mesenteric vein near the point of origin of the portal vein. Care must be taken to avoid tearing these structures during the mobilization of the vein. Once hemorrhage occurs, it is difficult to control.

The coronary (left gastric) vein (5) returns blood from the lower esophageal segment and the lesser curvature of the stomach. It runs parallel to the left gastric artery and then courses retroperitoneally downward and medially to enter the portal vein behind the pancreas. It anastomoses freely with the right gastric vein (6), and both vessels drain into the portal vein to produce a complete venous circle. It has a significance in portal hypertension in that the branches of the coronary vein, along with the short gastric veins (7), produce the varicosities in the fundus of the stomach and lower esophagus.

The other major venous channel in the area is the splenic vein (3), which lies deep and parallel to the splenic artery along the superior aspect of the pancreas. The splenic vein also receives venous drainage from the greater curvature of the stomach and the pancreas, as well as from the colon, through the inferior mesenteric vein (8). When a splenorenal shunt is performed, meticulous dissection of this vein from the pancreas with ligation of the numerous small vessels is necessary. As the dissection proceeds, the splenic vein comes into closer proximity with the left renal vein where anastomosis can be performed. The point of anastomosis is proximal to the entrance of the inferior mesenteric vein.

The colon has been displaced inferiorly as indicated by the arrow to allow visualization of the portal vein in the hepatoduodenal ligament and the venous drainage of stomach, head of the pancreas, and duodenum. The venous configuration on the gastric wall is relatively constant. In performing a conservative hemigastrectomy, venous landmarks can be used to locate the proximal line of resection. On the lesser curvature of the stomach, the third branch (5a) of the coronary vein down from the esophagocardiac junction is used as a point for transection. On the greater curvature of the stomach the landmark is where the left gastroepiploic vein (9) most closely approximates the gastric wall (9a). Transection is carried out between these two landmarks (5a, 9a).

The anterior and posterior pancreaticoduodenal veins (10) produce an extensive venous network about the head of the pancreas. They empty into the superior mesenteric or hepatic portal vein. The anterior surface of the head of the pancreas is relatively free of vascular structures, and blunt dissection may be carried out here without difficulty. There is, however, a small anastomotic vein (11) between the right gastroepiploic (12) and the middle colic vein (13). This vein, if not recognized, can produce troublesome bleeding in the mobilization of the greater curvature of the stomach, as well as of the hepatic flexure of the colon. The pancreaticoduodenal veins have assumed new importance with the advent of transhepatic venous sampling and hormonal assays for localization of endocrine-secreting tumors of the pancreas and duodenum.

In executing the Kocher maneuver, no vessels are encountered unless the maneuver is carried inferiorly along the third portion of the duodenum. At this point the middle colic vessels (13) cross the superior aspect of the duodenum to enter the transverse mesocolon. Unless care is taken in doing an extensive Kocher maneuver, this vein may be injured.

The lymphatic drainage of the upper abdominal viscera is extensive. Lymph nodes are found along the course of all major venous structures. For convenience of reference, there are four major zones of lymph node aggregations. The superior gastric lymph nodes (A) are located about the celiac axis and receive the lymphatic channels from the lower esophageal segment and the major portion of the lesser curvature of the stomach, as well as from the pancreas. The suprapyloric lymph nodes (B) about the portal vein drain the remaining portion of the lesser curvature and the superior aspect of the pancreas. The inferior gastric subpyloric group (C), which is found anterior to the head of the pancreas, receives the lymph drainage from the greater curvature of the stomach, the head of the pancreas, and the duodenum. The last major group is the pancreaticolienal nodes (D), which are found at the hilus of the spleen and drain the tail of the pancreas, the fundus of the stomach, and the spleen. There are extensive communications among all these groups of lymph nodes. The major lymphatic depot, the cisterna chyli, is found in the retroperitoneal space. This communicates with the systemic venous system by way of the thoracic duct into the left subclavian vein. This gives the anatomic explanation for the involvement of Virchow's node in malignant diseases involving the upper abdominal viscera. ■

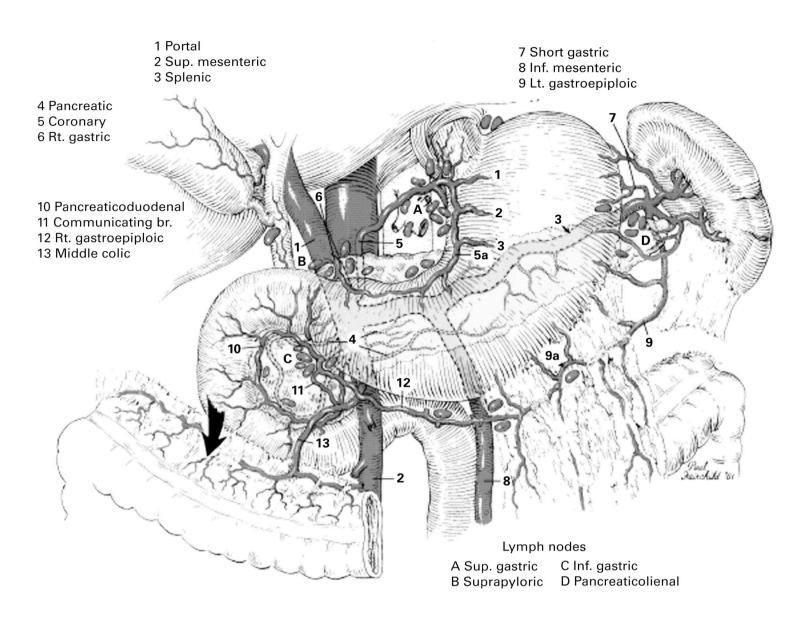

1 Portal
2 Sup. mesenteric
3 Splenic

4 Pancreatic
5 Coronary
6 Rt. gastric

10 Pancreaticoduodenal
11 Communicating br.
12 Rt. gastroepiploic
13 Middle colic

7 Short gastric
8 Inf. mesenteric
9 Lt. gastroepiploic

Lymph nodes
A Sup. gastric   C Inf. gastric
B Suprapyloric   D Pancreaticolienal

Because of its embryologic development from both the midgut and hindgut, the colon has two main sources of blood supply: the superior mesenteric (1) and the inferior mesenteric arteries (2). The superior mesenteric artery (1) supplies the right colon, the appendix, and small intestine. The middle colic artery (3) is the most prominent branch of the superior mesenteric artery. It arises after the pancreaticoduodenal vessels (see Chapter 5). The middle colic artery branches into a right and left division. The right division anastomoses with the right colic (4) and the ileocolic (5) arteries. The left branch communicates with the marginal artery of Drummond (6). The middle and right colic and ileocolic arteries are doubly ligated near their origin when a right colectomy is performed for malignancy. The ileocolic artery reaches the mesentery of the appendix from beneath the terminal ileum. Angulation or obstruction of the terminal ileum should be avoided following the ligation of the appendiceal artery (7) in the presence of a short mesentery.

The inferior mesenteric artery arises from the aorta just below the ligament of Treitz. Its major branches include the left colic (8), one or more sigmoid branches (9, 10), and the superior hemorrhoidal artery (11). Following ligation of the inferior mesenteric artery at its origin, the viability of the colon is maintained through the marginal artery of Drummond (6) by way of the left branch of the middle colic artery.

The third blood supply to the large intestine arises from the middle and inferior hemorrhoidal vessels. The middle hemorrhoidal vessels (12) arise from the internal iliac (hypogastric) (13), either directly or from one of its major branches. They enter the rectum along with the suspensory ligament on either side. These are relatively small vessels, but they should be ligated.

The blood supply to the anus is from the inferior hemorrhoidal (14) vessels, a branch of the internal pudendal artery (15). In low-lying lesions wide excision of the area is necessary with ligation of the individual bleeders as they are encountered.

The venous drainage of the right colon parallels the arterial supply and drains directly into the superior mesenteric vein (1). The inferior mesenteric vein, in the region of the bifurcation of the aorta, deviates to the left and upward as it courses beneath the pancreas to join the splenic vein. High ligation of the inferior mesenteric vein (16) should be carried out before extensive manipulation of a malignant tumor of the left colon or sigmoid in order to avoid the vascular spread of tumor cells.

The right colon can be extensively mobilized and derotated to the left side without interference with its blood supply. The mobilization is accomplished by dividing the avascular lateral peritoneal attachments of the mesentery of the appendix, cecum, and ascending colon. Blood vessels of a size requiring ligation are usually present only at the peritoneal attachments of the hepatic and splenic flexures. The transverse colon and splenic flexure can be mobilized by separating the greater omentum from its loose attachment to the transverse colon (see Chapter 26). Traction on the splenic flexure should be avoided lest troublesome bleeding could result from a tear in the adjacent splenic capsule. The abdominal incision should be extended high enough to allow direct visualization of the splenic flexure when it is necessary to mobilize the entire left colon. The left colon can be mobilized toward the midline by division of the lateral peritoneal attachment. There are few, if any, vessels that will require ligation in this area.

The descending colon and sigmoid can be mobilized medially by division of the avascular peritoneal reflection in the left lumbar gutter. The sigmoid is commonly quite closely adherent to the peritoneum in the left iliac fossa. The peritoneal attachment is avascular, but because of the proximity of the spermatic or ovarian vessels, as well as the left ureter, careful identification of these structures is required. Following the division of the peritoneal attachment and the greater omentum, further mobilization and elongation of the colon can be accomplished by division of the individual branches (8, 9, 10) of the inferior mesenteric artery. This ligation must not encroach on the marginal vessels of Drummond (6).

The posterior wall of the rectum can be bluntly dissected from the hollow of the sacrum without dividing important vessels. The blood supply of the rectum is in the mesentery adjacent to the posterior rectal wall. Following division of the peritoneal attachment to the rectum and division of the suspensory ligaments on either side, the rectum can be straightened with the resultant gain of considerable distance (Chapter 57). The pouch of Douglas, which may initially appear to be quite deep in the pelvis, can be mobilized well up into the operative field.

The lymphatic supply follows the vascular channels, especially the venous system. Accordingly, all of the major blood supplies of the colon should be ligated near their points of origin. These vessels should be ligated before a malignant tumor is manipulated. Complete removal of the lymphatic drainage from lesions of the left colon requires ligation of the inferior mesenteric artery (2) near its point of origin from the aorta.

Low-lying malignant rectal lesions may extend laterally along the middle hemorrhoidal vessels (12) as well as along the levator ani muscles. They may also extend cephalad along the superior hemorrhoidal vessels (11). The lymphatic drainage of the anus follows the same pathway but may include spread to the superficial inguinal lymph nodes (17). The lower the lesion, the greater the danger of multiple spread from the several lymphatic systems involved. ■

5 Ileocolic art. and vein
6 marginal vessels of Drummond

1 Sup. mesenteric art. and vein
2 Inf. mesenteric art.
3 Middle colic art. and vein
4 Rt. colic art. and vein

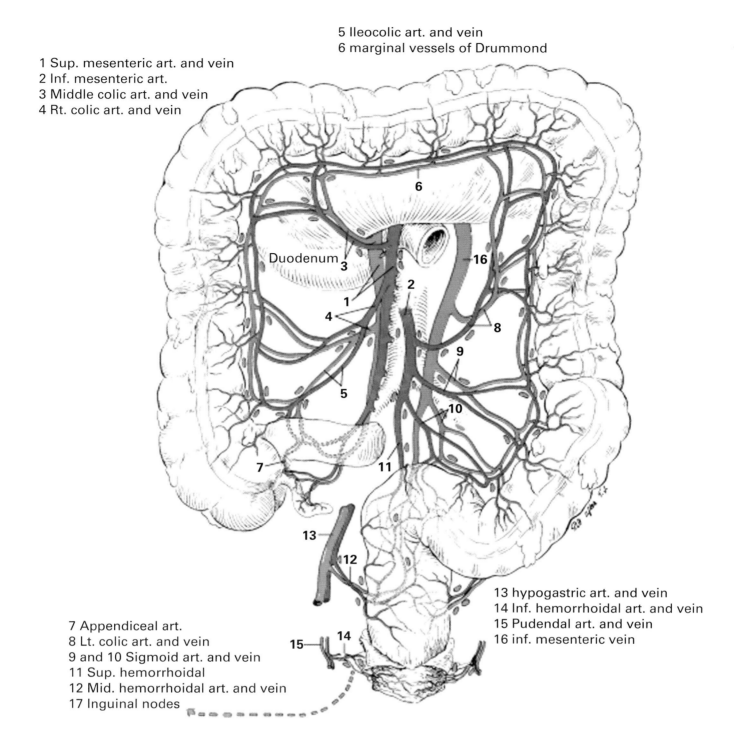

13 hypogastric art. and vein
14 Inf. hemorrhoidal art. and vein
15 Pudendal art. and vein
16 inf. mesenteric vein

7 Appendiceal art.
8 Lt. colic art. and vein
9 and 10 Sigmoid art. and vein
11 Sup. hemorrhoidal
12 Mid. hemorrhoidal art. and vein
17 Inguinal nodes

CHAPTER 8

ANATOMY OF THE ABDOMINAL AORTA AND INFERIOR VENA CAVA

The various vascular procedures that are carried out on the major vessels in the retroperitoneal area of the abdominal cavity make familiarity with these structures essential. Likewise, surgery of the adrenal glands and the genitourinary system invariably involves one or more of the branches of the abdominal aorta and inferior vena cava.

The blood supply to the adrenals is complicated and different on the two sides. The superior arterial supply branches from the inferior phrenic artery (1) on both sides. The left adrenal receives a branch directly from the adjacent aorta. A similar branch also may pass behind the vena cava to the right side, but the more prominent arterial supply arises from the right renal artery. The major venous return (3) on the left side is directly to the left renal vein. On the right side, the venous supply may be more obscure, as the adrenal is in close proximity to the vena cava and the venous system (2) drains directly into the latter structure.

The celiac axis (A) is one of the major arterial divisions of the abdominal aorta. It divides into the left gastric, splenic, and common hepatic arteries. Immediately below this is the superior mesenteric artery (B), which provides the blood supply to that portion of the gastrointestinal tract arising from the foregut and midgut. The renal arteries arise laterally from the aorta on either side. The left renal vein crosses the aorta from the left kidney and usually demarcates the upper limits of arteriosclerotic abdominal aneurysms. The left ovarian (or spermatic) vein (13) enters the left renal vein, but this vessel on the right side (5) drains directly into the vena cava.

In removing an abdominal aortic aneurysm, it is necessary to ligate the pair of ovarian (or spermatic) arteries (4), as well as the inferior mesenteric artery (C). In addition, there are four pairs of lumbar vessels that arise from the posterior wall of the abdominal aorta (14). The middle sacral vessels will also require ligation (12). Because of the inflammatory reaction associated with the aneurysm, this portion of the aorta may be intimately attached to the adjacent vena cava.

The blood supply to the ureters is variable and difficult to identify. The arterial supply (6, 7, 8) arises from the renal vessels, directly from the aorta, and from the gonadal vessels, as well as from the hypogastric arteries (11). Although these vessels may be small and their ligation necessary, the ureters should not be denuded of their blood supply any further than is absolutely necessary.

The aorta terminates by dividing into the common iliac arteries (9), which in turn divide into the external iliac (10) and the internal iliac (hypogastric) (11) arteries. From the bifurcation of the aorta, the middle sacral vessel (12) descends along the anterior surface of the sacrum. There is a concomitant vein that usually empties into the left common iliac vein at this point (12).

The ovarian arteries (4) arise from the anterolateral wall of the aorta below the renal vessels. They descend retroperitoneally across the ureters and through the infundibulopelvic ligament to supply the ovary and salpinx (15). They terminate by anastomosing with the uterine artery (16),

which descends in the broad ligament. The spermatic arteries and veins follow a retroperitoneal course before entering the inguinal canal to supply the testis in the scrotum.

The uterine vessels (16) arise from the anterior division of the internal iliac (hypogastric) arteries (11) and proceed medially to the edge of the vaginal vault opposite the cervix. At this point, the artery crosses over the ureter ("water under the bridge") (17). The uterine vein, in most instances, does not accompany the artery at this point but passes behind the ureter. In a hysterectomy, the occluding vascular clamps must be applied close to the wall of the uterus to avoid damage to the ureter. The uterine vessels then ascend along the lateral wall of the uterus and turn laterally into the broad ligament to anastomose with the ovarian vessels.

The lymphatic networks of the abdominal viscera and retroperitoneal organs frequently end in lymph nodes found along the entire abdominal aorta and inferior vena cava. Lymph nodes about the celiac axis (A) are commonly involved with metastatic cancer arising from the stomach and the body and tail of the pancreas. The para-aortic lymph nodes, which surround the origin of the renal vessels, receive the lymphatic drainage from the adrenals and kidneys.

The lymphatic drainage of the female genital organs forms an extensive network in the pelvis with a diversity of drainage. The lymphatic vessels of the ovary drain laterally through the broad ligament and follow the course of the ovarian vessels (4, 5) to the preaortic and lateroaortic lymph nodes on the right and the precaval and laterocaval lymph nodes on the left. The fallopian tubes and the uterus have lymphatic continuity with the ovary, and communication of lymphatics from one ovary to the other has also been demonstrated.

Lymphatics of the body and fundus of the uterus may drain laterally along the ovarian vessels in the broad ligament with wide anastomoses with the lymphatics of the tube and ovary. Lateral drainage to a lesser extent follows a transverse direction and ends in the external iliac lymph nodes (18). Less frequently, tumor spread occurs by lymphatic trunks, which follow the round ligament from its insertion in the fundus of the uterus to the inguinal canal and end in the superficial inguinal lymph nodes (22).

The principal lymphatic drainage of the cervix of the uterus is the preureteral chain of lymphatics, which follow the course of the uterine artery (16) in front of the ureters and drain into the external iliac (18), the common iliac (19), and obturator lymph nodes. Lesser drainage is by way of the retroureteral lymphatics, which follow the course of the uterine vein, pass behind the ureter, and end in the internal iliac (hypogastric) lymph nodes (20). The posterior lymphatics of the cervix, less constant than the other two, follow an anteroposterior direction on each side of the rectum to end in the para-aortic lymph nodes found at the aortic bifurcation (21).

The lymphatics of the prostate and bladder, like those of the cervix, are drained particularly by nodes of the external iliac chain (18) and occasionally also by the hypogastric (20) and common iliac lymph nodes (19). ■

1 Inferior phrenic arteries
2 Rt. adrenal vein
3 lt. adrenal vein

4 Ovarian art.
5 Rt. ovarian vein
6, 7, and 8 Blood supply
   to ureter
9 Com. iliac art.
10 Ext. iliac art.
11 Hypogastric art.
12 Sacral art. and vein

13 Lt. ovarian vein
14 Lumbar arteries
   posteriorly

A - Celiac axis
B - Sup. mesenteric art.
C - Inf. mesenteric art.

13 Lt. ovarian vein
14 Lumbar arteries
   posteriorly

15 Tube and ovary
16 Uterine art. and vein
17 Ureter "Water under the bridge"

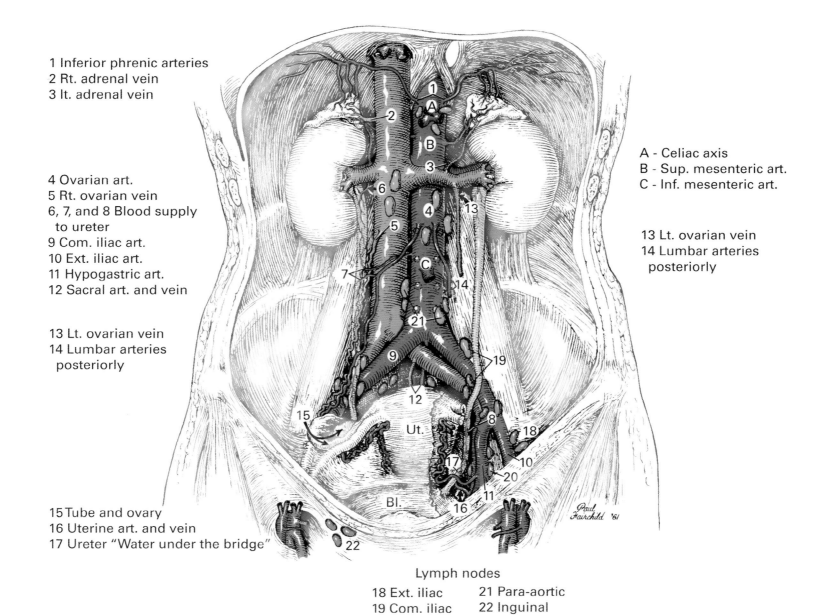

Lymph nodes
18 Ext. iliac   21 Para-aortic
19 Com. iliac   22 Inguinal
20 Int. iliac

The gross anatomic features of both the lungs are shown in FIGURE 1. On the right side the major division between the right lower (inferior) lobe (3) and the two others is a major fissure (2) which parallels the course of the fourth rib. The height to which the superior segment extends posteriorly behind the right upper (superior) lobe (1) should be noted, since the presence of the right lower lobe at this high level is important in interpreting x-rays. Of similar importance is the position of the right middle lobe (4), whose upper margin is demarcated by the approximately horizontal fissure (5). Accordingly, the middle lobe is entirely in the anterior half of the chest. In the left lung, the superior segment of the left lower (inferior) lobe (9) extends to a similarly high posterior level beneath the left oblique fissure (7) separating the left upper (superior) (6) and lower (inferior) lobes (9). The lingula (8) is, however, incorporated with the upper lobe and occupies a relatively narrow, wedge-shaped area along the anteroinferior border of that lobe.

After removal of the entire right lung, the thoracic cavity and mediastinum might appear as in FIGURE 2. Superiorly, the mediastinum contains the superior vena cava (1A) with the phrenic nerve (2) and the vagus nerve (3), which enters between the superior cava and innominate artery (4) and then crosses the trachea (5) to proceed along the lateral border of the esophagus (6). After received intercostal tributaries, the azygos vein (7) ascends lateral to the esophagus and then loops about the hilus of the right lung to join the superior vena cava near its junction with the right atrium. The investing visceral pleura about the hilus of the lung is shown as a cut edge as it joins the mediastinum and pericardium. Inferiorly this pleura forms the interior pulmonary ligament (8), which contains an occasional lymph node. This enclosed space of the hilum contains the right mainstem bronchus (9) in its posterosuperior position. Directly anterior to this is the right pulmonary artery (10), and then inferiorly are the right superior (11) and right inferior pulmonary veins (12), as well as a few hilar nodes. Other important nodes are those about the azygos vein (7) and the right phrenic nerve (2) on the superior vena cava. On the posterolateral chest wall are shown the intercostal neurovascular bundies (13) proceeding in their sheltered locations in grooves along the inferior border of each rib. The thoracic sympathetic nerve chain (14) is shown with its ganglia and with the origins of both the greater (15) and lesser splanchnic nerves (16).

The left thoracic cavity with the lung removed appears as in FIGURE 3. Arising from the arch of the aorta (17) are the innominate (4), the left common carotid (18), and left subclavian arteries (19). In close proximity to the innominate we see the left phrenic nerve (20), artery, and vein, which course down over the arch of the aorta and then along the anterolateral border of the pericardium before innervating the diaphragm (21). The internal mammary artery and vein (22) are found along the anteromedial aspect of the chest wall. The left vagus (23) accompanies the left common carotid through the mediastinum and proceeds laterally over the arch of the aorta where it gives off the recurrent laryngeal nerve (24) lateral to the ductus arteriosum. The vagus then continues down along the esophagus (6). The venous drainage of the left chest wall is different from that on the right. A superior intercostal vein (25) receives tributaries from the first few intercostal veins and then joins an accessory hemiazygos vein (26) and the hemiazygos vein (27), which crosses posteriorly to join the azygos (7). The left thoracic sympathetic trunk with its ganglia (28) and the branches to the greater (29) and lesser splanchnic nerves (30) are quite similar to those on the right side.

The structures of the left hilus are enclosed within the visceral pleura, which extends to the diaphragm as to the left inferior pulmonary ligament (31). In contrast to the right side, the left main pulmonary bronchus (32) is directly posterior but in the midportion of the hilus. Superior and anterior to this bronchus is the left main pulmonary artery (33), while the superior (34) and inferior (35) pulmonary veins on the left are anterior and inferior, respectively, to this bronchus. There are occasional lymph nodes in the inferior pulmonary ligament, but the principal node areas about this hilus are near the ductus arteriosum (36) where the recurrent laryngeal nerve may be involved. Other nodes are found along the esophagus and trachea, but in general the lymphatic chain on this side tends toward the anterior mediastinum. ■

LOBES OF THE LUNGS

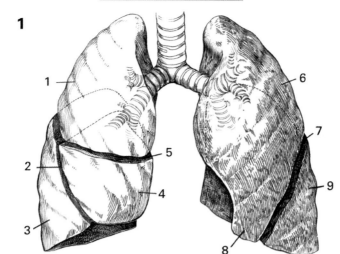

THE LUNG Figure 1

1. Right upper (superior) lobe
2. Right oblique fissure
3. Right lower (inferior) lobe
4. Right middle lobe
5. Horizontal fissure
6. Left upper (superior) lobe
7. Left oblique fissure
8. Lingula
9. Left lower (inferior) lobe

THE THORACIC WALL AND MEDIASTINUM Figures 2 and 3

1. Vena cava
   A. Superior
   B. Inferior
2. Right phrenic nerve and vessels
3. Right vagus nerve
4. Innominate artery
5. Trachea
6. Esophagus
7. Azygos vein
8. Right inferior pulmonary ligament
9. Right main bronchus
10. Right pulmonary artery
11. Right superior pulmonary vein

12. Right inferior pulmonary vein
13. Intercostal neurovascular bundle
14. Right thoracic sympathetic trunk with ganglia
15. Right greater splanchnic nerve
16. Right lesser splanchnic nerve
17. Aortic arch
18. Left common carotid artery
19. Left subclavian artery
20. Left phrenic nerve and vessels
21. Diaphragm
22. Left internal mammary artery and vein
23. Left vagus nerve
24. Left recurrent laryngeal nerve

25. Superior intercostal vein
26. Accessory hemiazygos vein
27. Hemiazygos vein
28. Left thoracic sympathetic trunk with ganglia
29. Left greater splanchnic nerve
30. Left lesser splanchnic nerve
31. Left inferior pulmonary ligament
32. Left main bronchus
33. Left pulmonary artery
34. Left superior pulmonary vein
35. Left inferior pulmonary vein
36. Ligamentum arteriosum

RIGHT MEDIASTINUM

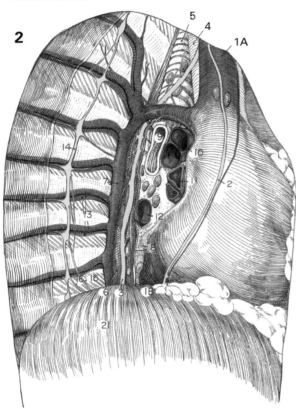

LEFT MEDIASTINUM

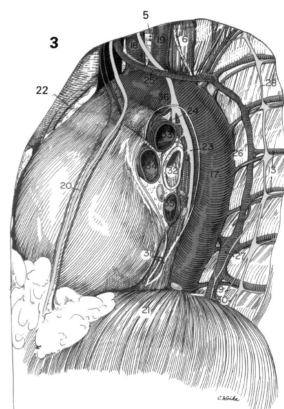

SECTION III
GENERAL ABDOMEN AND THORAX

PREOPERATIVE PREPARATION Prior to bringing the patient to the operating room, the surgical site is marked with the patient's co-operation by the operating surgeon to ensure correct site surgery. The patient is carefully positioned on the operating table while taking into consideration the need for special equipment such as heating pads, electrocautery grounding plates, sequential compression stockings, and anesthesia monitoring devices. The arms may be positioned at the side or at right angles on arm boards, which allows the anesthesiologist better access to intravenous lines and other monitoring devices. It is important that the patient be positioned without pressure over the elbows, heels, or other bony prominences; neither should the shoulders be stretched in hyperabduction. The arms, upper chest, and legs are covered with a thermal blanket. Simple cloth loop restraints may be placed loosely about the wrists, whereas a safety belt is usually passed over the thighs and around the operating table. The entire abdomen is shaved with clippers, as is the lower chest when an upper abdominal procedure is planned. In hirsute individuals, the thigh may also require hair removal with clippers for effective application of an electrocautery grounding pad. The grounding pad should not be placed in the region of metal orthopedic implants or cardiac pacemakers. Loose hair may be picked up with adhesive tape, and the umbilicus may require cleaning out with a cotton-tipped applicator. The first assistant scrubs, puts on sterile gloves, and then places sterile towels well beyond the upper and lower limits of the operative field so as to wall off the unsterile areas. The assistant vigorously cleanses the abdominal field with gauze sponges saturated with antiseptic solution (see Chapter 1). Some prefer iodinated solution for skin preparation. Prophylactic antibiotics are administered intravenously within 1 hour of the incision.

After positioning, skin preparation, and draping, a **TIME OUT** is performed as described in Chapter 3, TABLE 1.

The incision should be carefully planned before the anatomic landmarks are hidden by the sterile drapes. Although cosmetic considerations may dictate placing the incision in the lines of skin cleavage (Langer's lines) in an effort to minimize subsequent scar, other factors are of greater importance. The incision should be varied to fit the anatomic contour of the patient. It must provide maximum exposure for the technical procedure and of the anticipated pathology, while creating minimal injury to the abdominal wall, especially in the presence of one or more scars from previous surgical procedures. The most commonly used incision is a midline one that goes between the two rectus abdominis muscles, around the umbilicus, and through the linea alba (FIGURE 1). For procedures in the pelvis, the incision is extended to the pubis; whereas for upper abdominal operations, the incision may extend up and over the xiphoid. Following preparation, the abdomen is walled off with sterile towels placed transversely at the xiphoid and pubis and longitudinally about either rectus muscle. Some surgeons prefer further to seal the field with an adhesive plastic drape that may be impregnated with an antiseptic solution. This technique is particularly useful in patients who have pre-existing intestinal stomas, tubes, or other processes that may contaminate the operative field.

INCISION AND EXPOSURE In making the incision, the operator should hold the scalpel with the thumb on one side and the fingers on the other. The distal portion of the handle rests against the ulnar aspect of the palm. Some prefer to rest the index finger on top of the knife handle as a sensitive means of guiding the pressure being applied to the blade. The primary incision may be made in three ways. First, the surgeon may take a sterile gauze pad in his or her left hand and pull the skin superiorly at the upper end of the incision. The taut skin immediately below the surgeon's left hand is cut. As the incision progresses, the gauze is shifted down the incision, always keeping the skin taut such that the knife makes a clean incision. Second,

the surgeon may prefer to make the skin taut from side to side with the forefinger and thumb (FIGURE 2) as he or she progresses sequentially down the abdomen. Third, the gauze-covered left hand of the surgeon and that of the first assistant may exert lateral tension on the skin, thus permitting the scalpel to create a clean incision. The compressing fingers should be separated and flexed to exert a mild downward and outward pull; however, it is essential that the line of incision not be pulled to one side or the other (i.e., off the true midline). This technique allows the surgeon to have a full view of the operative area as he or she cuts evenly through the taut skin along the length of the incision.

The incision is carried down to the underlying linea alba, which may be difficult to find in the obese patient. A most useful technique is for the surgeon and first assistant to apply strong lateral traction to the subcutaneous fat which will then split (FIGURE 3) directly down to the linea alba. This maneuver may be the only way to find the midline in morbidly obese patients; however, it works equally well in most patients. The linea alba should be freed of fat (FIGURE 4) for a width of approximately 1 cm such that the margins can be easily identified at the time of closure. Bleeding vessels are clamped carefully with small hemostats and are either ligated or cauterized. As soon as hemostasis in the superficial fat layer has been accomplished, moistened large gauze pads are placed in the incision such that the fatty layer is protected from further desiccation or injury. This also aids in providing a clear view of the underlying parietes.

The linea alba is incised in the midline (FIGURE 5). Preperitoneal fat may require division to expose the peritoneum. The surgeon and first assistant alternatively pick up and release the peritoneum to be certain that no viscus is included in their grasp. Using toothed forceps which lift the peritoneum upward, the surgeon makes a small opening in the side of the tent of elevated peritoneum rather than in its vertex (FIGURE 6). Usually, the tent formation has pulled the peritoneum away from the underlying tissue, and the side opening allows air to enter such that adjacent structures fall away. A culture is taken at this time if abnormal fluid is encountered. Large collections of ascites within the abdomen may be removed by suctioning. The volume of ascites should be recorded, and it may be kept within a special bottle trap if cytologic studies are planned to determine whether it is a malignant ascites.

The edges of the linea alba fascia and the adjacent peritoneum are grasped with Kocher clamps. Care is taken to prevent inclusion and injury to underlying viscera. By continuously elevating the tissues that are to be cut, the surgeon may enlarge the opening with scissors (FIGURE 7). In cutting the peritoneum and fascia with scissors, it is wise to insert only as much of the blade as can be clearly visualized, so as to avoid cutting any internal structures such as bowel that may be adherent to the parietal peritoneum. Tilting the points of the scissors upward may afford a better visualization of the lower blade. Having extended the incision to its uppermost limits, the operator may insert the index and middle fingers of the left hand beneath the peritoneum heading toward the pelvis. The linea alba and peritoneum may be divided with a scalpel (FIGURE 8) or scissors. Care must be taken in the region of the umbilicus as there are often one or two significant blood vessels in the fatty layer between the fascia and peritoneum. These may be grasped with hemostats and ligated. Additional care must be taken at the extreme lower end of the opening where the bladder comes superiorly. The peritoneal incision must stop just short of the bladder, which is seen and identified as a palpable thickening. In general, the peritoneal incision should not be as long as the facial opening since undercutting may make the closure difficult. Small incisions may be preferred by the patient; however, an inadequate incision may result in a prolonged and more difficult procedure for the surgeon. **CONTINUES ▶**

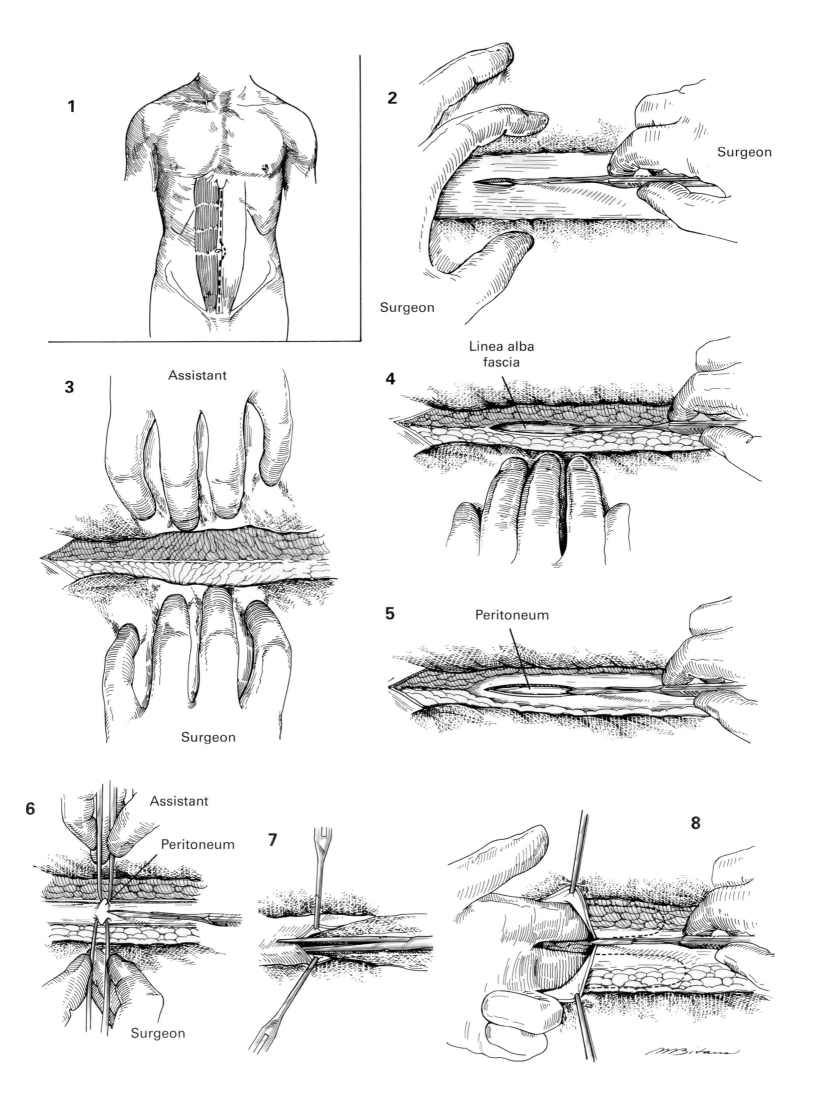

1

2 Surgeon

Surgeon

3 Assistant

Surgeon

4 Linea alba fascia

5 Peritoneum

6 Assistant

Peritoneum

Surgeon

7

8

CLOSURE ‹CONTINUED› More or less the same steps for closure are carried out whether the incision is midline or transverse. If the peritoneum and linea alba fascia are separate, the fascial edge may be grasped with toothed forceps (FIGURE 9), exposing the edge of the peritoneum, which is grasped with Kocher's clamps. The closure sutures may be absorbable or nonabsorbable. The technique may use interrupted or continuous sutures that approximate the peritoneum and linea alba either as separate layers, or as a combined unified one. If a continuous suture is used, it is technically easier to close from the lower end of the incision upward, particularly if the surgeon stands on the right side of the patient. The suture is anchored in the peritoneum just below on the end of the incision (FIGURE 10). The needle is passed through the peritoneum and run superiorly in a continuous manner. A medium width metal ribbon is often placed beneath the peritoneum to ensure a clear zone for suturing and to avoid incorporation of visceral or other structures into the suture line. The placement of the continuous suture is made easier if the assistant crisscrosses the two leading Kocher clamps (FIGURE 11) to approximate the peritoneum. At the superior end of the incision, the looped and free ends of the suture are knotted together across the line of incision (FIGURE 12). The type of knot and the number of throws are determined by the characteristics of the suture material.

The linea alba fascia may be closed, beginning at either end of the incision. Simple interrupted sutures may be placed (FIGURE 13) or figure-of-eight sutures (FIGURE 19, page 37) may be used. The sutures are placed about 1 to 2 cm apart whether interrupted or continuous (FIGURE 14) technique is used.

Alternatively, the linea alba and peritoneum may be closed as a single unified layer with either interrupted or continuous suture. The most expeditious closure may be made with a heavy looped suture on a single needle. The suture material may be either synthetic absorbable or a nonabsorbable in a 0 or #1 size. The suture begins with the transverse placement through the peritoneum and fascia across the lower end of the incision (FIGURE 15). The needle is then brought through the eye of the loop (FIGURE 16). Upon tightening, the suture is secured without the need of tying a knot. CONTINUES›

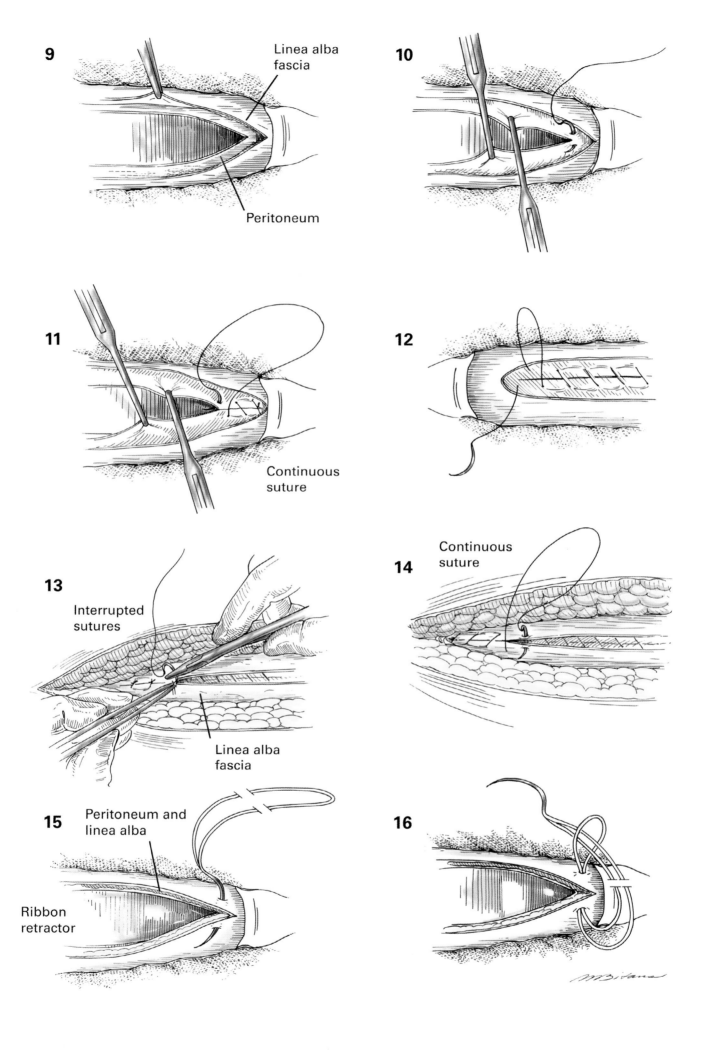

9   Linea alba fascia

Peritoneum

10

11   Continuous suture

12

13   Interrupted sutures

Linea alba fascia

14   Continuous suture

15   Peritoneum and linea alba

Ribbon retractor

16

CLOSURE ◄CONTINUED The double loop suture is run in a continuous manner taking full thickness of the linea alba fascia and peritoneum on either side of the incision (FIGURE 17). After placement of the final stitch superiorly, the needle is cut off and one limb of the suture retracted back across the incision. This allows the two cut ends to be tied along one side of the incision.

Some surgeons prefer to use the figure-of-eight, or the so-called eight-pound stitch, when closing fascia with the interrupted sutures. A full-thickness horizontal bite is taken that enters the linea alba on the far side at **A** and exits at **B** (FIGURE 18). The suture is advanced for a centimeter or two, and an additional transverse full-thickness bite is taken that enters at **C** and exits at **D**. When the two ends of the suture are tied, a crisscrossing, horizontal figure-of-eight is created (FIGURE 19). The knot should be tied to one side. In general, the figure-of-eight suture is placed snugly rather than tightly where it may cut through the tissue with any postoperative swelling.

After each knot is tied during the closure, the ends of the suture are held under tension by the assistant and are cut. Silk sutures may be cut within 2 mm of the knot, whereas many absorbable or synthetic sutures require several millimeters be left, as the knots may slip. As the suture is held nearly perpendicular to the incision by the assistant, the scissors are slid down to the knot and rotated a quarter turn (FIGURES 20 and 21). Closure of the scissors at this level allows the suture to be cut near the knot without destroying it. In general, the scissors are only opened slightly such that the cutting occurs near the tips. Additional fine control of the scissors may be obtained by supporting the midportion of the scissor on the outstretched index, and middle fingers of the opposite hand just as the rest supports the chisel on a wood-turning lathe. Following closure of the fascia, some surgeons reapproximate Scarpa's fascia with a few interrupted 3/0 absorbable sutures (FIGURE 22), whereas others proceed directly to skin closure, the details of which are shown later in this chapter.

Occasionally, it is necessary to use a retention or through-and-through suture. This is especially true in debilitated patients who have risk factors for dehiscence such as advanced age, malnutrition, malignancy, or contaminated wounds. The most frequent use of retention sutures, however, is for a secondary reclosure of a postoperative evisceration or full-thickness disruption of the abdominal wall. Through-and-through #2 nonabsorbable sutures on very large needles may be placed through all layers of the abdominal wall as a simple suture or as a far-near/near-far stitch (FIGURE 27). In this technique, the fascia is grasped with Kocher clamps and a metal ribbon retractor is used to protect the viscera. The surgeon places the first suture full thickness through the far side abdominal wall. The needle is then brought through the near linea alba or fascia about 1 cm back from the cut edge with the path going from peritoneal surface toward the skin (FIGURE 23). The suture then crosses the midline to penetrate the far side fascia in a superficial to deep manner (FIGURE 24). The free intraperitoneal suture is then continued full thickness through the near abdominal wall (FIGURE 25). As seen in cross section (FIGURE 26), it is important that the abdominal wall full-thickness bites taken at the beginning and end of this placement are not positioned so laterally as to include the epigastric vessels within the rectus abdominis muscles. Compression of these vessels when the suture is tied may lead to abdominal wall necrosis. In addition, the intraperitoneal exposure of this suture should be small so as to minimize the possibility of a loop of intestine becoming entrapped when the retention is tied. In general, the entrance and exit sites are approximately 1.5 or 2 inches back from the cut edge of the skin (FIGURE 27). Many surgeons use retention suture bolsters or simple 2-inches sections of sterilized red rubber tubing in order to minimize the cutting of the suture into the skin during the inevitable postoperative swelling. Because of this swelling, the retention sutures should be tied loosely rather than snugly such that the surgeon can still pass a finger between the retention suture and the skin of the abdominal wall. CONTINUES►

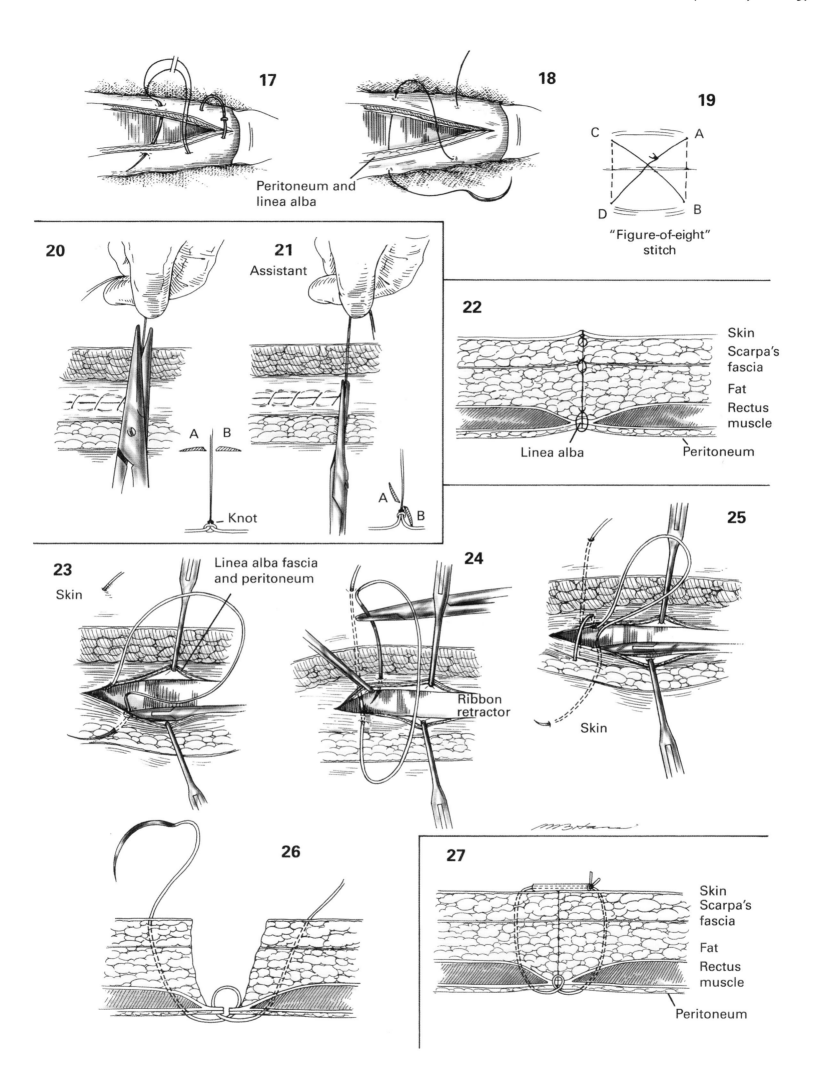

17

18

Peritoneum and linea alba

19

C ······ A

D ······ B

"Figure-of-eight" stitch

20

21
Assistant

A B

Knot

A

B

22

Skin
Scarpa's fascia

Fat
Rectus muscle

Linea alba

Peritoneum

23
Skin

Linea alba fascia and peritoneum

24

Ribbon retractor

25

Skin

26

27

Skin
Scarpa's fascia

Fat
Rectus muscle

Peritoneum

CLOSURE ◁CONTINUED▷ Following closure of the peritoneum and the linea alba, Scarpa's fascia may be approximated with 3/0 absorbable suture. Many feel this lessens the subcutaneous dead space within the fat (FIGURE 28). In thin patients, this suture may be placed in an inverted manner (as shown), with the knot at the bottom of the loop. However, in most patients, these sutures are placed upright with the knot on top.

The skin may be closed with interrupted fine 3/0 or 4/0 nonabsorbable sutures using a curved cutting needle (FIGURE 29). The skin edge is elevated with forceps in such a manner that the needle is introduced perpendicular to the skin on the one side and exits perpendicularly on the opposite. The sutures are spaced such that the distance between them is approximately equal to their width. This creates a pleasing uniform pattern. As the individual sutures are tied, the skin will rise, creating a slight ridge. When all sutures are tied, they are held in the surgeon's left hand and then sequentially cut with the scissors (FIGURE 30). Some surgeons prefer an interrupted vertical mattress suture for skin closure. The vertical mattress suture is especially well suited for circumstances where the skin edges do not lie in level approximation. The skin is grasped with the toothed forceps. A wide lateral base is created as the needle enters the skin about 1 cm or so lateral to the cut edge (FIGURE 31). The opposite skin edge is then grasped with forceps and the needle brought through in a symmetric manner (FIGURE 32). A careful approximation of the skin edges at equal levels is accomplished by a returning small bite that is approximately a millimeter or two from the skin edge and only a millimeter or two deep. A symmetric bite on the proximal skin edge completes the stitch (FIGURE 33). This stitch is tied loosely, producing a gentle ridge effect (FIGURE 34).

The skin may also be closed with interrupted fine 4/0 or 5/0 synthetic absorbable subcuticular sutures. With this method, the suture must lie in the deepest layers of the corium. The skin edge is grasped with toothed forceps and the suture is placed by either the continuous or interrupted horizontal mattress technique. Multiple interrupted sutures are preferred for short incisions, whereas continuous sutures are more suitable for incisions that are more than a few centimeters long. In this technique, small horizontal bites are taken in opposite sides of the skin margins (FIGURES 35 and 36). When the knot is tied, a perfect approximation occurs (FIGURE 37). After tying, the sutures are cut as close to the knot as possible. Thereafter, the skin is cleaned of the preparative antiseptic solution and a benzoin-like skin protector is applied. When this becomes tacky, porous adhesive paper tapes are applied transversely (FIGURE 38). This relieves tension in the incision and provides a simple covering.

Conversely, some surgeons use metal staples for skin closure. Their advantage is speed of application (FIGURE 39) and ease of removal (FIGURE 40). Special care must be taken, however, to approximate carefully the everted skin margins with a pair of fine-toothed forceps. The stapling instrument should not press into the skin. A gentle light application will result in the desired mounding up that keeps the two skin edges in good approximation. Some prefer to place these staples widely and use the adhesive paper tapes between them. Finally, a covering gauze dressing is necessary so as to absorb the small amount of serum and blood that evacuates in the postoperative period. In general, staples should be removed sooner rather than later as they penetrate the skin and can result in localized inflammations. ■

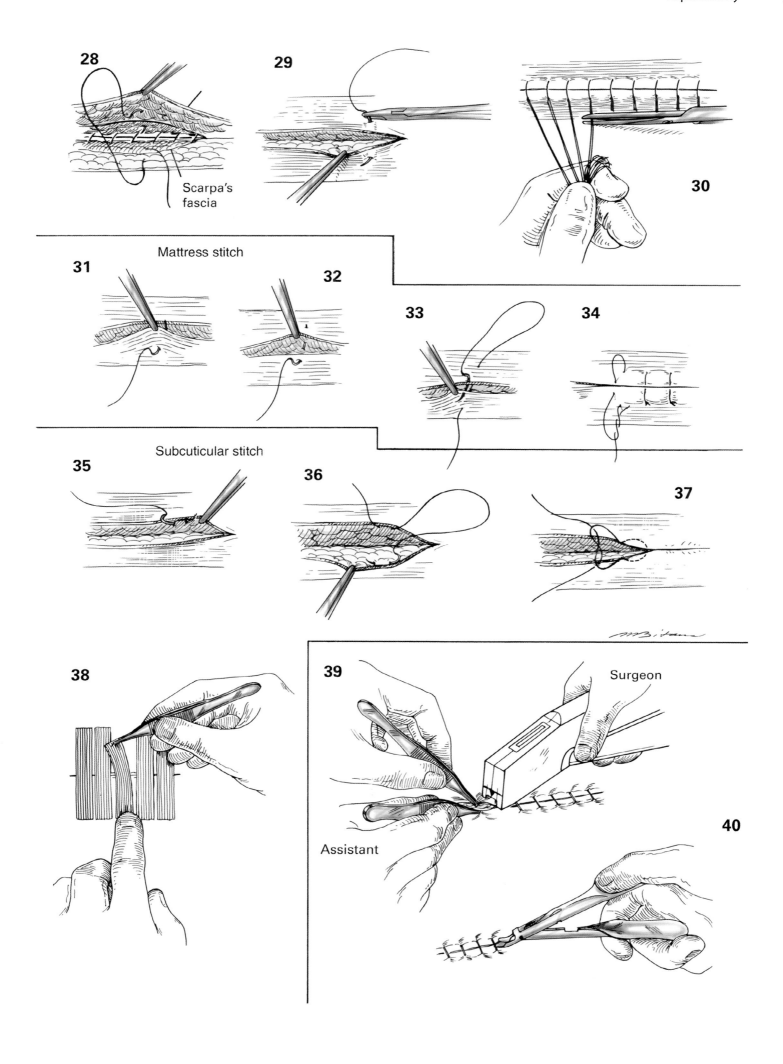

28

Scarpa's fascia

29

30

Mattress stitch

31   **32**

33   **34**

Subcuticular stitch

35   **36**   **37**

38

39   Surgeon

Assistant

40

Hasson Open Technique for Laparoscopic Access

INDICATIONS The first step in most abdominal laparoscopic procedures is insufflation of the intraperitoneal space with CO_2 gas and the introduction of the videoscope system. The original and the most established technique uses the Veress needle, described in the following Chapter 12, page 42. The Veress needle can be placed in any quadrant of the abdomen, but is most frequently inserted just below the umbilicus, where a skin incision has been made for the introduction of a large 10-mm port for the videoscope. General surgeons, however, have been cautious in adopting this technique of blind puncture, as their training has emphasized the importance of complete visualization of anatomy and of the planned action of their surgical instruments. Accordingly, the open or Hasson technique for entering the abdomen under direct vision has become more popular and safer. This technique can be used to enter into any quadrant of the abdomen but is most commonly employed at the central umbilical site (FIGURE 1). A vertical or transverse skin incision approximately 10 to 12 mm in length is made just below (FIGURE 2) or above the umbilicus. The choice of site may be based on the surgeon's preference or the presence of a previous regional incision that may have adhesions. The subcutaneous fat and tissues are bluntly dissected apart using small narrow finger retractors or a Kelly hemostat. The white linea alba is visualized and grasped on either side with hemostats. The linea alba is elevated with the hemostats and a vertical 10-mm incision is made through the fascia (FIGURE 2). Further dissection with a hemostat will reveal the thickened white peritoneum, which is grasped with a pair of laterally placed hemostats. The peritoneum is elevated and opened cautiously with a scalpel. A dark, empty peritoneal space is seen and a pair of lateral stay sutures are placed (FIGURE 3). These sutures incorporate the peritoneum and linea alba and are later used to secure the Hasson port.

The next step is to verify that the intraperitoneal space has been entered freely. The surgeon's fifth finger is inserted (FIGURE 4). This maneuver sizes the hole for the port and allows the surgeon to palpate the region. Usually this space is clear, but occasionally there are some filmy omental adhesions that can be swept away. The Hasson port with its blunt, rounded-tip obturator is introduced into the abdomen (FIGURE 5). The spiral collar is screwed into the fascia so as to provide a snug gas seal, and the lateral stay sutures are secured to the notches on the collar. The obturator is removed. The CO_2 line is attached and the stopcock opened. The surgeon sets the rates of CO_2 flow and maximum pressure (15 mm Hg). He or she observes the intra-abdominal pressure and the total volume of CO_2 infused as the abdomen enlarges and becomes tympanitic. The videoscope is white-balanced and focused. The optical end of the instrument is coated with antifog solution. The videoscope is introduced into the port and advanced into the peritoneal space. If an angled optical instrument, typically 30 degrees, is used, it is important for the operator of the videoscope to establish the correct orientation of the optics and the video head. Typically, the optical bevel is downward-viewing (6 o'clock) when the fiberoptic light cable is vertical

(12 o'clock). The video head is correctly oriented when its cable is positioned at 6 o'clock posteriorly. Rotation of either instrument from these positions will produce a rotated view on the TV monitor.

In the presence of omental adhesions or an enlarged falciform ligament, the intraperitoneal space may not easily be entered as the videoscope comes to the end of the Hasson port. If this area was clear to palpation with the surgeon's fifth finger, careful angulation and rotation of the videoscope usually finds the right opening. When the opening cannot be found, the port is removed and a repeat finger palpation is performed before reinsertion of the Hasson port. In extreme cases, when finger palpation cannot find an easy intraperitoneal entrance because of dense adhesions, an alternative site for the Hasson port should be used.

The usual alternative sites (FIGURE 1) are in the four quadrants of the abdomen, although the Hasson port can also be placed through the midline linea alba in the epigastric or suprapubic regions. A transverse skin incision is made and the subcutaneous fat spread with narrow finger retractors or a Kelly hemostat. The fascia of the external oblique muscle is incised with a scalpel. Further deep dissection is performed through the internal oblique and transversus muscles, whose thin fascia usually does not require incision. The white peritoneum is grasped between hemostats and elevated. A scalpel incises the peritoneum and a clear entry into the intraperitoneal space is verified by the deep passage of a Kelly hemostat. A pair of lateral stay sutures incorporating the peritoneum and fascia are placed. The remainder of this procedure is performed as described for the umbilical site.

SUTURE OF PORT SITE Most 5-mm port sites do not require suture closure of the fascia, especially if the port is passed originally in a zigzag or oblique manner through the muscle layers of the abdominal wall. On occasion, however, a blood vessel of the intra-abdominal wall that was not seen with transillumination may be cut by the trocar during the placement of a port. Most small vessels will stop bleeding. However, some may continue to drip into the intraperitoneal space and obscure visualization. A technique for the control of these vessels or for closure of a fascial defect is shown (FIGURE 6). A 00 delayed absorbable suture is placed into the tip of a special suturing needle. The needle and suture are passed through the inner abdominal wall about 1 cm beyond the edge of the port entry site (FIGURE 6A). The suture is released from the needle tip with a long free end showing within the abdomen. The special suturing needle is removed and reinserted about 1 cm beyond the opposite edge of the port entry site. The needle tip is opened and the suture is grasped (FIGURE 6B). The free end of the suture and the needle are withdrawn. The suture is tied down through the skin opening. This technique produces a mattress suture that can secure abdominal wall blood vessels or close fascial defects created by the placement of large ports. Both maneuvers are done under direct visualization using the videoscope. ■

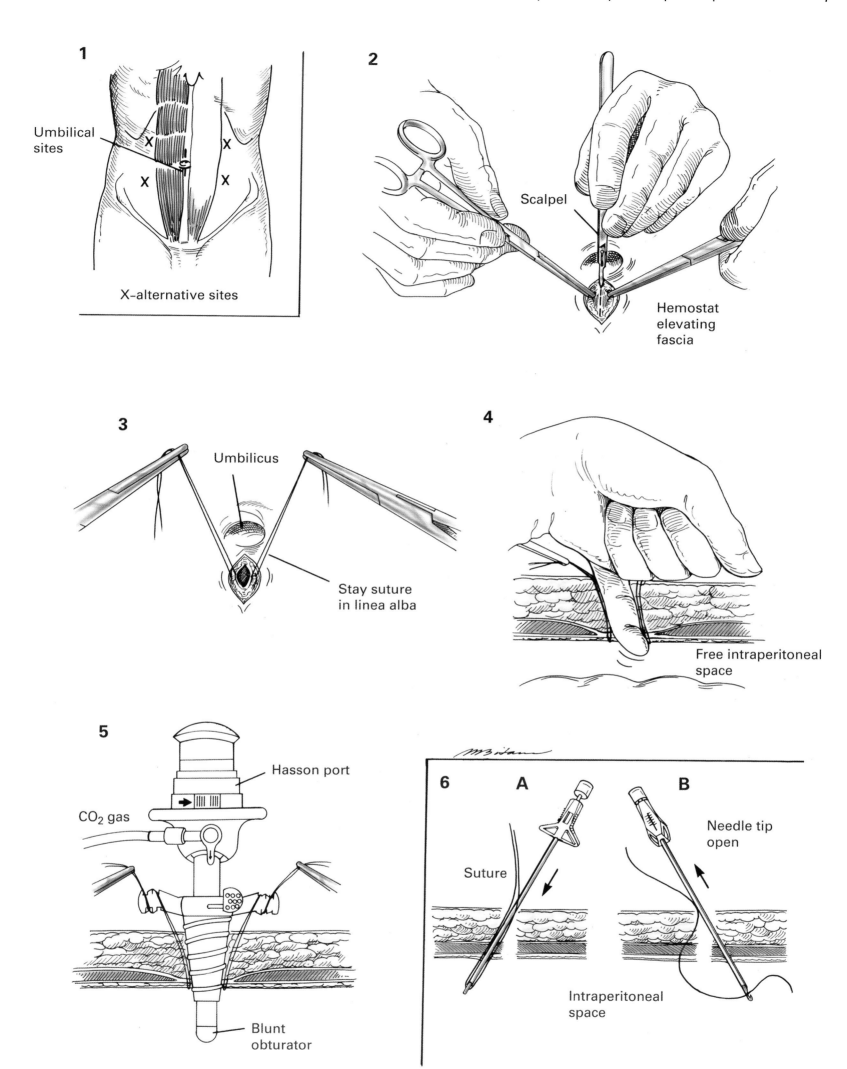

1

Umbilical sites

X–alternative sites

2

Scalpel

Hemostat elevating fascia

3

Umbilicus

Stay suture in linea alba

4

Free intraperitoneal space

5

Hasson port

CO_2 gas

Blunt obturator

6

A

Suture

B

Needle tip open

Intraperitoneal space

VERESS NEEDLE TECHNIQUE

ANESTHESIA General anesthesia with endotracheal intubation is recommended. Preoperative prophylactic antibiotics for anticipated bile pathogens are administered such that adequate tissue levels exist.

POSITION As laparoscopic cholecystectomy makes extensive use of supporting equipment, it is important to position this equipment such that it is easily visualized by all members of the surgical team (FIGURE 1).

OPERATIVE PREPARATION The skin of the entire abdomen and lower anterior chest is prepared in the routine manner.

INCISION AND EXPOSURE The abdomen is palpated to find the liver edge or unsuspected intra-abdominal masses. The patient is placed in a mild Trendelenburg position and an appropriate site for the creation of the pneumoperitoneum is chosen. The initial port may be placed by an open or Hasson technique which is preferred. Alternatively, a Veress needle technique is used as described below. In the unoperated abdomen this is usually at the level of the umbilicus (FIGURE 2); however, previous laparotomy incisions with presumed adhesions may suggest a more lateral approach site which avoids the epigastric vessels (FIGURE 2 at X). A 1-cm vertical or horizontal skin incision is made and the abdominal wall on either side of the umbilicus is grasped by the surgeon and first assistant either by thumb and forefinger or by towel clips so as to elevate the abdominal wall (FIGURE 3). A Veress needle is held like a pencil by the surgeon who inserts it through the linea alba and peritoneum where a characteristic popping sensation is felt (FIGURE 4). An unobstructed free intraperitoneal position for the Veress needle is verified by easy irrigation of *clear* saline in and out of the peritoneal space (FIGURE 5) and by the hanging drop method where the saline in the translucent hub of the Veress needle is drawn into the peritoneal space when the abdominal wall is lifted.

If one does not obtain a free flow or an unobstructed saline irrigation, then the Veress needle may be removed and reinserted. In general it is safer to convert the umbilical site into the Hasson open approach (Chapter 11) if any difficulty is experienced with the placement, irrigation, or insufflation of the Veress needle. The appropriate tubing and cables for the CO_2 insufflation, the fiber optic light source, and the laparoscopic videoscope with its sterile sheath are positioned as are the lines for the cautery or laser, suction, and saline irrigation. The pneumoperitoneum begins with a low flow of about 1 or 2 L/min with a low-pressure limit of approximately 5 to 7 cm H_2O. Once 1 to 2 L of CO_2 are in, the abdomen should be hyperresonant to percussion. The flow rate may be increased; however, the pressure should be limited to 15 cm H_2O. Three to four liters of CO_2 are required to fully inflate the abdomen and the Veress needle is removed. After grasping either side of the umbilicus, a 10-mm trocar port is inserted with a twisting motion, aiming toward the pelvis (FIGURE 6). If a disposable trocar port is used, it is important to be certain that the safety sheath is cocked. A characteristic popping sensation is felt as the trocar enters the peritoneal space. The trocar is removed and the escape of free CO_2 gas is verified.

Although the Veress needle technique has a long history and is preferred by some, most general surgeons use the Hasson technique, as shown in the preceding Chapter 11. ■

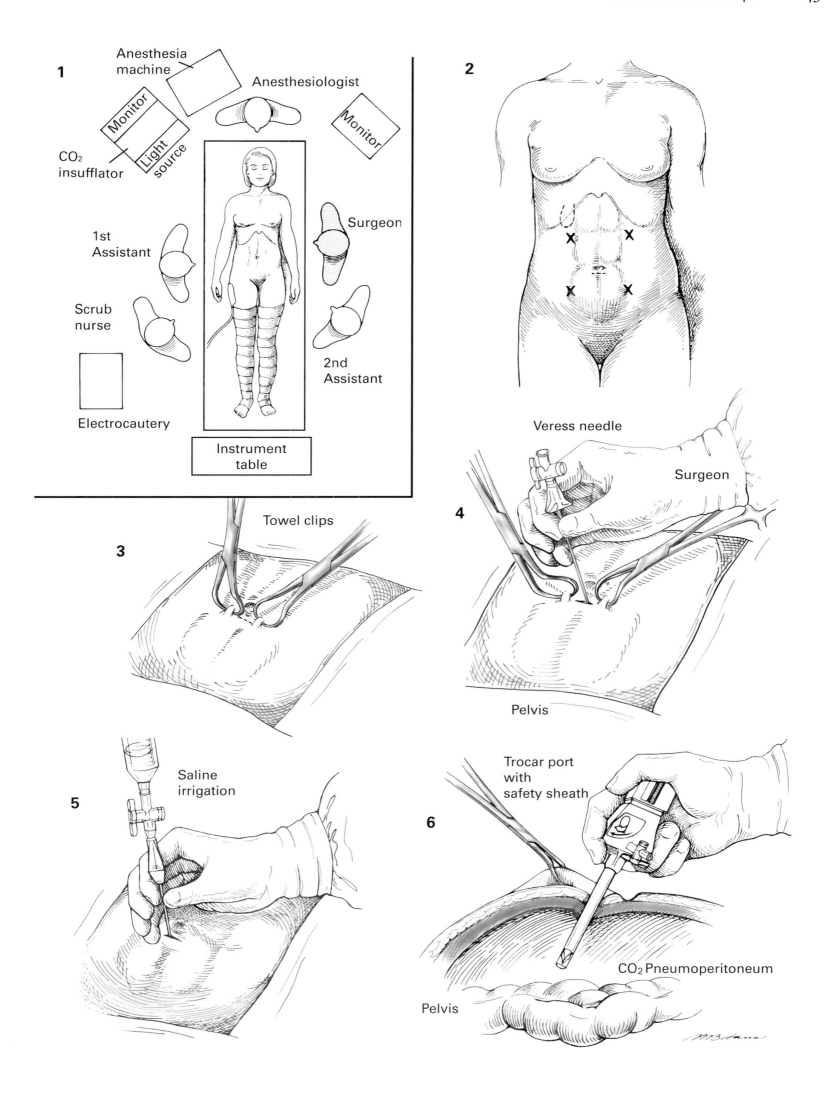

1 Anesthesia machine · Anesthesiologist · Monitor · CO_2 insufflator · Light source · Monitor · Surgeon · 1st Assistant · Scrub nurse · 2nd Assistant · Electrocautery · Instrument table

2

3 Towel clips

4 Veress needle · Surgeon · Pelvis

5 Saline irrigation

6 Trocar port with safety sheath · CO_2 Pneumoperitoneum · Pelvis

DIAGNOSTIC LAPAROSCOPY

INDICATIONS Indications for diagnostic laparoscopy can be divided into three broad groups. Gynecologic conditions include infertility, endometriosis, primary amenorrhea, pelvic pain in the female, and to rule out appendicitis in women with pelvic pain. In an effort to accurately diagnose or stage cancer, patients with gastric, esophageal, or pancreatic cancer may undergo diagnostic laparoscopy to stage the disease and determine resectability or direct further treatment. In patients with intra-abdominal lymphadenopathy where lymphoma is a possibility, diagnostic laparoscopy is indicated to biopsy a representative lymph node to make the diagnosis. Benign conditions represent the third group whom may benefit from diagnostic laparoscopy. Patients (typically those who have undergone previous abdominal procedures) with chronic abdominal pain and intermittent partial small bowel obstructions may benefit from diagnostic laparoscopy and adhesiolysis. Patients with symptoms suggestive of an inguinal hernia but lack a clear inguinal hernia on physical examination may benefit from diagnostic laparoscopy. These may then be repaired laparoscopically. In patients with a unilateral inguinal hernia, laparoscopy can diagnose an inguinal hernia on the contralateral side to rule out a contralateral hernia. The laparoscopic incisions cause less pain and there is a faster return to normal activities or work in the event no therapeutic maneuvers are undertaken.

PREOPERATIVE PREPARATION The patient must be optimized prior to undergoing an operative procedure. Respiratory function should be optimized with cessation of smoking and appropriate pulmonary function evaluation if indicated. A discussion with the patient should occur preoperatively as the findings at diagnostic laparoscopy may dictate further surgery and consent should be obtained for these potential additional procedures prior to undergoing anesthesia. In the event the diagnostic laparoscopy is for adhesiolysis after previous abdominal procedures, the preceding operative note, should be reviewed.

ANESTHESIA A general anesthetic with an endotracheal tube is required. The patient should be relaxed or chemically paralyzed with paralytics to facilitate relaxation of the abdominal wall and visualization with insufflation.

POSITION The patient is placed in a supine position with a pillow placed to produce mild flexion of the hips and knees. This helps to relax the abdominal wall. If visualization of the upper abdomen is required (gastric, esophageal, or pancreatic cancers), the arms should be left "out" at 90 degrees. Video screens should be placed at the head of the bed just over the patients' shoulders for viewing by the surgeons on the contralateral side (FIGURE 1). Patients undergoing laparoscopy of the pelvis should have their arms tucked at their side to facilitate the position of the surgeon to view the video screen(s) placed at the foot of the bed (FIGURE 2).

OPERATIVE PREPARATION The patient is given perioperative antibiotics. An orogastric tube is passed for gastric decompression. For pelvic laparoscopy, a Foley catheter is placed and pneumatic sequential stockings are applied. The skin is prepared in the routine manner.

INCISION AND EXPOSURE Typically placement of a 5- or 10-mm videoscope port and two 5-mm operating ports are a function of what region of the abdomen wishes to be explored and the preference of the surgeon (FIGURES 1 and 2). The general principle is that of triangulation. The ports should be about a hand's breadth or more apart from each other and the two operating ports should be placed as widely apart as possible. One of the operating ports should be 10-mm in size if a 5-mm videoscope is not available.

The videoscope port is placed first, using the open Hasson technique or an optical trocar may be used after preinsufflation of the abdomen using a Veress needle when accessing the abdominal cavity laterally. In patients undergoing upper abdominal exploration, an infraumbilical Hasson cannula (FIGURE 1) is appropriate while patients undergoing pelvic or lower abdominal exploration a supra-umbilical point of access should be undertaken (FIGURE 2). After the abdomen is entered safely and the port secured with stay sutures, the intraperitoneal space is inflated with carbon dioxide. The surgeon sets the gas flow rate and the maximum pressure ($\leq$15 mm Hg). The rising intra-abdominal pressure and total volume of gas infused is observed as the abdomen distends. The videoscope is white-balanced and focused. The optical end, typically a 30-degree angle, is coated with antifog solution and the scope is advanced down the port into the abdomen under direct vision. All four quadrants of the abdomen are explored visually (FIGURES 3 to 5). Omental and other adhesions to the abdominal and anterior abdominal wall in the region to be explored are visualized and taken down bluntly or with sharp dissection. Placement of the operating ports begins with the infiltration of the skin with a long-acting local anesthetic. The local needle may be passed perpendicularly full thickness through the abdominal wall and its entry site verified with the videoscope. The skin is incised and the subcutaneous tissues are dilated with a small hemostat. The abdominal

wall is transilluminated with the videoscope to show any regional vessels within the abdominal musculature. The 5-mm operating ports are placed in a location to facilitate dissection and exposure of the upper or lower abdomen with visualization of their clean entry into the intraperitoneal space.

DETAILS OF PROCEDURE In patients who have undergone previous abdominal procedures or who present with chronic abdominal pain and intermittent partial small bowel obstruction, the omentum or bowel will have formed some adhesions to the abdominal wall and must be taken down. Attention should be directed to the area in which the patient is experiencing the pain as the adhesions in this location may be the etiology of the pain and should be taken down completely. Placing the patient in reverse Trendelenburg position will facilitate visualization of the upper abdomen bringing the abdominal contents down from the diaphragm. Conversely, placing the patient in Trendelenburg position will facilitate dissection and exposure of the pelvic organs. Rotation of the operating table side to side to bring the patients' left or right side up will also allow the surgeon to visualize the lateral abdominal wall and lateral areas of the abdomen that need to be explored. For this reason, the patient should be secured to the bed with belt(s) or a foot rest in the event steep reverse Trendelenburg is required. The omentum is grasped near the abdominal wall with a blunt atraumatic instrument and gentle traction is applied. Using laparoscopic scissors, the surgeon sharply incises the junction of the omentum with the peritoneum of the abdominal wall. After each cut, a blunt sweeping motion in the same area will open up the next zone for sharp dissection. There should be minimal bleeding. Electrocautery or other heat-generating coagulating systems (ultrasonic dissectors) should be used sparingly and only with full visualization so as to minimize the chance of thermal injury to the bowel. Extensive dense adhesions or an enterotomy that is not easily repaired laparoscopically require conversion to an open laparotomy and repair if necessary. Throughout this dissection, the surgeon must be vigilant for the appearance of a loop of bowel hidden within adhesions. Small and large bowel may also be cautiously cut away from the abdominal wall but less sweeping and traction is applied, lest an enterotomy should occur. The appearance of bile or succus demands a search for the source, which may be repaired laparoscopically or after conversion to an open laparotomy.

Once adhesiolysis is complete and exposure optimized, the region of the abdomen in question is explored. The anterior surfaces of the liver and the diaphragm are examined. It is important for the diaphragm to be inspected in patients with suspected or proven gastrointestinal or pancreatic cancer as this is a common site of metastatic disease. The undersurface of the liver is exposed by lifting the liver upward with a blunt forceps (FIGURE 4). Biopsy of the liver can be obtained using laparoscopic instrumentation, or a "tru-cut" needle can be passed through the abdominal wall under direct laparoscopic visualization to the site/area to be biopsied. The biopsy of diaphragmatic lesions is best performed with a biopsy forceps or the lesion may be sharply excised with laparoscopic scissors. Biopsies can be obtained and sent for frozen or permanent section as desired.

Atraumatic/blunt instruments can be used to "run" the bowel to visualize areas in question (FIGURE 5). The small bowel may be run by using atraumatic instruments by passing the grasped intestine from one hand to the other. Again, rotation or "airplaning" of the table can facilitate exposure. Therapy can be instituted as directed by findings at laparoscopy.

For examination of the pelvis the patient should be placed in the Trendelenburg position. This allows the bowel to move to the upper abdomen facilitating exposure of the pelvic organs (FIGURE 6). The ovaries are exposed by lifting the uterus upward. The peritoneal surface of the pelvis is examined carefully in cases of suspected malignancy. Biopsies of suspicious lesions should be obtained as described above.

Upon completion of the procedure, the abdomen is lavaged with the suction irrigator and aspirated. Careful inspection is made for any bleeding sites and bile or succus the source of which must be identified. Each of the operating ports is removed under direct vision to be certain that there are no bleeding sites in the abdominal wall. The fascia of any 10-mm port site is closed with 00 delayed absorbable sutures. Any 5-mm port sites do not require fascial closure, only skin. The skin is approximated with fine 4-0 subcuticular sutures. Adhesive skin strips and dry sterile dressings are applied.

POSTOPERATIVE CARE The orogastric tube is removed before the patient awakens and the Foley catheter is discontinued as indicated. Patients may experience a moderate amount of pain for a few days. The diet is advanced as tolerated. Depending on the findings and therapy delivered at the time of laparoscopy the patient may be discharged home the same day or require inpatient admission. ■

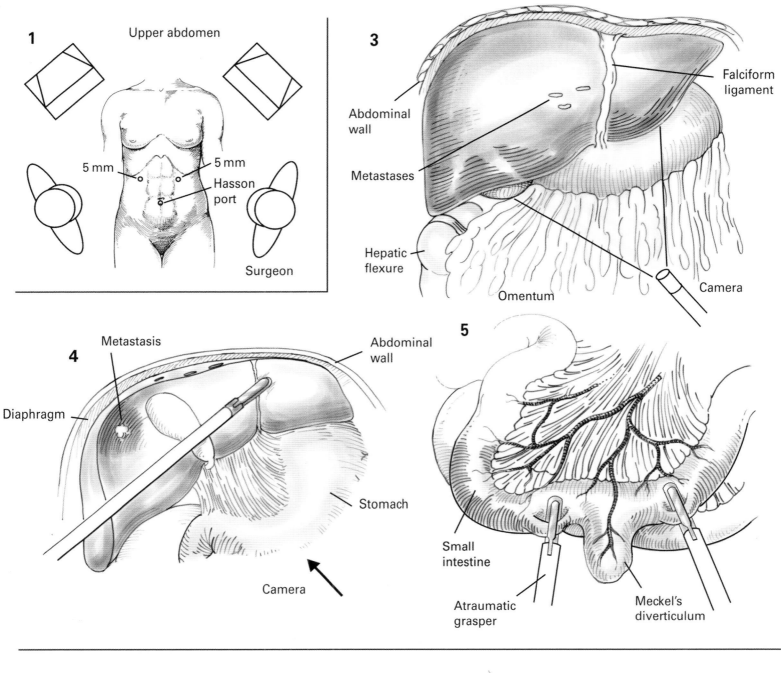

1 Upper abdomen

5 mm   5 mm   Hasson port

Surgeon

3 Abdominal wall

Metastases

Hepatic flexure

Omentum

Falciform ligament

Camera

4 Metastasis

Abdominal wall

Diaphragm

Stomach

Camera

5 Small intestine

Atraumatic grasper

Meckel's diverticulum

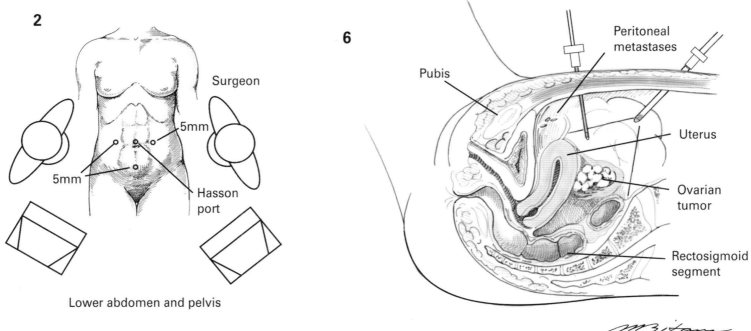

2 Surgeon

5mm

5mm

Hasson port

Lower abdomen and pelvis

6 Pubis

Peritoneal metastases

Uterus

Ovarian tumor

Rectosigmoid segment

CHAPTER 14

CHRONIC AMBULATORY PERITONEAL DIALYSIS CATHETER INSERTION

INDICATIONS Placement of a chronic ambulatory peritoneal dialysis (CAPD) catheter is usually indicated largely for patients with chronic kidney disease (CKD) stages 4 or 5 or with a reduced glomerular filtration rate of less than 20 to 30 cc/min. Such patients will have discussed the suitability of peritoneal dialysis versus hemodialysis with their nephrologist. In general, peritoneal dialysis is preferred over hemodialysis for patients with poor cardiac function, prosthetic heart valves, significant vascular disease, hemodialysis vascular access failure, difficult access to a hemodialysis center, and young age OR small body habitus that makes vascular access for hemodialysis challenging. Candidates for CAPD insertion should be deemed capable of maintaining appropriate sterile techniques when using the catheter to avoid developing bacterial peritonitis due to contamination of the catheter. Intra-abdominal adhesions resulting from previous abdominal surgeries or peritonitis can complicate successful CAPD insertion.

PREOPERATIVE PREPARATION The day of surgery the patient should have electrolytes checked to verify the absence of hyperkalemia. Diabetic patients should have their blood glucose checked prior to initiation of the procedure, as well as during the procedure with correction of hyperglycemia when identified. Antibiotic prophylaxis directed at covering skin flora is administered within 1 hour of the procedure. Determination of the catheter exit site is made with the patient standing to ensure the exit site can be seen by the patient for ease of daily exit site care (especially important in the obese patient) and to avoid the beltline.

ANESTHESIA Local anesthesia accompanied by sedation is adequate for most patients. General anesthesia can be used for patients unwilling or unable to tolerate local anesthesia.

POSITION The patient is placed supine on the operating room table with their arms extended out from the table 90 degrees allowing for easy access to IV sites in the upper extremities and to facilitate the surgeon access to the abdomen without interference from an arm that is tucked to the patient's side.

OPERATIVE PREPARATION The surgeon first verifies that the necessary catheter and stylet are available (FIGURE 1). Any hair within the surgical field is removed with clippers immediately prior to the procedure. The abdomen is prepped from the symphysis pubis to midway between the umbilicus and xiphoid process (or more cephalad), and laterally to the midaxillary line.

INCISION AND EXPOSURE A 3- to 5-cm midline, generally infraumbilical skin incision (midline approach), or paramedian skin incision (paramedian approach) in made and dissection is carried down to the fascia. A 2- to 3-cm incision is made through the fascia at the midline (midline approach FIGURE 2A) or through the anterior and posterior rectus sheath with splitting of the rectus muscle (paramedian approach FIGURE 2B). The peritoneum beneath the fascia is tented up and a small hole created, taking great care to avoid injury to intra-abdominal structures.

DETAILS OF PROCEDURE Once a small hole, sized to permit insertion of the CAPD catheter has been created, a purse-string suture of 4-0 absorbable suture is placed in the peritoneum around the opening. The stylet (FIGURE 1) is placed into the catheter, ensuring the end with multiple side holes will be placed within the abdominal cavity. The catheter with stylet is then inserted through the peritoneal opening and the catheter is ideally directed into the pelvis to the right side of the rectum (FIGURE 2A). Care should be taken to limit the force used to insert the catheter to avoid injury to adjacent structures. Avoidance of advancing the stylet tip beyond the end of the catheter tip will also minimize adjacent structure injury. Irrigating the lumen of the catheter with saline prior to stylet insertion will aid in stylet removal and avoidance of altering the catheter position after proper placement within the pelvis. The peritoneal purse-string suture is then cinched around the catheter just below the deep dacron cuff closest to the abdominal cavity (FIGURE 2B). Alternatively, if the catheter has a silastic ball or cuff, the peritoneal purse string is cinched just above this, leaving the silastic attachment within the abdominal cavity. The fascia is closed snugly around the catheter using a single layer of interrupted #1 nonabsorbable suture immediately above the deep Dacron cuff (midline facial incision FIGURES 2A and 6), or using two layers of #1 nonabsorbable suture for the anterior and posterior rectus sheaths, closed snugly below and above the deep Dacron cuff (FIGURE 2B), respectively. Saline is injected into the catheter and allowed to drain to verify functionality.

A subcutaneous tunnel is created between the catheter insertion site and the usual right lower quadrant skin exit using a long narrow hemostat (FIGURE 3). A heavy silk suture is grasped in the hemostat and it is secured to the proximal free end of the catheter (FIGURE 4) which is tunneled subcutaneously to the skin exit site leaving the second or superficial Dacron cuff 1 to 2 cm deep to the skin. The catheter is anchored to the skin at the exit site with a 3-0 nonabsorbable monofilament suture placed snugly around the catheter without constricting the internal lumen (FIGURE 5). The catheter cap adapter and clamp are placed on the exteriorized end of the catheter (FIGURE 5). Cross-sectional views for the final positions of the one and two cuff catheters and their securing sutures are shown in the inset FIGURES 2A,B and 6. The catheter is flushed with heparinized saline (500–1,000 units/cc) to avoid fibrin clot formation within the catheter.

POSTOPERATIVE CARE The patient is discharged from the operative facility the day of the procedure. The catheter anchoring suture at the skin exit site is removed 2 weeks after the procedure. The surgical site is allowed to heal for 2 weeks prior to CAPD catheter use. Premature catheter use increases the risk of hernia formation and dialysate leakage around the catheter, potentially precipitating wound infection. The patient is instructed in daily exit site care and appropriate catheter use and maintenance. ■

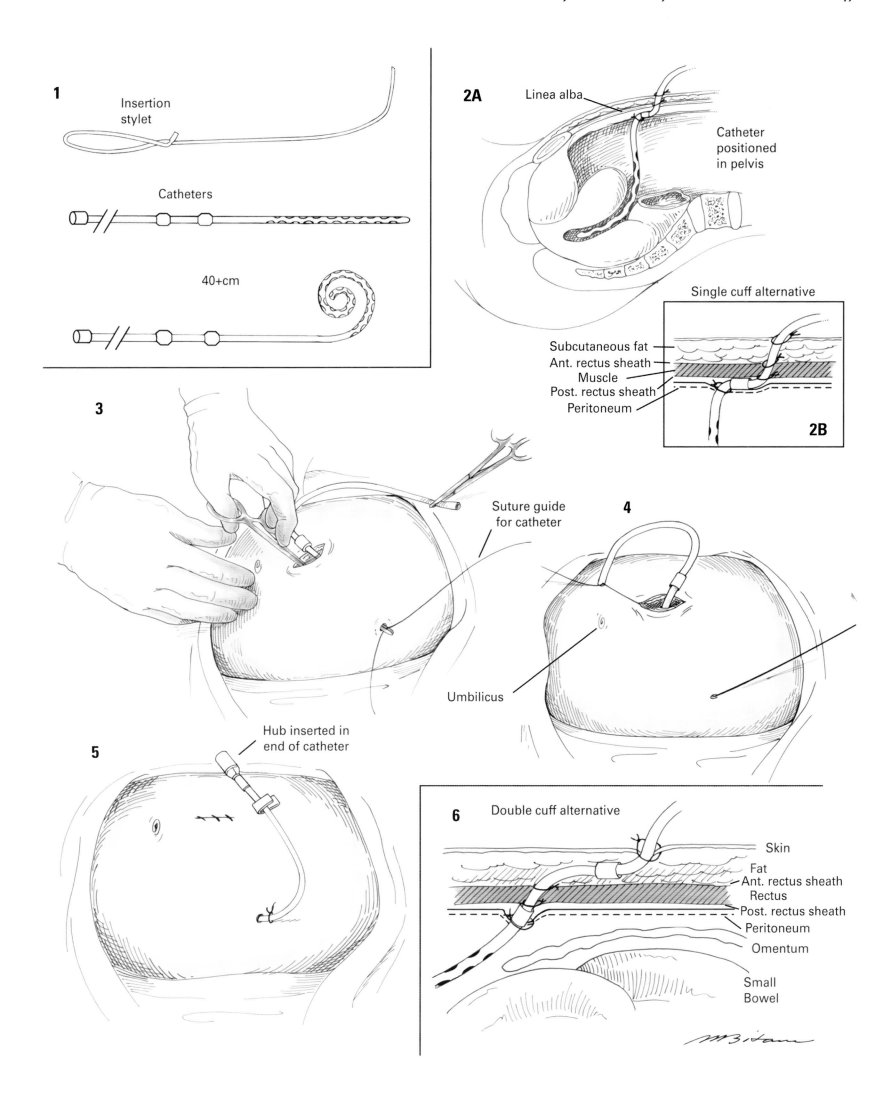

1
Insertion stylet

Catheters

40+cm

2A
Linea alba

Catheter positioned in pelvis

Single cuff alternative

Subcutaneous fat
Ant. rectus sheath
Muscle
Post. rectus sheath
Peritoneum

2B

3
Suture guide for catheter

Umbilicus

4

5
Hub inserted in end of catheter

6   Double cuff alternative

Skin
Fat
Ant. rectus sheath
Rectus
Post. rectus sheath
Peritoneum
Omentum
Small Bowel

THORACOTOMY INCISION

INDICATIONS This incision is ideal for a wide variety of elective as well as emergency procedures. Through the left side, the left lung, heart, descending aorta, lower esophagus, vagus nerves, and diaphragmatic hiatus are well exposed, whereas both the vena cavas, the right lung, the superior exposure of the hepatic veins, and the upper esophagus are approached through the right chest.

The height of the incision on the chest wall varies with the nature of the procedure to obtain optimum exposure of either the apex, the middle, or the basal portions of the chest cavity. One or more ribs may be divided posteriorly and occasionally removed, depending on the mobility of the chest wall and the exposure required. For optimum exposure of the upper portion of the chest cavity, such as in closure of a patent ductus or resection of a coarctation, the chest is entered at the level of the fifth rib. This may be divided posteriorly, along with the fourth rib, if necessary. For procedures on the diaphragm and lower esophagus, the thoracic cavity should be entered at the level of the sixth or seventh rib. If still wider exposure is desired, one or two ribs above and below may be transected at the neck.

PREOPERATIVE PREPARATION Preventative spirometry is preferably started preoperatively to improve compliance postoperatively. Patients should be advised not to smoke for several weeks before an elective operation. Pulmonary functions studies and a room air arterial blood gas analysis should be performed on all patients being considered for thoracotomy. A further evaluation can be obtained by noting the patient's tolerance to climbing stairs. For practical purposes, any patient able to walk up three flights of stairs will tolerate a thoracotomy. When a patient has borderline pulmonary function, aggressive preoperative pulmonary rehabilitation may be appropriate. Because technical difficulties may arise necessitating more extensive resection than planned, the surgeon must be thoroughly familiar with the patient's respiratory reserve.

ANESTHESIA Prior to undergoing a thoracotomy, all patients should undergo fibro-optic bronchoscopy at the beginning of the case via a single-lumen endotracheal tube to remove any secretions, verify the endobronchial anatomy, and survey for endobronchial masses. All thoracotomies require thoracic anesthetic expertise and include the insertion of a thoracic epidural for adequate pain control, an arterial line, and the capacity to perform single lung ventilation. Single lung ventilation can normally be achieved by way of a double-lumen endotracheal tube appropriately positioned or an endobronchial blocker. The position of the double-lumen tube or the endobronchial blocker must be verified prior to deployment with a fibro-optic bronchoscope.

POSITION The patient is placed in a lateral decubitus position with the hips secured to the table by wide adhesive tape (FIGURE 1). The lower leg is flexed at the knee, and a pillow is placed between it and the upper leg, which is extended. A rolled sheet or blanket is placed under the axilla, referred to as an "axillary roll" to support the shoulder and upper thorax. The arm on the side of the thoracotomy is extended forward and upward and placed in a padded grooved arm holder in line with the head, permitting access to the veins. The lower arm is extended forward and rested on an arm board perpendicular to the operating table.

OPERATIVE PREPARATION The skin is cleaned with antiseptic, and the area of incision is either draped with towels or covered with an adhesive plastic drape, followed by the large sterile thoracotomy sheet.

INCISION AND EXPOSURE (POSTEROLATERAL) The surgeon makes the incision while standing posterior to the patient, with the first assistant on the other side of the table across from the surgeon. The incision begins midway between the medial border of the scapula and the spine, proceeding downward parallel to these two structures for the first few inches and then curving in a gentle S one fingerbreadth below the tip of the scapula, and finally extending down into or just below the submammary crease, if necessary. In exposures of the fourth or fifth interspace, the medial end of the incision is extended transversely toward the sternum. For lower openings of the seventh or eighth interspace, or ones involving transection of the costal cartilages for maximum exposure, the medial end of this incision curves gently toward or into the epigastrium. The surgeon then carries the incision directly down through the latissimus dorsi and the serratus anterior muscles (FIGURE 2). During this process, each of the muscles may be elevated individually by the surgeon's index and middle fingers. This is accomplished by entering the auscultatory triangle formed by the superior border of the latissimus dorsi, the inferior border of the trapezius, and the medial border of the scapula.

The incision is extended anteriorly and posteriorly through the borders of the trapezius and rhomboid muscles. Care must be taken to make this posterior incision parallel to the spinal column and thus lessen the chance of dividing the spinal accessory nerve, which innervates the trapezius. Bleeders are cauterized as they appear. By palpating the widened interspace between the first and second ribs and the insertion of the posterior scalene muscle on the first rib, the surgeon may count down to the appropriate rib level (FIGURE 3). The pleural space should be entered just over the superior part of the rib to eliminate the potential for injury to the neurovascular bundle (FIGURE 4). The periosteum is incised directly over the midportion of the rib (FIGURE 4). The sacrospinalis muscle and fascia are elevated by a periosteal elevator, and a retractor is inserted in this space. A Coryllos periosteal elevator is swept anteriorly along the upper half of the rib (FIGURE 5). The Hedblom periosteal elevator is then inserted under the bared portion of the rib and slipped upward along the rib, stripping the remaining periosteum from the upper half of the rib in a posterior-to-anterior direction (FIGURE 6). After ensuring that the patient is on single lung ventilation (i.e., no ventilation to the side being operated upon), a small incision is made entering the pleura (FIGURE 7). The lung drops away, thus allowing the incision to be extended for the desired length. A cross section of this approach is shown beneath FIGURE 5. CONTINUES

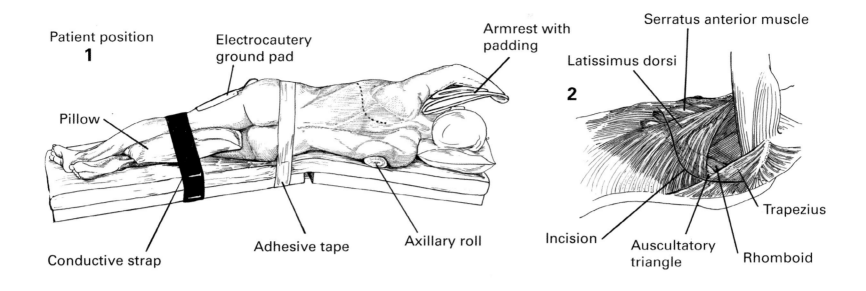

Patient position
1

Pillow

Conductive strap

Electrocautery
ground pad

Adhesive tape

Armrest with
padding

Axillary roll

2

Latissimus dorsi

Serratus anterior muscle

Incision

Auscultatory
triangle

Trapezius

Rhomboid

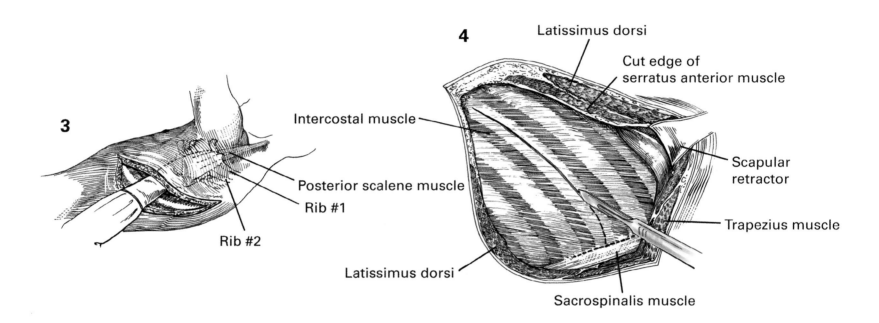

3

Intercostal muscle

Posterior scalene muscle

Rib #1

Rib #2

4   Latissimus dorsi

Cut edge of
serratus anterior muscle

Scapular
retractor

Trapezius muscle

Latissimus dorsi

Sacrospinalis muscle

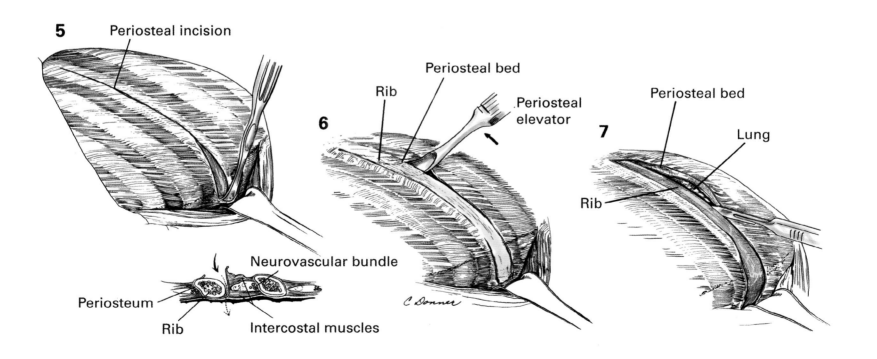

5   Periosteal incision

Periosteum

Rib

Neurovascular bundle

Intercostal muscles

6   Rib

Periosteal bed

Periosteal
elevator

7   Periosteal bed

Lung

Rib

C Donner

INCISION AND EXPOSURE (ANTEROLATERAL) CONTINUED An alternative method is direct incision into the intercostal space. The incision is made through the intercostal muscles along the superior border of the rib. Simple ligation of these is sufficient. Dissection is carried directly down and into the pleura. The incision in the pleura is extended anteriorly and posteriorly with cautery. The internal mammary vessels, which join the intercostals at the sternum, lie medial and deep to the costal cartilages and should not be injured during this incision (FIGURE 8). If additional exposure is required, a rib may be divided or resected. The periosteum along the lower border of the rib is stripped to isolate the neurovascular bundle, which is grasped between right-angled forceps, ligated, and divided. The rib is then transected at the costal cartilage of the neck with rib shears (FIGURE 9). A self-retaining retractor is inserted (FIGURE 10) and opened gradually.

CLOSURE The closure of the thoracotomy incision requires stabilization of the thorax for the entire length of the incision. Encircling no. 1 absorbable sutures (A) are placed and can be tied with or without a rib approximator to aid in the process (FIGURE 11A). If any ribs were transected or fractured during spreading, sutures (B) must encircle both ribs and immobilize all rib fragments (FIGURE 11B). Further hemostasis and stabilization of the transected rib are accomplished by placing a suture (C) through the sacrospinalis muscle, fixing it to the neck of the transected rib and the rib above (FIGURE 11C). The chest muscles are approximated using a running or interrupted absorbable suture as shown in FIGURE 12. Care must be taken to approximate each of the layers separately—that is, rhomboids and the serratus anterior above the trapezius and latissimus dorsi. Subcutaneous 000 nonabsorbable sutures will prevent disruption of the incision when the skin staples are removed in 7 or 8 days.

All patients undergoing thoracotomy should have postoperative drainage of the pleural space. The chest tube used must be of adequate size, and anything less than a 32 French catheter will obstruct with blood clots. It is often advantageous to have two chest tubes in the postoperative chest—one lying over the diaphragm muscle in the posterior gutter along the spine and the other directed anteriorly. The posterolateral chest tube is brought out through stab wounds in the skin as low as possible in a posterolateral position (FIGURE 12). The chest tubes are to be placed prior to the closure of the thoracotomy and should ideally be anterior to the midaxillary line for patient comfort and ease of drainage. Single, untied skin nonabsorbable sutures may be placed through the stab wound before the tube is inserted to aid in closing when the chest tubes are withdrawn. In placing the chest tube, the surgeon first grasps the lower cut edges of the latissimus dorsi and the serratus anterior, and the assistant retracts them superiorly. The surgeon forms a tunnel through the chest wall with Kelly forceps, grasps the chest tube, and draws it out through the wall. The catheter serves two main purposes: to remove escaping air from lung parenchymal injury and to remove blood or serum. The chest tubes are usually attached with underwater seal with or without sutures for as long as there is drainage from the pleural space or persistence of an air leak (FIGURE 13). Should excessive air leakage be present, another chest tube is placed in the second or third interspace anteriorly at the level of the midclavicular line (FIGURE 13). A smaller Silastic catheter will suffice and will be the last chest tube to be removed. The catheters allow expansion of the lung with approximation of pleural surfaces and thus prevent postoperative atelectasis and fluid accumulation with infection. The catheters are usually attached to an underwater-seal device with or without negative suction (FIGURE 14).

POSTOPERATIVE CARE The preoperative insertion of a thoracic epidural should help postoperative pain control. If an epidural is not possible due to coagulation defects or anesthesia preference, intercostal blocks above and below the incision using a long-acting local anesthetic can be placed at the end of surgery. Intercostal blocks combined with the use of a patient-controlled analgesic device are known to provide adequate pain control.

The patient should be encouraged to cough vigorously and use incentive spirometry. The patient should be helped in coughing by supporting his operative side with a pillow. The patient should be encouraged to change positions frequently. Ambulation should be early, and active exercise should be encouraged.

The chest tubes are usually removed when they have served their purpose, as evidenced by normal breathing sounds on the operative side and x-ray films showing complete expansion of the lung and the absence of air leak and fluid accumulation. This is usually on the second or third postoperative day. Persistent air leakage may indicate improper position of the catheter, leakage around the entrance of the thoracotomy tube, or large bronchial air leaks. In these circumstances, early bronchoscopy and radiologic imaging with plain films or computed tomography are encouraged. ■

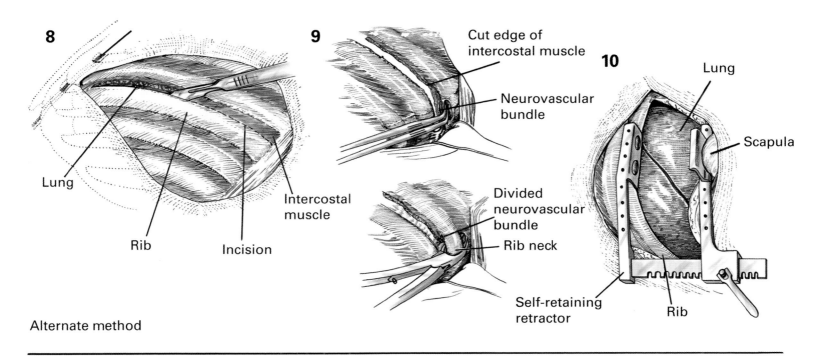

8

Lung

Rib

Incision

Intercostal muscle

9

Cut edge of intercostal muscle

Neurovascular bundle

Divided neurovascular bundle

Rib neck

10

Lung

Scapula

Self-retaining retractor

Rib

Alternate method

Thoracotomy closure

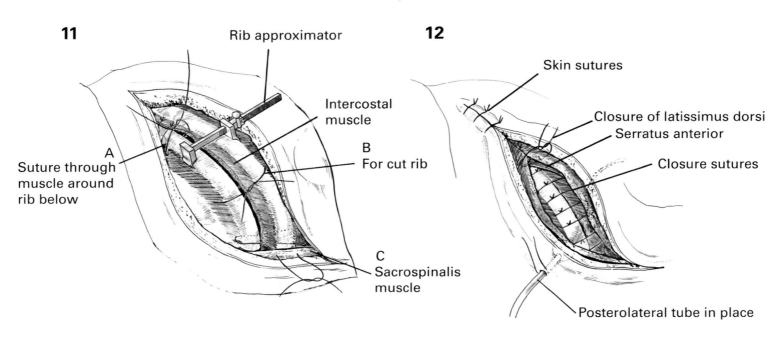

11

Rib approximator

Intercostal muscle

A

B
For cut rib

Suture through muscle around rib below

C
Sacrospinalis muscle

12

Skin sutures

Closure of latissimus dorsi

Serratus anterior

Closure sutures

Posterolateral tube in place

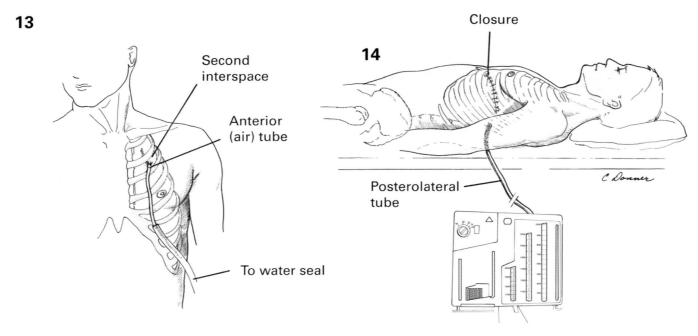

13

Second interspace

Anterior (air) tube

To water seal

14

Closure

Posterolateral tube

C Donner

CHAPTER 16 THORACOSCOPY

INDICATIONS This type of approach is ideal for a wide variety of elective and urgent procedures. Through this approach, the lung, mediastinum, pericardium, diaphragm, esophagus, sympathetic chain and chest wall are well visualized. Over the last decade, minimally invasive surgical techniques have gained widespread acceptance as technological improvements in imaging systems and instrumentation have occurred. Thoracoscopy has become the procedure of choice for the management of early-stage non–small-cell lung cancer, posterior and mediastinal masses biopsy or excision, primary spontaneous pneumothorax, fibropurulent empyema, evacuation of hemothorax, management of effusive pericardial disease, sympathetic chain ablation for hyperhidrosis, pleural biopsy, and recurrent pleural effusions. Depending on the indication, thoracoscopy can therefore be used both as a diagnostic and/or therapeutic intervention. For successful thoracoscopy, a sound understanding of surgical anatomy is essential due to limitation of viewing angles and reduction of tactile sense.

PREOPERATIVE PREPARATION Thoracoscopy is performed for the most part in elective, non-emergency situations. This allows for the pulmonary function to be optimized with preoperative incentive spirometry and smoking cessation. For thoracoscopy to be performed, the patient must be able to tolerate contralateral single lung ventilation which must be trialed prior to positioning the patient. Similarly, if the patient is on maximal ventilator support prior to the operation, it is unlikely that thoracoscopy will be well tolerated by the patient. A history of previous chest surgery including pleurodesis or empyema must be ascertained.

ANESTHESIA Prior to undergoing thoracoscopy, the patient should have bronchoscopy performed through a single-lumen tube. This will eliminate secretions, ensure normal anatomy, rule out endobronchial pathology, and ultimately facilitate the insertion of the double-lumen endotracheal tube by the anesthesiologist. Although thoracoscopic procedures are reported to be less painful, a thoracic epidural should be offered to the patient prior to the procedure and arterial blood pressure monitoring should be placed prior to induction. A double-lumen endotracheal tube is ideal for securing single lung ventilation, although an endobronchial blocker through a single-lumen endotracheal tube is a possible alternative. Prior to positioning the patient for thoracoscopy, the anesthesiologist should verify the position of the double-lumen tube or the endobronchial blocker and secure it well so it does not migrate during positioning. A trial of contralateral single lung ventilation should be attempted prior to positioning the patient. Relative contraindications to thoracoscopy include the presence of dense pleural adhesions or pleural symphysis as well as large intrathoracic tumors and hilar granulomatous disease that would preclude adequate visualization of the hilar vascular structures.

POSITION The patient is placed in a lateral decubitus position, facilitated by a bean bag on the operating room bed, with the hips secured to the table. The table is flexed so to expand the intercostal spaces. The lower leg is flexed at the knee and a pillow is placed between it and the upper leg which is extended. An axillary roll is placed under the axilla to protect the patient's upper thorax and brachial plexus. The patient's head may need to be supported by additional blankets after the flexing of the table. The arm, on the side of the operation, is extended forward and 90 degrees to the body and placed on two pillows or a grooved arm board (FIGURE 1).

OPERATIVE PREPARATION Prior to the operation, the appropriate surgical equipment must be assured for thoracoscopy. The equipment consists of both imaging systems and thoracoscopic instrumentation. Imaging systems consist of a video thoracoscope, processor, and imaging tower with screen. Zero- and 30-degree optical angulation scopes are most popular and applicable. The scopes can also be either 5 or 10 mm in diameter, with the smaller scope being for diagnostic as compared to therapeutic interventions. The basic set of thoracoscopic instruments includes an atraumatic lung grasper,

scissors, blunt dissection, and forceps. The skin is cleaned with antiseptic and the area of the incisions is draped with adhesive plastic drape and a large sterile thoracotomy sheet. The video monitors with screens should be positioned on either side of the patient near the head of the bed.

INCISION AND EXPOSURE For thoracoscopy procedures, the surgeon stands anterior to the patient and the assistant stands next to the surgeon (FIGURE 1). The assistant needs to be facing and operating in the same direction as the surgeon, thus avoiding mirror imaging. The placement of what is referred to as "ports" is critical, with the placement of the camera being most critical. When properly placed, the camera has a 180-degree viewing angle of the region of interest. The camera is usually positioned over the seventh rib, in the midaxillary line, after making a 1-cm incision that is slightly tunneled and entering directly into the pleural space (FIGURE 2). Once the camera is positioned, the other port sites can be placed under direct visualization. The additional port sites should be within the 180-degree viewing angle of the camera. The additional ports are placed at different levels from the thoracoscope so to allow for triangulation of the instruments. Depending on the complexity of the thoracoscopic procedure, one, two, or three more ports may be positioned and placed.

DETAILS OF THE PROCEDURE The placement of the thoracoscope is the first part of the procedure. The patient is placed on single lung ventilation. A small incision is made over the seventh rib that is approximately 1 cm in size (FIGURE 2). Local anesthetic can be instilled prior to incision, particularly if a thoracic epidural has not been placed. A small amount of tunneling is advised. This incision is carried down through the intercostal muscle using cautery and the pleura is entered under direct visualization. Once the chest cavity is entered, a finger should be gently placed to ensure that there are no dense adhesions that would prevent safe introduction of the port. If all clear, the port is placed then the camera is inserted. The camera is used to complete a surveillance of the entire chest so that an overall appreciation of the chest cavity is gained. Using the camera, the additional ports can be placed under direct visualization. These additional ports should create a triangle with the camera and be within the 180-degree viewing angle (FIGURE 3). Care should be taken to place the ports or instruments on top of the rib to avoid the intercostal vessels that course on the inferior portion of the rib. Their exact position will be dependent on the nature of the clinical problem, body habitus, and intrathoracic pathology. In general, a second port for instrumentation is placed over the sixth rib anteriorly and a third port is placed over the fourth rib anteriorly or posteriorly relative to the clinical scenario. FIGURE 2 illustrates port placement over the fourth and eighth ribs. Biopsies of superficial lesions may be obtained with a biopsy forceps or the lesion may be excised with a portion of lung using a linear stapler. At the completion of the surgical procedure, all operative sites must be visualized for hemostasis. In addition, all ports must be directly visualized so to ensure hemostasis prior to completion of the procedure. A single 32 French chest tube is placed through one of the ports and positioned to the apex under visualization (FIGURE 4). Concepts that must be remembered to minimize complications include: extraction of all tissue containing potential malignancy in a protected specimen bag, avoidance of instrument leveraging and large diameter instruments so to lessen intercostal nerve pressure, and a well-delineated preconceived plan for addressing potential vessel injury and bleeding.

POSTOPERATIVE CARE Most patients have a single chest tube placed at the completion of the thoracoscopy. This can often be removed within 24 hours when the pleural drainage is less than 300 mL. The incision sites are all small and are closed primarily, so wound care is minimal. Pain management is usually achieved with oral agents. Once the chest tube is removed and the patient is discharged, the patient can normally return to normal activities within 2 weeks. ∎

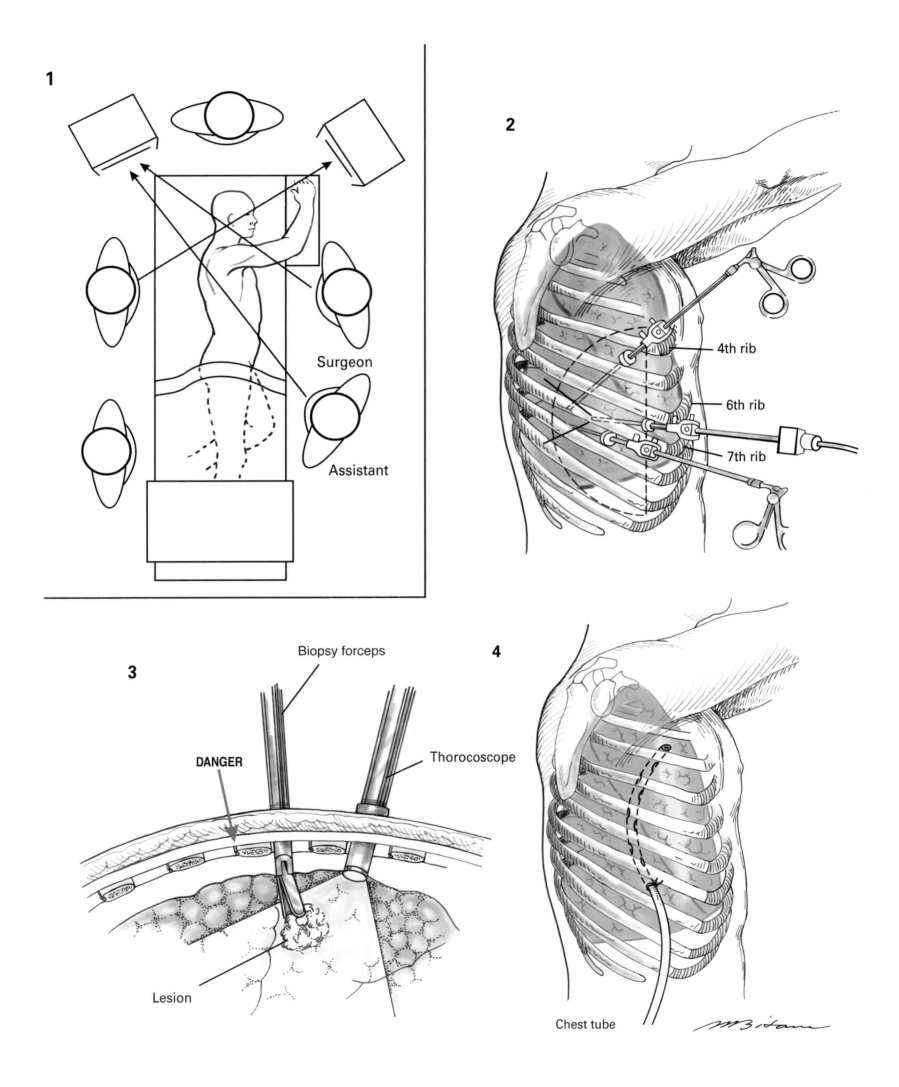

1

Surgeon

Assistant

2

4th rib

6th rib

7th rib

3

Biopsy forceps

DANGER

Thorocoscope

Lesion

4

Chest tube

SECTION IV
ESOPHAGUS AND STOMACH

INDICATIONS Gastrostomy is commonly utilized as a temporary procedure to avoid the discomfort of prolonged nasogastric suction following such major abdominal procedures as vagotomy and subtotal gastrectomy, colectomy, and so forth. This procedure should be considered during abdominal operation in those poor-risk or elderly patients prone to pulmonary difficulties or where postoperative nutritional difficulties are anticipated.

Gastrostomy is considered in the presence of obstruction of the esophagus, but it is most frequently employed as a palliative procedure in nonresectable lesions of the esophagus or as the preliminary step in treating the cause of the obstruction. A permanent type of gastrostomy may be considered for feeding purposes in the presence of almost complete obstruction of the esophagus due to nonresectable malignancy. The type of gastrostomy depends upon whether the opening is to be temporary or permanent.

As a temporary gastrostomy, the Witzel or the Stamm procedure is used frequently and is easily performed. A permanent type of gastrostomy, such as the Janeway and its variations, is best adapted to patients in whom it is essential to have an opening into the stomach for a prolonged period of time. Under these circumstances, the gastric mucosa must be anchored to the skin to ensure long-term patency of the opening. Furthermore, the construction of a mucosa-lined tube with valve-like control at the gastric end tends to prevent the regurgitation of the irritating gastric contents. This allows periodic intubation and frees the patient from the irritation of a constant indwelling tube.

PREOPERATIVE PREPARATION If the patient is dehydrated, fluid balance is brought to a satisfactory level by the intravenous administration of 5% dextrose in saline. Since these patients may be malnourished, parenteral nutrition may be warranted. Blood transfusion should be given if there is evidence of symptomatic, physiologically significant secondary anemia or for a hemoglobin <7 g/dL. No special preparation is required for the temporary gastrostomy since this is usually performed as a minor part of a primary surgical procedure.

ANESTHESIA Since some patients requiring a permanent gastrostomy are both anemic and cachectic, local infiltration or field block anesthesia is usually advisable. There is no special indication in anesthesia for a temporary gastrostomy, since this is usually a minor technical procedure that precedes the closure of the wound of a major operation.

POSITION The patient lies in a comfortable supine position with the feet lower than the head, so that the contracted stomach tends to drop below the costal margin.

OPERATIVE PREPARATION The skin is prepared in the routine manner.

INCISION AND EXPOSURE A small incision is made high in the left mid-rectus region, and the muscle is split with as little injury to the nerve supply as possible, if the gastrostomy is the lone surgical procedure planned (FIGURE 1). The high position is indicated since the stomach may be contracted because of the long-term starvation that the patient may have experienced. The usual temporary tube gastrostomy is brought out through a stab wound some distance from the primary incision and away from the costal margin. The site of the stab wound must correspond exactly to the area of the abdominal wall to which the underlying stomach can be attached without tension (FIGURE 1).

A. STAMM GASTROSTOMY

This type of gastrostomy is most commonly utilized as a temporary procedure. The mid anterior gastric wall is grasped with a Babcock forceps, and the ease with which the gastric wall approximates the overlying peritoneum is tested. A purse-string suture using oo nonabsorbable suture is placed in the mid anterior wall of the stomach (FIGURE 2). An incision is made in the central portion of the purse string at right angles to the long axis of the stomach is made in an effort to minimize the number of arterial bleeders. The incision with electrocautery, scissors, or a knife. A mushroom catheter of average size, 18 to 22 French, is introduced into the stomach for a distance of 10 to 15 cm. A Foley-type catheter also may be used. The purse-string suture is tied (FIGURE 3). The gastric wall about the tube is then inverted by a second purse-string suture of oo nonabsorbable suture (FIGURE 3) or with interrupted Lembert's stitches (oo nonabsorbable suture). The gastric wall should be inverted about the

tube to ensure rapid closure of the gastric opening when the catheter is removed (FIGURE 6).

A point is then selected some distance from the margins of the operative incision and the costal margin for the placement of the stab wound and subsequent passage of the tube through the anterior abdominal wall (FIGURE 4). The position of the catheter end should be checked to make certain that a sufficient amount extends into the gastric lumen to ensure efficient gastric drainage. The gastric wall is then anchored to the peritoneum about the tube (FIGURE 5) by four or five oo nonabsorbable sutures. Occasionally, additional sutures are necessary. The gastric wall must not be under undue tension at the completion of the procedure. The cross-sectional diagram in (FIGURE 6) shows the inversion of the gastric wall about the tube and the sealing of the gastric wall to the overlying peritoneum. The gastrostomy tube is snugged upward and then secured to the abdominal skin with a nonabsorbable suture.

B. JANEWAY GASTROSTOMY

This procedure is one of the many types of permanent gastrostomies utilized to avoid an inlying tube and prevent the regurgitation of irritant gastric contents. Such a mucosa-lined tube anchored to the skin tends to remain patent with a minimal tendency toward closure of the mucosal opening.

DETAILS OF PROCEDURE The operator visualizes the relation of the stomach to the anterior abdominal wall and then with Allis forceps outlines a rectangular flap, the base of which is placed near the greater curvature to ensure an adequate blood supply (FIGURE 7). Because the flap, when cut, contracts, it is made somewhat larger than would appear to be necessary to avoid subsequent interference with its blood supply when the flap is approximated about the catheter. The gastric wall is divided between the Allis clamps near the lesser curvature, and a rectangular flap is developed by extending the incision on either side toward the Allis clamps on the greater curvature. To prevent soiling from the gastric contents and to control bleeding, long, straight enterostomy clamps may be applied to the stomach both above and below the operative site. The flap of gastric wall is pulled downward, and the catheter is placed along the inner surface of the flap (FIGURE 8). The mucous membrane is closed with a continuous suture or interrupted 0000 nonabsorbable sutures (FIGURE 9). The outer layer, which includes the serosa and submucosa, is also closed either with continuous absorbable sutures or, preferably, by a series of interrupted nonabsorbable sutures (FIGURE 10). When this cone-shaped entrance to the stomach has been completed about the catheter, the anterior gastric wall is attached to the peritoneum at the suture line with additional nonabsorbable oo sutures (FIGURE 11). A gastric tube can be constructed with a stapling instrument.

CLOSURE After the pouch of gastric wall is lifted to the skin surface, the peritoneum is closed about the catheter. The catheter may be brought out through a small stab wound to the left of the major incision. The layers of the abdominal wall are closed about this, and the mucosa is anchored to the skin with a few sutures (FIGURE 12). Catheters are anchored to the skin with strips of adhesive tape in addition to a suture that has included a bite in the catheter.

POSTOPERATIVE CARE When the temporary Stamm type of gastrostomy is used in lieu of prolonged nasogastric suction, the usual principles of gastric decompression and fluid replacement are adhered to. Usually, the tube is clamped off as soon as normal bowel function returns. The temporary gastrostomy provides an invaluable method of fluid and nutritional replacement; compared to the more tedious and less-efficient intravenous route, it is the method of choice, especially in the elderly patient.

The temporary gastrostomy should not be removed for at least 14 to 28 days to ensure adequate peritoneal sealing. In addition, it should not be removed until alimentary function has returned to normal and all postoperative gastric secretory studies have been completed.

When a permanent gastrostomy is done because of esophageal obstruction, liquids such as water and milk may be injected safely into the catheter within 24 hours, while parenteral nutrition continues. Liquids of a high-calorie and high-vitamin value are added gradually, beginning with small volumes that are diluted so as to minimize osmotic changes or diarrhea. After a week or more, the catheter may be removed and cleaned, but it should be replaced immediately because of the tendency toward overly rapid closure of the sinus tract in the Janeway type of gastrostomy. ∎

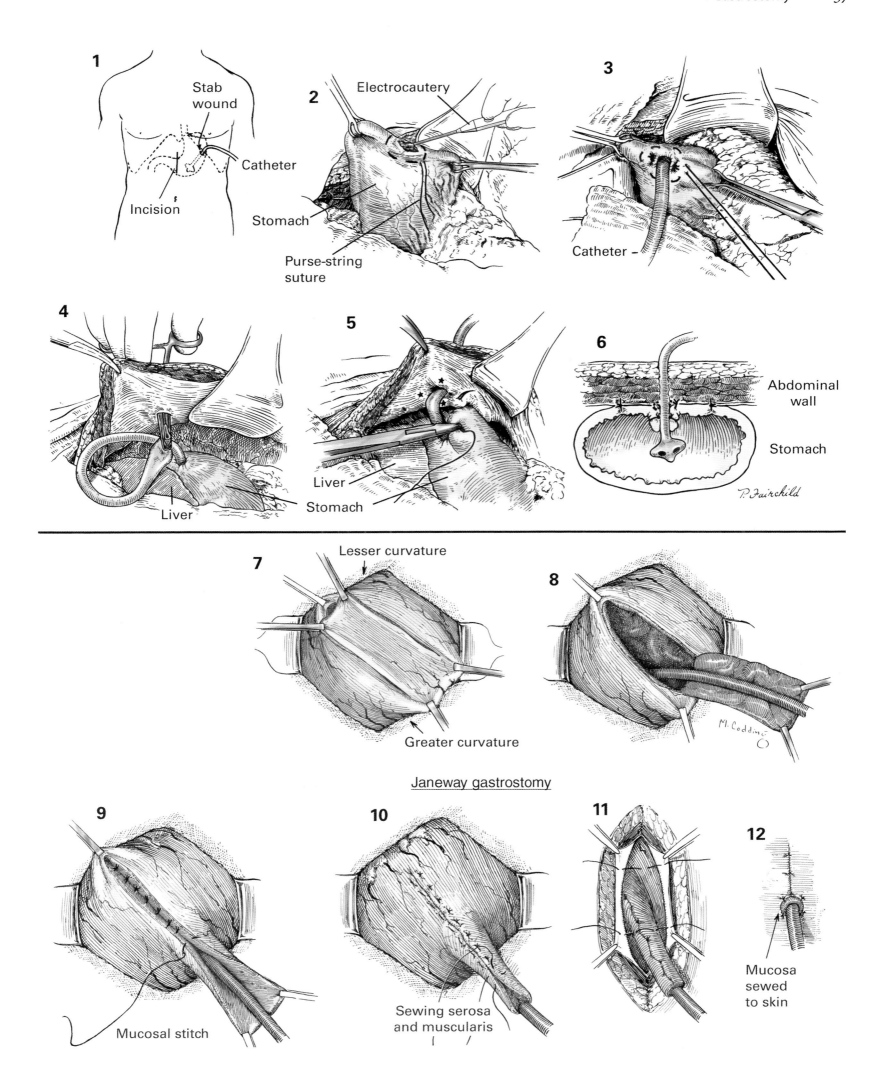

1
Stab wound
Catheter
Incision

2
Electrocautery
Stomach
Purse-string suture

3
Catheter

4
Liver

5
Liver
Stomach

6
Abdominal wall
Stomach

P. Fairchild

7
Lesser curvature
Greater curvature

8
M. Codding

Janeway gastrostomy

9
Mucosal stitch

10
Sewing serosa and muscularis

11

12
Mucosa sewed to skin

PERCUTANEOUS ENDOSCOPIC GASTROSTOMY

INDICATIONS The usual indications for gastrostomy include the need for feeding, decompression, or gastric access. In feeding situations, the gastrointestinal tract must be functional and the need for enteral feeding must be for a prolonged interval. Stamm gastrostomies are most commonly performed at the conclusion of some other major gastrointestinal procedure while the abdomen is open, however the percutaneous endoscopic gastrostomy (PEG) allows the placement of a gastrostomy in adults and children without laparotomy. This technique depends upon the safe passage of an endoscope into the stomach, which can be dilated with air. Inability to pass the endoscope safely and inability to identify the transabdominal lumination of the lighted endoscope tip within the dilated stomach are contraindications to the procedure. Ascites, partially corrected coagulopathy, and intra-abdominal infection are relative contraindications to the PEG method.

PREOPERATIVE PREPARATION The indications for the gastrostomy dictate the extent and type of preoperative preparation. Passage of a nasogastric tube for gastric decompression is usually not needed if the patient has been nothing by mouth (NPO) for several hours. A single dose of intravenous antibiotic may be given within 1 hour prior to the procedure because the peroral passage of the special catheter may contaminate the abdominal wall tract created as the catheter is brought out through the stomach.

ANESTHESIA A topical anesthesia for the oropharynx is needed for passage of the endoscope, and local anesthesia is used at the abdominal site where the special catheter will be placed. An intravenous needle or catheter is positioned for administration of sedatives.

POSITION The patient is usually supine while the topical anesthetic is sprayed into the oropharynx. He or she is allowed to gargle, swallow, or spit into a basin. After satisfactory anesthesia is obtained, the patient is positioned supine on the table with the head slightly elevated.

OPERATIVE PREPARATION In adults as well as children, the smallest possible gastroscope is used. After the endoscope is passed safely into the stomach, the skin of the abdomen and lower chest is prepared with antiseptic solutions in the usual manner. Sterile drapes are applied.

DETAILS OF PROCEDURE During the placement of the gastroscope, any pathology may be evaluated. The stomach is fully inflated with air. This displaces the colon inferiorly and places the anterior gastric wall against the abdominal wall over a large area. A suitable zone is selected and the endoscopist places the lighted gastroscope end firmly upward at this point. This is usually halfway between the costal margin and the umbilicus (FIGURE 1). The room lights are dimmed and the transilluminated site is identified. In very thin patients, the tip of the endoscope may be palpated. The area of transillumination is marked for incision (FIGURE 1). The endoscope is backed away from the anterior gastric wall, and the appropriateness of the site is verified as external palpation with a finger indents the chosen area.

Local anesthesia is injected and a 1-cm skin incision is made. The endoscopist visualizes the site as a 16-gauge smoothly tapered intravenous cannula/needle is introduced through the incision and abdominal and gastric walls and into the lumen of the stomach. This sequence should be done quickly so as to minimize the chance for displacement of the stomach away from the abdominal wall and peritoneum.

A guide wire is passed through the hollow outer cannula after the stiffening inner needle has been withdrawn. The wire is grasped with a polypectomy snare passed through the endoscope and then all are withdrawn through the patient's mouth (FIGURE 2). The PEG catheter (FIGURE 3) is secured to the wire. The catheter has a tapered end. The long wire and the catheter assembly are covered with a sterile water-soluble lubricant. Gentle, steady traction on the abdominal end of the long suture pulls the tapered end of the assembly down the esophagus and then through the gastric and abdominal wall (FIGURE 4).

The endoscope is reintroduced and the positioning of the intragastric end of the catheter is verified. An external crosspiece (FIGURE 5) or collar is applied, and a nonabsorbable suture is used to secure the catheter and crosspiece to the skin without pressure or tension that might cause necrosis of the skin or gastric wall. The small skin incision is left open, and topical antiseptic may be applied.

POSTOPERATIVE CARE The gastrostomy catheter is opened for decompression and gravity drainage for a day. Thereafter, feedings may start in a sequential manner. The catheter may be changed in a periodic manner or may be converted to a silastic prosthesis (button) after 4 weeks or more when the gastrostomy incision has solidly healed and the stomach has fused to the anterior abdominal wall. This prosthesis is stretched and thinned over an obturator (FIGURE 6) and inserted into the open gastrostomy tract (FIGURE 7). ■

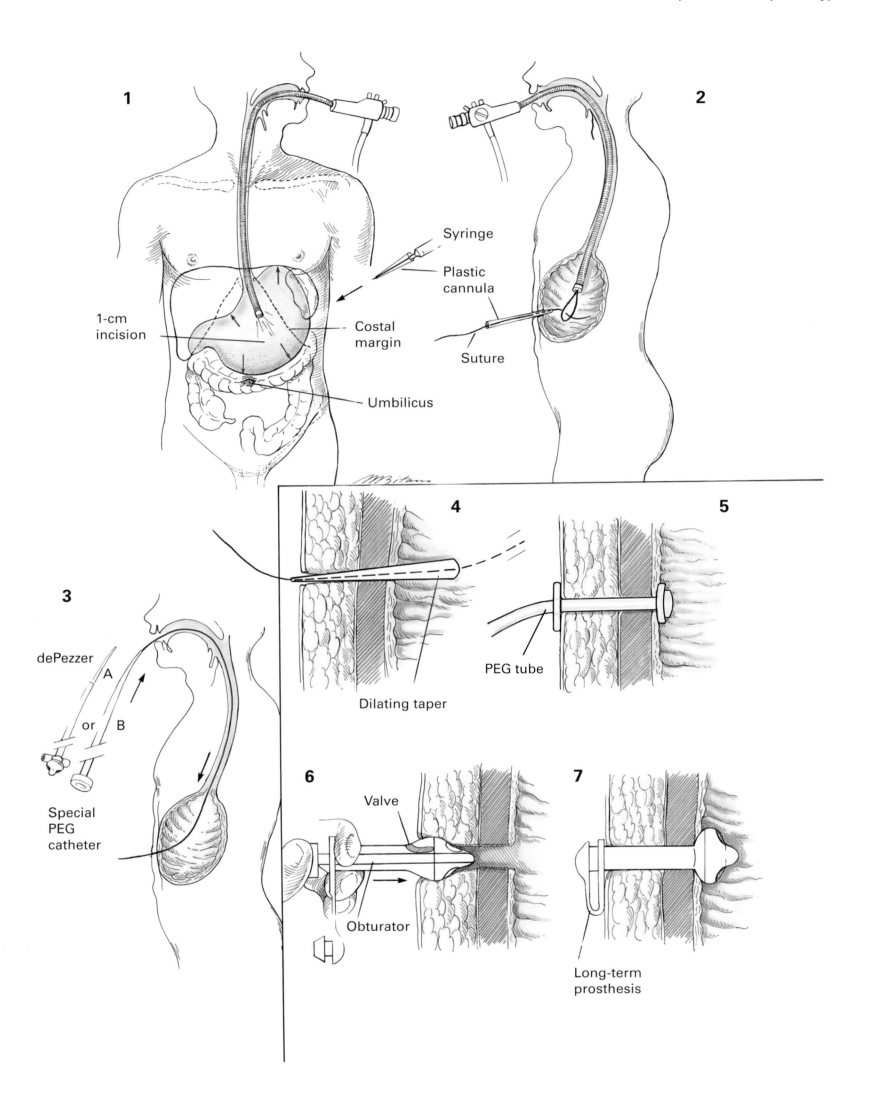

1

1-cm incision

Syringe

Plastic cannula

Costal margin

Umbilicus

2

Suture

3

dePezzer

A

or

B

Special PEG catheter

4

Dilating taper

5

PEG tube

6

Valve

Obturator

7

Long-term prosthesis

A. CLOSURE OF PERFORATION

INDICATIONS Perforation of an ulcer of the stomach or duodenum is a surgical emergency; however, before performing the operation, sufficient time should be allowed for the patient to recover from the initial shock (rarely severe or prolonged) and for the restoration of the fluid balance. The choice for closure of the perforation versus a definitive ulcer procedure depends upon the overall assessment of risk factors by the surgeon. Laparoscopic exploration with or without definitive repair is often preferred especially in the setting of anterior perforation of the duodenum with a plan for simple closure.

PREOPERATIVE PREPARATION A narcotic is used to control pain only after the diagnosis is established. The intravenous administration of appropriate type and volume of fluid is necessary, depending upon the patient's general condition and the length of time that has elapsed since perforation. The parenteral administration of antibiotics and the institution of constant gastric suction are routine.

ANESTHESIA General endotracheal anesthesia combined with muscle relaxants is preferred.

POSITION The patient is placed in a comfortable supine position with the feet slightly lower than the head to assist in bringing the field below the costal margin and to keep gastric leakage away from the subphrenic area.

OPERATIVE PREPARATION The skin is prepared in the usual manner.

INCISION AND EXPOSURE Since the majority of perforations occur in the anterior-superior surface of the first portion of the duodenum, a small, high, midline is made. A culture of the peritoneal fluid is taken, and as much exudate as possible is removed by suction. The liver is held upward with retractors, exposing the most frequent sites of perforation. The site may be walled off with omentum if the perforation has been present several hours; therefore, care is exercised in approaching the perforation to avoid unnecessary soiling.

DETAILS OF PROCEDURE The easiest method of closure consists of placing three sutures of fine silk through the submucosal layer on one side with extension through the region of the ulcer and then out a corresponding distance on the other side of the ulcer (FIGURE 1). Starting at the top of the ulcer, the sutures are tied very gently to prevent laceration of the friable tissues. The long ends are retained (FIGURE 2). The closure is reinforced with omentum by separating the long ends of the three previously tied sutures and placing a small portion of omentum along the suture line. The ends of these sutures are loosely tied, anchoring the omentum over the site of the ulcer (FIGURE 3).

The tissue may be so indurated that the ulcer cannot be closed successfully, making it necessary to seal the perforation by anchoring omentum directly over the ulcer.

In the presence of a perforated gastric ulcer, the area surrounding the ulcer can be completely excised often with a stapler and sent for frozen section to exclude malignancy. This is determined by the site of ulcer perforation. Alternatively, a small biopsy of the margin of the perforation is taken because of the possibility of malignancy (FIGURES 4 and 5). The omentum may be anchored over the suture line (FIGURE 6). Closure of a gastric ulcer may be reinforced with a layer of interrupted silk serosal sutures since there is little danger of obstruction.

In the presence of perforation of an obvious carcinoma, resection is preferred; however, in cases of high operative risk or metastatic disease requiring palliation, it may be acceptable to close the perforation, to be followed by resection upon recovery. If the patient's general condition is good and the perforation has lasted only a few hours, a gastric resection may be justified. Vagotomy and pyloroplasty or antrectomy for an early perforated duodenal ulcer in a good-risk patient is preferred by some surgeons.

CLOSURE All exudate and fluid are removed by suction. Repeated irrigation of the peritoneal cavity with saline should be considered when there is gross contamination by food particles. The wound is closed without drainage. A temporary Stamm gastrostomy (Chapter 17) can be considered since prolonged obstruction of the pylorus may occur.

POSTOPERATIVE CARE The patient, when conscious, is placed in Fowler's position. Nasogastric suction can be employed for the first 24 hours or as needed. The fluid balance is maintained by intravenous infusions. Antibiotics are continued. Proton pump inhibitors should be given IV until PO intake is started. Consideration should be given to eradicate *Helicobacter pylori* as well. Simple closure of the perforation has not cured the patient's ulcer or the patient's tendency to form another. It must be remembered that a subphrenic or a pelvic abscess may complicate the postoperative period.

B. SUBPHRENIC ABSCESS

INDICATIONS The most common origins of a subphrenic abscess are perforation of a peptic ulcer, perforation of the appendix, or acute infection of the gallbladder. It is to be suspected in an unsatisfactory recovery from any of these conditions. Intensive antibiotic therapy may mask the systemic reaction to the infection. Chest radiographs may show a pleural effusion and ultrasound or computed tomographic (CT) scans should be diagnostic. In addition, the CT scan may guide a fine-needle aspiration for culture or the placement of a catheter for drainage, if the pus is thin and the cavity is unilocular. It is rare that a surgical procedure is necessary and percutaneous transperitoneal drainage is acceptable. In some situations surgical drainage can be undertaken.

PREOPERATIVE PREPARATION The clinical data combined with radiologic studies usually indicate the location of the abscess. The location and extent of the abscess often can be defined by CT, which may also be used to guide needle aspiration or catheter drainage. Subphrenic abscesses occur much more frequently on the right side. Antibiotics, blood transfusions, and intravenous fluids are usually necessary because of the prolonged sepsis.

ANESTHESIA Local anesthesia by direct infiltration of the site of the incision is preferable for the poor-risk patient. Spinal or inhalation anesthesia also may be used, depending upon the patient's general condition.

POSITION For an anterior abscess, the patient is placed supine with the head of the table elevated. For a posterior abscess, the patient is placed on the side with the arm on the affected side pulled forward.

OPERATIVE PREPARATION The skin is prepared in the usual manner.

1. ANTERIOR ABSCESS

INCISION AND EXPOSURE The incision is placed one fingerbreadth below the costal margin and extended from the mid-rectus region laterally (FIGURE 7). The free peritoneal cavity is not opened.

DETAILS OF PROCEDURE The surgeon inserts the index finger upward between the peritoneum and diaphragm until the abscess cavity is encountered; extraperitoneal drainage is thus established (FIGURE 8).

2. POSTERIOR ABSCESS

INCISION AND EXPOSURE These can most often be drained with image-guided percutaneous approach. It may be desirable to drain the subphrenic abscess by the extraperitoneal route without rib resection whenever possible. On occasion, it may be desirable to approach the abscess through the bed of the 12th rib (FIGURE 9, Incision A). The entire 12th rib is resected. The erector spinae are retracted toward the midline, and a deep transverse incision is made at right angles to the vertebrae across the periosteal bed of the resected rib, opposite the transverse process of the first lumbar vertebra (FIGURE 9, Incision B).

DETAILS OF PROCEDURE Intraoperative ultrasound can be used to localize the abscess. The location of the abscess cavity is approached by the index finger of the surgeon, who separates the peritoneum from the undersurface of the diaphragm, thus ensuring dependent drainage without contamination of the peritoneal cavities (FIGURE 10). Once pus has been obtained, the abscess cavity can be entered and thoroughly evacuated, and rubber tissue drains or mushroom catheters can be inserted. Several cultures are taken routinely, and the sensitivity of the offending organism is determined. Some organisms, such as *Staphylococcus*, require isolating the patient to prevent spread of the organism to others.

CLOSURE Drains are inserted into the abscess cavity in numbers indicated by the size of the abscess. There is no further closure.

POSTOPERATIVE CARE The abscess cavity is carefully irrigated with normal saline each day, and the capacity of the cavity measured from time to time. The external opening is maintained, and the drains or tubes are removed sequentially as the cavity is obliterated. Vigorous pulmonary and nutritional support is given, and antibiotics are continued until sepsis is over.

If the chest is entered, closure of the opening with placement of a temporary chest tube is usually necessary. ■

Duodenal ulcer

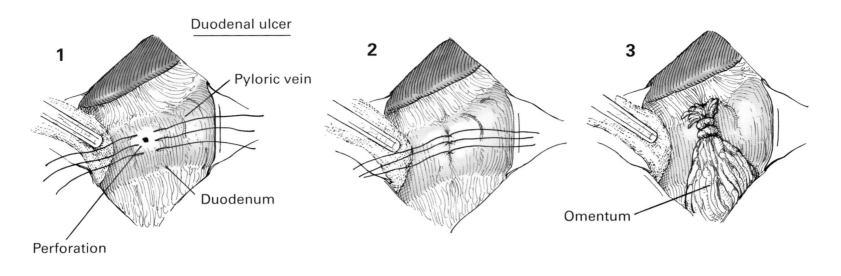

1 Pyloric vein — Duodenum — Perforation

2

3 Omentum

Prepyloric ulcer

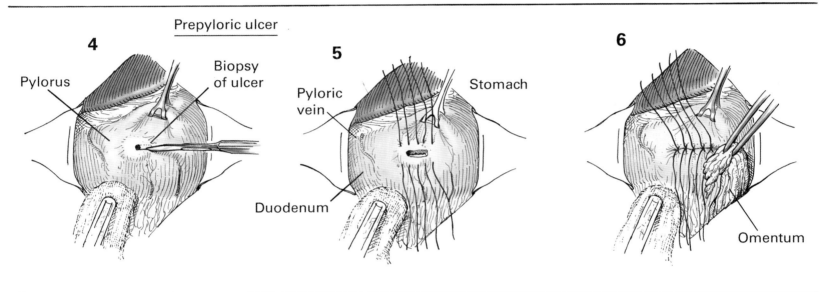

4 Pylorus — Biopsy of ulcer

5 Pyloric vein — Stomach — Duodenum

6 Omentum

Anterior abscess   Subphrenic abscess   Posterior abscess

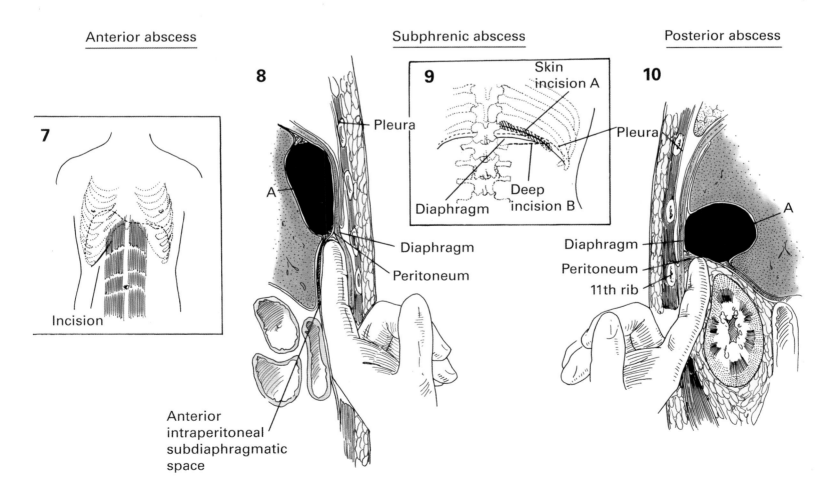

7 Incision

8 Pleura — A — Diaphragm — Peritoneum — Anterior intraperitoneal subdiaphragmatic space

9 Skin incision A — Deep incision B — Diaphragm

10 Pleura — A — Diaphragm — Peritoneum — 11th rib

CHAPTER 20 GASTROJEJUNOSTOMY

INDICATIONS Gastrojejunostomy is indicated for certain patients with duodenal ulcer complicated by pyloric obstruction. It is indicated also if technical difficulties prevent resection or make resection hazardous; if the patient is such a poor operative risk that only the safest surgical procedure should be carried out; or if a vagus nerve resection has been performed. It is occasionally indicated for the relief of pyloric obstruction in the presence of nonresectable malignancies of the stomach, duodenum, or head of the pancreas.

PREOPERATIVE PREPARATION The preoperative preparation must be varied, depending upon the duration and severity of the pyloric obstruction, the degree of secondary anemia, and the protein depletion. Obviously, electrolyte replacement and fluid resuscitation should be completed. Nasogastric suction should be implemented to allow an empty stomach where complete obstruction has occurred and to prevent aspiration with induction of anesthesia. Preoperative antibiotics should be given. Laparoscopy in these high-risk patients should be considered or at least a laparoscopic-assisted procedure allowing identification of the proximal jejunum and an extracorporeal anastomosis.

ANESTHESIA General anesthesia combined with endotracheal intubation is usually satisfactory.

POSITION The patient is placed in a comfortable supine position with the feet at least a foot lower than the head. In patients with an unusually high stomach, a more upright position may be of assistance. The optimum position can be obtained after the abdomen is opened and the exact location of the stomach is determined.

OPERATIVE PREPARATION The lower thorax and abdomen are prepared in the routine manner.

INCISION AND EXPOSURE As a rule, midline epigastric incision is made. The incision is extended upward to the xiphoid or to the costal margin and downward to the umbilicus. With the abdomen opened, a self-retaining retractor may be utilized; but since most of the structures involved in this operation are mobile, it is usually unnecessary to use any great amount of traction for adequate exposure.

DETAILS OF PROCEDURE The stomach and duodenum are visualized and palpated to determine the type and extent of the pathologic lesion present. A short loop of jejunum is utilized for gastrojejunostomy, with the proximal portion anchored to the lesser curvature. The stoma is made on the posterior gastric wall and extends from the lesser to the greater curvature, about two fingers in length. It is located at the most dependent part of the stomach (FIGURE 1A).

When the gastroenterostomy is performed with vagotomy in the treatment of duodenal ulcer, the location and size of the stoma are very important. In order to ensure adequate drainage of the paralyzed antrum and keep postoperative side effects to a minimum, a small stoma parallel to the greater curvature and near the pylorus is indicated (FIGURE 1B). The jejunum should be anchored for several centimeters to the gastric wall on either side of the stoma. This permits circular uncut muscles going away from the stoma to contract and improve gastric emptying. Special effort is required as a rule to ensure placement of the stoma within 3 to 5 cm of the pylorus because of the inflammation and fixation of the pylorus associated with duodenal ulceration. Accordingly, it may be impractical to perform an anastomosis on the greater curvature as shown in FIGURE 1B.

The location of the stoma is first outlined on the anterior gastric wall with Babcock forceps. The greater omentum may be brought outside the wound so that the contour of the stomach is not distorted, and the most dependent portion of the greater curvature may be more accurately determined (FIGURE 2). The Babcock forceps are left in place as the greater omentum is reflected upward over the stomach and the inferior aspect of the mesocolon is visualized (FIGURE 3). The transverse colon is held firmly by an assistant as the surgeon invaginates the Babcock forceps on the anterior gastric wall. This produces a bulge in the mesentery of the colon at the point through which the stomach is to be drawn (FIGURE 3). The mesocolon is carefully incised to the left of the middle colic vessels and near the ligament of Treitz, great care being taken to avoid any of the large vessels in the arcade. Four to six guide sutures (sutures a, b, c, d, e, and f) are placed in the margins of the incised mesocolon to be utilized after the anastomosis to the stomach at the proper level. The presenting posterior wall of the stomach is grasped with a Babcock forceps (FIGURE 4A and B) adjacent to the lesser and greater curvatures, and opposite the points of counter pressure from the similarly placed forceps on the anterior gastric wall (FIGURE 4). A portion of the gastric wall is pulled through the opening. In many instances, the inflammatory reaction associated with the duodenal ulcer may anchor the posterior surface of the antrum to the capsule of the pancreas. Sharp and blunt dissection may be required to mobilize the stomach in order to ensure placement of the stoma sufficiently near the pylorus. Some surgeons prefer to anchor the mesocolon to the stomach at this time. The forceps on the greater curvature is swung toward the operator on the patient's right side, while the forceps on the lesser curvature is rotated to a position opposite the first assistant.

The ligament of Treitz is identified, and a loop of jejunum 10 to 15 cm distal to this fixed point is delivered into the wound. The jejunum at this point is held with Babcock forceps and stay sutures placed (FIGURE 5). The orientation of the bowel is shown in FIGURE 6. The technique of the anastomosis is shown in the continuing FIGURES 7 through 22 of this Chapter. CONTINUES ▶

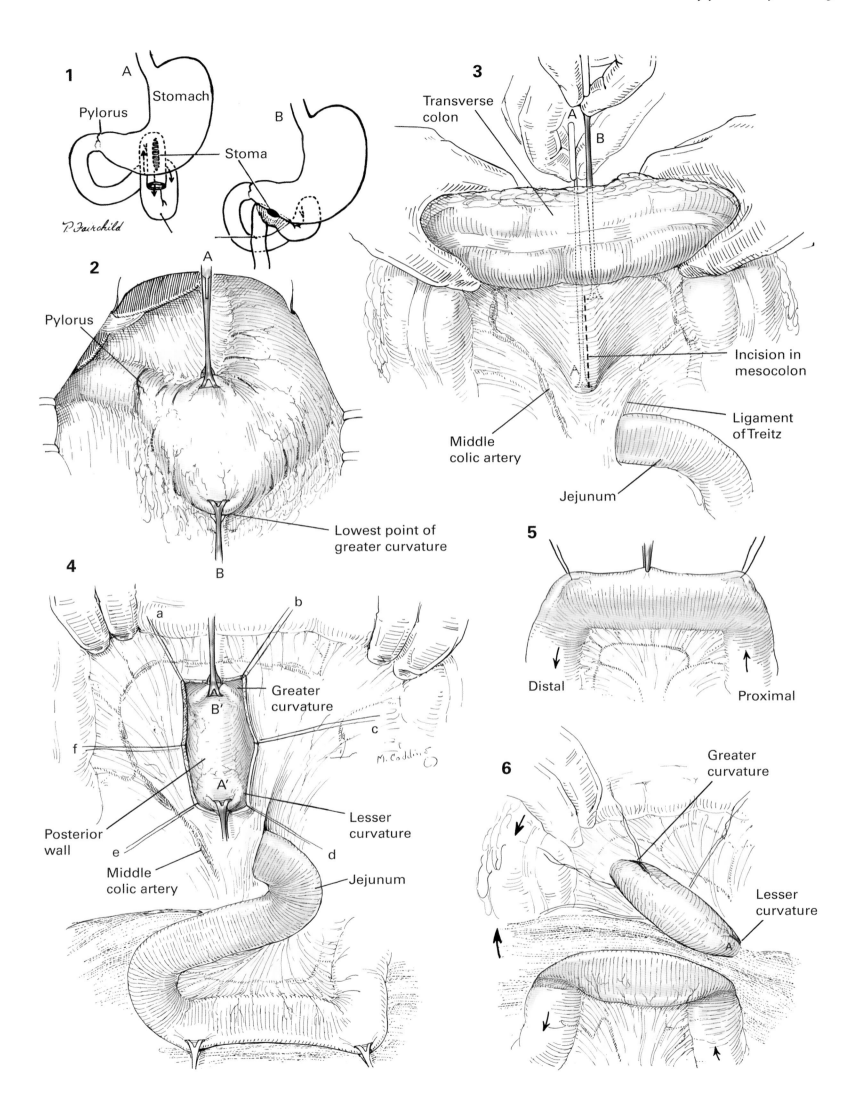

1

A

Stomach

Pylorus

Stoma

B

P. Fairchild

2

A

Pylorus

Lowest point of
greater curvature

B

3

Transverse
colon

A

B

Incision in
mesocolon

Ligament
of Treitz

Middle
colic artery

Jejunum

4

a   b

Greater
curvature

A'
B'

c

f

A'

Lesser
curvature

Posterior
wall

e

d

Middle
colic artery

Jejunum

M. Codding

5

Distal

Proximal

6

Greater
curvature

Lesser
curvature

A

DETAILS OF PROCEDURE ◄CONTINUED The large intestine and omentum are returned within the abdomen above the stomach. The clamps and the anastomotic site usually can be delivered outside the peritoneal cavity, which should be entirely protected with gauze. Retraction on the edges of the abdominal wound is discontinued while the anastomosis is being performed. This mobilization is usually impossible when the stoma must be made within 3 to 5 cm of the pylorus following vagotomy. Under these circumstances, the anastomosis must be made within the peritoneal cavity, lest the stoma be made too far to the left, with recurrent ulcer difficulties due to hormone stimulation from the distended antrum inducing gastric hypersecretion.

Stay sutures are placed to facilitate exposure. Scudder clamps, which are nontraumatic, may be placed on the afferent and efferent limbs to prevent to minimize contamination. The posterior serosal sutures are now begun by placing a mattress suture of 000 silk at either angle (FIGURE 7). The surgeon depresses the presenting portions of the stomach and jejunum with the index and middle fingers as the posterior row of interrupted mattress sutures in the serosa (FIGURE 8). Alternate bites of jejunum and stomach are taken; these include the submucosa but do not enter the lumen of the bowel. Each suture is taken close to the preceding one to ensure a complete closure. It is best to tie them after all have been placed.

An incision is made in the stomach. The serosal incision may be made with a knife (FIGURE 9) but the majority of surgeons use electrocautery. If this incision is too far from the serosal layer, too large a cuff of inverted bowel may result. In making these incisions, the operator should be careful to cut the bowel wall perpendicular to its surface, since there is always a tendency to incise the intestine obliquely, thereby leaving an irregular and unequalized mucosal layer for the next suture line (FIGURE 10). The incision in the jejunum is made slightly shorter than that made in the stomach (FIGURE 11). With the stomach and intestine opened and cleaned, a continuous absorbable suture is started in the midportion of the posterior mucosal layers (FIGURE 12). Swedged on curved needles are most commonly used. As the operator sews away from himself or herself, he or she uses a simple over-and-over suture or a lock stitch, which pulls together the mucosal layers (FIGURE 13). Since this suture is also used to control the blood supply, it must be kept under a tension sufficient for accurate approximation and prevention of hemorrhage, yet not completely strangulating the blood supply and hindering healing. This is a critical step. Interrupted sutures are placed to secure any bleeding points that have not been controlled by the continuous suture. When the operator reaches the angle of the wound, a Connell suture, which allows inversion of the structures as they are sewn, is substituted (FIGURE 14). In FIGURE 14, for example, the needle has just entered the gastric side. It comes out on the gastric side 2 or 3 mm from its point of entrance (FIGURE 15). It is then crossed over, inserted through the jejunal wall from outside as in FIGURE 16, and comes back out through the jejunal wall before being reinserted through the gastric wall (FIGURE 17). After this angle has been closed, the other end, B, of the continuous suture is used to close the opposite angle in a similar fashion (FIGURE 18). The continuous sutures, A and B, finally meet along the anterior surface. The final bite of each suture brings it to the inner wall of the stomach and jejunum (FIGURE 19). The two ends are tied together with the final knot on the inside. If slight oozing persists, additional interrupted sutures may be taken to supplement the anterior mucosal layer.

Approximation of the anterior serosal layer is carried out with interrupted 000 silk sutures (FIGURE 20). These are placed approximately 6 to 8 mm apart. Additional interrupted sutures of fine silk are placed at the angles of the anastomosis for reinforcement so that any strain at this point avoids the original suture line (FIGURE 21). The patency and size of the stoma should be determined by palpation. A secure anastomosis is desirable with a stoma approximately the size of the end of the thumb or two fingers.

The stomach is anchored to the mesocolon, with sutures b, c, and d (FIGURE 21) adjacent to the anastomosis in order to close the opening and thus prevent a potential internal hernia. This also prevents any torsion of the jejunum near the anastomosis, which might result if the stoma retracts above the mesocolon (FIGURE 22).

Occasionally, in the presence of extensive inflammation about the pylorus, marked obesity, or extensive malignancy, it may be impossible to mobilize the posterior gastric wall sufficiently for an anastomosis that allows adequate drainage of the antrum. Under these circumstances, anterior gastrostomy or enterostomy should be considered following vagotomy to ensure adequate drainage of the antrum or proximal drainage of an inoperable gastric malignancy. In order to avoid the possibility of poor emptying following anterior gastrojejunostomy, the thick omentum should be divided to permit the upper jejunum to be easily brought up over the transverse colon. Some prefer to clear the greater curvature near the pylorus for 5 to 8 cm and place the gastrojejunal stoma in this area. The antecolic efferent jejunal loop should be anchored to the anterior gastric wall for approximately 3 cm beyond the anastomosis to provide uncut circular muscle contractions to assist in gastric emptying. A Stamm-type gastrostomy should be considered to ensure patient comfort and provide an efficient and readily available method of gastric decompression until gastric emptying is satisfactory.

CLOSURE The wound is closed in the routine manner. It is not drained.

POSTOPERATIVE CARE The use of fluids, glucose, vitamins, and parenteral alimentation depends upon daily clinical and laboratory evaluation. Water in sips is given within 24 hours, and the fluid and food intake is increased gradually thereafter. Six small feedings per day are gradually replaced by a full diet as tolerated. ∎

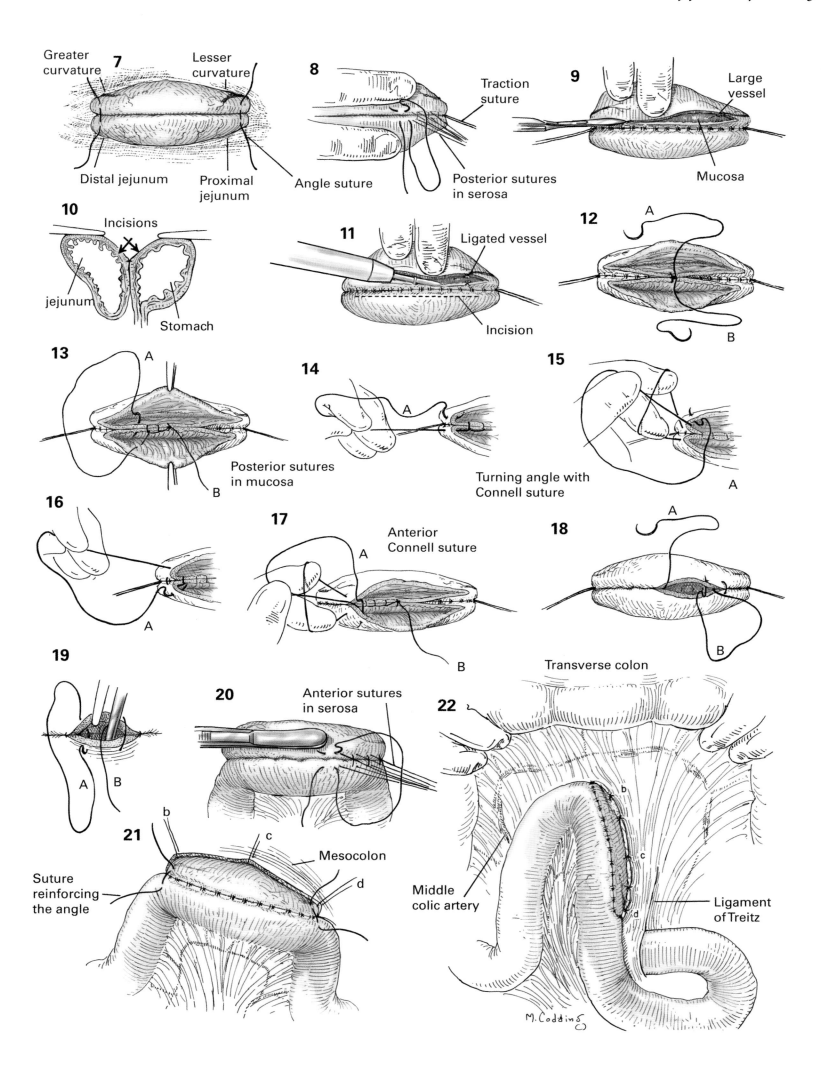

7 Greater curvature   Lesser curvature   Distal jejunum   Proximal jejunum   Angle suture

8 Traction suture   Posterior sutures in serosa

9 Large vessel   Mucosa

10 Incisions   jejunum   Stomach

11 Ligated vessel   Incision

12 A   B

13 A   B   Posterior sutures in mucosa

14 A

15 Turning angle with Connell suture   A

16 A

17 Anterior Connell suture   A   B

18 A   B   Transverse colon

19 A   B

20 Anterior sutures in serosa

21 b   c   Mesocolon   d   Suture reinforcing the angle

22 Middle colic artery   b   c   d   Ligament of Treitz

M. Codding

INDICATIONS These procedures may be used when the vagus innervation of the stomach has been interrupted either by truncal vagotomy, selective vagotomy, or division of the vagus nerves associated with esophagogastric resection and re-establishment of esophagogastric continuity. The pyloroplasty ensures drainage of the gastric antrum following vagotomy and, therefore, partially eliminates the antral phase of gastric secretion. It does not alter the continuity of the gastrointestinal tract and decreases the possibility of marginal ulceration occasionally seen after gastrojejunostomy. Pyloroplasty carries a low surgical morbidity and mortality rate because of its technical simplicity. Two types of pyloroplasty are commonly used: the Heineke–Mikulicz pyloroplasty (FIGURE A) and the Finney pyloroplasty (FIGURE B). Pyloroplasty should be avoided in the presence of a marked inflammatory reaction or severe scarring and deformity on the duodenal side of the gastric outlet. Under these circumstances, the Jaboulay procedure (FIGURE C) should be considered or a gastroenterostomy located within 3 cm of the pylorus on the greater curvature. Gastrin levels should be determined. The Jaboulay reconstruction should be considered when a long incision is made in the anterior wall of the duodenum during the search for very small mucosal gastrinomas.

HEINEKE–MIKULICZ PYLOROPLASTY The pylorus is identified with the pyloric vein as the landmark. A Kocher maneuver (Chapter 26, page 83) is then carried out to mobilize the duodenum for good exposure and relaxation of tension on the subsequent transverse suture line. Traction sutures of oo silk are placed and tied at the superior and inferior margins of the pyloric ring for anatomic orientation. Efforts should be made to include the pyloric vein in these sutures in order to partially control the subsequent bleeding. A longitudinal incision is made approximately 2 to 3 cm on each side of the pyloric ring through all layers of the anterior wall (FIGURE 1). In the presence of marked deformity, it may be advisable to incise the midportion of the duodenum and then, with a hemostat directed up through the constricted pyloric canal as a guide, make the incision in the midportion of the pylorus, across the midportion of the anterior duodenal wall, and across the midpoint of the pyloric wall into the gastric side. Bleeding is controlled with electrocautery.

Traction on the angle sutures draws the longitudinal incision apart until it becomes first diamond shaped (FIGURE 1) and then transverse (FIGURE 2). Active bleeders tend to occur in the divided duodenal wall and in the region of the divided pyloric sphincter. Inverting sutures of interrupted silk are passed through all layers to approximate the mucosa. Some prefer a one-layer closure (FIGURE 2) in order to minimize the encroachment on the pyloric lumen resulting from the inversion that follows a two-layer closure. The one-layer, the Gambee suture, is shown in cross section. This is placed in four passes, with the second and third bites involving only the gastric or duodenal mucosa (FIGURE 3). The result is complete inversion with good serosa-to-serosa approximation. After the closure is completed, the thumb and index finger are used to palpate the newly formed lumen by invagination of the gastric and duodenal walls on each side of the transverse closure. A temporary gastrostomy may be performed (Chapter 17).

FINNEY U-SHAPED PYLOROPLASTY The pylorus is identified by noting the overlying pyloric vein. Freeing all interfering adhesions and mobilizing the pyloric end of the stomach, the pylorus, and the first and second portions of the duodenum by use of an extensive Kocher maneuver are essential (Chapter 26, page 83). A traction suture is placed in the superior margin of the mid pylorus, and a second suture joins a point approximately 5 cm proximal to the pyloric ring on the greater curvature of the stomach to a point 5 cm distal to the pyloric ring on the duodenal wall (FIGURE B). The walls of the stomach and duodenum are sutured together with interrupted oo or ooo silk as in the start of the usual two layer gastrointestinal anastomosis. These sutures should be placed as near the greater curvature margins of the stomach and the inner margin of the duodenum as possible to ensure adequate room for subsequent closure. A U-shaped incision is then made into the stomach from a point just above the traction suture, around through the pylorus, and down a similar distance on the duodenal wall adjacent to the suture line. If an ulcer is present on the anterior wall, it may be excised. Electrocautery is used to control bleeding. A wedge of the pyloric sphincter may be removed from either side to facilitate the mucosal closure. The posterior mucosal septum between the stomach and duodenum is united with a running absorbable suture in a standard fashion for a side to side anastomosis. These sutures run from the superior aspect and include all layers of the septum (FIGURE 4). The anterior mucosal layer is approximated with inverting interrupted sutures of ooo silk.

As seen in FIGURE 5, a second layer of sutures starts superiorly and brings together the seromuscular layers of the anterior walls of the stomach and duodenum. A portion of the omentum may be sutured over the anastomosis. A temporary gastrostomy may be performed (Chapter 17) or constant nasogastric suction maintained until the stomach empties satisfactorily.

JABOULAY GASTRODUODENOSTOMY It is advisable to carry out a very extensive Kocher maneuver (Chapter 26, page 83) with complete mobilization of the second and third parts of the duodenum. When this procedure is carried out, it is wise to visualize the middle colic vessels, which sometimes tend to swing down over the duodenum and appear rather unexpectedly during the dissection. It is also advisable to attempt a limited mobilization of the inner surface of the duodenum without interference with its blood supply. The gastric wall, however, adjacent to the pylorus and downward for 6 to 8 cm may be freed of its blood supply and tested for mobility over to the duodenal wall. A suture is taken between the gastric wall and duodenum as near the pylorus as practical, and a second suture is taken between the gastric wall and the second part of the duodenum as near the inner duodenal border as possible to provide for approximation of 6 to 8 cm of the gastric wall and duodenum (FIGURE C).

The procedure varies little from that described for Finney Pyloroplasty. Sutures of oo interrupted silk are used on the serosa. An incision is made in the gastric wall as well as in the duodenal wall adjacent to the serosal suture line. The pylorus is left intact (FIGURE 6). All active bleeding points on both the gastric and duodenal sides should be controlled. The mucosa is approximated with either interrupted sutures of ooo silk or a continuous absorbable suture layer. Interrupted sutures of oo or ooo silk are placed to approximate the seromuscular coat as a second layer (FIGURE 7). The inferior angle between the second part of the duodenum and greater curvature of the stomach may require several additional interrupted sutures of oo silk to assure complete sealing of the angle. ■

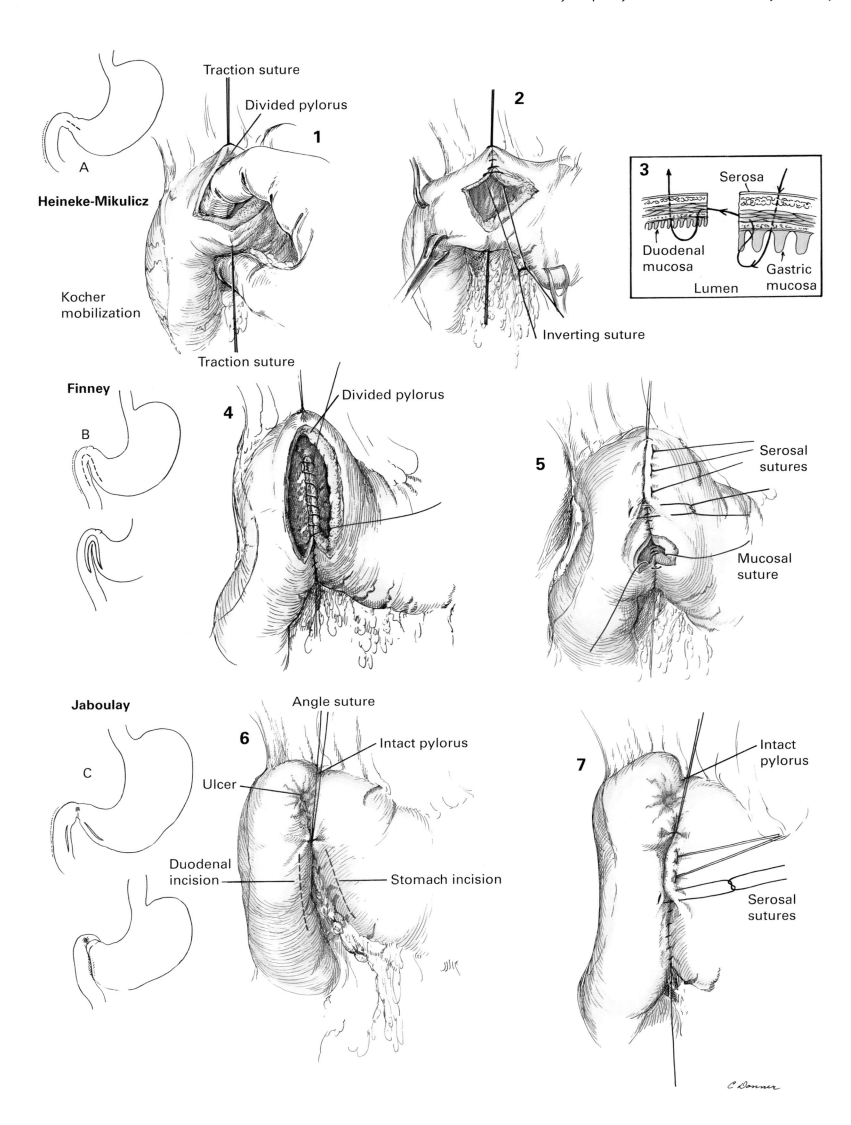

Heineke-Mikulicz

A

Kocher
mobilization

Traction suture

Divided pylorus

1

Traction suture

2

Inverting suture

3

Serosa

Duodenal
mucosa

Gastric
mucosa

Lumen

Finney

B

4

Divided pylorus

5

Serosal
sutures

Mucosal
suture

Jaboulay

C

6

Angle suture

Intact pylorus

Ulcer

Duodenal
incision

Stomach incision

7

Intact
pylorus

Serosal
sutures

C Donner

Bilateral resection of segments of the vagus nerves in the region of the lower esophagus is a key component in treating intractable duodenal or gastrojejunal ulcers, refractory to antisecretory medicine or when intervening situation is not optimized. The motor paralysis and resultant gastric retention that may follow truncal vagotomy alone make it mandatory that a concomitant gastric resection or drainage procedure, such as pyloroplasty or an antrally placed gastroenterostomy, be performed. Gastrojejunal or stomal ulcers following a previous gastrectomy or gastrojejunostomy show a favorable response to vagotomy. The use of vagotomy to control the cephalic phase of secretion is preferred when it is desirable to retain as much gastric capacity as possible because of the preoperative nutritional status of the patient with duodenal ulcer. In those individuals below their ideal weight preoperatively, controlling the acid factor by vagotomy followed by pyloroplasty, posterior gastroenterostomy, or hemigastrectomy should be seriously considered. In many patients laparoscopy provides excellent exposure of the vagal trunks and mobilization of the distal esophagus can be straightforward. In patients with scarring or previous operation consideration could be given to a transthoracic thoracoscopic approach via the left chest to the GE junction. There are two vagal trunks—the anterior or left vagus nerve, which lies along the anterior wall of the esophagus, and the posterior or right vagus nerve, which is sometimes overlooked since it is more easily separated from the esophagus. The vagus nerves may be divided 5 to 7 cm above the esophageal junction (truncal vagotomy), divided below the celiac and hepatic branches (selective vagotomy), or divided so that only the branches to the upper two-thirds of the stomach are interrupted, while the nerves of Latarjet, innervating the antrum or lower one-third, as well as the celiac and hepatic branches, are retained (proximal gastric vagotomy).

TRUNCAL VAGOTOMY A good exposure of the lower end of the esophagus is essential and sometimes requires removal of the xiphoid as well as mobilization of the left lobe of the liver. The vagal nerves should be identified and divided as far from the esophagogastric junction as possible (FIGURE 1). Sections of these trunks should be sent to the pathologist for microscopic evidence that at least two vagus nerves have been divided. Whether silver clips or ligatures are applied to both ends of each nerve is the choice of the individual surgeon. It may be advisable to ligate the posterior nerve to control possible oozing that may take place in the mediastinum. The esophagus should be carefully inspected, and the area behind the esophagus, in particular, should be searched as the esophagus is retracted upward to make sure that the posterior vagus nerve is not overlooked. In most instances, the cephalic phase of secretion will not be controlled if vagotomy has been incomplete. Some prefer to combine the vagotomy with a hemigastrectomy in order to control the gastric phase of secretion as well as the cephalic phase. Drainage of the antrum is essential by pyloroplasty, gastroenterostomy, or gastroduodenostomy (see Chapters 20–21). The increased incidence of recurrent ulceration following vagotomy and antral drainage by pyloroplasty or gastroenterostomy must be weighed against a somewhat higher mortality following vagotomy and hemigastrectomy.

SELECTIVE VAGOTOMY This procedure has been suggested as a means of decreasing the incidence of dumping by maintaining the vagal innervation of the liver and small intestine. It is not widely utilized because of the success of antisecretory medicines in most patients and the difficult technical aspects. The vagus nerves are carefully isolated from the esophagus and divided beyond the point where they give off branches to the liver and to the celiac ganglion (FIGURE 2). It is necessary to visualize clearly the lower end of the esophagus and to follow the anterior nerve down over the esophagogastric junction with identification of the hepatic branch. The nerve is divided beyond the hepatic branch, as shown in FIGURE 2. The posterior vagus nerve is likewise very carefully identified as it courses down over the esophagogastric junction, and the branch going to the celiac ganglion is

identified. The nerve is divided beyond that point in order to make certain that the vagus nerve supply to the small intestine has not been interrupted. Following this, some type of decompression procedure or resection is done.

PROXIMAL GASTRIC VAGOTOMY This procedure, also known as highly selective vagotomy, selective proximal vagotomy, or parietal cell vagotomy, is illustrated in FIGURE 3. It attempts to control the cephalic phase of secretion while maintaining the celiac branch, the hepatic branch, and the anterior and posterior nerves of Latarjet to the distal antrum (FIGURE 3). In this procedure, the vagal denervation is confined to the upper two-thirds of the stomach, while innervation is left intact to the lower third as well as to the biliary tract and small intestine. With superselective vagotomy it is anticipated that a drainage procedure will not be required since the pyloric sphincter retains its normal function. As a result, the incidence of disagreeable side effects associated with dumping should be decreased. This procedure is not widely utilized as well, mostly because of the high recurrence rate in patients with ulcer disease refractory to medical treatment.

It has been pointed out that the nerves of Latarjet send out branches in a crow's-foot pattern over the terminal 6 or 7 cm of the antrum. All other branches of the vagus nerves on either side of the lesser curvature are divided up to and around the esophagus (FIGURE 3). This may be a time-consuming and difficult technical procedure, particularly when the exposure is limited and the patient obese. Some prefer to identify the anterior and posterior vagus nerves at the lower end of the esophagus and place them under traction with carefully placed sutures or nerve hooks that serve as retractors, thus ensuring that the vagal nerve trunks will not be damaged and at the same time helping define the branches going to the stomach. The dissection is usually started about 6 cm from the pylorus on the anterior wall of the stomach (FIGURE 4A). Small hemostats are used in pairs to clamp carefully and divide the blood vessels and vagal branches as the dissection progresses up the anterior surface of the gastric wall along the lesser curvature (FIGURE 4B).

Special care must be taken as the dissection reaches the area where the left gastric artery reaches the lesser curvature of the stomach. The anterior nerve of Latarjet must be identified frequently as the dissection approaches the esophagogastric junction. The peritoneum over the lower end of the esophagus is divided carefully to permit identification of the vagal branches as the dissection is carried around the anterior portion of the esophagogastric junction. Finger dissection may be used to push gently both the anterior as well as the posterior vagus nerves away from the esophageal wall. After the finger has encircled the esophagus, a rubber tissue drain or a rubber catheter is introduced around the esophagus to provide traction. Upward traction on the esophagus provides easier identification of the top branches of the posterior nerve of Latarjet as they course over to the lesser curvature to provide innervation to the posterior gastric wall (FIGURE 5). The lower 5 cm of the esophagus should be completely cleared to avoid overlooking small fibers. The posterior branches are carefully identified and divided between pairs of small curved hemostats, similar to the procedure utilized on the anterior wall. A rubber tissue drain can be passed around the mobilized lesser omentum, including the nerves of Latarjet, to provide better exposure of the divided lesser curvature. A final search is made for any overlooked vagal branches, incomplete hemostasis, or possible injury to the nerves of Latarjet. Some prefer to peritonealize the lesser curvature by approximating the anterior and posterior gastric walls with a series of interrupted sutures. This approximation ensures control of any small bleeding points and provides insurance against possible necrosis with perforation along the denuded lesser curvature. Since the innervation to the antrum is retained, it is unnecessary to provide antral drainage by either pyloroplasty or gastroenterostomy, provided the duodenal outlet is not obstructed by scarring or a marked inflammatory reaction. ■

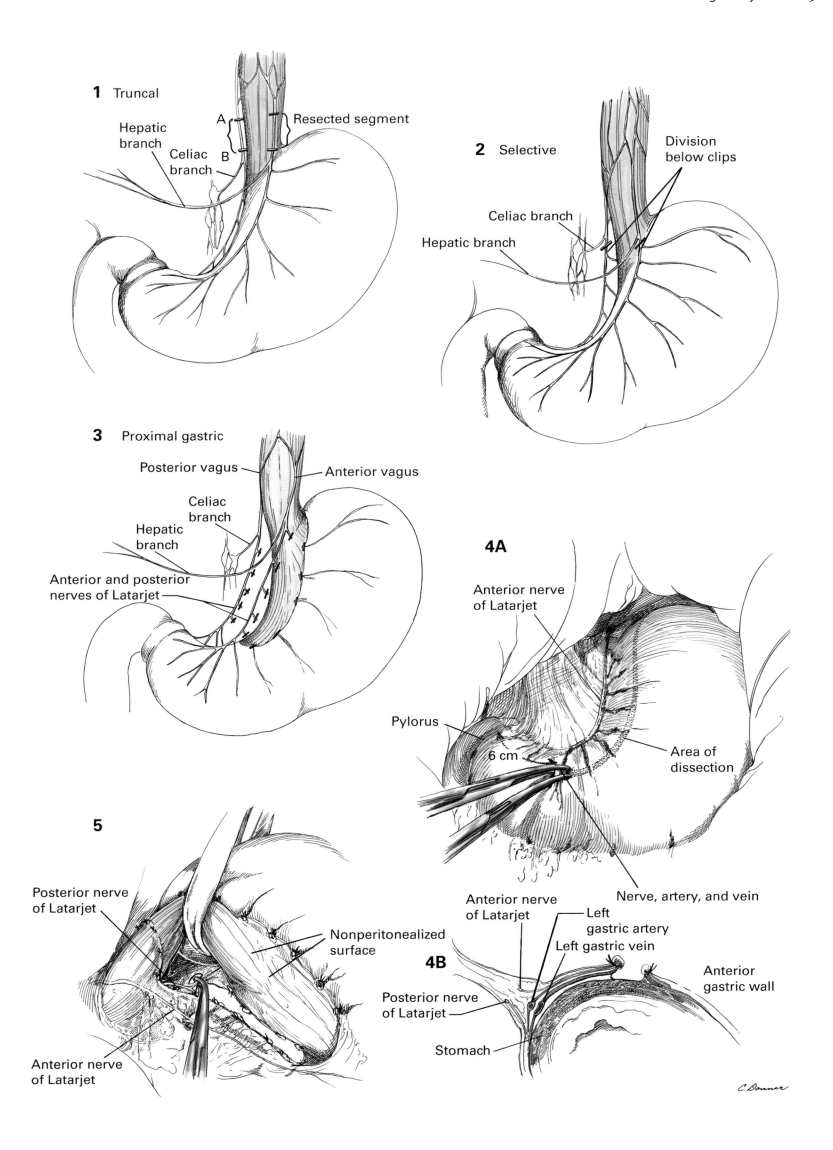

1 Truncal

Hepatic branch

Celiac branch

A

B

Resected segment

2 Selective

Division below clips

Celiac branch

Hepatic branch

3 Proximal gastric

Posterior vagus

Anterior vagus

Celiac branch

Hepatic branch

Anterior and posterior nerves of Latarjet

4A

Anterior nerve of Latarjet

Pylorus

6 cm

Area of dissection

Nerve, artery, and vein

5

Posterior nerve of Latarjet

Nonperitonealized surface

Anterior nerve of Latarjet

4B

Anterior nerve of Latarjet

Posterior nerve of Latarjet

Left gastric artery

Left gastric vein

Stomach

Anterior gastric wall

C Donner

VAGOTOMY, SUBDIAPHRAGMATIC APPROACH

INDICATIONS The long-term results of vagotomy are closely related to the completeness of the vagotomy and to efficient drainage or resection of the antrum (see Chapter 22).

PREOPERATIVE PREPARATION A careful evaluation of the adequacy and extent of the medical management is made. Proton pump inhibitors are effective in most patients and smoking cessation and *Helicobacter Pylori* eradication are important steps in medical management prior to operation. Obtaining fasting serum gastrin levels may be indicated. Persistent ulcer despite appropriate therapy may indicate the need for surgery. The laparoscopic approach is straightforward and should be considered.

ANESTHESIA General anesthesia with muscle relaxation is necessary. The insertion of an endotracheal tube provides smoother operating conditions for the surgeon and easy control of the airway for the anesthesiologist. An orogastric or nasogastric tube should be inserted to empty the stomach and allow palpation for the esophagus.

POSITION The patient is placed flat on the operating table, with the foot of the table lowered to permit the contents of the abdomen to gravitate toward the pelvis.

OPERATIVE PREPARATION The skin is prepared in the usual manner.

INCISION AND EXPOSURE A high midline incision is extended up over the xiphoid and down to the region of the umbilicus. In some patients the exposure is greatly enhanced by removal of a long xiphoid process. A thorough exploration of the abdomen is carried out, including visualization of the site of the ulcer. The location of the ulcer, especially if it is near the common duct, the extent of the inflammatory reaction, and the patient's general condition should all be taken into consideration in evaluating the risk of gastric resection in comparison to a more conservative drainage procedure. The anatomy of the vagus nerve is shown in FIGURE 1.

It may be necessary to mobilize the left lobe of the liver, alternatively a mechanical retractor (padded by a gauze sponge) can retract the left lobe superiorly. Mobilization is especially useful in obese patients where good exposure enhances the probability of complete vagotomy. If the operator stands on the right side of the patient, it is usually easier to grasp the left lobe of the liver with the right hand and with the index finger to define the limits of the thin, relatively avascular left triangular ligament of the left lobe of the liver. In many instances the tip of the left lobe extends quite far to the left

(FIGURE 2). By downward traction on the left lobe of the liver, and with the index finger beneath the triangular ligament to define its limits and to protect the underlying structures, the triangular ligament is divided with a long electrocautery probe or curved scissors. The assistant stands on the patient's left side and can usually do this more easily than the surgeon (FIGURE 3). The left lobe of the liver is then folded either downward or upward so that the region of the esophagus is clearly exposed (FIGURE 4). A gauze pad is placed over the liver, and a retractor is inserted to maintain even pressure throughout the rest of the procedure (FIGURE 5). In many instances the exposure is adequate without mobilization of the left lobe of the liver.

DETAILS OF PROCEDURE The region of the esophagus is palpated. The peritoneum immediately over the esophagus is grasped with a forceps, and an incision is made in the peritoneum at right angles to the long axis of the esophagus (FIGURE 5). The incision may be extended laterally to ensure mobilization of the fundus of the stomach. Curved scissors are then directed gently upward to free the anterior surface of the esophagus from the surrounding tissue. This can be done by blunt dissection, using the index finger (FIGURE 6). The dissection should carry posteriorly and laterally along both crura as far as necessary to allow the posterior esophagus to be dissected. Sometimes it is helpful to divide the left side of the crura and the proximal attachments to the stomach. After an inch or more of the anterior wall of the esophagus has been freed from the surrounding structures, the index finger should be introduced beneath the esophagus from the left side. It is frequently necessary to loosen some adhesions in this area by sharp dissection. Usually, little difficulty is encountered in gently passing the index finger beneath the esophagus and its indwelling nasogastric tube and completely freeing it from the surrounding structures. Just to the right of the esophagus, the index finger will usually encounter resistance from the uppermost limit of the hepatogastric ligament (FIGURE 7). This portion of the structure should be divided, since its division affords more mobilization of the esophagus and tends to provide exposure of the posterior or right vagus nerve. The major portion of the hepatogastric ligament in this area is quite avascular and thin, so that it can be perforated easily with scissors or electrocautery. If electrocautery is not available then a pair of right-angle clamps is then applied to the uppermost portion of the ligament, and the contents of these clamps divided with long, curved scissors (FIGURE 8). This exposes the region posterior to the esophagus and ensures adequate exposure of the hiatal region. CONTINUES ▶

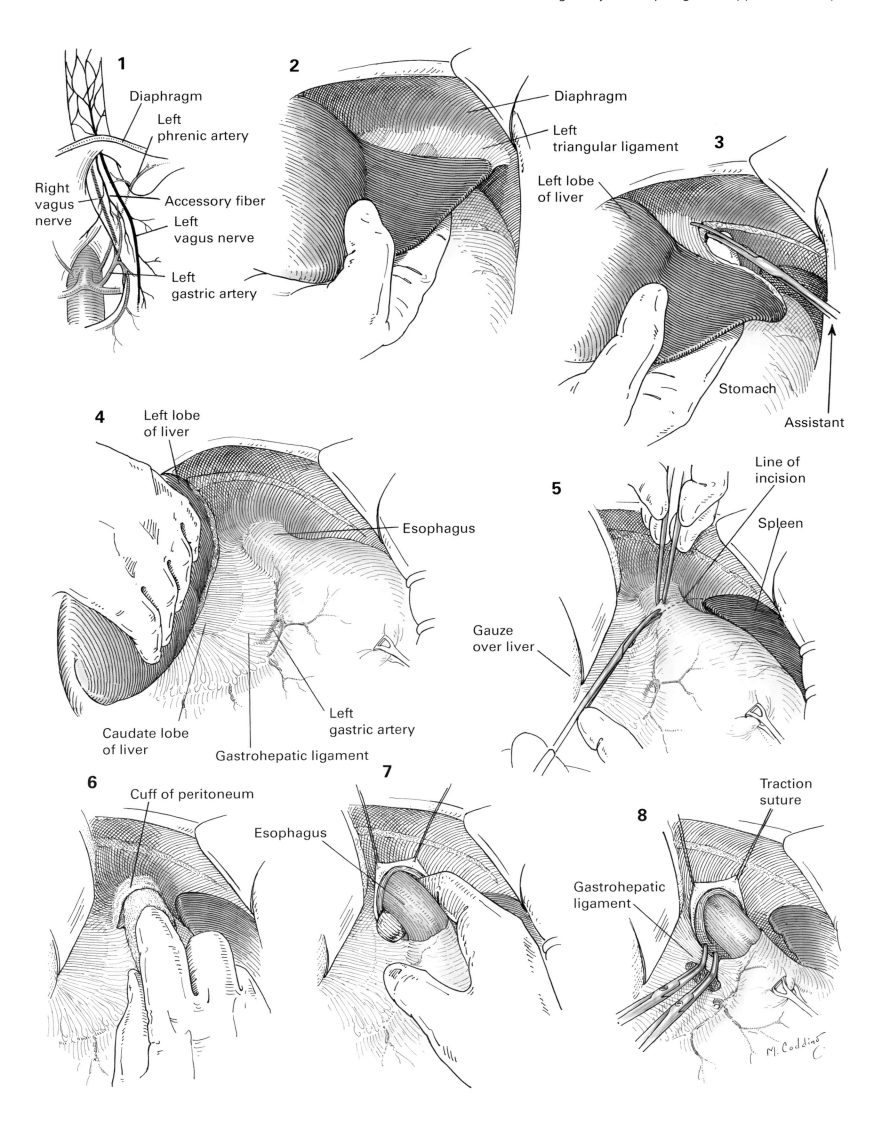

1

Diaphragm

Left
phrenic artery

Right
vagus
nerve

Accessory fiber

Left
vagus nerve

Left
gastric artery

2

Diaphragm

Left
triangular ligament

3

Left lobe
of liver

Stomach

Assistant

4

Left lobe
of liver

Esophagus

Caudate lobe
of liver

Gastrohepatic ligament

Left
gastric artery

5

Line of
incision

Spleen

Gauze
over liver

6

Cuff of peritoneum

Esophagus

7

8

Traction
suture

Gastrohepatic
ligament

M. Codding

DETAILS OF PROCEDURE ◂CONTINUED▸ Downward traction is maintained on the esophagus while it is further freed from the surrounding structures by blunt dissection with the index finger. The vagus nerves are not always easily identified, and their location is more quickly discovered by palpation (FIGURE 9). As the tip of the index finger is passed over the esophagus, the tense wirelike structure of the nerve is easily identified. It should be remembered that one or more smaller nerves may be found, both anteriorly and posteriorly, in addition to the large left and right vagus nerves. Additional small filaments may be seen crossing over the surface of the esophagus in its long axis. The left vagus nerve is usually located on the anterior surface of the esophagus, a little to the left of the midline, while the right vagus nerve is usually located a little to the right of the midline, posteriorly (FIGURES 10 and 10A). The left vagus is then grasped with a fine clamp, and is dissected free from the adjacent structures (FIGURE 11). The nerve can be separated from the esophagus easily by blunt dissection with the surgeon's index finger. It is usually possible to free at least 6 cm of the nerve (FIGURE 12). The nerve is clipped and is divided with long, curved scissors as high as possible. It is usually necessary to ligate the gastric ends of the vagus nerve as well. (FIGURE 13). The use of clips at the point where the vagus nerves divide minimized bleeding and serves to identify the procedures on subsequent roentgenograms. After the left vagus nerve has been resected, the esophagus is rotated slightly, and the traction is directed more to the left. It is usually not difficult to dissect free the right or posterior vagus nerve with the index finger or nerve hook (FIGURE 14). In some instances it has been found that the nerve has been separated from the esophagus at the time it was initially freed from the surrounding structures. The nerve, in such instances, appears to be resting against the posterior wall of the esophageal hiatus. The tendency to displace the right vagus nerve posteriorly during the blind process of freeing the esophagus no doubt accounts for the fact that this large nerve may be overlooked while all filaments about the esophagus are meticulously divided. This is the nerve most commonly found to be intact at the time of secondary exploration for a clinical failure of the vagotomy. A careful search should be made for additional nerves, since it is not uncommon to find more than one. A minimum of 6 cm of the right or posterior vagus nerve should be resected (FIGURE 15). Although the nerves may be clearly identified, the surgeon should not be satisfied until another careful search has been made completely around the esophagus. By traction on the esophagus and by direct palpation, any constricting band should be freed and resected, and a careful inspection should be made throughout the circumference of the esophagus. The operator will find that many of the little filaments that he dissects, in the belief that they are nerves, will prove to be small blood vessels that will require ligation. A final survey should always be made to be absolutely certain that the large right vagus nerve has not been displaced posteriorly, thus escaping division. A frozen section examination may be obtained to verify that both nerves have been removed. Traction should be released and the esophagus allowed to return to its normal position. The area should be carefully inspected for bleeding. No effort is made to reapproximate the peritoneal cuff over the esophagus to the cuff of peritoneum at the junction of the esophagus with the stomach. Finally, the esophagus is retracted upward and to the left by a narrow S retractor in order to expose the crus of the diaphragm. Two to three of nonabsorbable sutures may be placed sut to approximate the crus of the diaphragm as in the repair of a hiatus hernia if the hiatus appears patulous (FIGURES 16 and 17). Sufficient space about the esophagus must be retained to admit one finger or the passage of a 54 French or larger esophageal dilator into the stomach. All packs are removed from the abdomen, and the left lobe of the liver is returned to its normal position. It is not necessary to reapproximate the triangular ligament of the left lobe.

Vagotomy must always be accompanied either by a gastric resection or drainage of the antrum by posterior gastroenterostomy or division of the pylorus by pyloroplasty. Since gastric emptying may be unduly delayed following vagotomy, efficient gastric drainage by gastrostomy should be considered.

POSTOPERATIVE CARE Gastric suction is maintained until it has been determined that the stomach is emptying satisfactorily. If evidence of gastric dilatation develops, constant gastric suction is instituted. Occasionally, a moderate diarrhea will develop, which may be temporarily troublesome. The general care is that of any major upper abdominal procedure. Inability to swallow solid food because of temporary cardiospasm may occur for a few days in the early postoperative period. Six small feedings consistent with an ulcer diet should be recommended in order to combat the distention that may occur with an atonic stomach. The return to an unrestricted diet is determined by the patient's progress. ∎

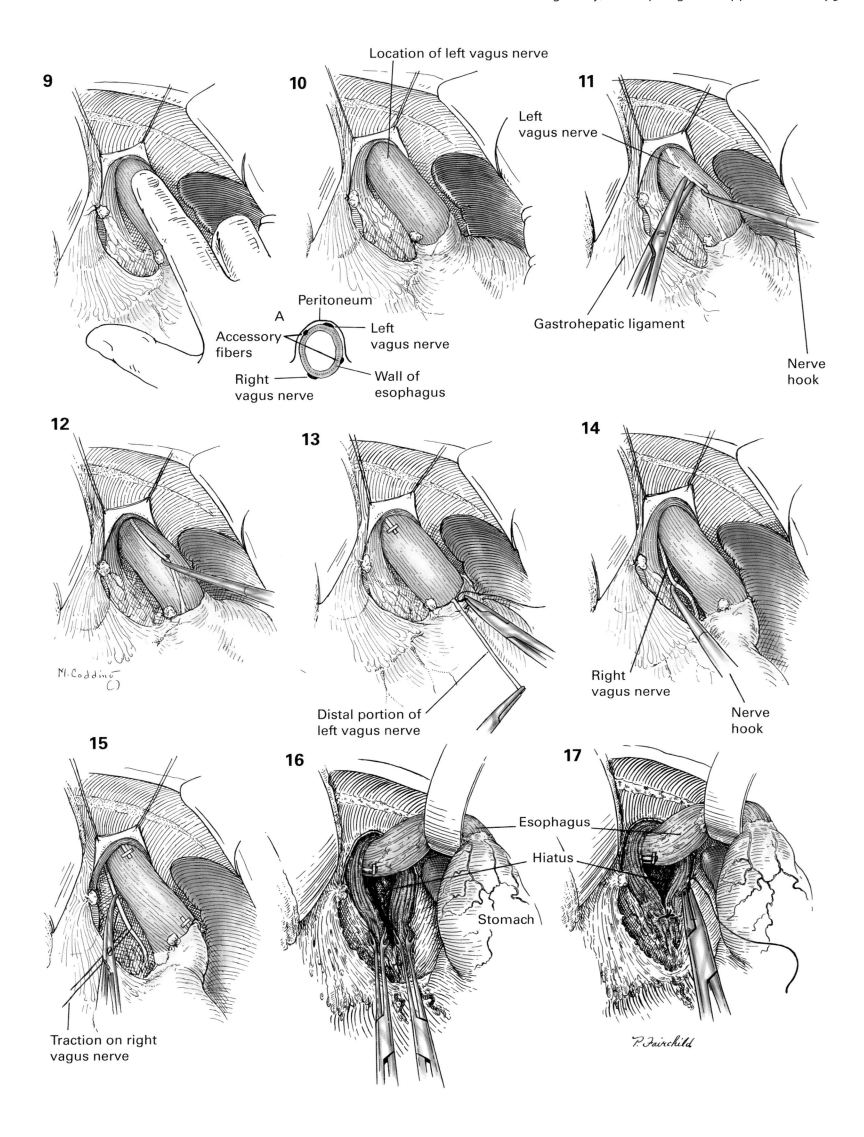

9

10
Location of left vagus nerve

11
Left vagus nerve

Gastrohepatic ligament

Nerve hook

A
Peritoneum
Accessory fibers
Left vagus nerve
Right vagus nerve
Wall of esophagus

12
M. Codding

13
Distal portion of left vagus nerve

14
Right vagus nerve

Nerve hook

15
Traction on right vagus nerve

16
Esophagus

Stomach

17
Esophagus
Hiatus

P. Fairchild

HEMIGASTRECTOMY, BILLROTH I METHOD

INDICATIONS The Billroth I procedure for gastroduodenostomy is the most physiologic type of gastric resection, since it restores normal continuity. Although long preferred by some in the treatment of gastric ulcer or antral carcinoma, its use for duodenal ulcer has been less popular. Control of acid secretion by vagotomy and antrectomy has permitted retention of approximately 50% of the stomach while ensuring the lowest ulcer recurrence rate of all procedures (FIGURE 1). This allows an easy anastomosis without tension, providing both stomach and duodenum have been thoroughly mobilized. Furthermore, the poorly nourished patient has an adequate gastric capacity for maintaining a proper nutritional status postoperatively. Purposeful constriction of the gastric outlet to the size of the pylorus tends to delay gastric emptying and decrease postgastrectomy complaints.

PREOPERATIVE PREPARATION The patient's eating habits should be evaluated, and the relationship between his or her preoperative and ideal weight should be determined.

ANESTHESIA General anesthesia via an endotracheal tube is used.

POSITION The patient is laid supine on the flat table, the legs being slightly lower than the head. If the stomach is high, a more erect position is preferable.

OPERATIVE PREPARATION The skin is prepared in a routine manner.

INCISION AND EXPOSURE A midline incision is usually made. If the distance between the xiphoid and the umbilicus is relatively short, or if the xiphoid is quite long and pronounced, the xiphoid is excised. Sufficient room must be provided to extend the incision up over the surface of the liver, because vagotomy is routinely performed with hemigastrectomy and the Billroth I type of anastomosis, especially in the presence of duodenal ulcer.

DETAILS OF PROCEDURE The Billroth I procedure requires extensive mobilization of the gastric pouch as well as the duodenum. This mobilization should include an extensive Kocher maneuver for mobilization of the duodenum. In addition, the greater omentum should be detached from the transverse colon, including the region of the flexures. In many instances the splenorenal ligament is divided, as well as the attachments between the fundus of the stomach and the diaphragm. Additional mobility is gained following the division of the vagus nerves and the uppermost portion of the gastrohepatic ligament. The stomach is mobilized so that it can be readily divided at its midpoint. The halfway point can be estimated by selecting a point on the greater curvature where the left gastroepiploic artery most nearly approximates the greater curvature wall (FIGURE 1). The stomach on the lesser curvature is divided just distal to the third prominent vein on the lesser curvature.

Extensive mobilization of the duodenum is essential in the performance of the Billroth I procedure. Should there be a marked inflammatory reaction, especially in the region of the common duct, a more conservative procedure, such as a pyloroplasty or gastroenterostomy and vagotomy, should be considered. If it appears that the duodenum, especially in the region of the ulcer, can be well mobilized, the peritoneum is incised along the lateral border of the duodenum and the Kocher maneuver is carried out. Usually it is unnecessary to ligate any bleeding points in this peritoneal reflection. With blunt dissection the peritoneum can be swept away from the duodenal surface as the duodenum is grasped in the left hand and reflected medially (FIGURE 2). It is important to remember that the middle colic vessels tend to course over the second part of the duodenum and are many times encountered rather suddenly and unexpectedly. For this reason the hepatic flexure of the colon should be directed downward and medially and the middle colic vessels identified early (FIGURE 2). As the posterior wall of the duodenum and head of the pancreas are exposed, the inferior vena cava readily comes into view. The firm, white, avascular ligamentous attachments between the second and third parts of the duodenum and the posterior parietal wall are divided with curved scissors, down through and almost including the region of the ligament of Treitz (FIGURE 2). This extensive mobilization is carried downward in order to ensure a very thorough mobilization of the duodenum. Following this, the omentum is separated from the colon, as described in Chapter 27. In obese patients it is usually much easier to start the mobilization by dividing the attachment between the splenic flexure of the colon and the parietes (FIGURE 3). An incision is made along the superior surface of the splenic flexure of the colon as the next step in freeing up the omentum. This should be done in an avascular cleavage plane. The lesser sac is entered from the left side. Care should be taken not to apply undue traction upon the tissues extending up to the spleen, since the splenic capsule may be torn, and troublesome bleeding, even to the point of requiring splenectomy, may be encountered. The omentum is then dissected free throughout the course of the transverse colon.

A truncal vagotomy is carried out as described in Chapter 17. At this point considerable distance can be gained if the peritoneum attaching the fundus of the stomach to the base of the diaphragm is divided up to and around the superior aspect of the spleen. If the exposure appears difficult, it is advisable for the surgeon to retract the spleen downward with his right hand and, using long curved scissors in his left hand, divide the avascular splenorenal ligament (Chapter 90, FIGURES 5 and 6). It must be admitted that sometimes troublesome bleeding does occur, which requires an incidental splenectomy, but in general great mobilization of the stomach is accomplished by this maneuver. Any bleeding from the splenic capsule should be controlled by conservative measures to minimize the need for splenectomy.

So far, the surgeon is not committed to any particular type of gastric resection but has ensured an extensive mobilization of the stomach and duodenum. The omentum should be reflected upward and the posterior wall of the stomach dissected free from the capsule of the pancreas, should any adhesions be found in this area. In the presence of a gastric ulcer, penetration through to the capsule of the pancreas may be encountered. These adhesions can be pinched off between the thumb and index finger of the surgeon and the ulcer crater allowed to remain on the capsule of the pancreas. A biopsy for frozen section study should be taken of any gastric ulcer since malignancy must be ruled out. The colon is returned to the peritoneal cavity. The right gastric and gastroepiploic arteries are doubly ligated (Chapter 26, FIGURES 12 to 16), and the duodenum distal to the ulcer divided.

At least 1 or 1.5 cm of the superior as well as the inferior margins of the duodenum must be thoroughly cleared of fat and blood vessels at the point of resection of the stomach is decided upon (FIGURE 4). The duodenum can be divided with a linear cutting or closed with a noncutting stapler.

In many instances, especially in the obese patient, it is advisable to further mobilize the stomach by dividing the thickened, lowermost portion of the gastrosplenic ligament without dividing the left gastroepiploic vessels. Considerable mobilization of the greater curvature of the stomach without traction on the spleen can be obtained if time is taken to divide carefully the extra heavy layer of adipose tissue that is commonly present in this area. Following this further mobilization of the greater curvature, a point is selected where the left gastroepiploic vessel appears to come nearer the gastric wall. This is the point in the greater curvature selected for the anastomosis, and the omentum is divided up to this point with freeing of the serosa of fat and vessels for the distance of the surgeon's finger (FIGURE 4). Traction sutures are applied to mark the proposed site of anastomosis. A site on the lesser curvature is selected just distal to the third prominent vein on the lesser curvature (FIGURE 1). Again, two traction sutures are applied, separated by the width of the surgeon's finger. This distance of about a centimeter on both curvatures assures a good serosal surface for closure of the angles.

It makes little difference how the stomach is divided, although there is some advantage to using a linear cutting or noncutting stapling instrument (FIGURE 4). Before the stomach is divided, a row of interrupted 000 silk sutures may be placed almost through the entire gastric wall in order to (1) control the bleeding from the subsequent cut surface of the gastric wall, (2) fix the mucosa to the seromuscular coat, and (3) pucker and constrict the end of the stomach to create a pseudopylorus (FIGURE 5). **CONTINUES▶**

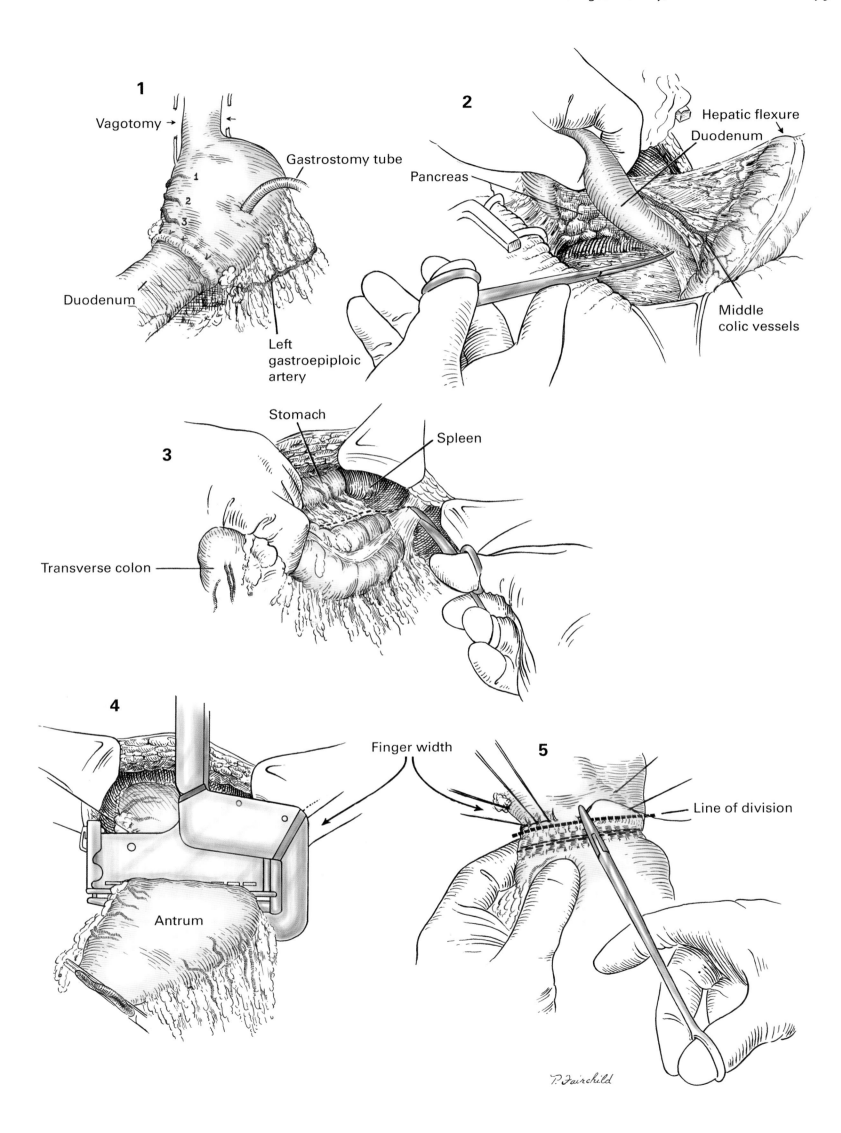

P. Fairchild

DETAILS OF PROCEDURE CONTINUED The staple line can be oversewn omitting the point of anastomosis along the lesser curvature. This opening should be approximately 2.5 to 3 cm wide (FIGURE 6). These sutures are then cut in anticipation of a direct end-to-end anastomosis with the duodenum (FIGURE 7). If the margins of the lesser and greater curvatures of the stomach as well as the superior and inferior margins of the duodenum have been properly prepared, it is relatively easy to insert angle sutures of oo silk. Successful closure of the angles depends upon starting the suture on the anterior gastric as well as the anterior duodenal wall rather than more posteriorly. Interrupted sutures of oo silk are then taken to close the stomach and duodenum together. Slightly bigger bites are necessary on the gastric side as a rule rather than on the duodenal side, depending upon the discrepancy in size between the two openings (FIGURE 8). The sutures should be tied, starting at the lesser curvature and progressing downward to the greater curvature. The angle sutures are retained while additional ooo silk or fine absorbable synthetic sutures are placed to approximate the mucosa (FIGURE 9, A–A′ and B–B′). Some prefer a continuous synthetic absorbable suture to approximate the mucosa. The anterior mucosal layer is closed with a series of interrupted sutures of ooo silk or a continuous synthetic absorbable suture. The seromuscular coat is then approximated to the duodenal wall with a layer of interrupted sutures (FIGURE 10). It has been found that a cuff of gastric wall can be brought over the duodenum, resulting in a "pseudopylorus," if two bites are taken on the gastric side and one bite on the duodenal side. When this suture is tied (FIGURE 10), the gastric wall is pulled over the initial mucosal suture line.

The vascular pedicles on the gastric side are anchored to the ligated right gastric pedicle along the top surface of the duodenum as well as the ligated right gastroepiploic artery pedicle (FIGURE 10, A and B). A and B are then tied together to seal the greater curvature angle (FIGURE 11). A similar type of approximation is effected along the superior surface in order to seal the angle and remove all tension from the anastomosis (FIGURE 11). The stoma should admit one finger relatively easily. There should be no tension whatsoever on the suture line.

The upper quadrant is inspected for oozing and thoroughly irrigated with saline.

POSTOPERATIVE CARE Intravenous administration of a balanced electrolyte solution is continued until bowel function has returned and an oral diet is tolerated. A nasogastric tube may be used. When bowel activity has resumed, clear liquids are given by mouth. If there is no evidence of retention, a progressive feeding regimen is begun. This consists of five or six small feedings per day of soft food, moderately restricted in volume, high in protein, and relatively low in carbohydrate. Eventually, the only limitations to the individual's diet are those imposed by his or her own intolerance. ■

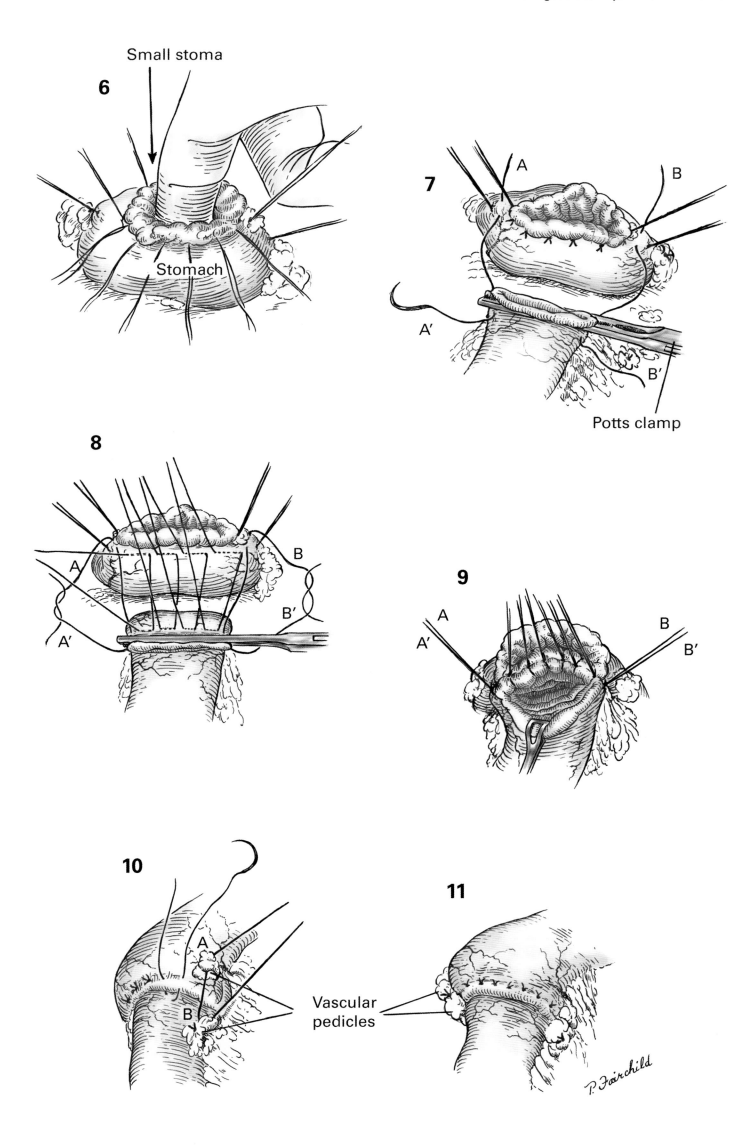

HEMIGASTRECTOMY, BILLROTH I STAPLED

INDICATIONS The Billroth I gastric resection along with truncal vagotomy is frequently performed for intractable duodenal ulcer or benign gastric ulcer. The procedure may be performed when hemigastrectomy is carried out for a variety of other reasons. It is hoped that this reconstruction to a normal configuration will result postoperatively in few symptoms and improved nutrition.

PREOPERATIVE PREPARATION The stomach is aspirated preoperatively, and nasogastric suction is maintained. Antibiotics are given to patients with achlorhydria, since they may have significant bacterial colonization of the duodenum or stomach.

ANESTHESIA Routine general anesthesia is given via a cuffed endotracheal tube.

POSITION The patient is placed supine on the table in a modest reverse Trendelenburg position.

OPERATIVE PREPARATION The skin of the lower chest and upper abdomen is shaved and prepared in the routine manner with antiseptic solutions.

DETAILS OF PROCEDURE When there is evidence of malignancy, the stomach should be resected with the width of the hand (7.5–10 cm) beyond the upper margins of the tumor. When the lesion is near the pylorus, at least 2.5 cm of the duodenum should be resected, along with the omentum and any lymph nodes about the right gastroepiploic veins.

The Billroth I procedure for control of peptic ulcer should include vagotomy (Chapters 22 and 23) as well as hemigastrectomy. The stomach is transected at the third vein on the lesser curvature and on the greater curvature where the gastroepiploic arterial blood supply is nearest the greater curvature (Chapter 26, FIGURE 1). These anatomic landmarks ensure a complete antrectomy with control of the hormonal phase of gastric secretion.

As shown in Chapter 26, the duodenum and stomach are mobilized. A modified Furniss clamp is placed across the duodenum at the appropriate level, and a purse-string suture of monofilament polypropylene on a straight needle is introduced (FIGURE 1). This automatically creates a purse string on the duodenal stump. The duodenum is divided and the previously selected site for division of the stomach should be cleared of fat in order to ensure good approximation of the anterior and posterior walls of the stomach by the noncutting linear stapler. The longer staples are usually needed for the thick walls of the stomach. Any bleeding points are controlled with additional sutures.

A gastrotomy is made with a cutting linear stapler (FIGURE 1) or electrocautery for the intragastric introduction of the circular stapler instrument through the anterior gastric wall at right angles to and about 3 to 5 cm proximal to the staple line closure of the distal stomach (FIGURE 2).

The closed end of the stomach is reflected to the left, and the posterior gastric wall is grasped with a Babcock forceps 3 to 5 cm from the midportion of the staple line closing the distal stomach. The circular stapler of the appropriate size is entered into the stomach with its detachable pointed plastic trocar exiting the back wall of the stomach. The plastic trocar is removed and replaced with the metal anvil cap (FIGURE 2). The cap is screwed onto the tip of the center rod and it is inserted into the duodenum (FIGURE 3). The monofilament polypropylene purse string around the end of the duodenum is snugged and securely tied (FIGURE 4). The wing nut on the near end of the circular stapler handle is turned until the stomach and the duodenum are firmly approximated. The safe zone indicator is checked to be certain that the thickness of the combined stomach and duodenum are within correct range of the staples. The safety is released, and the outside handles are squeezed. A double staggered, circular tow of staples is created, and an internal circular knife cuts the bowel walls within the staple lines simultaneously. The wing nut is loosened so that the anvils open, and the stapling instrument is gently removed (FIGURE 5). The doughnuts of tissue are carefully inspected to be certain there is no defect or discontinuity in the anastomosis. Several additional interrupted sutures may be placed to reinforce the anastomosis. The outer-wall gastrotomy opening is closed with a mucosa-to-mucosa noncutting linear stapler (FIGURE 6). **CONTINUES** ▶

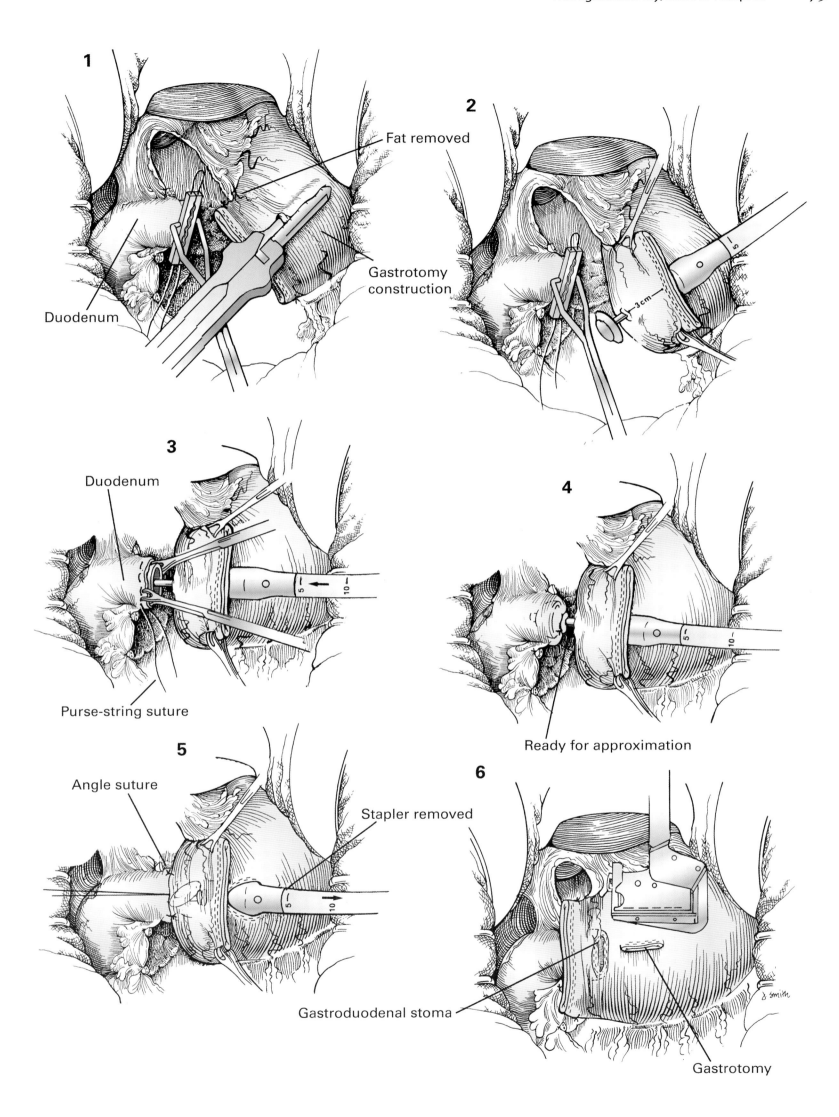

1

Fat removed

Duodenum

Gastrotomy construction

2

—3 cm—

3

Duodenum

Purse-string suture

4

Ready for approximation

5

Angle suture

Stapler removed

6

Gastroduodenal stoma

Gastrotomy

DETAILS OF PROCEDURE ‹CONTINUED› Alternatively, some prefer to introduce the circular stapler into the open distal end of the stomach prior to its removal (FIGURE 7) and direct the rod through the center of a previously placed purse-string suture in the posterior gastric wall approximately 3 cm from the proposed line of resection. The duodenal opening is checked with a sizing instrument; the 28-mm circular stapler is most commonly used. The cap is applied to the rod, and it is introduced into the open end of the transected duodenum (FIGURE 8). The monofilament polypropylene purse-string suture around the duodenal wall is tied tightly (FIGURE 9). The anvil and cap are approximated and the instrument is fired. The stapler is opened and then gently rocked back and forth and the line of staples stabilized with one hand as the tilted head of the instrument is slowly removed. Additional interrupted sutures may be indicated about the staple line (FIGURE 10). The posterior wall of the stomach may be opened longitudinally for a short distance to obtain better visualization of the suture line. Thereafter, the non-cutting linear stapler (TA 90) with the longer gastric staples is applied to transect the avascular distal antrum of the stomach (FIGURE 11). This may be the preferred method, since the anterior-wall suture line created by the gastrotomy for introduction of the stapler is avoided (FIGURE 12).

CLOSURE A small nasogastric (NG) tube may be inserted for decompression and later feedings. The incision is closed in a routine manner.

POSTOPERATIVE CARE Daily weight, fluid, and electrolyte measurements are recorded until the patient is taking adequate fluids and nutrition by mouth. Clear liquids may be permitted on the first postoperative day. Oral intake should be restricted if there is a feeling of fullness or if vomiting occurs. ∎

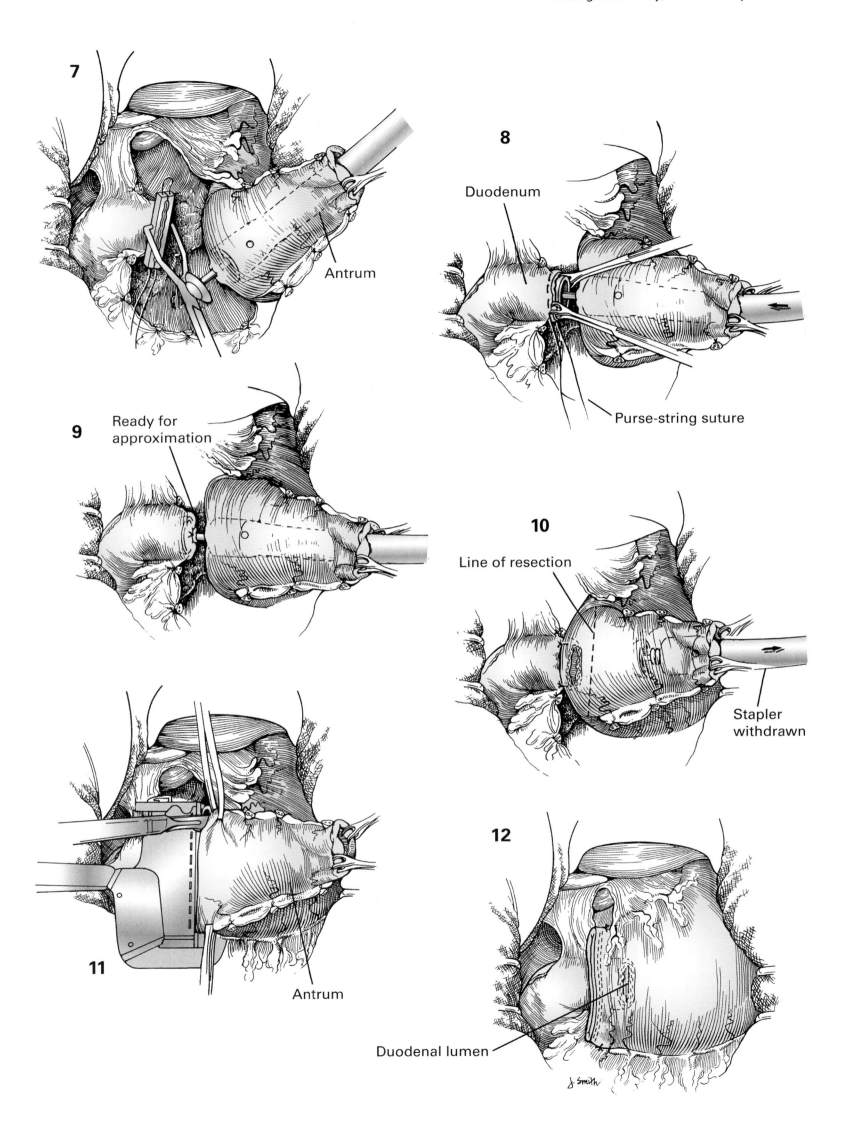

7

Antrum

8

Duodenum

Purse-string suture

9 Ready for approximation

10

Line of resection

Stapler withdrawn

11

Antrum

12

Duodenal lumen

J. Smith

GASTRECTOMY, SUBTOTAL

INDICATIONS Subtotal gastrectomy is indicated in the presence of malignancy; in the presence of gastric ulcer that persists despite intensive medical therapy; and sometimes in the presence of pernicious anemia, suspicious cells by gastric cytology, or equivocal evidence for and against malignancy by repeated gastroscopic observation with direct biopsy. It may be utilized to control acid secretion in cases of intractable duodenal ulcer. A more conservative procedure should be considered in underweight patients with duodenal ulcer, especially females. Likewise, block excision of a gastric ulcer with multicentric frozen section studies should be made for proof of malignancy before performing a radical resection on the assumption the lesion may be malignant.

PREOPERATIVE PREPARATION The preoperative preparation will be determined largely by the type of lesion presented and by the complication it produces. Sufficient time should be taken to improve the patient's nutrition if possible, especially if there has been considerable weight loss in a patient with obstruction. The fluid and electrolyte normalization should be treated with intravenous fluids and electrolytes as necessary. The increased incidence of pulmonary complications associated with upper abdominal surgery makes it imperative that elective gastric surgery be carried out only in the absence of respiratory infection, and active pulmonary physiotherapy with possible bronchodilators, expectorants, and incentive spirometry should be started in all patients but especially those with chronic lung disease. Preoperative antibiotics should be given.

ANESTHESIA General anesthesia with endotracheal intubation should be used. Excellent muscular relaxation without deep general anesthesia can be attained by utilizing muscle relaxants. Epidural catheter placement may be considered for analgesia and after surgery.

POSITION As a rule, the patient is laid supine on a flat table, the feet being slightly lower than the head. If the stomach is high, a more erect position is preferable.

OPERATIVE PREPARATION The skin is prepared in the routine manner.

INCISION AND EXPOSURE A midline incision extending from the xiphoid to the umbilicus may be used. Additional exposure can be obtained by excising the xiphoid using electrocautery. Placement of a self-retaining retractor or a broad-bladed, fairly deep retractor placed against the liver down to the gastrohepatic ligament will aid in visualization.

DETAILS OF PROCEDURE The surgeon should focus his or her attention on the arterial blood supply (FIGURE 1). Although the stomach will retain viability despite extensive interference with its blood supply, the duodenum lacks such a liberal anastomotic blood supply, and great care must be exercised in the latter instance to prevent postoperative necrosis in the duodenal stump. The blood supply to the lesser curvature of the stomach can be totally interrupted, and the retained fundus will be nourished by the small vessels in the gastrosplenic ligament in the region of the fundus. Importantly, if it is desirable to mobilize the stomach into the chest, its viability can be retained if only the right gastric artery is left intact. In such instances, however, the gastrocolic ligament should be divided some distance from the greater curvature to prevent interference with the right and the left gastroepiploic vessels.

The blood supply may also be used as landmarks in designating the extent of the gastric resection. Approximately 50% of the stomach is resected where the line of division extends from the region of the third large vein on the lesser curvature down from the esophagus to a point on the greater curvature where the left gastroepiploic vessels most nearly approach the gastric wall. Approximately 75% resection can be assumed when the line of resection includes most of the lesser curvature with extra gastric ligation of both the left gastric and left gastroepiploic vessel.

The surgeon likewise should be familiar with the major lymphatic drainage of the stomach in determining the presence or absence of metastasis if malignancy is suspected. Under such circumstances it is advisable to keep the dissection as far away as possible from both curvatures in order to retain all involved lymph nodes with the specimen. There is a tendency for metastases to involve distant lymph nodes of the lesser curvature (A) and the lymph nodes beneath the pylorus (B) as well as those of the greater omentum (C) (FIGURE 1).

In general, it is desirable to move the greater omentum, most of the lesser curve to the esophagus, and about 2.5 cm of the duodenum (including subpyloric lymph nodes), and the greater curvature. It is rarely necessary to remove the spleen unless there is direct extension of a gastric cancer into the spleen. Extended radical dissection of the preaortic (FIGURE 1 D and Chapter 31 FIGURES 2, 4 and 11) and portal area lymph nodes (not in the Chapter) has been shown to be beneficial in the Japanese experience; however, the utility of these dissections remains controversial.

Prior to operation, external (CT, MRI, PET) imaging and internal endoscopic transluminal ultrasound evaluations may show an inoperable extension of the malignancy. In addition, many potential candidates for a cancer resection are first evaluated with diagnostic laparoscopy (see Chapter 13 page 44, 45) and biopsy, as up to 40% of patients may have occult distant spread. Such findings preclude curative resection but not necessarily a gastric procedure for relief of obstruction and bleeding.

If the exploratory peritoneoscopy does not reveal contraindications to resection, the abdomen is opened and a careful regional inspection with palpation is performed. It must also be determined whether there have been direct extension and fixation to adjacent structures, such as the pancreas, liver, or spleen. Additional information may be obtained as to the extent and fixation of the tumor mass by exploring the lesser omental cavity through an opening made in the relatively avascular gastrohepatic ligament (FIGURE 2). Evidence of fixation of the posterior gastric wall with the pancreas or involvement of the tissues about the middle colic vessels should be sought. However, in the absence of visible or palpable distance metastases, it may be feasible to excise the stomach, en masse, along with the spleen and portions of the left lobe of the liver, or tail and body of the pancreas, if the involvement is by direct extension of the tumor. If there is widespread metastatic involvement with impending pyloric obstruction, it may be wiser to avoid radical surgery and to carry out the simple procedure of anterior or posterior gastrojejunostomy.

After evaluation indicates that a subtotal gastrectomy is practicable, it has been found that preliminary mobilization of the duodenum by the Kocher maneuver may facilitate some of the subsequent steps necessary in the procedure (FIGURES 3 to 5). The duodenum is grasped with Babcock forceps in the region of the pylorus, and traction is sustained downward (FIGURE 3). Any avascular adhesive bands that appear to be fixing the duodenum in the region of the hepatoduodenal ligament should be severed. The common duct is exposed so that it can be identified easily from time to time as the duodenum is divided and the stump is inverted (FIGURE 6).

After the duodenum and region of the pylorus have been mobilized by freeing all the avascular attachments, the index finger of the right hand is passed through an avascular portion of the gastrohepatic ligament above the pylorus to facilitate the introduction of a Penrose drain or gauze tape, which is brought up through an avascular space along the greater curvature and is used for traction (FIGURE 7). **CONTINUES** ▶

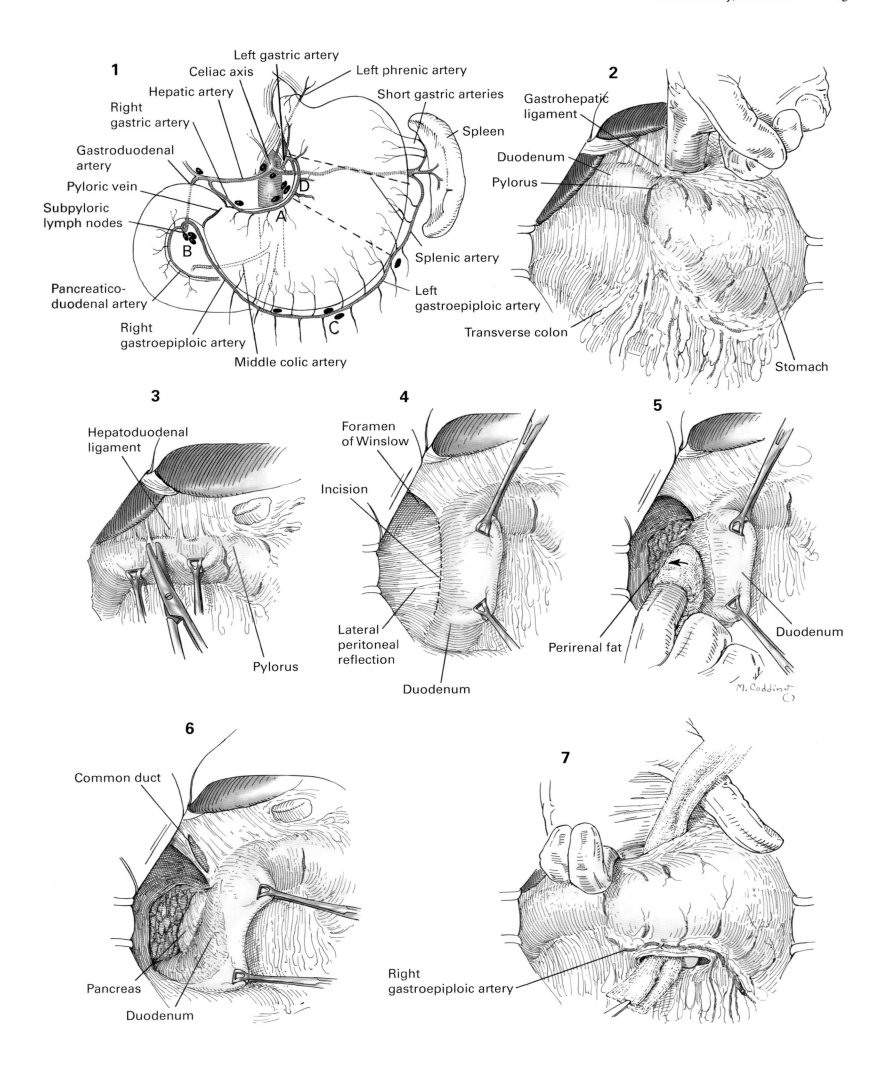

1
Left gastric artery
Celiac axis
Hepatic artery
Right gastric artery
Gastroduodenal artery
Pyloric vein
Subpyloric lymph nodes
Pancreatico-duodenal artery
Right gastroepiploic artery
Middle colic artery
Left phrenic artery
Short gastric arteries
Spleen
Splenic artery
Left gastroepiploic artery
A
B
C
D

2
Gastrohepatic ligament
Duodenum
Pylorus
Transverse colon
Stomach

3
Hepatoduodenal ligament
Pylorus

4
Foramen of Winslow
Incision
Lateral peritoneal reflection
Duodenum

5
Perirenal fat
Duodenum
M. Codding

6
Common duct
Pancreas
Duodenum

7
Right gastroepiploic artery

DETAILS OF PROCEDURE [CONTINUED] The gastrocolic ligament is divided near the epiploic vessels along the greater curvature, if there is no evidence of malignancy. The stomach is retracted upward, and the surgeon's left hand is introduced behind the stomach to avoid the possibility of damaging the middle colic vessels when the gastrocolic ligament is divided, since these vessels may be very near (FIGURE 8). Furthermore, by spreading the fingers apart beneath the gastrocolic ligament along the greater curvature, it is easier to identify the individual vessels so that they can be more accurately clamped and divided between pairs of small curved clamps (FIGURE 9). The dissection is carried around to the region of the gastrosplenic ligament, and a portion of this structure may also be removed, depending upon the amount of stomach to be resected. It is necessary to free the greater curvature to this extent to accomplish a 75% to 80% resection of the stomach. This usually demands the sacrifice of the left gastroepiploic artery and one or two of the short gastric arteries in the gastrosplenic ligament. The nutrition of the remaining fundus of the stomach depends upon the remaining short gastric arteries (FIGURE 10) when the left gastric artery has been ligated at its base. When hemigastrectomy is planned, the greater curvature is divided in the area where the left gastroepiploic artery most nearly approximates the gastric wall. On the lesser curvature the third large vein on the anterior gastric wall is used as the approximate point of division to ensure a hemigastrectomy (FIGURE 1).

In the obese patient the gastrosplenic ligament may be quite thickened and the identification of the vessels for ligation more difficult than elsewhere. However, fewer vessels require ligation if the omentum is removed, as in Chapter 27, rather than repeatedly clamping and tying the blood vessels in the gastrocolic ligament near the greater curvature. The division of the usual attachments of the omentum to the lateral abdominal wall about the splenic flexure of the colon will further mobilize the greater curvature of the stomach. Undue traction on the stomach or omentum may result in troublesome bleeding from the spleen, especially if the small strands of tissue extending up to the anterior margin are torn along with some of the splenic capsule. Under such circumstances splenectomy may be safer than depending on a hemostatic sponge or splenorrhaphy to control the troublesome and persistent bleeding. However, every effort should be made to repair the torn capsule, either by the use of coagulant or by the use of sutures, which may include the omentum when tied, in order to conserve the spleen, especially in younger patients. Alternatively, topical hemostatic agents can be applied and packed off for a period of time to establish excellent control. The greater curvature can be further mobilized into the field of operation if the relatively avascular splenocolic ligament is divided (Chapter 90 FIGURES 5–7). Indeed, the spleen may be quite extensively mobilized by dividing the splenorenal ligament laterally, permitting it, along with the fundus of the stomach, to be presented into the field of operation. This procedure ensures an easier exposure

for the gastrojejunal anastomosis following a very high gastric resection. Any bleeding points in the splenic bed should be carefully controlled with electrocautery.

At this time it is desirable to prepare the greater curvature for subsequent anastomosis. The serosa should be dissected free of fat for approximately the width of the index finger. A transfixing silk suture is placed in the greater curvature in this area to serve as a guide suture at the time the clamps or staplers are finally applied for division of the stomach (FIGURE 11, page 85 and FIGURE 30, page 89 in this Chapter). In addition, such a transfixing suture tends to prevent damage to the adjacent blood supply from subsequent manipulation of the stomach while preparing it for anastomosis (FIGURE 11).

Upward retraction of the stomach is maintained as the gastrocolic ligament is divided up to the region of the pylorus. If there is a possibility of malignancy within the area, care should be taken to stay about 3 to 5 cm from the pylorus in order to include the subpyloric nodes with the specimen. At the same time large, blind bites with hemostats in the neighborhood of the inferior portion of the duodenum should be avoided because of possible damage to the pancreaticoduodenal artery. It should be remembered that since the duodenum does not have a rich anastomotic blood supply but is supplied from end arteries, it is necessary to guard its blood supply carefully. The right gastroepiploic vessels should be carefully isolated from the surrounding fat and securely ligated (FIGURE 12).

After the blood supply of the greater curvature of the stomach has been divided and tied, the vascular supply and ligamentous attachments to the superior portion of the first part of the duodenum can be divided. Freeing the pylorus and the upper portion of the duodenum may be one of the most difficult steps in the operation, especially in the presence of a large, penetrating ulcer. One cannot state beforehand whether the attack should begin at the upper or lower border of the duodenum. In the presence of gastric malignancy extending to the pylorus, it is essential to remove at least 3 cm of the duodenum because of the possibility of infiltration of carcinoma for some distance within the wall of the duodenum itself. In addition, a more extensive lymph node dissection is accomplished of the area beneath the pylorus and the periportal area along with an omentectomy (see Chapter 27). The most medial portion of the hepatoduodenal ligament, which includes the right gastric artery, is divided. It is better to take small bites in this area with a small curved hemostat and re-apply the clamps repeatedly than to attempt mass ligation (FIGURE 13). The location of the common duct and adjacent vessels within the hepatoduodenal ligament should be accurately identified before these clamps are applied. The mobilization of the duodenum is facilitated by the division and ligation of the contents of these clamps. The vascular pedicles from the duodenal side of the anastomosis are clearly defined. [CONTINUES]

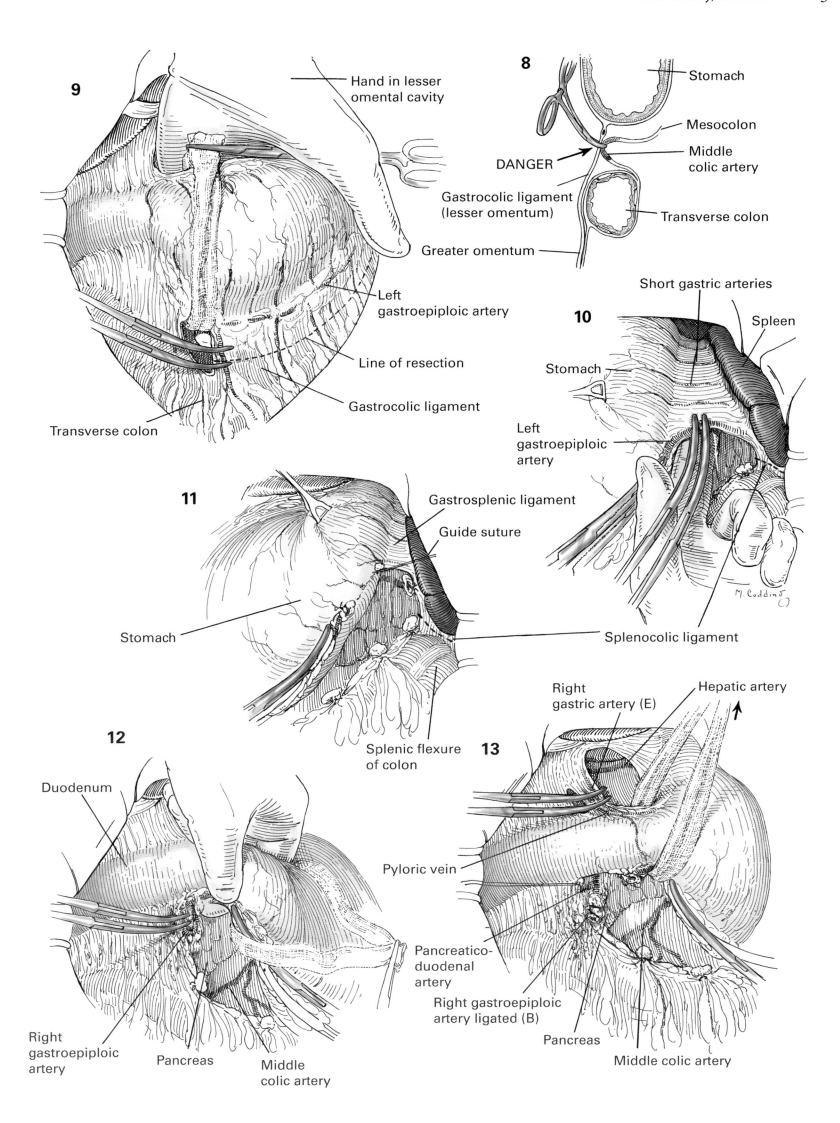

9

Hand in lesser omental cavity

Left gastroepiploic artery

Line of resection

Gastrocolic ligament

Transverse colon

8

Stomach

Mesocolon

Middle colic artery

DANGER

Gastrocolic ligament (lesser omentum)

Transverse colon

Greater omentum

10

Short gastric arteries

Spleen

Stomach

Left gastroepiploic artery

Gastrosplenic ligament

Guide suture

Splenocolic ligament

M. Codding

11

Stomach

Splenic flexure of colon

12

Duodenum

Right gastroepiploic artery

Pancreas

Middle colic artery

13

Right gastric artery (E)

Hepatic artery

Pyloric vein

Pancreatico-duodenal artery

Right gastroepiploic artery ligated (B)

Pancreas

Middle colic artery

DETAILS OF PROCEDURE CONTINUED Transfixing silk traction sutures are applied to the superior and inferior borders of the duodenum adjacent to its retained blood supply (FIGURE 14). These traction sutures are helpful when passing a linear stapler or the narrow crushing large vascular clamp is applied to the duodenum. The duodenal stump can be closed with a cutting linear stapler, noncutting linear stapler or as shown with sutures in a single or double layer. After the blood supply about the pylorus has been divided and tied, the stomach is held upward in order to free any adhesions between the first portion of the duodenum and the pancreas (FIGURE 14). At this time the transverse colon can be returned to the abdomen and retracted out of the operating field.

A thin-bladed, noncrushing clamp of the vascular type (Potts) can then be applied across the duodenum at the prepared level or it can be stapled with a linear cutting or noncutting stapler (FIGURE 15). A large clamp is applied to the gastric side to prevent spilling when necessary. There should be at least 1 cm of cleansed serosal surface at either border of the duodenum, between the noncrushing clamp and the traction sutures when this technique is used. This amount of prepared duodenal wall is necessary to ensure a safe subsequent closure of the duodenal stump. If the adjacent ligature does not permit 1 cm of cleared serosa between it and the margin of the clamp, small served clamps should be applied to the interfering vascular attachments, and such attachments should be divided and ligated. The duodenum is divided with a knife, and the stomach is retracted to one side. The duodenal stump is then retracted laterally in order to determine whether a sufficient amount of the serosa of the posterior wall has been cleared away to permit a safe closure of the duodenal stump. At least 1 cm distal to the clamp, the duodenum should be freed from the pancreas in order that subsequent sutures in the serosa may be placed under full vision. Individual clamping and subsequent ligation of the small vascular attachments must be carried out without damaging the gastroduodenal artery (FIGURE 16). The placement of deep sutures to control bleeding should be rigorously avoided in this area because of the potential danger of pancreatitis.

There are many ways of closing the duodenal stump. However, it should be remembered that a very firm closure is necessary, since blowing-out of the duodenal stump is not an uncommon fatal complication of gastric surgery which may be caused by failure to clear a sufficient amount of duodenum, especially along the upper border but more often is related to technical difficulties from inflammation caused by chronic ulcer disease. The tendency of the "cloverleaf" deformity associated with the ulcer to produce a diverticulum-like extension beyond the superior margin must be corrected in many instances to ensure a closure of the stump in this area. Failure to free up and excise this deformity tends to make inversion of the mucosal layer very difficult. The superior margin as well as the inferior margin of the duodenum adjacent to the clamp may be grasped with Babcock forceps preliminary to removal of the noncrushing clamp (FIGURE 17). As the noncrushing clamp is removed, the bleeding margin of the duodenal stump is grasped with two or three Babcock or Allis forceps (FIGURE 18). The duodenum is then closed with interrupted 0000 silk sutures or a continuous absorbable suture (FIGURE 19). The mucosal suture line should then be inverted by applying a row of interrupted mattress sutures of 00 silk, which tends to pull the anterior wall downward toward the pancreas (FIGURE 20). A cleaned serosal surface should be available at both the superior and inferior margins when this layer of interrupted serosal sutures is finally inverted.

As a final safety measure to reinforce the closure, interrupted sutures may be taken in the anterior wall of the duodenum and, superficially, in the capsule of the pancreas, especially in situations where a posterior ulcer has caused inflammation (FIGURES 21 and 22). While the duodenal stump is being closed, the common duct should be visualized and its relationship determined from time to time, so that there is no possibility of its accidental angulation, injury, or obstruction as a result of inverting the duodenal stump. CONTINUES

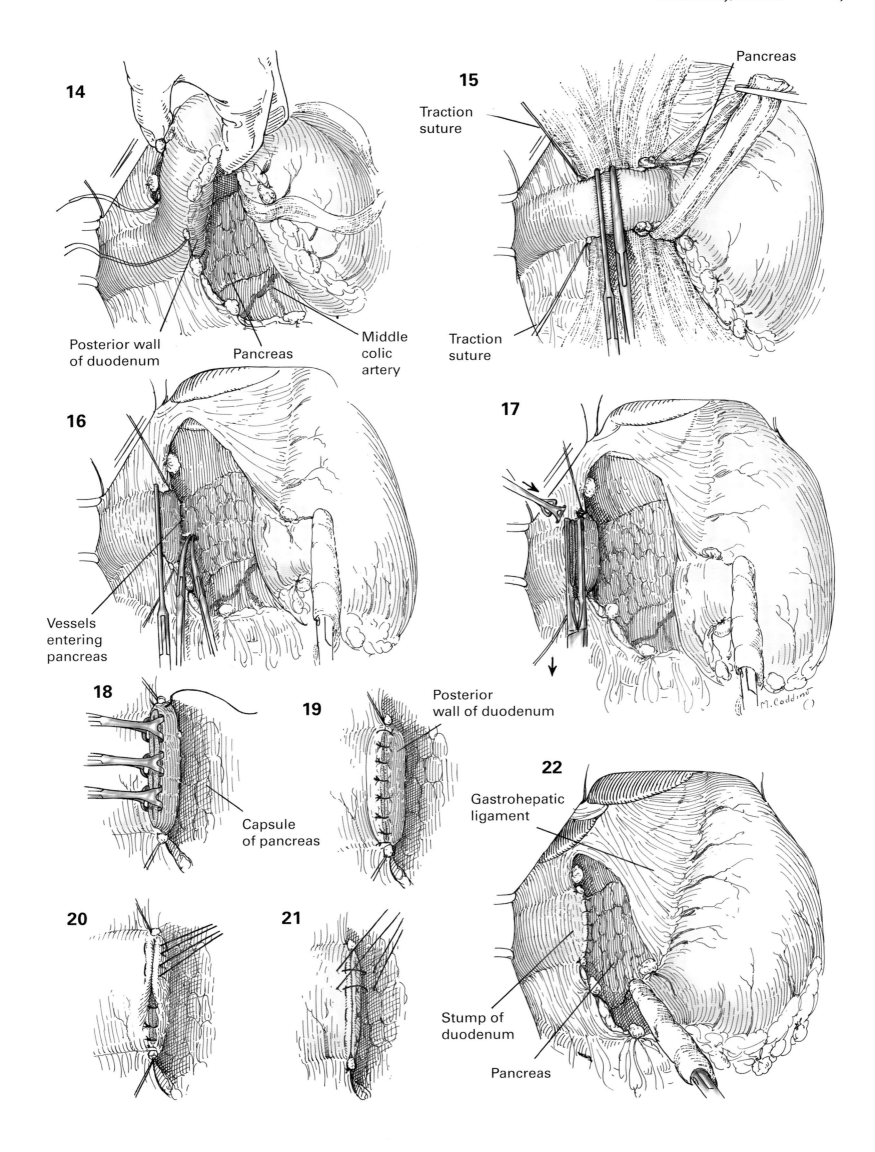

14

Posterior wall
of duodenum

Pancreas

Middle
colic
artery

15

Pancreas

Traction
suture

Traction
suture

16

Vessels
entering
pancreas

17

18

19

Capsule
of pancreas

Posterior
wall of duodenum

20

21

22

Gastrohepatic
ligament

Stump of
duodenum

Pancreas

M. Coddino

DETAILS OF PROCEDURE ◀ CONTINUED One of the important steps in gastric resection is the preparation of the lesser curvature. Frequently, the gastrohepatic ligament is quite thin and avascular at some distance from the lesser curvature. It is divided between pairs of small curved forceps (FIGURE 23). In the presence of malignancy the division of the gastrohepatic ligament should be as near the liver as possible and carried up almost to the esophagus to make certain that all involved nodes along the lesser curvature are removed. The uppermost portion of the gastrohepatic ligament may be clamped before division, since it may contain a sizable artery that requires ligation. The division of the gastrohepatic ligament does not involve a division of the left gastric artery, which comes up from the celiac axis directly to the stomach (FIGURES 24 and 25). Whether the left gastric artery is ligated depends upon how extensive a resection is indicated. A radical gastric resection is usually interpreted as one in which the left gastric artery has been ligated and the stomach divided at this level or higher. Attempts at mass ligation, especially in the obese, of the fat and blood vessels along the lesser curvature are dangerous and do not ensure a lesser curvature properly prepared for closure or anastomosis, as the case may be. The left gastric vessels divide as they reach the stomach, extending paired branches to either side of the curvature to enter the gastric wall (FIGURE 24). An effort should be made to surround an individual vessel before its division and ligation (FIGURE 25). The main vessels on either side of the curvature should be ligated as well as the individual tributaries that run down over the gastric wall (FIGURES 26 and 27). In a thin patient, a mass ligation may be carried out without difficulty by passing a small curved clamp from front to back, being careful to avoid the blood vessels extending downward over both anterior and posterior surfaces of the stomach. Following this, a transfixing suture, A (FIGURE 27), is placed to approximate the serosa of the anterior gastric wall to the serosa of the posterior gastric wall, so that when it is tied, a firm peritonealized surface is provided for the important subsequent sutures to be placed in this area. The lesser curvature should be freed of attached fat for several centimeters, and the larger blood vessels should be clamped and tied on the gastric wall. A smooth serosal surface is essential for a safe anasto-mosis (FIGURE 27). Further celiac and preaortic lymph node dissections for malignancy may be done now or after high division of the left gastric artery (FIGURE 28). Proximal vessel division and vascular control can also be obtained with linear cutting or noncutting staplers with appropriate vascular staple lengths.

When a very high resection is indicated, especially in the presence of malignancy, it is desirable to divide the left gastric artery as far away from the lesser curvature as possible (FIGURE 29). Care should be taken to isolate the surrounding tissue from the pillar that includes the left gastric vessels. Since these are large vessels, they are doubly clamped on the proximal side and transfixing sutures are used. It is frequently much simpler to ligate the left gastric artery near its point of origin rather than to attempt to ligate its individual branches as they divide along the lesser curvature. When the left gastric artery has been ligated, it is essential that the lesser curvature be prepared for anastomosis relatively near the gastroesophageal junction (FIGURE 29). It is possible to mobilize the small gastric pouch into the field by dividing the vagus nerves and incising the peritoneal attachments to the fundus as well as to the splenorenal ligament. The blood supply to the remaining stomach will be adequate through the short gastric vessels and in some patients a posterior gastric artery that originates from the splenic artery. Such mobilization facilitates the anastomosis when the exposure is otherwise difficult.

Regardless of the method used, it is important that the serosa be properly cleared for about the width of the index finger adjacent to the traction sutures, A and B, and either curvature (FIGURE 30). One or more additional sutures are usually required to adequately approximate the serosal surfaces along the lesser curvature. The stomach is now ready for the application of a stapling instrument preparatory to division of the stomach. It is important to stabilize the lesser as well as the greater curvature of the stomach by means of either Allis or Babcock forceps, lest the gastric wall be distorted as the crushing or sewing clamps are applied across the areas of both curvatures that have been previously prepared (FIGURE 30). Various methods of reconstruction may then employed as shown in Chapters 28, 29 and 30, however Roux-en-y gastrojejunostomy (Chapter 33) is preferred. ∎

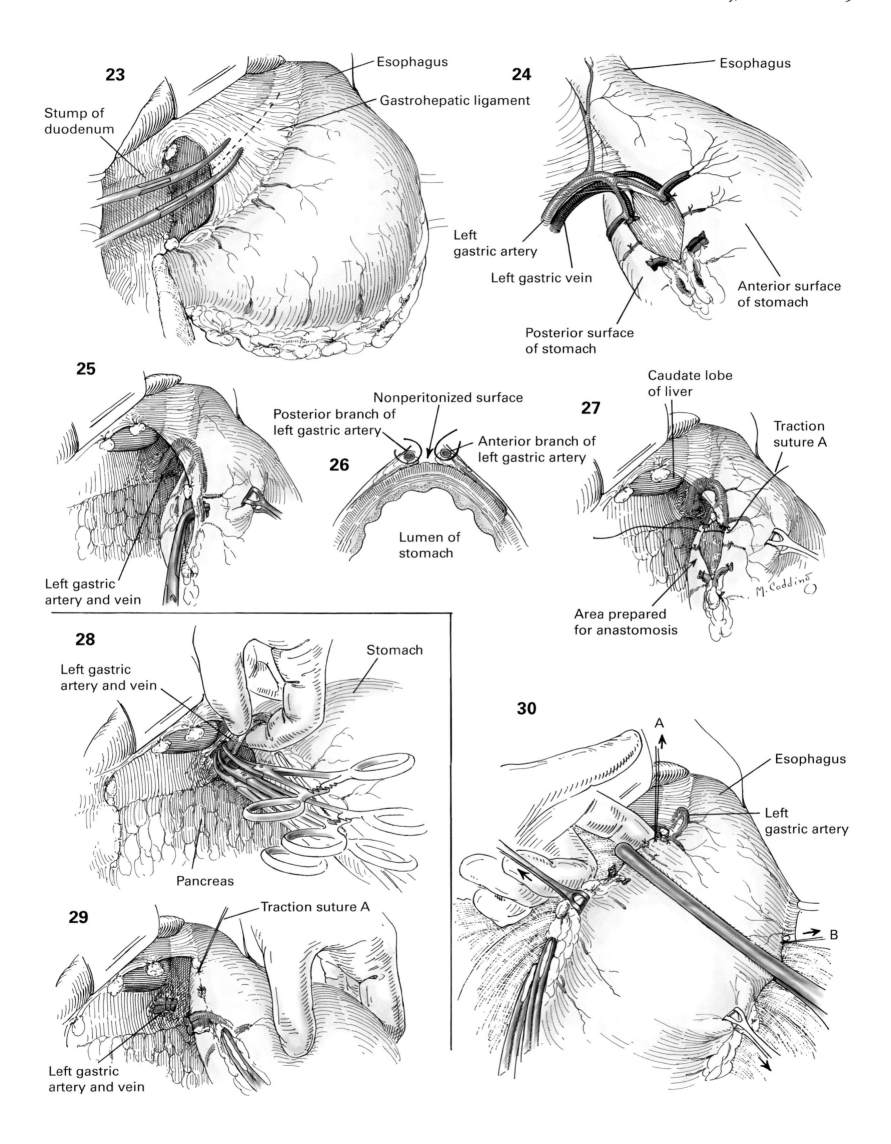

23

Stump of duodenum

Esophagus

Gastrohepatic ligament

24

Esophagus

Left gastric artery

Left gastric vein

Posterior surface of stomach

Anterior surface of stomach

25

Left gastric artery and vein

26

Posterior branch of left gastric artery

Nonperitonized surface

Anterior branch of left gastric artery

Lumen of stomach

27

Caudate lobe of liver

Traction suture A

Area prepared for anastomosis

M. Codding

28

Left gastric artery and vein

Stomach

Pancreas

29

Traction suture A

Left gastric artery and vein

30

A

Esophagus

Left gastric artery

B

REMOVAL OF OMENTUM

DETAILS OF PROCEDURE In cases of malignancy of the stomach, it is desirable to resect the greater omentum, because it allows for improved removal of lymph nodes along the greater curvature of the stomach and because of the possibility of metastatic implants in this structure. Removing the omentum is not difficult and can commonly be effected with less technical effort than dividing the gastrocolic ligament adjacent to the greater curvature of the stomach (see Chapter 26, FIGURES 8 to 10). For this reason, some prefer to use this procedure rather routinely, regardless of the indication for subtotal gastrectomy. The transverse colon is brought out of the wound, and the omentum is held sharply upward by the operator and assistants (FIGURE 1). Using scissors of the Metzenbaum type, dissection is started at the right side, adjacent to the posterior taenia of the colon. In many instances the peritoneal attachment can more easily be divided with a scalpel or electrocautery than with scissors. A thin and relatively avascular peritoneal layer can be seen, which can be rapidly divided (FIGURES 1 to 3). Upward traction is maintained on the omentum as blunt gauze dissection is utilized to sweep the colon downward, freeing it from the omentum (FIGURE 2). As the dissection progresses, a few small blood vessels in the region of the anterior taenia of the colon may require division and ligation. Finally, the thin, avascular peritoneal layer can be seen above the colon. This is incised, giving direct entrance into the lesser omental sac (FIGURES 4 and 5). In the obese individual it may be easier to divide the attachments of the omentum to the lateral abdominal wall just below the spleen as a preliminary step. If the upper margin of the splenic flexure can be visualized clearly, the splenocolic ligament is divided and the lesser sac entered from the left side rather than from above the transverse colon, as shown in FIGURE 6. The surgeon should be on guard constantly to avoid injuring the splenic capsule of the middle colic vessels, since the mesentery of the transverse colon may be intimately attached to the gastrocolic ligament, especially on the right side. As the dissection progresses toward the left, the gastrocolic omentum is divided, and the greater curvature of the stomach is separated from its blood supply to the desired level (FIGURE 6). In some instances it may be easier to ligate the splenic artery and vein along the superior surface of the pancreas and remove the spleen, especially if there is a malignant growth in this location. It should be remembered that if the left gastric artery has been ligated proximal to its bifurcation, and the spleen has been removed, the blood supply to the stomach has been so compromised that the surgeon is committed to total gastrectomy.

In the presence of malignancy the omentum over the head of the pancreas is removed, as well as the subpyloric lymph nodes (FIGURE 7). Small, curved clamps should be utilized as the wall of the duodenum is approached, and the middle colic vessels, which may be adherent to the gastrocolic ligament in this location, should be carefully visualized and avoided before the clamps are applied. Unless care is exercised, troublesome hemorrhage and a compromised blood supply to the colon may result. ■

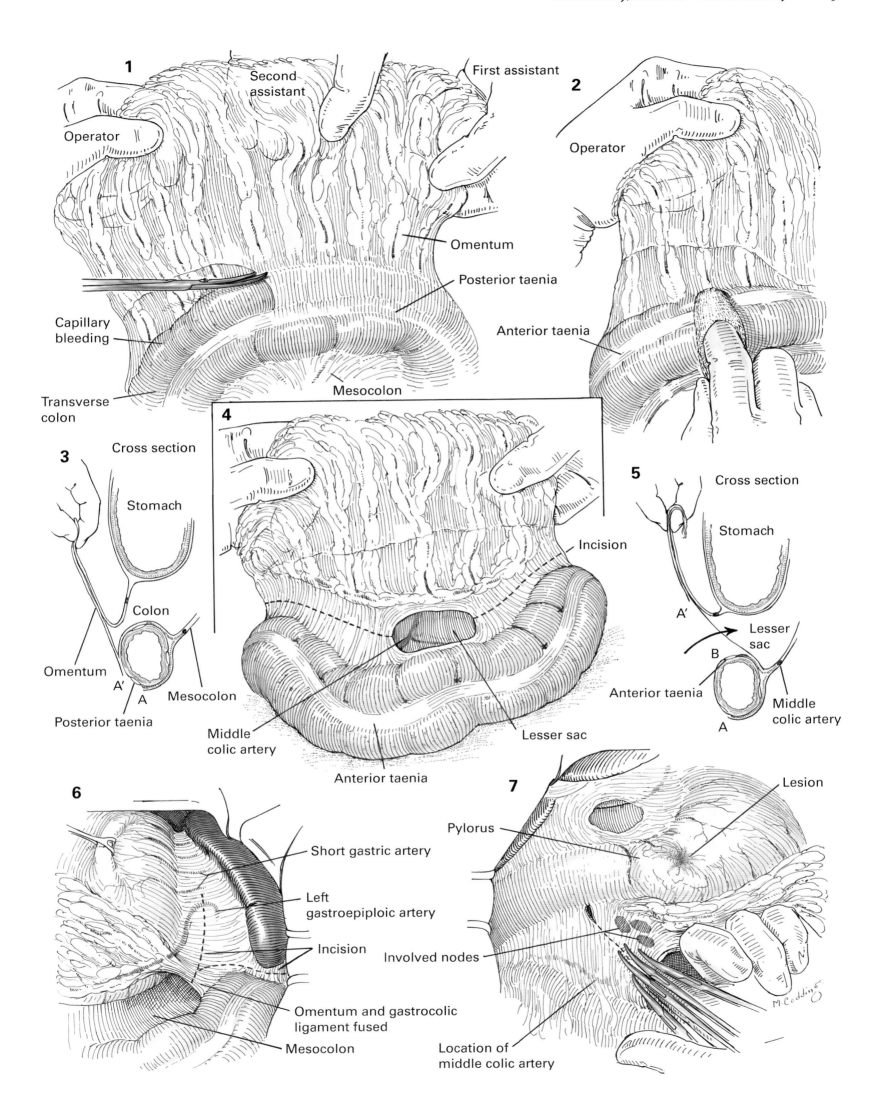

1

Operator

Second assistant

First assistant

Omentum

Posterior taenia

Capillary bleeding

Transverse colon

Mesocolon

2

Operator

Anterior taenia

3   Cross section

Stomach

Colon

Omentum

Posterior taenia

A'

A

Mesocolon

4

Incision

Middle colic artery

Lesser sac

Anterior taenia

5   Cross section

Stomach

A'

Lesser sac

B

Anterior taenia

A

Middle colic artery

6

Short gastric artery

Left gastroepiploic artery

Incision

Omentum and gastrocolic ligament fused

Mesocolon

7

Pylorus

Lesion

Involved nodes

Location of middle colic artery

M. Codding

CHAPTER 28 · GASTRECTOMY, POLYA METHOD

INDICATIONS The Polya procedure, or a modification of it, is one of the safest and most widely used repairs after extensive gastric resections have been performed, whether for ulcer or cancer.

DETAILS OF PROCEDURE The schematic drawing (FIGURE 1) shows the position of the viscera after this operation is completed, which in principle consists of uniting the jejunum to the open end of the stomach. The jejunum may be anastomosed either behind or in front of the colon. In the retrocolic anastomosis, a loop of jejunum is brought through a rent in the mesentery of the colon to the left of the middle colic vessels and near the ligament of Treitz (FIGURE 2). In the antecolic anastomosis, a longer loop must be used in order to pass in front of the colon freed of fatty omentum. If the resection has been done for ulcer to control the acid factor, it is important that the afferent jejunal loop be made reasonably short, since long loops are more prone to subsequent marginal ulceration. The jejunum is grasped with Babcock forceps and brought up through the opening made in the mesocolon, with the proximal portion in juxtaposition to the lesser curvature of the stomach (FIGURE 2). With the Polya technique the gastrojejunostomy uses the entire length of the stomach and jejunum for the anastomosis. The Hofmeister technique shown in Chapter 29 is an alternative in which only a portion of the gastric length is used for the anastomosis (Chapter 29, FIGURE 1). The jejunal loop is approximated to the posterior surface of the stomach adjacent to the staple line by a layer of closely placed, interrupted 00 silk mattress sutures (FIGURE 3). This posterior row should include both the greater curvature and the lesser curvature of the stomach. Otherwise, subsequent closure of the angles may be insecure. The ends of the sutures are cut, except those at the lesser and greater curvatures, B and A, which are retained for purposes of traction (FIGURE 4). The border of the stomach is cut away with scissors or electrocautery. An opening is made lengthwise in the jejunum, approximating in size the opening in the stomach. The fingers hold the jejunum down flat, and the incision is made close to the suture line (FIGURE 5).

The mucous membranes of the stomach and jejunum are approximated by a continuous mucosal absorbable synthetic suture as the opposing surfaces are approximated by Allis clamps applied to either angle (FIGURE 6).

A continuous suture is started in the middle and is carried toward either angle as a running suture or as an interlocking continuous suture, if preferred. The corners are inverted with a Connell-type suture that is continued anteriorly, and the final knot is tied on the inside of the midline (FIGURE 7). Some prefer to approximate the mucosa with multiple interrupted 000 silk sutures. The anterior layer is closed with the knots on the inside by using an interrupted Connell-type suture. The anterior serosal layers are then approximated with interrupted 00 silk sutures (FIGURE 8). Finally, at the upper and lower angles of the new stoma, additional sutures are placed so that any strain exerted on the stoma is met by these additional reinforcing serosal sutures and not by the sutures of the anastomosis (FIGURE 9). In the retrocolic anastomosis the new stoma is anchored to the mesocolon with interrupted sutures, care being taken to avoid blood vessels in the mesocolon and prevent the small bowel from herniating through the mesocolon (FIGURE 10).

CLOSURE The closure is performed in a routine manner without drainage.

POSTOPERATIVE CARE The patient is placed in a semi-Fowler's position when conscious. Any significant deficiencies resulting from the measured blood loss during surgery should be corrected by transfusions.

Pulmonary complications are common; therefore the patient is encouraged to cough and sit upright. If the patient's condition warrants, he or she may be out of bed on the first day after operation. Water in sips is allowed 24 hours after operation. Constant gastric suction is maintained during the procedure and for a few days after operation. It may be discontinued when clinical signs of GI function return. After the nasal tube is removed, the patient may be placed on a postgastrectomy diet regimen that progresses gradually from bland liquids to six small feedings per day. Beverages containing caffeine, excessive sugar, or carbonation should be avoided. An additional daily intake of fats should be encouraged for those patients well below their ideal body weight. Frequent evaluation of the patient's dietary intake and weight trends is strongly advised during the first year after surgery and at longer intervals thereafter for at least 5 years. ■

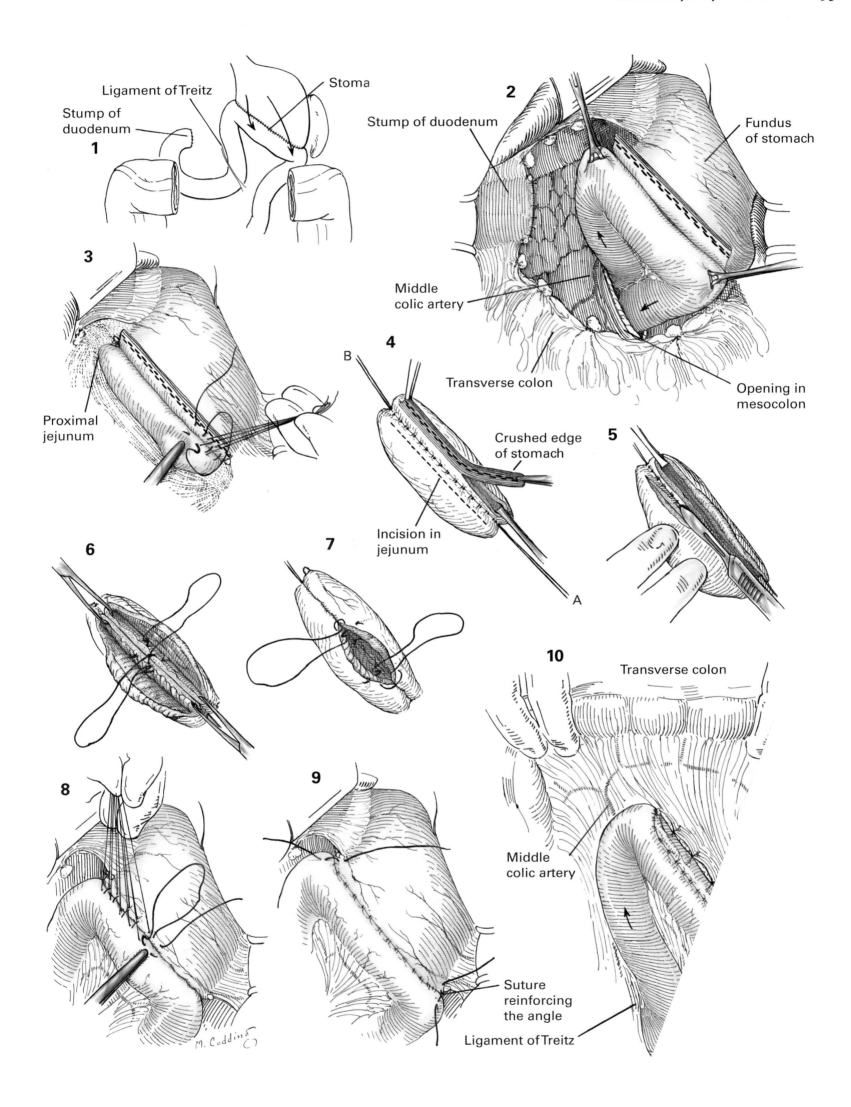

1
Stump of duodenum
Ligament of Treitz
Stoma

2
Stump of duodenum
Fundus of stomach
Middle colic artery
Transverse colon
Opening in mesocolon

3
Proximal jejunum

4
B
Crushed edge of stomach
Incision in jejunum
A

5

6

7

8

9
Suture reinforcing the angle
Ligament of Treitz

10
Transverse colon
Middle colic artery
Ligament of Treitz

M. Codding

GASTRECTOMY, HOFMEISTER METHOD

DETAILS OF PROCEDURE The schematic drawing shows the position of the viscera after this operation is completed, along with the alternative antecolic placement of the jejunal loop. In principle, this technique consists of closing about one-half of the gastric outlet adjacent to the lesser curvature and performing a gastrojejunal anastomosis adjacent to the greater curvature, with approximation of the jejunum to the entire end of the gastric remnant (FIGURE 1). Alternatively a Roux-en-Y reconstruction should be considered in some cases to avoid significant bile reflux that can occur with a small gastric pouch. This operation is favored when very high resections are indicated, because it provides a safer closure of the lesser curvature. It may also retard sudden overdistention of the jejunum after eating. The jejunum may be brought up either anterior to the colon or through an opening in the mesocolon to the left of the middle colic vessels (Chapter 28, FIGURE 2).

There are many ways of closing the opening of the stomach adjacent to the lesser curvature. Linear cutting or noncutting staplers are most commonly used as the staple line can be cut off at the site of the anastomosis. The older but effective Payr clamp is shown (FIGURE 2), as it provides a protruding cuff of gastric wall in situations where stapling instruments are not available.

The Staple line adjacent to the greater curvature is grasped with Babcock forceps to ensure a stoma approximately two fingers wide. A continuous absorbable synthetic material on a curved needle is started in the mucosa, which protrudes beyond the clamp in the region of the lesser curvature, and is carried downward toward the greater curvature until the Babcock forceps defining the upper end of the stoma is encountered (FIGURE 3). Some prefer to approximate the mucosa with interrupted ooo silk sutures. The crushing clamp is then removed, and an enterostomy clamp is applied to the gastric wall. A layer of interrupted mattress sutures of oo silk is placed to invert either the mucosal suture line or the stapled gastric wall (FIGURE 4). It should be carefully ascertained that a good serosal surface approximation has been effected at the very top of the lesser curvature. The sutures are not cut but may be retained and subsequently utilized to anchor the jejunum to the anterior gastric wall along the closed end of the gastric pouch.

A loop of jejunum adjacent to the ligament of Treitz is brought up anterior to the colon or posteriorly through the mesocolon in order to approximate it to the remaining stomach. The jejunal loop should be as short as possible but must reach the line of anastomosis without tension when the anastomosis is completed. An enterostomy clamp is applied to the portion of jejunum to be used in making the anastomosis. The proximal portion of the jejunum is anchored to the lesser curvature of the stomach. An enterostomy clamp is maintained on the gastric remnant unless this is impossible because of its high location. Under these circumstances it is necessary to make the anastomosis without applying clamps to the stomach.

The posterior serosal layer of interrupted mattress sutures of oo silk anchors the jejunum to the entire remaining end of the stomach. This is done to avoid undue angulation of the jejunum; it removes strain from the site of the stoma and reinforces the closed upper half of the stomach posteriorly (FIGURE 5). Following this, the crushed or stapled gastric wall still retained in the Babcock forceps is excised with scissors, and any active bleeding points are tied (FIGURE 6). The contents of the stomach are aspirated by suction unless it has been possible to apply an enterostomy clamp on the gastric side. The mucosa of the stomach and the jejunum toward the greater curvature are approximated by a continuous fine double ended absorbable suture on an atraumatic needle (FIGURE 7). Some prefer interrupted sutures of ooo silk. A Connell-type stitch is used to invert the angles and the anterior mucosal layer (FIGURE 8). A layer of interrupted mattress sutures is continued anteriorly from the closed portion to the margin at the greater curvature. Both the angles of the lesser and greater curvatures are reinforced with additional interrupted sutures. The long tails retained from closing the upper portion of the stomach are rethreaded on a spring-eye French needle (if still available to the surgeon). Otherwise, new nonabsorbable sutures are placed (FIGURE 9). These sutures are utilized to anchor the jejunum to the anterior gastric wall and buttress the closed end of the stomach anteriorly, as was previously done on the posterior surface. The stoma is tested for patency as well as for the degree of tension placed on the mesentery of the jejunum. The transverse colon is adjusted behind the jejunal loops going to and from the anastomosis. If a retrocolic anastomosis has been performed, the margins of the mesocolon are anchored to the stomach about the anastomosis (Chapter 28, FIGURE 10).

CLOSURE The wound is closed in the routine manner. Retention sutures should be used in emaciated or cachectic patients.

POSTOPERATIVE CARE See postoperative care, Chapter 28. ■

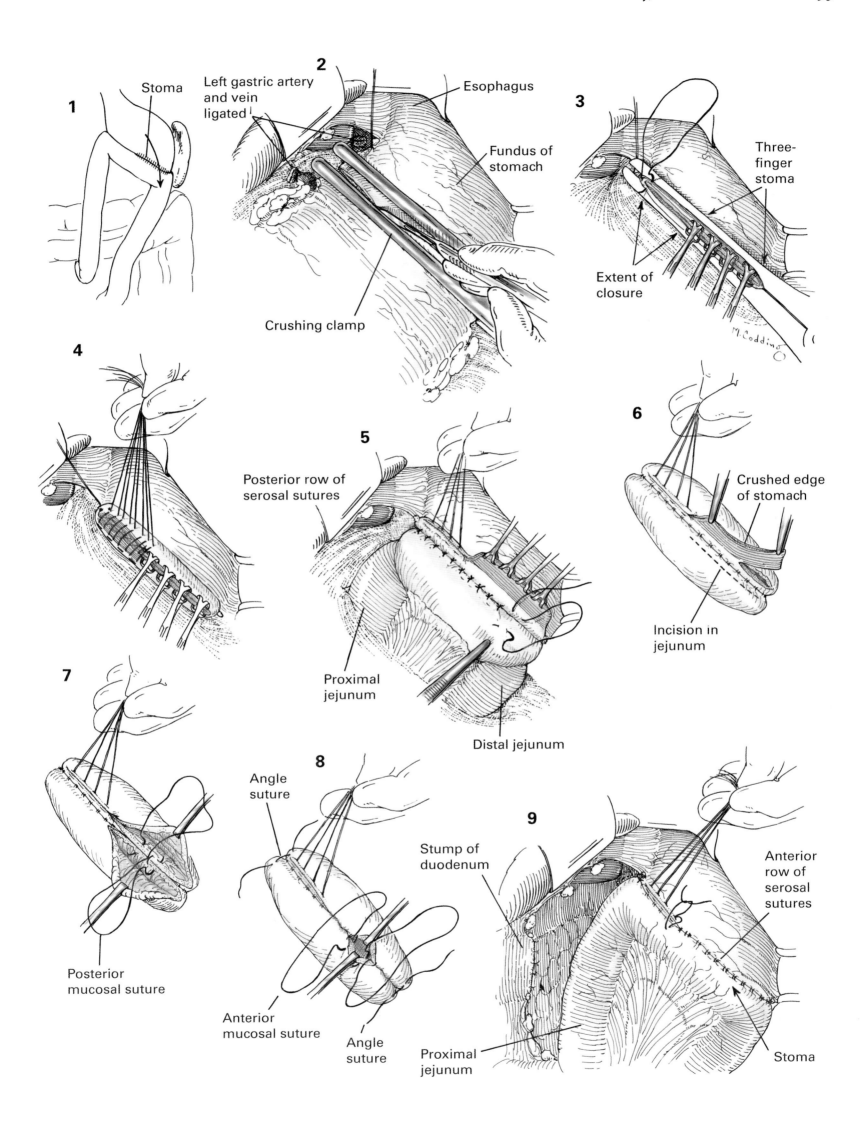

1 Stoma

2 Left gastric artery and vein ligated | Esophagus | Fundus of stomach | Crushing clamp

3 Three-finger stoma | Extent of closure | M. Codding

4

5 Posterior row of serosal sutures | Proximal jejunum | Distal jejunum

6 Crushed edge of stomach | Incision in jejunum

7 Posterior mucosal suture

8 Angle suture | Anterior mucosal suture | Angle suture

9 Stump of duodenum | Proximal jejunum | Anterior row of serosal sutures | Stoma

HEMIGASTRECTOMY, BILLROTH II STAPLED

INDICATIONS The Billroth II gastric resection is one of the most commonly performed procedures for malignancy of the stomach or for the control of gastric hypersecretion in the treatment of ulcer. The extent of the resection varies, with a two-thirds to three-fourths resection being the most common. When the left gastric vessels are ligated, 75% or more of the stomach is resected with the major blood supply coming from the gastrosplenic circulation. In the presence of carcinoma involving the body of the stomach, all the lymph nodes along the lesser curvature up to the esophagus are resected. The greater omentum is also removed, along with any lymph nodes about the right gastroepiploic vessels. When a malignancy is near the pylorus, 2 to 3 cm at least of the duodenum distal to the pylorus should be resected (see discussion in Chapter 26). Sometimes only a rim of gastric mucosa remains attached to the esophagus, which may require reconstruction with sutures rather than with the stapler. Consideration should be made for laparoscopic resection in cases without a contraindication such as extensive previous operations or large bulky tumors.

PREOPERATIVE PREPARATION General anesthesia is administered endotracheally.

POSITION The patient is placed supine on the table in a modest reverse Trendelenburg position.

OPERATIVE PREPARATION The skin of the lower chest and upper abdomen is shaved and prepared in a routine manner with antiseptic solutions. Preoperative antibiotics are administered.

INCISION AND EXPOSURE An upper midline incision is made. If a high resection is indicated, the xiphoid process is resected and the left lobe of the liver may be freed and folded toward the right side after dividing the triangular ligament.

DETAILS OF PROCEDURE The entire omentum is usually freed from the transverse colon, including both flexures in the presence of malignancy (see Chapter 27, Omentectomy). It is technically easy to remove the greater omentum by the technique shown in Chapter 27, FIGURES 1 to 5. The superior and inferior borders of the duodenum are partially freed to permit mobilization and ligation of the duodenal opening by a non-cutting linear stapler or a cutting linear stapler if there is adequate length. A Kocher clamp is applied across the pyloric end of the stomach or duodenum just beyond the point where the staple line is divided with a knife if using a non-cutting linear stapler (FIGURE 1). The duodenum should be disturbed as little as possible when a posterior penetrating ulcer is known to be present, lest perforation into the ulcer crater occur with subsequent leakage.

The lesser and greater curvatures at the level selected for resection are freed of fat in preparation for the placement of the linear stapler in a similar fashion, using staples of adequate length for a thickened or edematous stomach (FIGURE 1). The nasogastric tube is retracted before the stapler is applied. Straight Kocher clamps are applied on the specimen side from either curvature, and the stomach is divided with a scalpel applied against the stapler if a non-cutting stapler is used. Additional sutures may be required to control bleeding in the staple line. The extent of stomach removed and the performance of vagotomy are both related to the indications for the resection.

The jejunum just beyond the ligament of Treitz is selected for the anastomosis. It must be sufficiently long to easily reach the gastric pouch, but extra-long loops are avoided. While the loop of jejunum may be brought up through an opening made in the avascular portion of the transverse mesocolon to the left of the middle colic vessels (retrocolic position), many bring the loop of jejunum up over the transverse colon (antecolic position). A thick, fat omentum should either be resected or split to permit the shortest loop of bowel to be used.

There are various options for performing the anastomosis between the gastric pouch and the jejunum. The anastomosis may span the full width of the stomach, with the stoma made either anterior or posterior to the suture line closing the stomach. Usually the proximal jejunum is anchored to the lesser curvature (FIGURE 2). An anastomosis to the posterior gastric wall is commonly made as illustrated. The jejunum is anchored to the full width of the posterior gastric wall, perhaps 3 cm proximal to the line of staples occluding the stomach. Babcock forceps or sutures can be used to fix the jejunum in place parallel to the gastric wall. Stab wounds are made either with a scalpel or cautery on the greater curvature end and the distal end of the jejunum limb to permit the introduction of the cutting linear stapler blades (FIGURE 2). The size of the anastomosis is governed by the depth to which the blades are inserted (FIGURE 3). When the cutting linear stapler is removed, the staple lines are inspected for bleeding, which may require a few sutures for control. Finally, the stab wounds are approximated with traction sutures (FIGURE 4) or Allis clamps and stapled shut with the non-cutting stapler (FIGURE 5). Additional interrupted sutures are added when bleeding is present, and the jejunum may be anchored to the lesser curve to remove any possible tension on the suture lines. The patency of the stoma is tested by finger palpation (FIGURE 6). The nasogastric catheter is then passed for some distance into the distal jejunum to provide early decompression followed within a day or two by the administration of liquid diet upon resumption of peristaltic activity of the gastrointestinal tract.

CLOSURE Routine closing of the incision is used.

POSTOPERATIVE CARE Fluid and electrolyte balances are maintained and the blood volume is restored. Liquids in small amounts are permitted within 24 hours. Early ambulation is encouraged. The stomach tube is removed as soon as there is clinical evidence of gastric emptying. ■

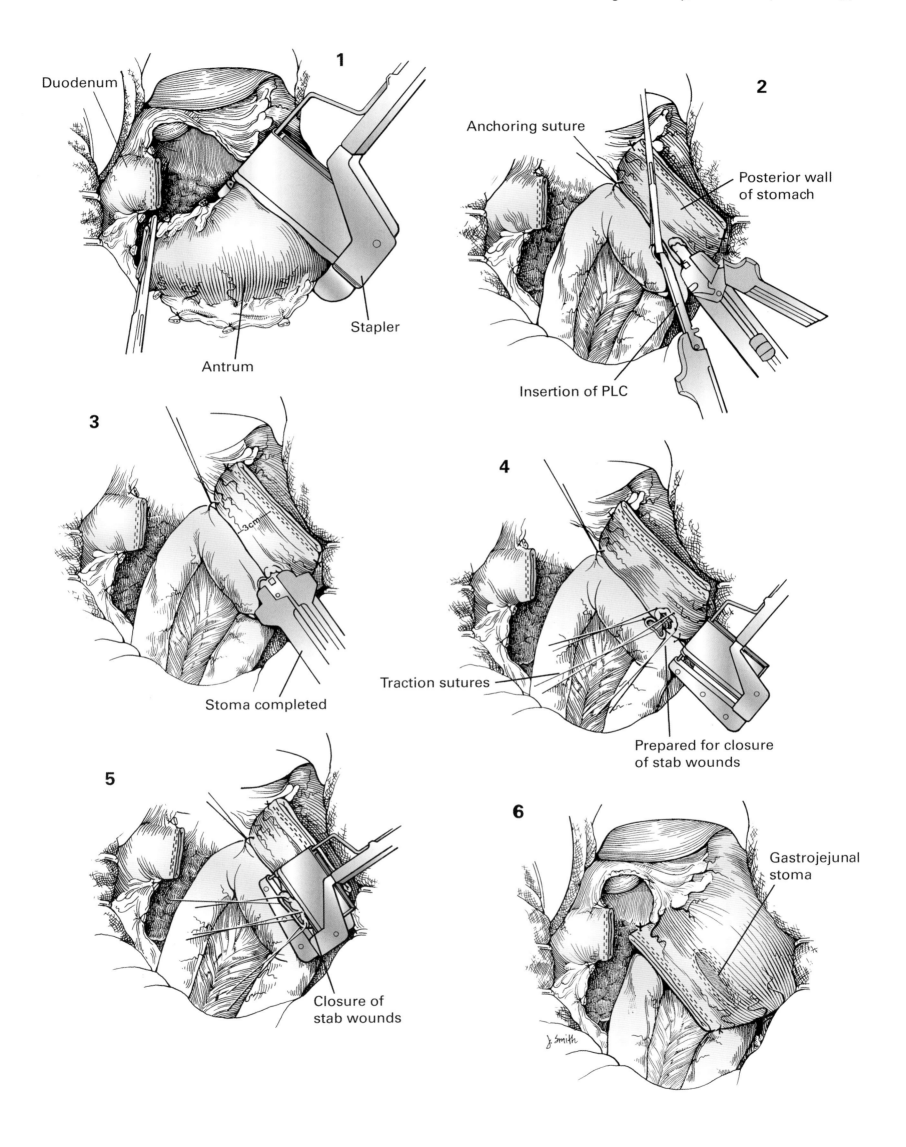

1

Duodenum

Stapler

Antrum

2

Anchoring suture

Posterior wall of stomach

Insertion of PLC

3

3cm

Stoma completed

4

Traction sutures

Prepared for closure of stab wounds

5

Closure of stab wounds

6

Gastrojejunal stoma

J. Smith

TOTAL GASTRECTOMY

INDICATIONS Total gastrectomy may be indicated in treating extensive stomach malignancies. This radical procedure is not performed when carcinoma with distant metastasis to the liver or pouch of Douglas or seeding throughout the peritoneal cavity is present. It may be performed in association with the extirpation of adjacent organs including the spleen, body and tail of the pancreas, or a portion of the transverse colon. It is also the procedure of choice in controlling the intractable ulcer diathesis associated with non-beta islet cell tumors of the pancreas when pancreatic tumor or metastases remain that cannot be controlled medically.

PREOPERATIVE PREPARATION Electrolyte replacement and fluid resuscitation should be complete. If colonic involvement is anticipated, the colon should be emptied with appropriate mechanical preparation. Blood should be readily available for transfusion.

ANESTHESIA General anesthesia with endotracheal intubation is used.

POSITION The patient is placed in a comfortable supine position on the table with the feet slightly lower than the head.

OPERATIVE PREPARATION The area of the chest from above the nipple downward to the symphysis is shaved. The skin over the sternum, lower chest wall, and entire abdomen is cleansed with the appropriate antiseptic solution. Preparation should extend sufficiently high and to the left on the chest for a midsternal or left thoracoabdominal incision if necessary.

INCISION AND EXPOSURE A diagnostic laparoscopy is often performed first to rule out inoperable spread of a malignancy (Chapter 13). If this view is clear, then a limited incision is made in the midline (FIGURE 1, A–A₁) between the xiphoid and umbilicus. The initial opening is only to permit inspection of the stomach and liver and to introduce the hand for general exploration of the abdomen. Because of the high incidence of metastases, a more liberal incision extending up to the region of the xiphoid and down to the umbilicus, or beyond it on the left side, is not made until it has been determined that there is no contraindication to total or subtotal gastrectomy (FIGURE 1). Additional exposure is allowed by removal of the xiphoid. Active bleeding points in the xiphocostal angle are transfixed with oo silk sutures, and bone wax may be applied to the end of the sternum. Some

prefer to split the lower sternum in the midline and extend the incision to the left into the fourth intercostal space. Adequate exposure is mandatory for a safe anastomosis between the esophagus and jejunum.

DETAILS OF PROCEDURE Total gastrectomy should be considered for malignancy high on the lesser curvature if there is no metastasis to the liver or seeding over the general peritoneal cavity, particularly in the pouch of Douglas (FIGURE 2). Before the surgeon is committed to a total gastrectomy, he or she must have a clear view of the posterior aspect of the stomach to determine whether the growth has extended into the adjacent structures including the pancreas, mesocolon, or major vessels (FIGURE 3). This can be assessed by reflecting the greater omentum upward, withdrawing the transverse colon from the peritoneal cavity, and searching the transverse mesocolon for evidence of invasion. By palpation the surgeon should determine that there is free mobility of the growth without involvement of fixation to the underlying pancreas or major vessels, especially in the region of the left gastric vessels (FIGURE 4).

The entire transverse colon, including the hepatic and splenic flexures, should be freed from the omentum and retracted downward. As the omentum is retracted cephalad and the transverse colon caudad, the venous branch between the right gastroepiploic and middle colic veins is visualized and ligated to avoid troublesome bleeding. The greater omentum in the region of the head of the pancreas and the hepatic flexure of the colon is freed so that it can be entirely mobilized from the underlying head of the pancreas and duodenum.

Following the exploration of the lesser sac, the surgeon further mobilizes the stomach. If the tumor appears to be localized, even if it is large and involves the tail of the pancreas, colon, and kidney, a very radical extirpation may be carried out. Resection of the left lobe of the liver may occasionally be necessary.

To ensure complete removal of the neoplasm, at least 2.5–3 cm of duodenum distal to the pyloric veins should be resected (FIGURE 2). Since it is not uncommon to have metastasis to the infrapyloric lymph nodes, they should be included in the resection. This is accomplished by doubly ligating the right gastroepiploic vessels as far away from the interior surface of the duodenum as possible (FIGURE 5). **CONTINUES ▶**

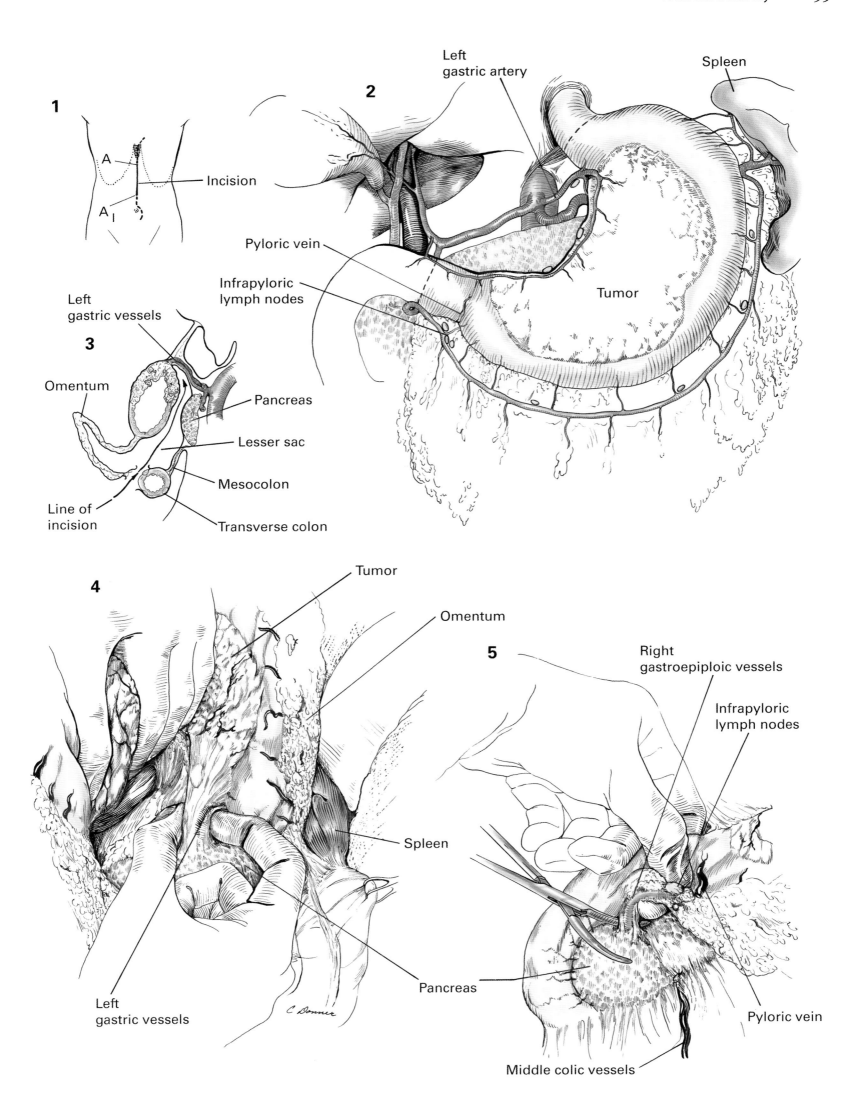

1

A

A

Incision

2

Left
gastric artery

Spleen

Pyloric vein

Infrapyloric
lymph nodes

Tumor

3

Left
gastric vessels

Omentum

Pancreas

Lesser sac

Mesocolon

Transverse colon

Line of
incision

4

Tumor

Omentum

Spleen

Pancreas

Left
gastric vessels

5

Right
gastroepiploic vessels

Infrapyloric
lymph nodes

Pyloric vein

Middle colic vessels

C Donner

DETAILS OF PROCEDURE CONTINUED The right gastric vessels along the superior margin of the first part of the duodenum are isolated and doubly ligated some distance from the duodenal wall (FIGURE 6). Palpation for potentially involved lymph nodes in the portal area is performed. If dissection is to be done, the surgeon must carefully identify and preserve the common hepatic and gastroduodenal arteries as well as the portal vein and common bile duct. The gastrohepatic ligament is divided as near the liver as possible up to the thickened portion, which contains a branch of the inferior phrenic artery.

The duodenum is divided with noncrushing straight forceps on the duodenal side and a crushing clamp, such as a Kocher, on the gastric side, or it may be divided with a linear cutting or non-cutting stapler (FIGURE 7). When clamps are used, the duodenum is divided with a scalpel. A sufficient amount of the posterior wall of the duodenum should be freed from the adjacent pancreas, especially inferiorly, where a few vessels may enter the wall of the duodenum (FIGURE 8). Even if it is extensively mobile, the duodenal stump should not be anastomosed to the esophagus because of subsequent esophagitis from the regurgitation of duodenal juices. If not stapled, the duodenal stump can be closed with sutures in a single or double layer. If stapled some surgeons prefer to oversew the staple line on the duodenum.

The region of the esophagus and fundus is next exposed and mobilized medially. The avascular suspensory ligament supporting the left lobe of the liver is divided, and the surgeon grasps the left lobe with the right hand and defines the limits of the avascular suspensory ligament from underneath by upward pressure with the index finger (FIGURE 9). Occasionally, a suture will be required to control oozing from the very tip of the mobilized left lobe of the liver. The left lobe should be carefully palpated for evidence of metastatic nodules deep within the substance of the liver. The mobilized left lobe of the liver is folded upward and covered with a moist pack, over which a large S retractor is placed. At this time the need for upward extension of the incision, or removal of the xiphoid process should be considered. The uppermost portion of the gastrohepatic ligament, which includes a branch of the inferior phrenic vessel, is isolated by blunt dissection. Two right-angle clamps are applied to the thickened tissues as near the liver as possible. The tissues between the clamps are divided and the contents of the clamps ligated with transfixing sutures of 00 silk (FIGURE 10). The incision in the peritoneum over the esophagus and between the fundus of the stomach and base of the diaphragm is outlined in FIGURE 10. CONTINUES

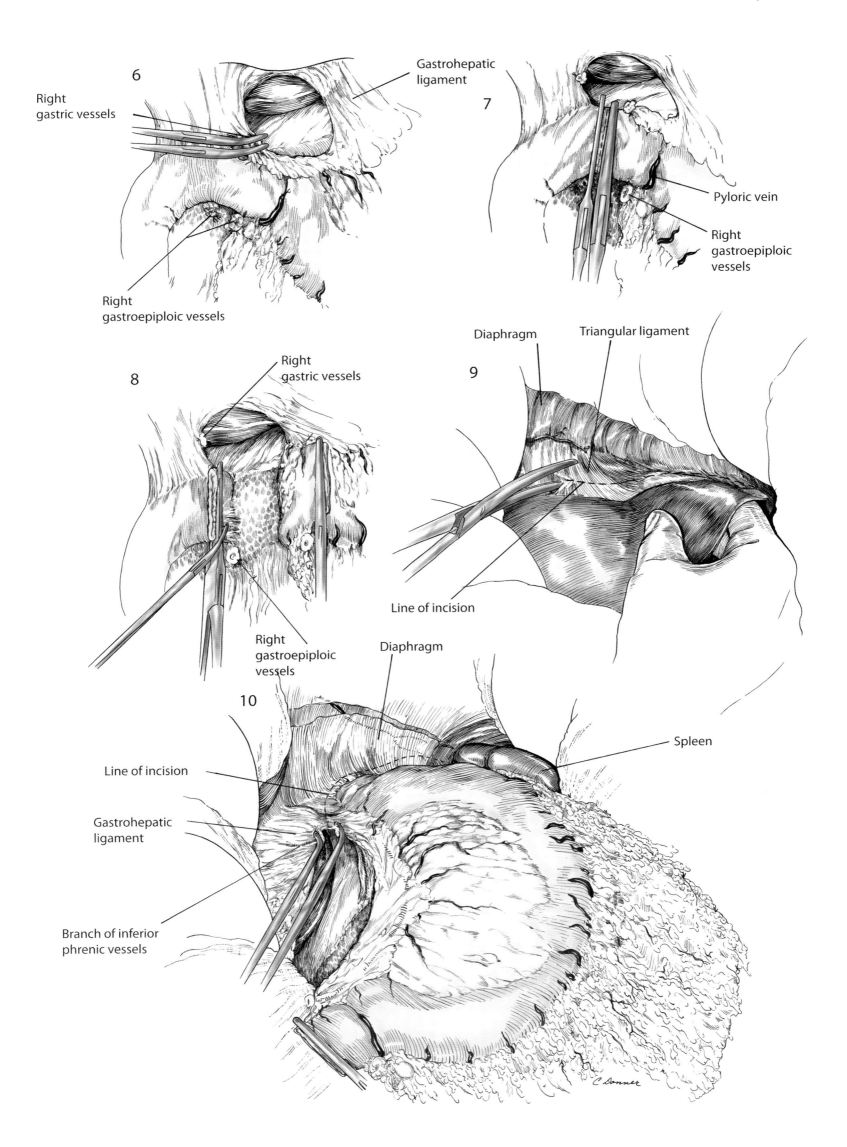

6

Right
gastric vessels

Gastrohepatic
ligament

Right
gastroepiploic vessels

7

Pyloric vein

Right
gastroepiploic
vessels

8

Right
gastric vessels

Right
gastroepiploic
vessels

9

Diaphragm

Triangular ligament

Line of incision

10

Diaphragm

Line of incision

Spleen

Gastrohepatic
ligament

Branch of inferior
phrenic vessels

C Donner

DETAILS OF PROCEDURE `CONTINUED` The peritoneum over the esophagus is divided and all bleeding points are carefully ligated. Several small vessels may require ligation when the peritoneum between the gastric fundus and base of the diaphragm is separated. The lower esophagus is freed by finger dissection similar to the technique of vagotomy (Chapter 23). The vagus nerves are divided to further mobilize the esophagus into the peritoneal cavity. By blunt and sharp dissection, the left gastric vessels are isolated from adjacent tissues (FIGURE 11). These vessels should be encircled with the surgeon's index finger and carefully palpated for evidence of metastatic lymph nodes. A pair of clamps, such as curved half-lengths, should be applied as close as possible to the point of origin of the left gastric artery, and a third clamp applied nearer the gastric wall. The contents of these clamps are first ligated and then transfixed distally. Alternatively, these vessels may be ligated using a vascular cutting linear stapler. Likewise, the left gastric vessels on the lesser curvature should be ligated to enhance the subsequent exposure of the esophagogastric junction. Depending on the location of the tumor and the findings on palpation, the surgeon may decide upon further celiac and preaortic lymph node dissection.

When the tumor is near the greater curvature in the midportion of the stomach, it may be desirable to remove the spleen and tail of the pancreas to assure an *en bloc* dissection of the immediate regional lymphatic drainage zone. The location and extent of the tumor, as well as the presence or absence of adhesions or tears in the capsule, determine whether the spleen should be removed. If the spleen is to remain, the gastroplenic ligament is divided as described for splenectomy (Chapter 90). The left gastroepiploic vessel is doubly tied. The greater curvature is freed up to the esophagus. Several vessels are usually encountered entering the posterior wall of the fundus near the greater curvature.

The anesthetist should aspirate the gastric contents from time to time to prevent possible regurgitation from the stomach as it is retracted upward, as well as peritoneal soiling when the esophagus is divided.

The duodenum is closed in two layers (see Chapter 26, FIGURE 19). The walls of the duodenum are closed with a first layer of interrupted 000 silk sutures. These are invaginated with a second layer of 000 silk mattress sutures. Alternatively, the duodenum may be closed with a stapling device.

One of the numerous methods that have been devised for reconstructing gastrointestinal continuity following total gastrectomy is selected.

The surgeon should keep in mind certain anatomic differences of the esophagus, which make its management more difficult than that of the rest of the gastrointestinal tract. First, since the esophagus is not covered by serosa, the longitudinal and circular muscle layers tend to tear when sutured. Second, the esophagus, while at first appearing to extend well down into the abdominal cavity, may retract into the thorax when divided from the stomach, leaving the surgeon hard-pressed for adequate length. It should be mentioned, however, that if the exposure is inadequate, the surgeon should not hesitate to remove more of the xiphoid or to split the sternum with potential extension into the left fourth intercostal space. Adequate and free exposure must be obtained to secure a safe anastomosis.

The wall of the esophagus can be lightly anchored to the crus of the diaphragm on both sides, as well as anteriorly and posteriorly (FIGURE 12), to prevent rotation of the esophagus or upward retraction. These sutures must not enter the lumen of the esophagus. Two or three 0 silk sutures are placed posterior to the esophagus to approximate the crus of the diaphragm (FIGURE 12).

Many methods have been devised for facilitating the esophagojejunal anastomosis. Some prefer to leave the stomach attached as a retractor until the posterior layers have been completed. The posterior wall of the esophagus may be divided and the posterior layers closed before the stomach is removed by dividing the anterior esophageal wall. In another method a noncrushing vascular clamp of the modified Pace–Potts type can be applied to the esophagus. Because the esophageal wall tends to tear easily, it is helpful to give substance to the wall of the esophagus and prevent fraying of the muscle layers by fixing the mucosa to the muscle coats proximal to the point of division. A series of encircling mattress sutures of 0000 silk can be inserted and tied, using a surgeon's knot (FIGURE 13). These sutures include the full thickness of the esophagus (FIGURE 14). The angle sutures, A and B, are used to prevent rotation of the esophagus when it is anchored to the jejunum (FIGURE 14).

The esophagus is then divided between this suture line and the gastric wall itself (FIGURE 15). Soiling should be prevented by suction on the nasogastric tube as it is withdrawn up into the lower esophagus and a clamp is placed across the esophagus on the gastric side. In the presence of a very high tumor that reaches the gastroesophageal junction, several centimeters of esophagus should be resected above the tumor. If 2.5 cm or more of esophagus does not protrude beyond the crus of the diaphragm, the lower mediastinum should be exposed in order to ensure a secure anastomosis without tension. `CONTINUES`

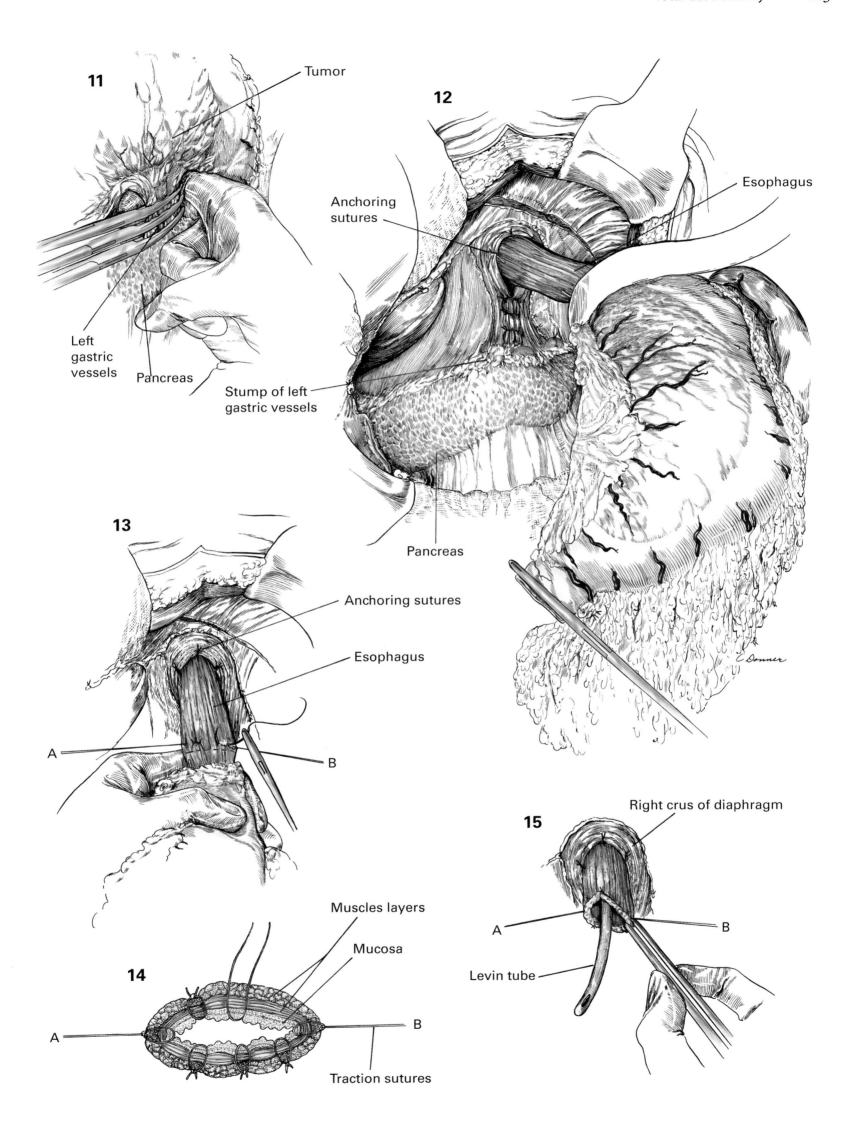

11

Tumor

Left gastric vessels

Pancreas

12

Anchoring sutures

Stump of left gastric vessels

Esophagus

Pancreas

13

Anchoring sutures

Esophagus

A

B

14

Muscles layers

Mucosa

A

B

Traction sutures

15

Right crus of diaphragm

A

B

Levin tube

DETAILS OF PROCEDURE CONTINUED The next step consists of mobilizing a long loop of jejunum, redundant enough so that it extends easily to the open esophagus. The jejunal loop is brought up through an opening in the mesocolon just to the left of the middle colic vessels. The region about the ligament of Treitz may need to be mobilized to ensure that the jejunum will reach to the diaphragm for easy approximation with the esophagus. The surgeon should be sure that the mesentery is truly adequate for the completion of all the layers of the anastomosis.

Various methods have been used to assure better postoperative nutrition and fewer symptoms following the complete removal of the stomach. A large loop of jejunum with an enteroenterostomy has been commonly used. However, bile reflux and ensuing alkaline esophagitis may be lessened by the Roux-en-Y reconstruction. Interposition of jejunal segments between the esophagus and duodenum, including reversed short segments, has not been found to be very satisfactory, and hence is uncommonly used.

Roux-en-Y reconstruction begins with division of the jejunum approximately 30 cm beyond the ligament of Treitz. With the jejunum held outside the abdomen, the arcades of blood vessels can be clearly defined by transillumination (FIGURE 16). Two or more arcades of blood vessels are divided and a short segment of devascularized intestine may need to be resected (FIGURE 17). The arm of the distal segment of jejunum is passed through the opening in the mesocolon to the left of the middle colic vessels. Additional mesentery is divided if the end segment of the jejunum does not easily extend up to and parallel with the crus of the diaphragm behind the esophagus. When the adequate length has been assured, the decision is made whether to perform an end-to-end anastomosis or an end-to-side anastomosis with the esophagus. If the end-to-side anastomosis is selected, the end of the jejunum is closed with two layers of ooo silk sutures or stapled (FIGURES 18 and 19). The end of the jejunum is then pulled through the opening made in the mesocolon to the left of the middle colic vessels (FIGURE 20). Care must be taken to avoid angulating or twisting the mesentery of the jejunum as it is pulled through. The jejunal wall is anchored about the margins of the hole in the mesocolon. All openings in the mesocolon should be occluded to avoid the possibility of an internal hernia. The opening created beneath the free margin of the mesentery and the posterior parietes should be obliterated by interrupted sutures placed superficially, avoiding injury to blood vessels.

The length of jejunum should again be tested to make certain that the mesenteric border can be approximated easily for 5 to 6 cm or more to the base of the diaphragm behind the esophagus (FIGURE 21). Additional mobilization of the jejunal limb for a distance of 4 or 5 cm may be secured by making relaxing incisions in the posterior parietal peritoneum around the base of the mesentery. Additional distance may be gained by very carefully incising the peritoneum both above and below the vascular arcade along with a few short radial incisions toward the mesenteric border. The closed end of the jejunum is shown directed to the right, but more commonly it is directed toward the left. CONTINUES

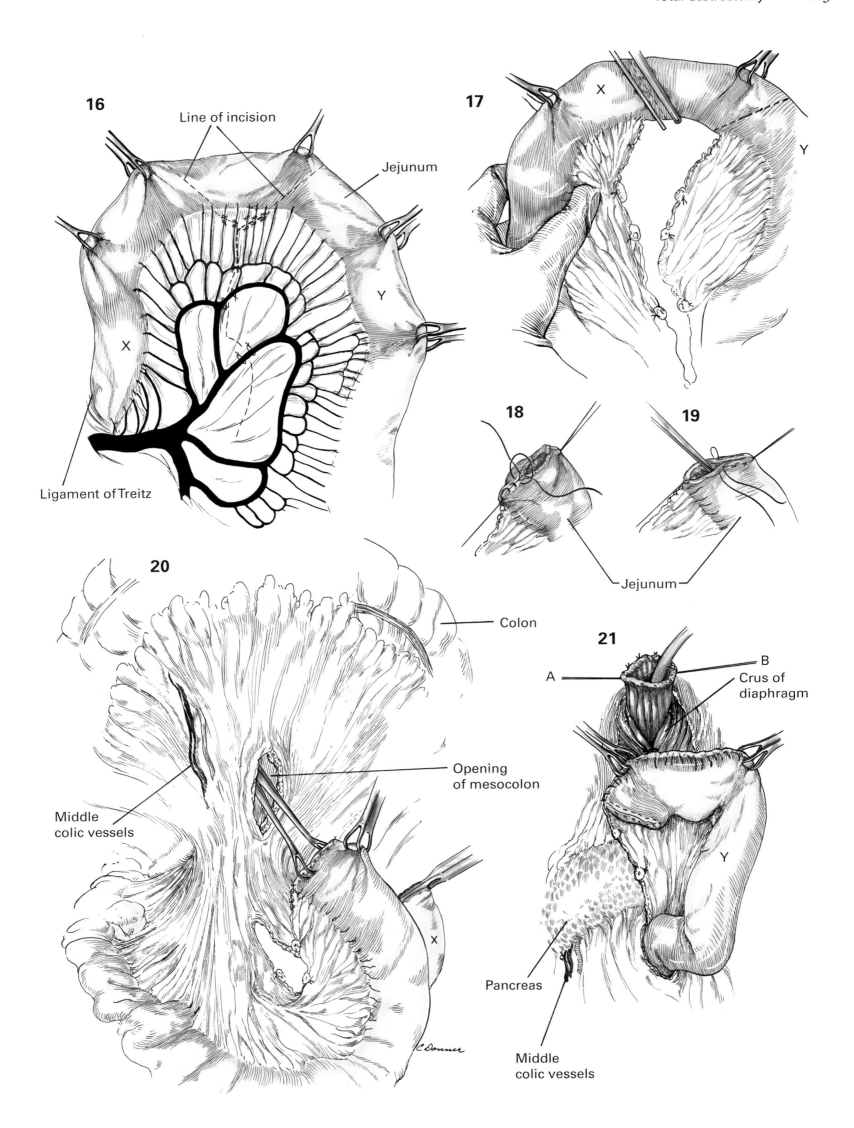

16

Line of incision

Jejunum

X

Y

Ligament of Treitz

17

X

Y

18

19

Jejunum

20

Colon

Opening
of mesocolon

Middle
colic vessels

X

21

A

B

Crus of
diaphragm

Y

Pancreas

Middle
colic vessels

DETAILS OF PROCEDURE <CONTINUED> A row of interrupted 00 silk sutures is placed to approximate the jejunum to the diaphragm on either side of the esophagus, as well as directly behind it (FIGURE 22). It is necessary to emphasize that the arm of jejunum is anchored to the diaphragm to remove tension from the subsequent anastomosis of the esophagus. After these anchor sutures are tied, angle sutures are placed in either side of the esophagus and jejunum (FIGURE 23, C, D). The esophageal wall should be anchored to the upper side of the jejunum. An effort should be made to keep the interrupted sutures close to the mesenteric side of the jejunum, since there is a tendency to use all the presenting surface of the jejunum in the subsequent layers of closure. Three or four additional interrupted 00 silk mattress sutures, which include a bite of the esophageal wall with the serosa of the bowel, are required to complete the closure between the angle sutures, C and D (FIGURE 24). A small opening is then made into the adjacent bowel wall with the jejunum under traction so that during the procedure there is no redundancy of the mucosa from too large an incision. There is a tendency to make too large an opening in the jejunum with prolapse and irregularity of the mucosa, making an accurate anastomosis with the mucosa of the esophagus rather difficult. A layer of interrupted 0000 silk sutures is used to close the mucosal layer, starting at either end of the jejunal incision with angle sutures (FIGURE 25, E, F). The posterior mucosal layer is closed with a row of interrupted 0000 silk sutures (FIGURE 26). The Levin tube may be directed downward into the jejunum (FIGURE 27). The presence of the tube within the lumen tends to facilitate the placement of the interrupted Connell-type sutures closing the anterior mucosal layer (FIGURE 27). An additional layer will be added as carried out posteriorly. Therefore, when the jejunum is anchored to the diaphragm, the wall of the esophagus, and the mucosa of the esophagus, a three-layered closure is provided (FIGURE 28). <CONTINUES>

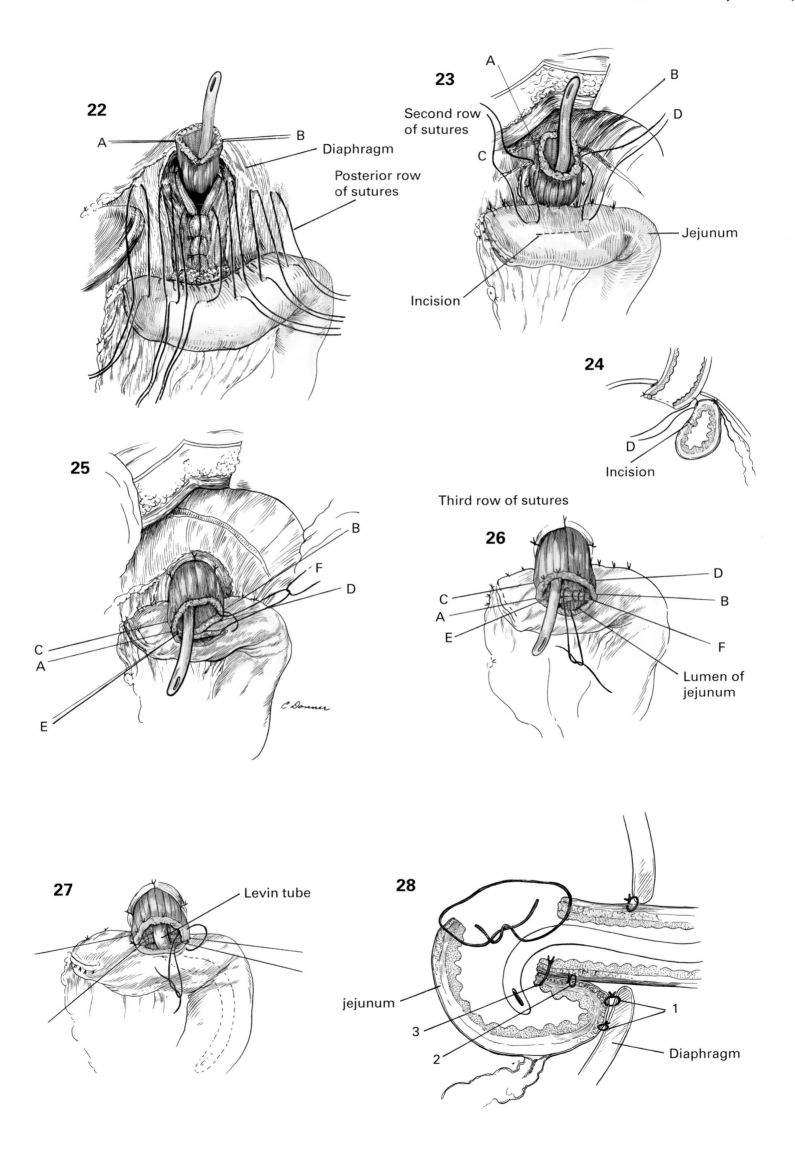

22

A — B

Diaphragm

Posterior row of sutures

23

A

Second row of sutures

C

B

D

Incision

Jejunum

24

D

Incision

25

B

F

D

C

A

E

C Donner

Third row of sutures

26

D

C

A

E

B

F

Lumen of jejunum

27

Levin tube

28

jejunum

3

2

1

Diaphragm

DETAILS OF PROCEDURE ◂CONTINUED▸ The second layer of interrupted 000 silk sutures is completed anteriorly (FIGURE 29). Next, the peritoneum, which has been initially incised to divide the vagus nerve and mobilize the esophagus, is brought down to cover the anastomosis and anchored with interrupted 000 silk sutures to the jejunum (FIGURE 30). This ensures a third layer of support that extends all the way anteriorly around the esophageal anastomosis and takes any tension off the delicate line of anastomosis (FIGURE 31). The catheter can be extended well down the jejunum through the opening in the mesocolon to prevent angulation of the bowel. A number of superficially placed fine sutures are taken to anchor the edge of the mesentery to the posterior parietes to prevent angulation and interference with the blood supply (FIGURE 31). These sutures should not include pancreatic tissues or vessels in the margin of the jejunal mesentery. The color of the arm of the jejunum should be checked from time to time to make sure the blood supply is adequate. The open end of the proximal jejunum (FIGURE 32, Y on FIGURE 16, 17 and 21 page 105) is then anastomosed at an appropriate point in the jejunum (FIGURE 32, X on FIGURE 16, 17 and 20 page 105) with two layers of 0000 silk, or a side-to-side linear stapled technique. The opening into the mesentery beneath the anastomosis is closed with interrupted sutures to prevent any subsequent herniation. FIGURE 32A is a diagram of the completed Roux-en-Y anastomosis. Some surgeons use closed suction external drains placed in proximity to the duodenal stump and the esophagojejunostomy.

POSTOPERATIVE CARE Suction is maintained through the nasojejunal tube, which has been threaded through and beyond the anastomosis. The patient is ambulated on the first postoperative day, and a gradual increase in activity is encouraged. Clear liquids may be given in limited amounts after 24 hours. Oral feedings are begun once the integrity of the anastomosis is established with a fluoroscopic water-soluble contrast study. These patients, of course, will need frequent small feedings, and adequate caloric intake may be a problem. This calls for careful collaboration between patient, surgeon, and dietitian. In addition, long-term supplemental vitamin B_{12} will be necessary, and oral iron and vitamins may be indicated for life.

Initially, scheduled reevaluations at intervals of 6 to 12 months are advisable to assess caloric intake. Stenosis of the suture line may require dilatations.

Total gastrectomy is rarely performed to control the hormonal effects of a gastrinoma. It is usually reserved for gastric acid hypersecretion refractory to medical treatment or patients with complications such as gastrocolic fistula. If the patient does have a gastrinoma, then serum gastrin levels are taken to evaluate the presence and progress of residual tumor or metastasis. Blood calcium levels are also advised to document hyperparathyroidism that may be present in multiple endocrine neoplasia type I. If hypercalcemia is present, the possibility of multiple endocrine neoplasia should be investigated in all members of the patient's family. Long-term follow-up studies should include determination of serial serum gastrin, calcium, parathormone, prolactin, cortisol, and catecholamine levels. Evidence of recurrent hyper-parathyroidism is not uncommon. Normal fasting serum gastrin levels may become elevated if residual gastrin-producing tumor is present. The presence of one endocrine tumor is an indication to search for others over the years of follow-up observation. ■

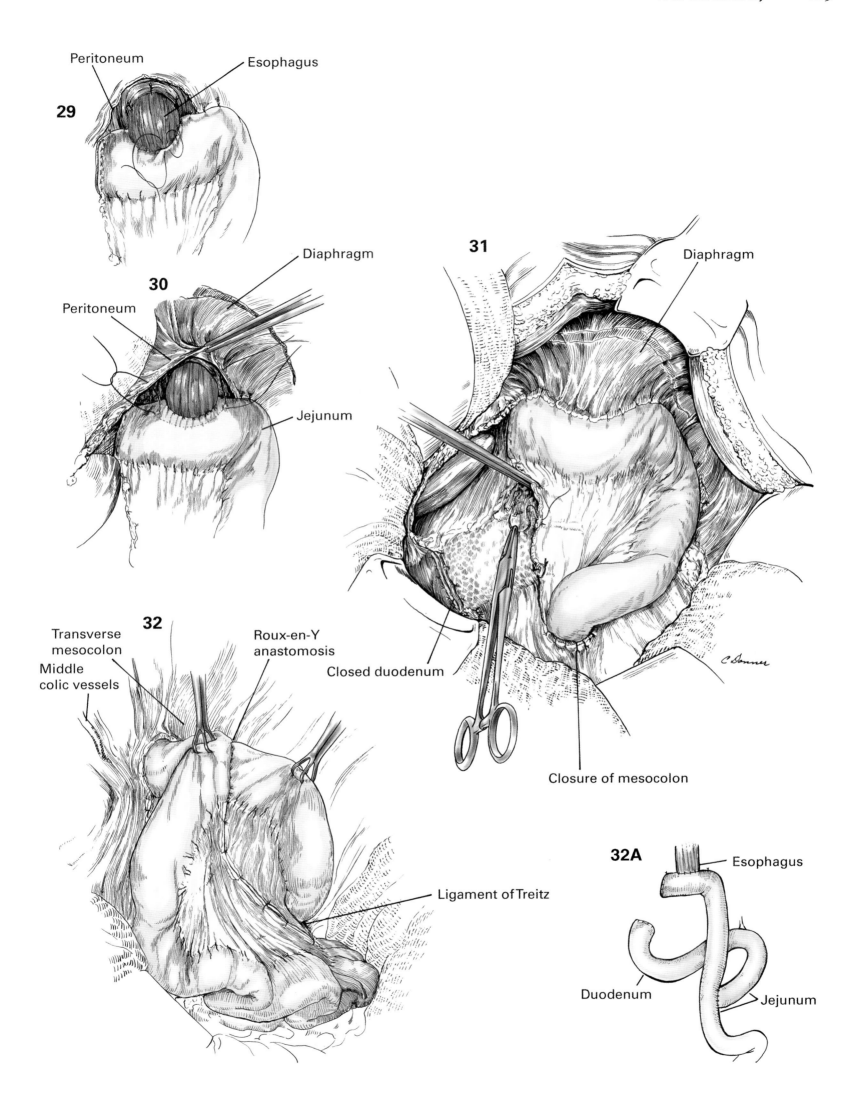

29

Peritoneum   Esophagus

30

Diaphragm

Peritoneum

Jejunum

31

Diaphragm

Closed duodenum

Closure of mesocolon

C. Denner

32

Transverse
mesocolon

Middle
colic vessels

Roux-en-Y
anastomosis

Ligament of Treitz

32A

Esophagus

Duodenum

Jejunum

CHAPTER 32   TOTAL GASTRECTOMY, STAPLED

INDICATIONS The indications and preoperative preparations are specific and are reviewed in Chapter 31, where the commonly used methods of reconstruction are shown with hand-sewn anastomoses. Many surgeons, however, prefer to use staples, because they simplify the anastomoses and lessen the total time of this operation.

ANESTHESIA General anesthesia is administered by endotracheal intubation.

POSITION Exposure is enhanced if the patient is placed in a reversed Trendelenburg position.

OPERATIVE PREPARATION The skin over the lower thorax as well as the abdomen is shaved and cleansed with the appropriate antiseptic solution.

INCISION AND EXPOSURE A diagnostic laparoscopy is often performed first to rule out inoperable spread of a malignancy. If this is clear, then a midline incision starting over the xiphoid and extending down to the umbilicus is made initially. This permits abdominal exploration and enables the surgeon to make a decision for or against proceeding with total gastrectomy. The incision is usually extended to the left and below the umbilicus if the decision is made to proceed with total gastrectomy. In the absence of metastases to the liver, peritoneum, omentum, and pelvis, the greater omentum is completely freed from the transverse colon. This permits evaluation of the posterior wall of the stomach as well as an evaluation for metastases about the left gastric vessels and attachments to the pancreas. Excision of the xiphoid provides a better exposure of the esophagogastric junction, along with medial mobilization of the left lobe of the liver following the division of the suspensory ligament to this lobe. An outline of a final reconstruction is shown in FIGURE 1.

DETAILS OF PROCEDURE As in Chapter 31, the region of the duodenum is first mobilized by the Kocher maneuver, and the blood supply about the pylorus ligated to prepare only the duodenal wall for the application of the stapler. The right gastroepigastric vessels are doubly ligated as far away from the duodenal wall as possible to ensure the inclusion of any possible lymph node metastases. The right gastric blood supply to the superior surface of the duodenum should also be divided and ligated to ensure the removal of 2.5 to 3 cm of duodenum distal to the pyloric vein, if the procedure is being performed for gastric carcinoma. The duodenum is closed with a non-cutting linear stapler. The duodenum is divided between the stapler and the Kocher clamp on the pyloric end of the duodenum. Alternatively the duodenum may be divided with a linear stapler. The entire stomach, along with the omentum and the gastric hepatic ligament, is then mobilized as shown in Chapter 31. The gastric vessels are divided and ligated in the presence of cancer of the fundus of the stomach. The spleen may also be resected, but this is indicated only if the spleen is involved with local spread of the tumor.

A good clear exposure of the lower esophagus is essential, along with the margins of the esophageal hiatus. Since the esophagus tends to retract upward when divided, it is helpful if the esophagus is pulled gently downward after vagotomy and anchored to the margins of the hiatus with four or five interrupted sutures that include only a modest bite of the esophageal wall (FIGURE 2). This ensures 5 or 8 cm of nonretractable esophagus below the hiatal opening. The crus of the diaphragm should be approximated posterior to the esophagus, allowing a reasonable-sized opening.

The nasogastric tube is retracted, and the modified Furniss clamp is applied to the esophagus above the gastric junction (FIGURE 2). The esophagus is divided against the clamp after a monofilament polypropylene suture on a straight needle has been inserted. This resection line must be close to the clamp to ensure a safe and secure closure by the stapler. It is also acceptable to divide the esophagus and place a purse-string freehand. The jejunum about 30 cm below the ligament of Treitz is exposed, and the blood supply in the mesentery studied to ensure a good blood supply to the mobilized arm of jejunum, which should be 50 to 60 cm long. The division of the jejunum and mesenteric blood vessels is demonstrated in FIGURES 16 and 17 in Chapter 31.

The divided jejunum is brought up through an opening in the avascular area to the left of the middle colic vessel. Special attention is required to avoid twisting the section of jejunum or in any way interfering with its blood supply. The jejunum is anchored to the margin of the opening, which must be closed to avoid internal herniation. The limb must extend easily up to the end of the esophagus as well as 5 to 8 cm beyond to provide entrance for the stapler to effect the esophagojejunal anastomosis (FIGURE 3).

The blood supply to the end of the jejunal limb is reconfirmed to be strong and adequate. The esophageal size is measured (FIGURE 4) with a calibrated sizing instrument. Some prefer to dilate the end of the esophagus by inserting a Foley catheter (size 16 French) into the lower esophagus and injecting 7 to 10 cm of saline, which gently dilates the end of the esophagus for the easier introduction of the anvil of the stapler. This may permit the introduction of a larger stapler. The appropriately sized circular stapler instrument is passed through the open end of the jejunum and directed toward the antimesenteric surface. The sharp plastic trocar on the end of the circular stapler instrument is passed through the antimesenteric surface of the small intestine. The tilting anvil is inserted through the opening made by the trocar and attached to the main portion of the circular stapler instrument. The tilted circular stapler cap is then carefully introduced into the esophagus (FIGURE 5). **CONTINUES** ▶

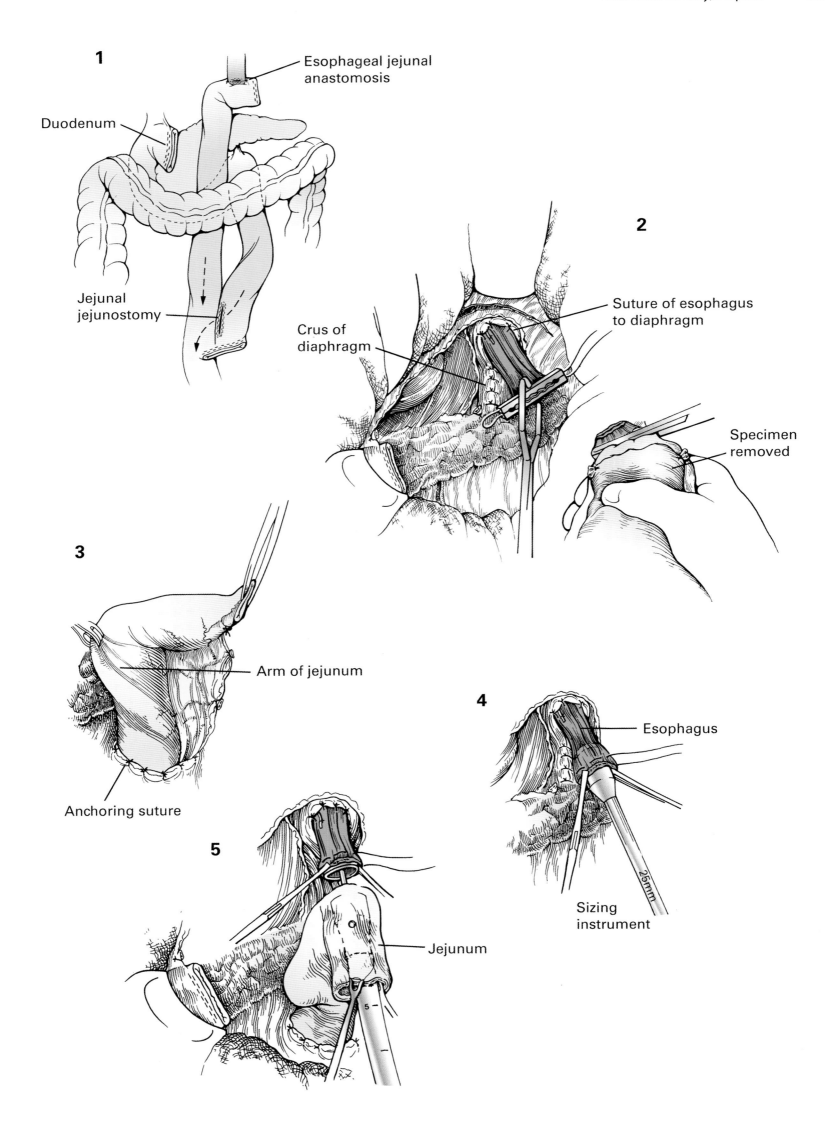

1

Esophageal jejunal anastomosis

Duodenum

Jejunal jejunostomy

2

Crus of diaphragm

Suture of esophagus to diaphragm

Specimen removed

3

Arm of jejunum

Anchoring suture

4

Esophagus

Sizing instrument

5

Jejunum

DETAILS OF PROCEDURE CONTINUED The security of the esophageal purse string should be evaluated before the handle and cartridge are approximated (FIGURE 6). After verifying that the combined thickness of the esophagus and jejunum is within the safe range of the staples, the circular stapler instrument is fired. Superficial interrupted sutures about the anastomosis are added after the instrument has been opened, gently rotated, and withdrawn. The nasogastric tube is passed beyond the anastomosis.

The open end of the jejunal limb is prepared for a stapled closure (FIGURE 7). Once again, the non-cutting linear stapler should be applied to serosa and at an angle to ensure an adequate blood supply to the antimesenteric border. Some prefer to place several sutures to anchor the arm of the jejunum posteriorly. This removes tension from the suture line and ensures against possible rotation.

The reestablishment of the gastrointestinal tract continuity beyond the ligament of Treitz can be accomplished in many ways. The afferent limb is connected to the Roux-en-Y jejunal loop approximately 25 cm from the ligament of Treitz and about 40 cm from the esophagojejunal anastomosis. A side-to-side anastomosis is performed, using a cutting linear stapler introduced into the antimesenteric sides of the jejunum (FIGURE 8). This anastomosis can be accomplished like the enteroenterostomy of a Roux-en-Y. The mucosal stab wounds are then closed with a non-cutting linear stapler (FIGURE 9).

The construction of a pouch below the esophagojejunal anastomosis does not seem to have a significantly beneficial effect on long-term nutrition.

The two jejunal limb mesenteries are approximated to eliminate potential internal hernia. The adequacy of the blood supply of each limb is verified, especially at the critical point near the anastomosis.

POSTOPERATIVE CARE Fluid and electrolyte balance are maintained during the initial postoperative period. Early ambulation is encouraged. Clear liquids are given in limited amounts after 24 hours. Oral feedings are begun once the integrity of the anastomosis is established with a fluoroscopic water-soluble contrast study. The patient is instructed in the value of six small feedings per day initially and is gradually advanced to three regular meals. The patient and family require reassurance that long-term problems concerning eating should be minimal. The weight should slowly increase, unless a diagnosis of extensive malignancy has been verified. Vitamin B_{12} injections must be given monthly along with a monthly dietary survey and nutritional evaluation. These monthly visits with reassurance can be helpful to the patient in returning the caloric intake toward normal during the first year after operation (see also discussion at Chapter 31). ■

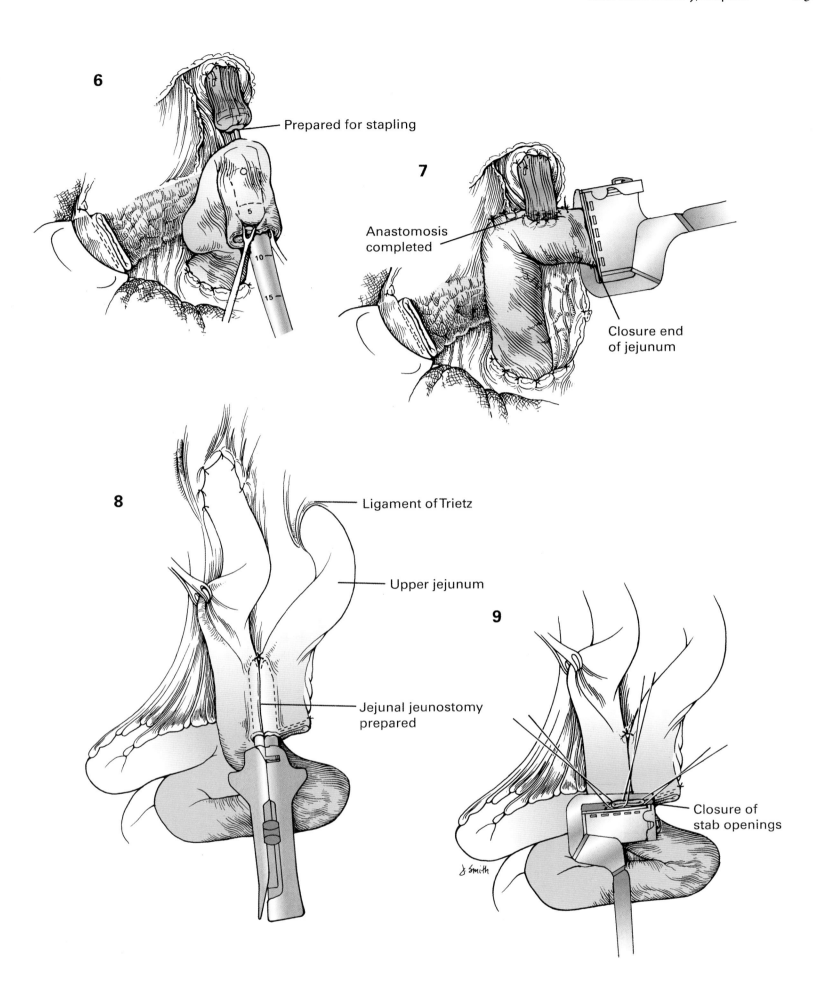

6

Prepared for stapling

7

Anastomosis completed

Closure end of jejunum

8

Ligament of Trietz

Upper jejunum

Jejunal jeunostomy prepared

9

Closure of stab openings

J Smith

Roux-en-Y Gastrojejunostomy

INDICATIONS The diversion of bile away from the gastric outlet that has been altered by pyloroplasty or some type of gastric resection may be indicated in an occasional patient with persistent and severe symptomatic bile gastritis.

PREOPERATIVE PREPARATION A firm diagnosis of postoperative reflux gastritis should be established. Endoscopic studies should demonstrate gross as well as microscopic evidence of severe gastritis of greater intensity than is routinely observed from the regurgitation of duodenal contents through an altered gastric outlet. A gastric analysis is performed in a search for evidence of previous complete vagotomy. Barium studies and serum gastrin determination are routinely performed. In addition to a firm clinical diagnosis of postoperative reflux bile gastritis, there should be evidence of persistent symptoms despite long-term intensive medical therapy. The operative procedure is designed to completely divert the duodenal contents away from the gastric outlet. Ulceration will occur unless the gastric acidity is controlled by a complete vagotomy combined with antrectomy.

Constant gastric suction by a nasogastric tube is maintained.

ANESTHESIA General anesthesia combined with endotracheal intubation is satisfactory.

POSITION The patient is placed in a supine position with the feet lower than the head.

OPERATIVE PREPARATION The skin of the lower thorax as well as the abdomen is prepared in a routine manner.

INCISION AND EXPOSURE The incision is made through the old scar of the previous gastric procedure. The incision should extend up over the xiphoid since exploration of the esophagogastric junction may be required to determine the adequacy of a previous vagotomy. Care is taken to avoid accidental opening of loops of intestine that may be adherent to the peritoneum.

Even when a previous vagotomy has been performed, it is advisable to search for overlooked vagal fibers, especially the posterior vagus nerves, unless firm adhesions between the undersurface of the left lobe of the liver and upper stomach make such a search too hazardous.

The site of the previous anastomosis is freed up to permit careful inspection and palpation for evidence of ulceration or stenosis, or evidence of a previous unphysiologic procedure such as a long loop, angulation, or partial obstruction of the jejunostomy. A patulous gastroduodenostomy may be found (FIGURE 1).

The extent of the previous resection must be determined to be certain that the antrum has been resected. A complete vagotomy as well as antrectomy is mandatory as a safeguard against recurrent ulceration.

DETAILS OF PROCEDURE When a Billroth I procedure is to be converted, it is essential to carefully isolate the anastomosis both anteriorly and posteriorly before applying straight Kocher clamps to either side of the anastomosis (FIGURE 2). Because a Kocher mobilization and medial rotation of the duodenum were previously made to ensure absence of tension in the suture line, it is important to sacrifice as little duodenum as possible (FIGURE 2). Unexpected injury to the accessory pancreatic duct or the common duct may occur if further mobilization of the first portion of the duodenum is carried out.

The end of the duodenum is closed with a row of interrupted sutures (FIGURE 3), although many surgeons prefer to close the duodenum with a double row of staples. This suture line is then reinforced with a second layer of interrupted silk sutures that bring the anterior duodenal wall down to the pancreatic capsule. The transverse colon is reflected upward, and the upper jejunum from the ligament of Treitz downward for at least 40 to 50 cm is freed from any adhesions that may have followed previous operations. An arm of jejunum (FIGURE 4) is mobilized as shown in Chapter 31, FIGURES 16–20. The end of the jejunum is closed with a double layer of sutures. This suture line is inverted by a second layer of interrupted oo silk sutures to evert the mucosal layer (FIGURE 6); the angles should be securely approximated. A retrocolic rather than an antecolic anastomosis is usually made (FIGURE 4) as the active limb is brought through an opening in the mesocolon to the left of the middle colic vessels. The open end of the Roux-en-Y loop is closed in two layers. The first is a running absorbable suture (FIGURE 5). Alternatively, this may have been stapled if the jejunum was divided with a cutting linear stapler instrument. A second layer of inverting interrupted silk mattress sutures may be placed FIGURE 6. **CONTINUES ▶**

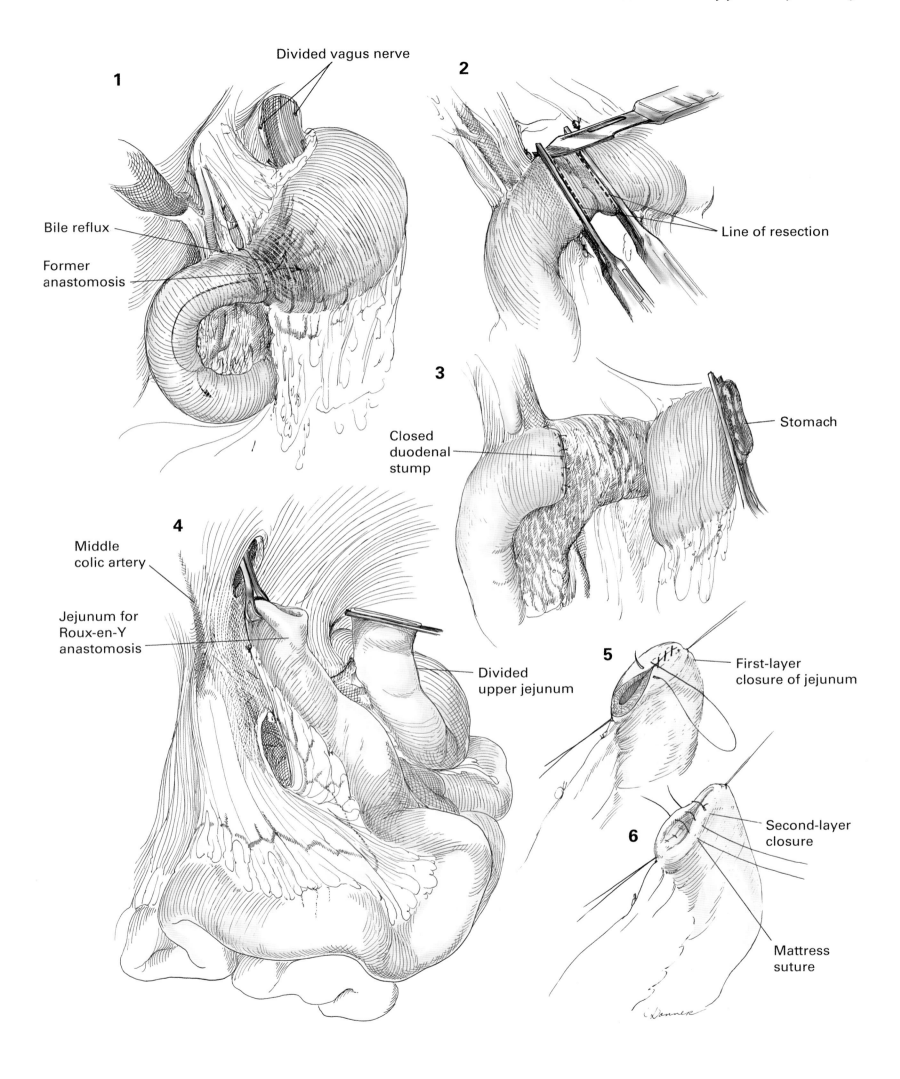

1

Divided vagus nerve

Bile reflux

Former anastomosis

2

Line of resection

3

Closed duodenal stump

Stomach

4

Middle colic artery

Jejunum for Roux-en-Y anastomosis

Divided upper jejunum

5

First-layer closure of jejunum

6

Second-layer closure

Mattress suture

DETAILS OF PROCEDURE ◄**CONTINUED** It is advisable to resect additional stomach to be certain that all of the antrum has been removed. A noncrushing clamp is applied across the gastric pouch to control bleeding and prevent gross soiling, as well as to fix the gastric wall for the placement of sutures (FIGURE 7). A two-layer anastomosis, end of stomach to side of jejunum, is made with the full width of the gastric outlet (FIGURE 8). The end of the jejunum should not extend more than 2 cm beyond the anastomosis (FIGURE 9). All openings in the mesocolon are closed with interrupted sutures to avoid a possible internal hernia and avoid a twist or angulation of the arm of jejunum.

A jejunojejunal anastomosis is done at least 40 cm from the gastrojejunal anastomosis (FIGURE 10). A two-layer anastomosis is performed, and all openings in the mesenteries are closed to avoid any chance of herniation or obstruction about the anastomosis (FIGURE 11). A long Levin tube is directed through the anastomosis and may be directed around into the duodenum to ensure decompression of the duodenal stump. After a thorough search for needles, instruments, and sponges, and affirming a correct count, the abdomen is closed.

CLOSURE The abdominal incision is closed in the routine manner.

POSTOPERATIVE CARE Fluid and electrolyte balance are maintained. Clear liquids are initiated on the first postoperative day, followed by gradual advancement of oral intake. Ultimately, six small feedings a day are permitted since slow gastric emptying is often a problem. Careful medical supervision is required to ensure a good result. ∎

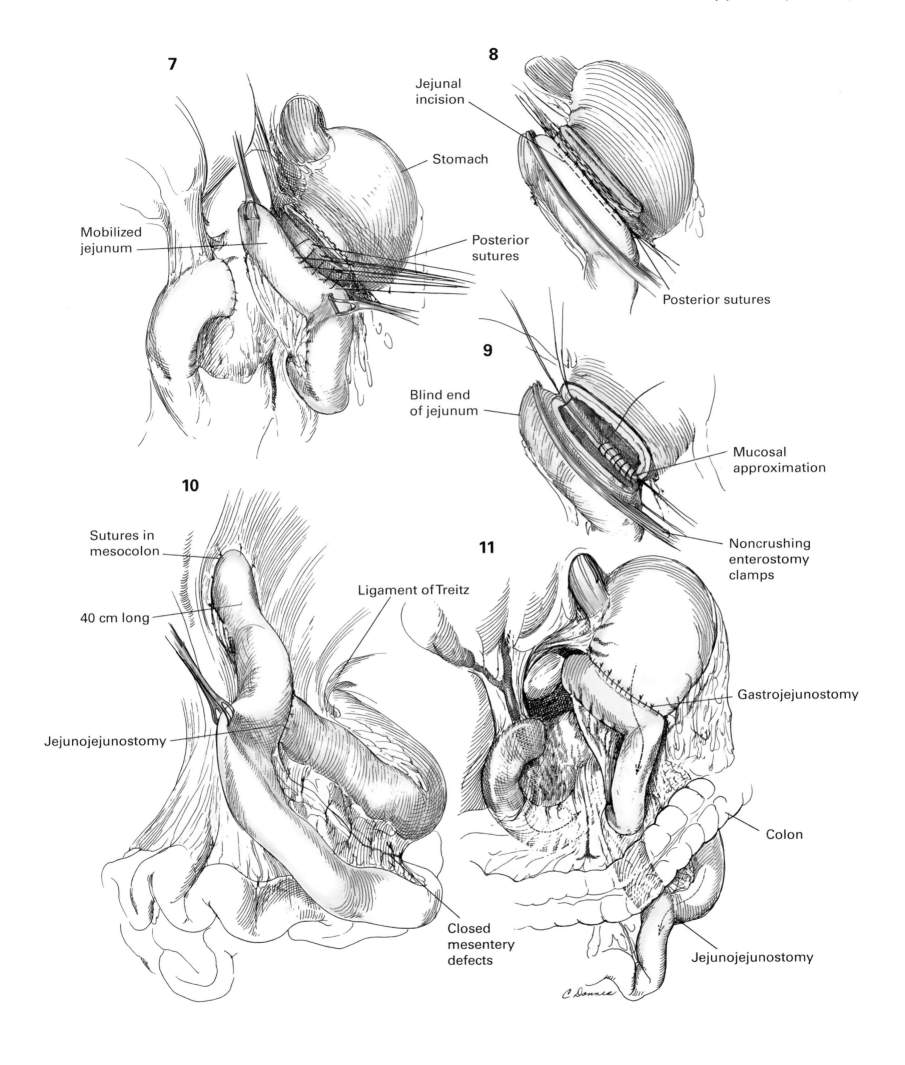

7

Mobilized jejunum

Stomach

Posterior sutures

8

Jejunal incision

Posterior sutures

9

Blind end of jejunum

Mucosal approximation

Noncrushing enterostomy clamps

10

Sutures in mesocolon

40 cm long

Jejunojejunostomy

Ligament of Treitz

Closed mesentery defects

11

Gastrojejunostomy

Colon

Jejunojejunostomy

C. Donner

FUNDOPLICATION

INDICATIONS Fundoplication may be considered in certain patients with symptomatic reflux gastritis associated with esophagitis or refractory to maximal medical therapy. Esophagitis with stricture and paraesophageal hernia are other common indications. A preliminary trial of repeated dilatations should be instituted when there is evidence of a stricture of the lower end of the esophagus prior to fundoplication.

Substernal pain, especially in the recumbent position, difficulty in swallowing, and recurrent bouts of aspiration pneumonia are commonly associated with gastroesophageal reflux. Esophagoscopy should be performed to assess for presence of hiatal hernia, esophagitis, esophageal stricture or mass, and Barrett's esophagus. Esophageal motility must be assessed by either manometry or video barium esophagram demonstrating normal motility. In the absence of erosive esophagitis, 24-hour pH monitoring should be performed to provide objective evidence of acid reflux.

Surgical procedures are designed to prevent acid peptic reflux and to restore normal sphincteric function. When reflux esophagitis is associated with duodenal ulcer, either parietal cell vagotomy or truncal vagotomy and pyloroplasty should be considered.

PREOPERATIVE PREPARATION Pulmonary function studies are indicated in patients with a history of aspiration pneumonia. Antacid therapy is maintained. Systemic antibiotics may be given. Nasogastric intubation should be instituted.

ANESTHESIA General anesthesia with endotracheal intubation is employed.

POSITION The patient is placed in a comfortable supine position on the table with the feet slightly lower than the head.

OPERATIVE PREPARATION The area from the nipples downward to the symphysis is shaved. The skin over the sternum, lower chest wall, and the entire abdomen is cleaned with the appropriate antiseptic solutions.

INCISION AND EXPOSURE A liberal incision starting over the xiphoid and extending down the midline to the umbilicus is made (FIGURE 1). When the xiphoid is elongated, it is removed to enhance the exposure of the esophagogastric junction. Active arterial bleeding in either xiphocostal angle is controlled with a transfixing suture of oo silk.

DETAILS OF PROCEDURE The peritoneum is opened and the abdomen explored with special attention given to the gallbladder, duodenal bulb, and the size of the esophageal hiatus. A considerable portion of the stomach may be up in the chest as a result of the enlarged hiatus opening.

It is important to develop good exposure of the margins of the esophageal hiatus. The exposure is improved by dividing the relatively avascular triangular ligament of the left lobe of the liver and rotating it toward the midline (FIGURE 2). It is retracted medially by a large S retractor applied to a moist pad placed over the mobilized left lobe (FIGURE 3).

The peritoneum over the esophagus is incised and the esophagus mobilized with the index finger of the right hand (Chapter 23, FIGURE 7). The vagus nerves are not divided unless the operative, laboratory, roentgenographic, and clinical studies verified gastric hypersecretion with evidence of duodenal deformity and a concurrent drainage procedure such as a pyloroplasty is also planned. It is important to divide and ligate the uppermost portion of the gastrohepatic ligament in order to provide exposure for the fundoplication. The uppermost portion of the gastrohepatic ligament is grasped by a long pair of right-angle clamps (FIGURE 3). The contents between the clamps are divided, and each side is tied with oo silk to ensure adequate control of the left phrenic artery (FIGURE 3). This may include the hepatic branch of the vagus nerve. The cuff of peritoneum at the esophagogastric junction may include considerable extra tissue due to trauma from the hiatus hernia. Additional sutures may be required to control bleeding in this area. Such sutures must not include the vagus nerves unless vagotomy is indicated by an associated duodenal ulcer and measured high acid values. The peritoneum to the left of the esophagogastric junction should be divided meticulously with great care to avoid tearing of the splenic capsule.

Downward traction with a rubber tissue (Penrose) drain about the esophagus is maintained to completely reduce the funds of the stomach into the peritoneal cavity. A small S retractor is introduced posterior to the esophagus to provide exposure to the hiatus (FIGURE 4). The margins of the hiatus are grasped with long Babcock forceps to facilitate the placement of two or three interrupted sutures of o silk for closure of the hiatus posterior to the esophagus (FIGURE 4). The hiatus is narrowed to the point where the index finger can be inserted easily alongside the esophagus. Alternatively, many surgeons prefer to size the opening with passage of a large esophageal dilator usually ranging between 56 and 60 French. **CONTINUES** ▶

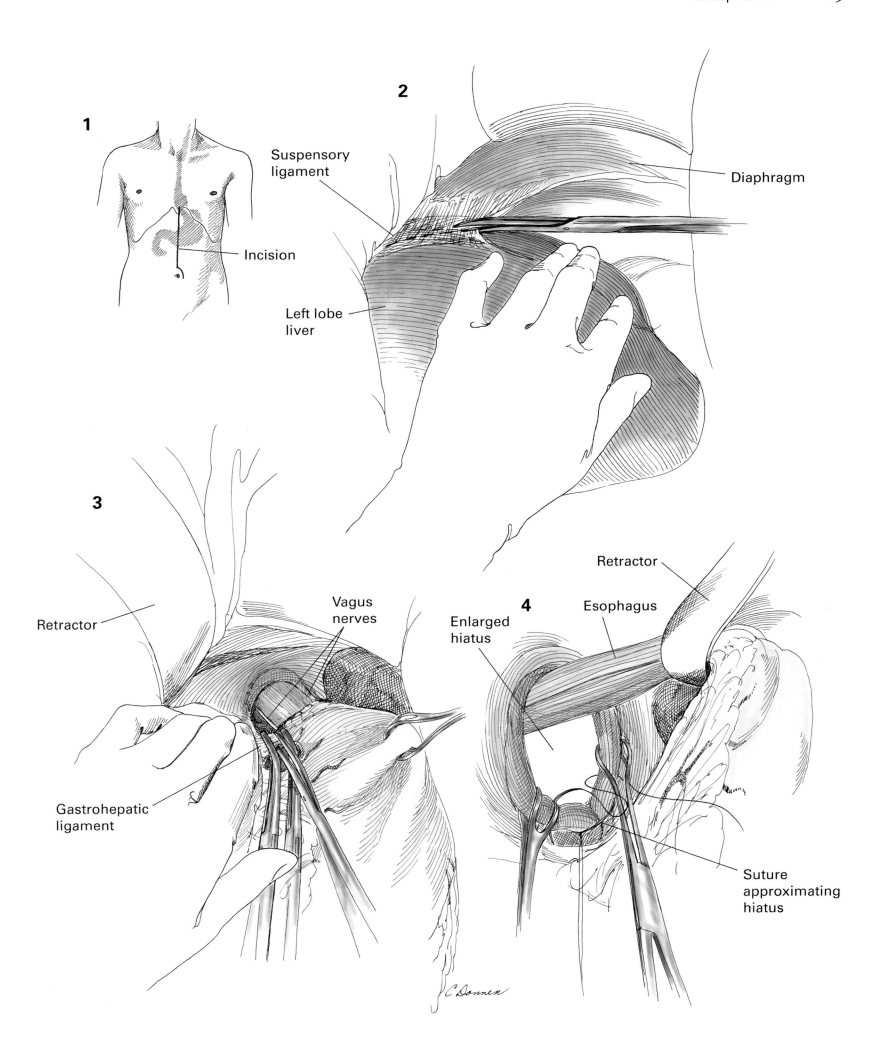

1

Suspensory ligament

Incision

2

Diaphragm

Left lobe liver

3

Retractor

Vagus nerves

Gastrohepatic ligament

4

Retractor

Esophagus

Enlarged hiatus

Suture approximating hiatus

C Donner

DETAILS OF PROCEDURE ◄**CONTINUED**] The effectiveness of the procedure depends upon the adequacy of the fundoplication. It is important to completely mobilize the fundus of the stomach by ligating the gastrosplenic (short gastric) vessels and posterior draining veins of the gastric fundus (FIGURE 5). This must be done carefully to avoid splenic injury. Some prefer to ligate the vessel on the gastric side by a transfixing suture that includes a portion of the gastric wall, alternatively a ultrasonic or bipolar ligating device may be used. A rubber tissue (Penrose) drain is placed around the esophagus to provide downward traction (FIGURE 6). A large (56–60 French) Maloney dilator is inserted into the esophagus before the procedure to prevent undue compression of the esophageal lumen and to ensure performance of a loose fundoplication. The right hand is introduced behind the fundus of the stomach to test the adequacy of the gastric mobilization (FIGURE 6). It is absolutely essential that sufficient fundus be freed up to permit an easy wrap around the lower esophagus. As downward traction is maintained on the esophagus with the rubber drain, the right hand holds the gastric wall around the esophagus. One or more long Babcock forceps are applied to the gastric wall on either side of the esophagus (FIGURE 7). Traction on both sets of forceps makes it unnecessary for the hand of the surgeon to be in the wound. The anterior and posterior gastric walls are approximated with interrupted sutures of oo silk (FIGURE 7). Three interrupted sutures are adequate along a 2- to 3-cm distance. Each suture should include a superficial bite in the esophageal wall and the gastric wall as insurance against the fundoplication "slipping" downward around the gastric cardia (FIGURE 8). In addition, many place an anchoring suture between the gastric wrap and the crus or lateral esophageal wall. This also prevents downward migration of the fundoplication. The large dilator in the esophagus prevents undue constriction of the esophagus. After the traction rubber drain and esophageal dilator are removed, the surgeon introduces the index finger or thumb upward under the plicated gastric wall. Neither undue constriction must exist nor further mobilization of the greater curvature of the fundus be provided. The area of the esophagus is finally inspected to be certain that the vagus nerves have not been injured. A pyloroplasty should be considered if the vagotomy is performed.

CLOSURE Routine closure of the abdominal wall is performed.

POSTOPERATIVE CARE Clear liquids are given in limited amounts on the first postoperative day, followed by a thick liquid diet for the first several days. Gradual return to a full diet occurs over a several week period. ∎

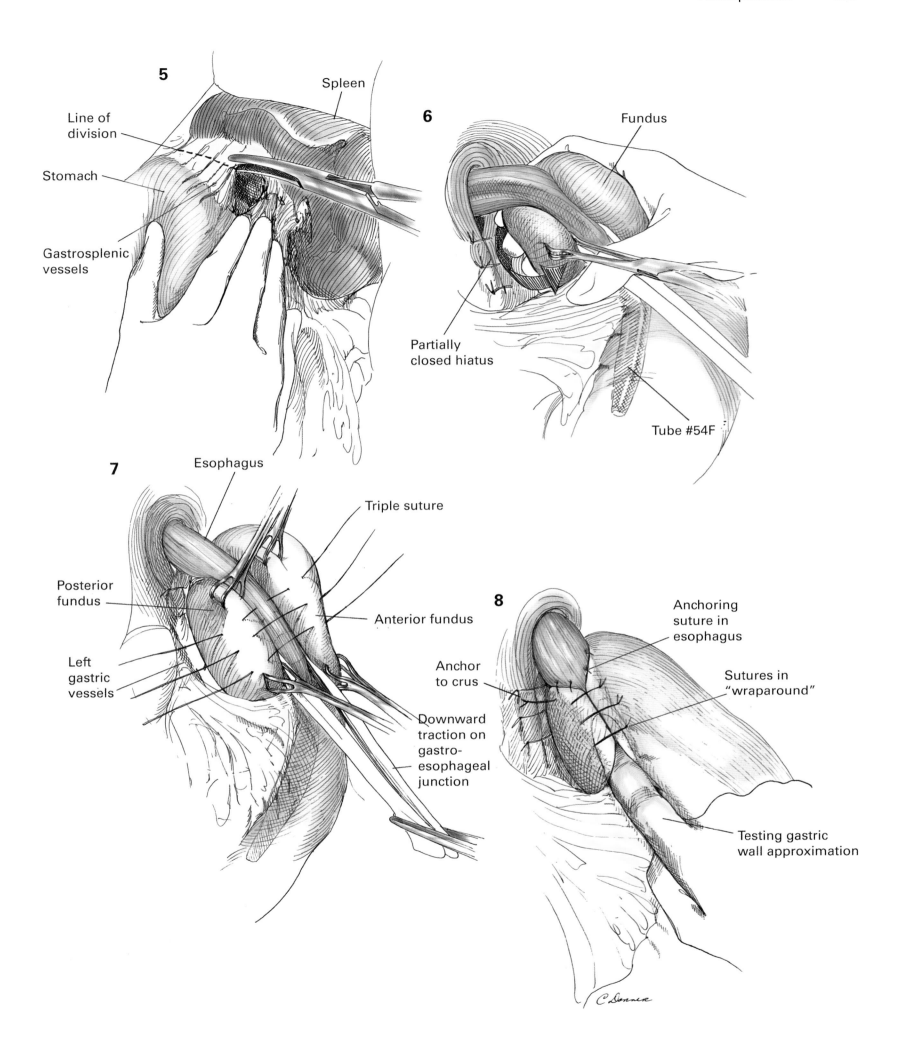

5

Spleen

Line of division

Stomach

Gastrosplenic vessels

6

Fundus

Partially closed hiatus

Tube #54F

7

Esophagus

Triple suture

Posterior fundus

Anterior fundus

Left gastric vessels

Downward traction on gastro-esophageal junction

8

Anchoring suture in esophagus

Anchor to crus

Sutures in "wraparound"

Testing gastric wall approximation

C. Denner

FUNDOPLICATION, LAPAROSCOPIC

INDICATIONS Symptomatic gastroesophageal reflux disease is the most common indication for laparoscopic fundoplication using the floppy 360-degree Nissen technique. The clinical presentation and diagnostic workup are described in detail in Chapter 34. Repeated episodes of aspiration pneumonia or asthma triggered by reflux are significant indications. Intolerance to medical management with proton pump inhibitors, noncompliance with recommended medication regimens, and the cost of lifelong medications represent additional indications for this procedure.

PREOPERATIVE PREPARATION A full general medical evaluation is performed and the usual preanesthesia testing is obtained. Esophageal function studies such as manometry or video esophagography are necessary in order to plan for a full or partial fundoplication and to detect underlying dysmotility not related to reflux. Special emphasis is placed upon the pulmonary workup. Pulmonary function studies are needed in high-risk patients, especially if recurrent episodes of aspiration pneumonia or asthma have occurred. Antacids, acid blockers, and proton pump inhibitors are continued. Perioperative antibiotic coverage is optional.

ANESTHESIA General anesthesia with endotracheal intubation is used. An orogastric (OG) tube is placed for gastric decompression.

POSITION The patient is placed in the supine split-legged or low lithotomy position with the arms out on arm boards or tucked in at the sides (FIGURE 1). The legs are spread sufficiently for the surgeon to be positioned, but the thighs are only partially elevated. Elastic stockings or pneumatic sequential compression stockings are put on the lower legs. The patient is placed in a reverse Trendelenburg position, with at least 30 degrees of elevation to the head of the table.

OPERATIVE PREPARATION The area from the nipples to the pubic symphysis is shaved. Routine skin preparation is performed.

INCISION AND EXPOSURE A combination of 5- and 10-mm ports are placed as shown (FIGURE 1). Following Veress needle access and peritoneal insufflation, a 5- or 10-mm camera port is placed just to the left of the midline, 15 cm caudal to the xiphoid process using a closed technique. Alternatively, an open Hasson technique may be used (Chapter 11). All four quadrants of the abdomen are explored visually. Placement of each of the other selected port sites begins with skin infiltration using a local anesthetic. The local needle can then be passed perpendicularly through the abdominal wall and its entry site verified. A 10-mm port is placed in the left midsubcostal position. Five-mm ports are placed in the epigastrium

just to the right of the midline and through the falciform ligament, and in the far left subcostal positions. In order to expose the esophageal hiatus, a self-retaining liver retractor may be placed in the subxiphoid position, or alternatively, via a right subcostal port (FIGURE 2).

DETAILS OF PROCEDURE The surgeon uses the right and left subcostal ports for the operating instruments (FIGURE 1). The assistant guides the videoscope while providing additional traction and exposure with an instrument passed through the left lateral subcostal port. If there is a hiatal hernia, it is gently reduced and the assistant provides retraction on the gastroesophageal fat pad. The dissection begins with the division of the pars flaccida of the lesser omentum using ultrasonic dissection (FIGURE 3). In thin patients, this is a minimal structure that is easily entered and contains few vessels. However, in overweight patients, the gastrohepatic ligament has significant fatty substance that requires a careful dissection. Exposure for the surgeon may be improved with a careful grasping and elevation of the cut hepatic edge of the ligament. Careful dissection is essential, as some patients may have an aberrant left hepatic artery in this region (FIGURE 4). This vessel must be identified and preserved. The peritoneum over the left crus muscle is carefully dissected and divided until the crus muscle bundle is clearly seen (FIGURE 5). The phrenoesophageal ligament is divided with the ultrasonic dissector to complete the anterior peritoneal dissection (FIGURE 5). With traction on the lesser curve of the stomach, the peritoneum over the right crus muscle is entered. This crus is cleaned posteriorly. The hiatal defect will appear behind the esophagus and the posterior "V" or fan-shaped fusion of the left and right crus will become apparent.

The mobilization of the fundus begins with the surgeon grasping the greater curvature of the stomach with an atraumatic clamp that retracts the stomach anteriorly and to the patient's right (FIGURE 6). The assistant grasps the lateral gastrosplenic ligament and retracts this ligament and spleen to the patient's left. The area of the gastrosplenic ligament is clearly visualized (FIGURE 6). A suitable zone is chosen and opened with blunt dissection. The ultrasonic dissector begins sequential division of the short gastric vessels about 1 cm out from the stomach so as to minimize thermal injury (FIGURE 6). The tissue grasped by the ultrasonic dissector must be clearly visualized, especially in its tip, so as not to partially transect the next short gastric vessel. A partially cut vessel results in bleeding that is difficult to isolate and control without conversion to an open abdominal operation. A better visualization of the lesser sac space and the path of the gastrosplenic ligament can be obtained if the stomach is sequentially grasped along its posterior wall beneath the cut short gastrics (FIGURE 6). **CONTINUES ▶**

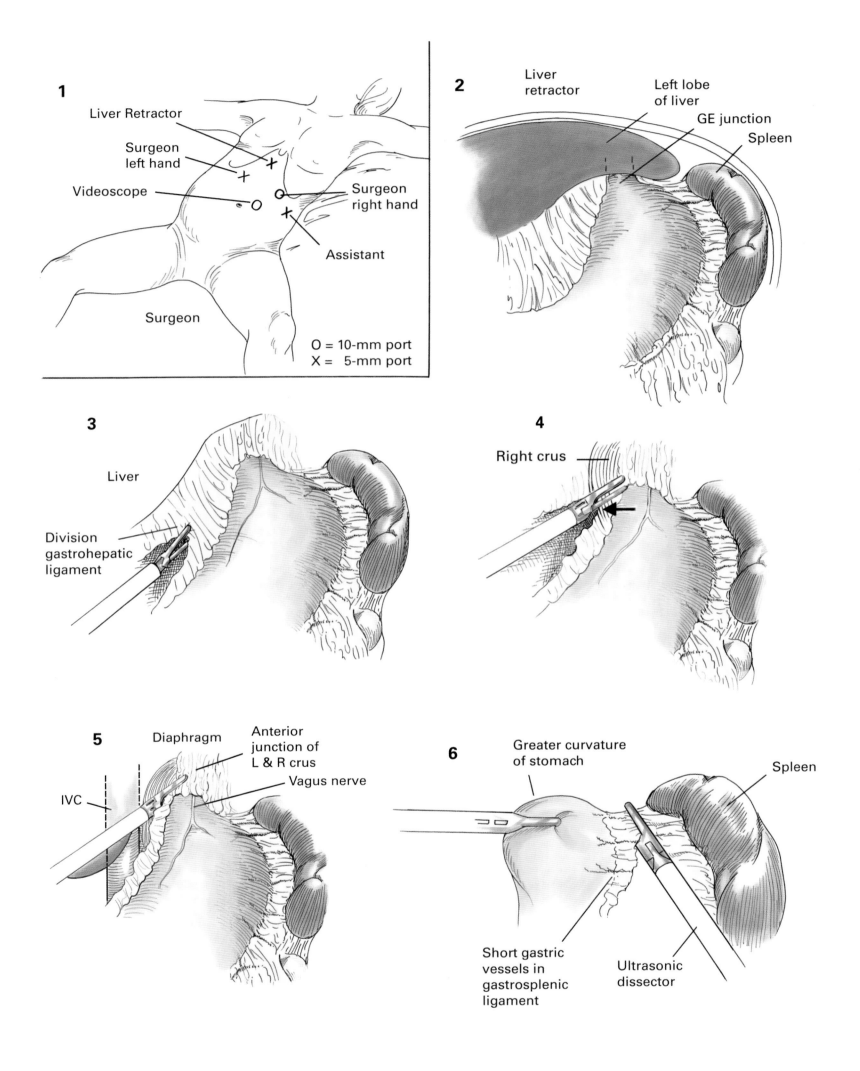

1 Liver Retractor / Surgeon left hand / Videoscope / Surgeon right hand / Assistant / Surgeon / O = 10-mm port / X = 5-mm port

2 Liver retractor / Left lobe of liver / GE junction / Spleen

3 Liver / Division gastrohepatic ligament

4 Right crus

5 Diaphragm / Anterior junction of L & R crus / Vagus nerve / IVC

6 Greater curvature of stomach / Spleen / Short gastric vessels in gastrosplenic ligament / Ultrasonic dissector

DETAILS OF PROCEDURE ◀CONTINUED▶ This ultrasonic dissection continues to divide the short gastrics superiorly until the spleen is free and the left crus of the diaphragm is visualized completing the circumferential esophageal dissection (FIGURE 7). Posterior peritoneal adhesions to the back of the stomach may need division and posterior draining veins should be divided with the ultrasonic dissector to ensure adequate mobility of the fundus. Care must be taken in this region to avoid the left gastric artery.

With the circumferential esophageal dissection achieved (FIGURE 8) a Penrose drain may be placed around the distal esophagus to facilitate caudal retraction (FIGURE 9). Alternatively, the gastroesophageal fat pad may be used to facilitate this retraction. The distal esophagus is mobilized within the mediastinum using blunt dissection to provide a minimum of 3 cm of tension free esophageal length below the diaphragm.

The esophagus is then mobilized further with careful preservation of the left anterior and right posterior vagus nerves. Two to three centimeters of the esophagus should extend into the abdomen without traction. This dissection is performed using gentle elevation and lateral retraction of the gastroesophageal junction with the shaft of an instrument. Dissection should not proceed blindly into the hiatus or above the superior or cephalad top of each crus, as a pleural opening may be created. This usually does not present a significant problem, as the positive-pressure endotracheal ventilation has greater pressure than the CO_2 inflation pressure within the abdomen.

With experience, most surgeons can estimate the extent of the hiatal opening that needs to be closed. In general, two sutures are required to join the two crus muscles posteriorly. This may be accomplished using intracorporeal sutures, (FIGURE 9) or a 10-mm endoscopic suturing instrument containing a 0 non-absorbable braided suture. The suture is passed through the left crus, then the right crus from the patient's left to right (FIGURE 10). A second suture in the crus is usually sufficient.

The floppy 360-degree wrap is created after first determining that there is sufficient gastric mobility. The upper greater curvature of the stomach is passed behind the esophagus. A pair of instruments grasp the stomach in the proposed wrap areas and a "shoeshine"-like maneuver from side to side is performed (FIGURE 11). It is verified that there is more than enough gastric mobility to create a tension-free loose wrap over a several-centimeter zone. This maneuver may reveal the need for further division of short gastric vessels along the lower aspect of the greater curvature of the stomach. The orogastric tube is withdrawn and the anesthesiologist passes a 56- to 60-French esophageal dilator (FIGURE 12). It is essential that the tapered tip of this dilator is passed fully into the stomach so as not to undersize the esophagus. With the dilator in place, the adequacy of the hiatal opening is verified by examining the posterior approximation of the right and left crus. In addition, the right and left gastric wraps are tested for sufficient length to cover a zone of 2 to 3 cm of intra-abdominal esophagus (FIGURE 12). Construction of the wrap requires three sutures that begin at the cephalad extent of the fundoplication (FIGURE 13). Each suture is placed as a triple bite (FIGURE 14A), the midportion of which includes a seromuscular partial-thickness component of the esophagus. A final suture anchors the wrap to the right crus (FIGURE 14) or lateral esophageal wall to prevent distal migration of the wrap around the gastric cardia.

CLOSURE The fascia of the 10-mm port sites are sutured with one or two delayed absorbable 00 sutures. The skin is approximated with fine absorbable subcuticular sutures. Adhesive skin strips and dry sterile dressings are placed.

POSTOPERATIVE CARE Gastric decompression with a nasogastric tube is usually not required. Clear liquids are given as tolerated and the diet is advanced to soft, easily chewed foods. Some patients may experience transient dysphagia, which can be controlled with dietary changes. ■

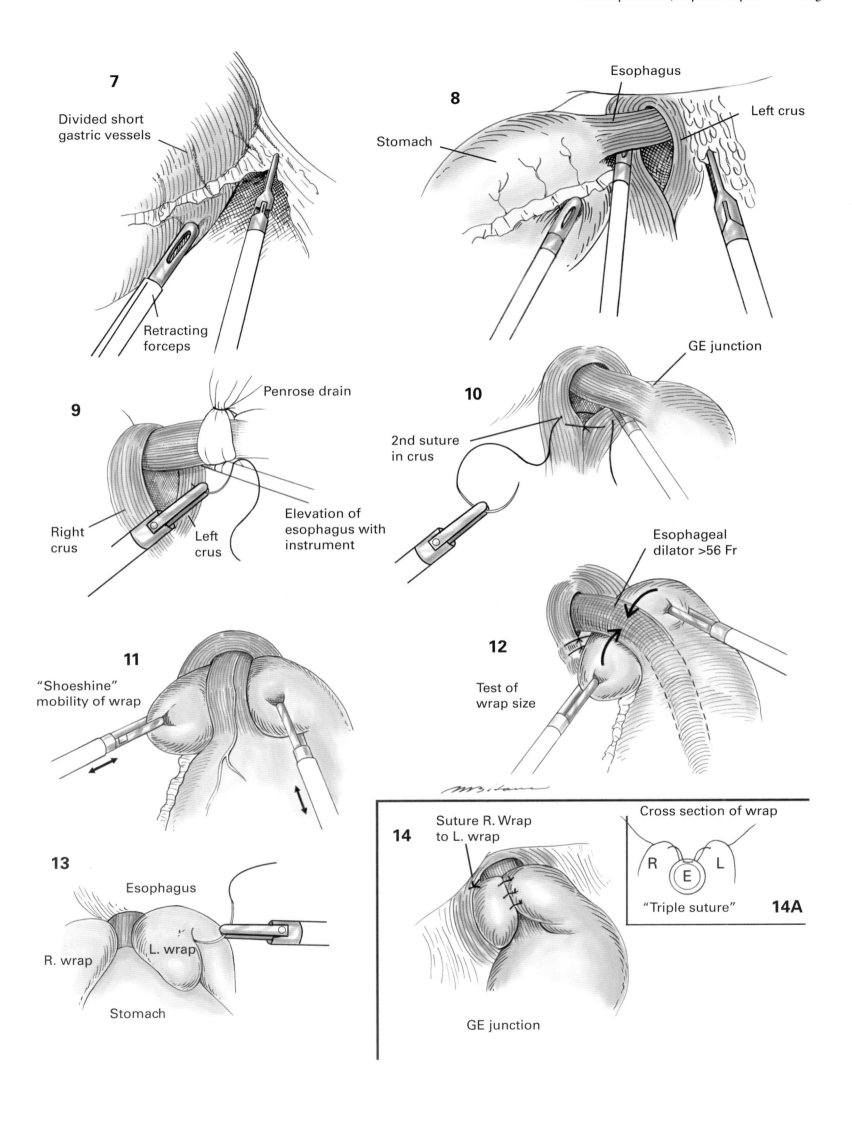

7

Divided short gastric vessels

Retracting forceps

8

Esophagus

Left crus

Stomach

9

Penrose drain

Elevation of esophagus with instrument

Right crus

Left crus

10

GE junction

2nd suture in crus

Esophageal dilator >56 Fr

11

"Shoeshine" mobility of wrap

12

Test of wrap size

13

Esophagus

R. wrap

L. wrap

Stomach

14

Suture R. Wrap to L. wrap

GE junction

Cross section of wrap

R   E   L

"Triple suture"   **14A**

ESOPHAGEAL MYOTOMY, LAPAROSCOPIC

INDICATIONS The manifestations of achalasia include chest pain, dysphagia, and in late situations malnutrition. Most patients have been treated for some length of time for the presumptive diagnosis of gastroesophageal reflux disease, however upon objective evaluation, the classic findings of aperistalsis of the esophagus and nonrelaxation of the lower esophageal sphincter are realized. Radiographic evidence may demonstrate long-standing disease and in some situations a dilated and distended esophagus.

The treatment of achalasia can be multidisciplinary. Endoscopic surveillance and exclusion of malignancy or mechanical obstruction is important. Injection of botulin toxin into the lower esophageal sphincter has shown to provide relief, although this relief is temporary and may further complicate later definitive therapy. Botox injection for the treatment of achalasia should only be considered as a temporizing measure or as palliative therapy in selected patients. Pneumatic dilatation of the lower esophageal sphincter with a 3- or 4-cm balloon can be considered. This should be done under fluoroscopic guidance and reports have demonstrated reasonable success rates, especially when combined with salvage therapy or recurrent dilation. Despite these successes, surgical intervention remains as the first-line therapy for most patients and is associated with good outcomes. Peroral endoscopic myotomy is an emerging therapy that allows for division of the circular muscle fibers alone via a transoral–transmucosal route and is under evaluation.

PREOPERATIVE PREPARATION Patients should be screened for other medical conditions, careful attention should be paid to the risk of pulmonary disease as chronic aspiration maybe a significant factor. Malnutrition likewise should be addressed. When a dilated esophagus is seen or a chronic disease is suspected, then careful preparation of the esophagus should be undertaken. Many patients will require a liquid only diet for several days prior to surgery to allow most of the solid contents of the esophagus to be gone at the time of induction of anesthesia and operative intervention. In planning the operative approach, the two standard approaches have been the left chest or through the abdomen. After extensive experience with laparoscopic exposure and laparoscopic manipulation of the gastroesophageal junction the preferred method is now a transabdominal laparoscopic Heller myotomy.

ANESTHESIA Patients are given a general anesthetic with careful attention to prevent aspiration upon induction.

POSITION Patients are placed in a supine position and can be in a leg split position with the arms extended, the operating surgeon can then stand between the patients' leg with an assistance on each side.

OPERATIVE PREPARATION The patient is kept NPO after midnight. Standard prophylactic antibiotics are administered within 1 hour of the incision. Prophylaxis for thromboembolism is administered.

DETAILS OF THE PROCEDURE A variable trocar positioning can be utilized, however standard approach would include a midline periumbilical camera trocar with four additional trocars placed in the hypochondrium for #1 retraction of the liver, #2 and #3 for operative manipulation, and port #4 is usually added after placement of the others (not shown in figure) for retraction of the stomach (FIGURE 1). After retraction of the left lobe of the liver anteriorly, the esophagus is approached through the gastrohepatic ligament (FIGURE 2). The dissection of the right crura (FIGURE 3B), is followed by the left and then circumferential dissection of the gastroesophageal junction is performed with mobilization of the distal esophagus into the abdomen. FIGURE 3A shows the anatomy of the vagus nerves which should be identified and preserved throughout the dissection. The placement of an atraumatic Penrose drain around the GE junction allows for gentle inferior traction aiding the mobilization of the proximal esophagus. The dissection should be carried into the mediastinum as high as practically possible, however rarely is further opening of the hiatus necessary. Some mobilization of the proximal stomach maybe necessary although division of the short gastric vessels is rarely needed.

After complete dissection, the fat pad overlying the gastroesophageal junction should be divided using careful electrocautery or ultrasonic dissection to allow complete visualization of the GE junction. The anterior and posterior vagus nerves should be identified and preserved throughout the course of the dissection. When approached laparoscopically, the myotomy can be made on the anterior or right anterolateral aspect of the esophagus parallel to the anterior vagus, preventing injury (FIGURE 4A). This section is started approximately 2 cm above the GE junction using a combination of blunt and judicious use of energy to identify first the longitudinal muscles, and then the circular muscles. Once the submucosal plane is entered, blunt dissection allows careful separation of the submucosa from the circular coat of fibers which then can be divided, first in a proximal fashion 6 to 8 cm above the gastroesophageal junction and then distally onto the stomach approximately 2 to 3 cm (FIGURE 4B). Caution should be used at the distal extent as the gastric mucosa can become adherent to the muscular fibers at this juncture. Following the careful myotomy, the area should be carefully inspected for injuries to the submucosa. Intraoperative endoscopy can be utilized to insufflate and check for leaks as well as to identify the Z line to ensure that the myotomy has been carried down well onto the stomach.

Partial fundoplication is a routine part of laparoscopic esophageal myotomy. A posterior Toupet fundoplication can be created by placing the redundant portion of the proximal stomach posterior to the esophagus, fixing it to the posterior crura, and then to the right side and left side of the cut myotomy (FIGURE 5). Alternatively, a Dor fundoplication or an anterior fundoplication can be created by taking a redundant portion of the fundus of the stomach and placing it anterior to the esophagus, placing sutures first on the left side of the cut myotomy (FIGURE 6A). Then the redundant portion of the stomach is placed over the myotomy anteriorly and secured by placing sutures on the right lateral aspect of the esophagus (FIGURE 6B). Trocar sites greater than 5 mL should be sutured in the fascia and the skin closed in a routine fashion.

POSTOPERATIVE CARE Most patients can be started on a full liquid diet on the evening of surgery. Early mobilization is encouraged, however heavy lifting and straining should be avoided. Patients should be advised that their dysphagia may improve slowly over the first few weeks following surgery as postoperative edema resolves. Surveillance endoscopy is important over the course of the patient's life or screening for malignancies. ■

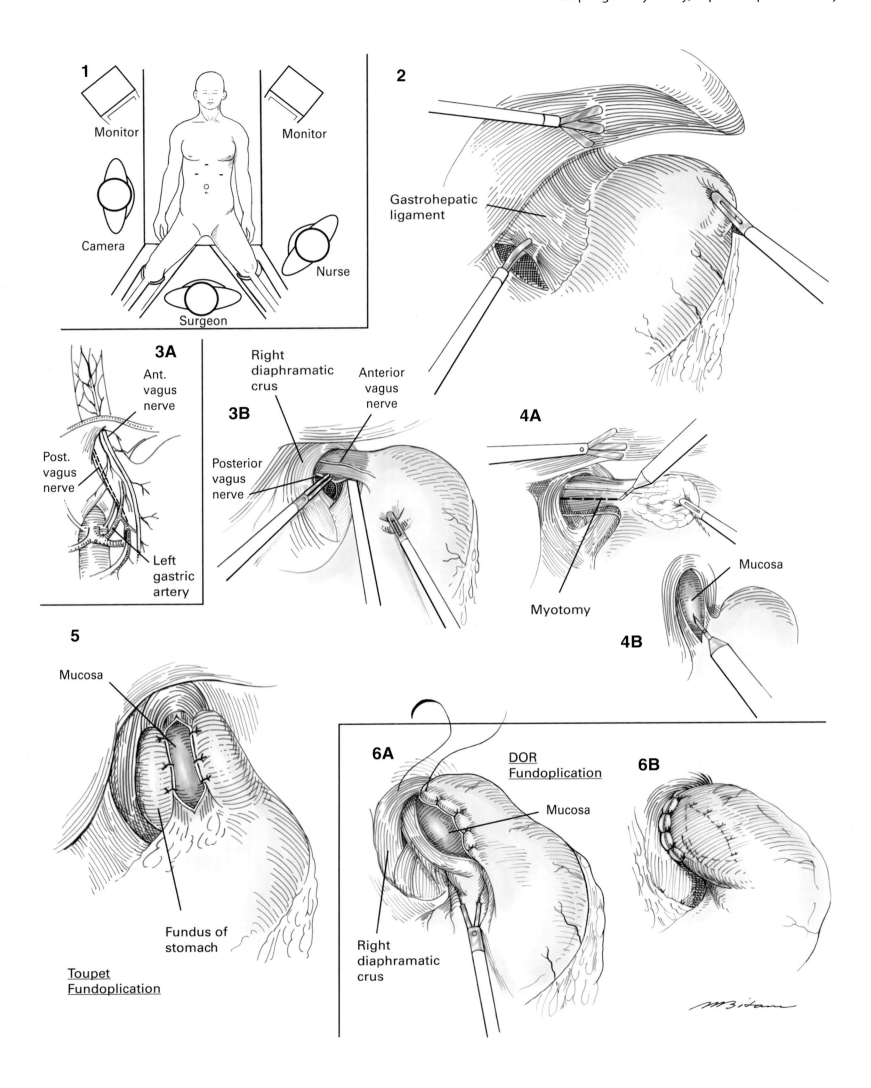

1

Monitor

Monitor

Camera

Nurse

Surgeon

2

Gastrohepatic ligament

3A

Ant. vagus nerve

Post. vagus nerve

Left gastric artery

3B

Right diaphramatic crus

Anterior vagus nerve

Posterior vagus nerve

4A

Myotomy

4B

Mucosa

5

Mucosa

Fundus of stomach

Toupet Fundoplication

6A

DOR Fundoplication

Mucosa

Right diaphramatic crus

6B

ROUX-EN-Y GASTRIC BYPASS, LAPAROSCOPIC

INDICATIONS Selection of patients for bariatric procedures is based on evidence-based guidelines. Patients must have failed dietary therapy and have a body mass index (BMI) greater than 40 kg/m² without associated medical conditions or a BMI greater than 35 kg/m² with associated medical condition(s). In addition, practical considerations for the patient to be a candidate for the procedure include psychiatric stability, a motivated attitude, and comprehension of the nature of the procedure and the changes in eating that will follow the procedure.

PREOPERATIVE PREPARATION A team approach is necessary for the optimal care of the patient with morbid obesity. Prior to the initial clinic visit, the patient must provide evidence of a medically supervised diet, counseling and referral from a primary care physician, and completion of a reading assignment to include a comprehensive review of bariatric surgery including the types of procedures, expected results, and possible complications or attendance at a seminar regarding the same. At the initial visit the patient is expected to attend a group session on bariatric surgery and a presentation by the nutritionalist on dietary issues preoperatively and postoperatively. In addition, the patient has individual assessment and counseling with the surgical team and the dietician. Subsequent evaluations may include, as indicated, a full psychological evaluation, specialty medical evaluation, ultrasound of the gallbladder, and a pulmonary evaluation including baseline arterial blood gases. Finally, preoperative assessment by anesthesiology is warranted.

ANESTHESIA General endotracheal tube anesthesia is required for the procedure. The anesthesiologist should be prepared for the potential of a difficult intubation including the availability of flexible bronchoscopy to assist placement of the endotracheal tube.

POSITION The patient is transferred to the operating room table with a lateral transfer device. The patient is placed in the supine position and secured to the operating room table with Velcro leg straps and a spindle sheet for the pelvis. The arms are placed on arm boards, and sometimes the left arm is tucked at the side. Additional securing of the patient to the table with tape may be appropriate. FIGURE 1A shows the room setup.

OPERATIVE PREPARATION Preoperative antibiotics are administered and venous thromboembolism prophylaxis is employed. Hair on the abdominal wall is removed with a clipper. A Foley catheter is placed and an orogastric tube is positioned.

INCISION AND DETAILS OF THE OPERATION The abdomen is prepared and draped in the standard surgical fashion. A small transverse skin incision is made in the left upper quadrant through which a Veress needle is inserted and pneumoperitoneum is established to a maximum pressure of 15 mm Hg. The Veress needle is withdrawn and a 12-mm port is placed. A 10-mm 30-degree laparoscope is inserted into the abdominal cavity and the peritoneal cavity and viscera inspected to ensure that there is no evidence of port insertion injury. Next, a supraumbilical 10-mm port, a right upper quadrant 15-mm port, and right and left upper quadrant 5-mm ports are placed under direct visualization (FIGURE 1B). The greater omentum is elevated, exposing the transverse colon and ligament of Treitz (FIGURE 2A).

In some centers, staple lines are reinforced with absorbable material such as polyglycolic/trimethylene carbonate copolymer fiber. The staple lines that may benefit from reinforcement are so indicated. The jejunum is divided approximately 30 cm from the ligament of Treitz with an endoscopic stapler (FIGURE 2B). The small bowel mesentery is divided with an endoscopic linear stapler with reinforcement to provide extra length to the Roux limb. It may be helpful to mark the proximal portion of the efferent limb of the Roux loop of the jejunum with a blue Penrose drain in order to avoid confusing the divided ends of the jejunum. This will be later anastomosed to the gastric pouch. The efferent Roux limb is then measured 150 cm from the division of the bowel (FIGURE 2B), at which point a side-to-side jejunojejunostomy is performed between the distal Roux limb and the biliopancreatic limb (FIGURE 3). The two small bowel segments are aligned along their antimesenteric surface with a 2-0 Polysorb suture. Two small enterotomies are made on the antimesenteric surface with an ultrasonic device. A side-to-side jejunojejunostomy is performed with an endoscopic linear stapler. The enterotomy is closed transversely with an endoscopic linear stapler.

A 2-0 nonabsorbable antitorsion suture is placed. The mesenteric defect at the jejunojejunostomy is closed with a running 2-0 nonabsorbable suture. The Roux limb is then traced back proximally to verify appropriate orientation. The greater omentum is divided with the ultrasonics device, taking care to avoid injury to the underlying transverse colon (FIGURE 2A). This provides space for passage of the Roux limb in an antecolic fashion to the gastric pouch.

The patient is placed in the reverse Trendelenburg position and the orogastric tube is removed. A liver retractor is inserted in one of the proximal ports. The left lateral segment of the liver is retracted anteriorly exposing the gastroesophageal junction. The pars flaccida is divided bluntly providing exposure to the lesser sac. The lesser omentum is divided with an endoscopic linear stapler with reinforcement to the lesser curvature approximately 4 cm from the gastroesophageal junction. Once this is completed, a distal gastrotomy is made with the ultrasonics device (FIGURE 4). A 25-mm circular stapler is usually employed for the gastrojejunostomy. This may be reinforced. The anvil of the stapler is inserted into the stomach through the distal gastrotomy. A second small gastrotomy is made along the lesser curvature approximately 4 cm distal to the gastroesophageal junction using an articulating dissector and an ultrasonics device (FIGURE 5). The tip of the anvil is delivered through the proximal gastrotomy (FIGURE 6). The distal gastrotomy is then closed with an endoscopic stapler.

Attention is then turned toward creation of a 30-mL gastric pouch (FIGURE 6). The first staple line is made transversely, closely approximating the anvil with a reinforced endoscopic linear stapler (3.8-mm staple). The next several staple lines are made longitudinally toward the angle of His with a reinforced endoscopic linear stapler. Complete division of the stomach is verified by laparoscopic visualization. Next, the proximal efferent Roux limb is brought in an antecolic fashion to the gastric pouch. If placed, the blue Penrose drain is removed and the proximal 3 cm of the mesentery is divided with an endo-GIA gray stapler. The jejunal staple line is opened with the ultrasonic device. The 25-mm circular stapler is inserted into the enterotomy of the Roux limb (FIGURE 7). The spike of the circular stapler is advanced through the antimesenteric surface of the jejunum. The anvil of the gastric pouch is connected to the stapler (FIGURE 7). A stapled gastrojejunostomy is performed (FIGURE 8). The jejunal enterotomy is closed with an endoscopic linear stapler resecting the distal 3 cm of the Roux limb that is passed from the field. A 2-0 absorbable antitension suture is placed at the gastrojejunal anastomosis.

Next, an intraoperative upper endoscopy is performed to determine patency of the gastrojejunal anastomosis and the presence of intraluminal bleeding. If bleeding is encountered, it may be controlled with a reinforcing suture. The gastric pouch is insufflated under saline. No bubbles should be identified, indicating absence of an anastomotic leak. If bubbles are seen, the staple line should be oversewn.

CLOSURE The liver retractor is removed. The fascia of the 12-mm port site is closed with two interrupted 0 absorbable sutures. It may be helpful to use a Carter-Thomason port closure device for this purpose. The remainder of the ports are withdrawn under direct visualization and inspected for evidence of bleeding. The camera is withdrawn and the abdomen is deflated. The subcutaneous tissues are irrigated with saline solution and all skin incisions are closed with 4-0 absorbable subcuticular sutures. The skin is cleaned and dried. Steri-Strips are applied.

POSTOPERATIVE CARE Appropriate fluid resuscitation is required and urine output monitored with a Foley catheter for the first 24 hours. A nasogastric tube is not necessary. A contrast study may be obtained on postoperative day 1 to determine the presence or absence of a leak from the gastrojejunostomy or obstruction. If there is no leak or obstruction, or in the absence of a contrast study, if the patient exhibits no tachycardia or temperature greater than 100°F, then a trial of water with advancement to liquids as tolerated may be started. The timing of discharge is usually 2 to 3 days but may be influenced by many factors. The patient is seen within 30 days to assess oral intake and wound healing. Patients with diabetes may experience decreasing insulin requirements and even hypoglycemic episodes that precede significant weight loss. Long-term follow-up is required in all patients. ■

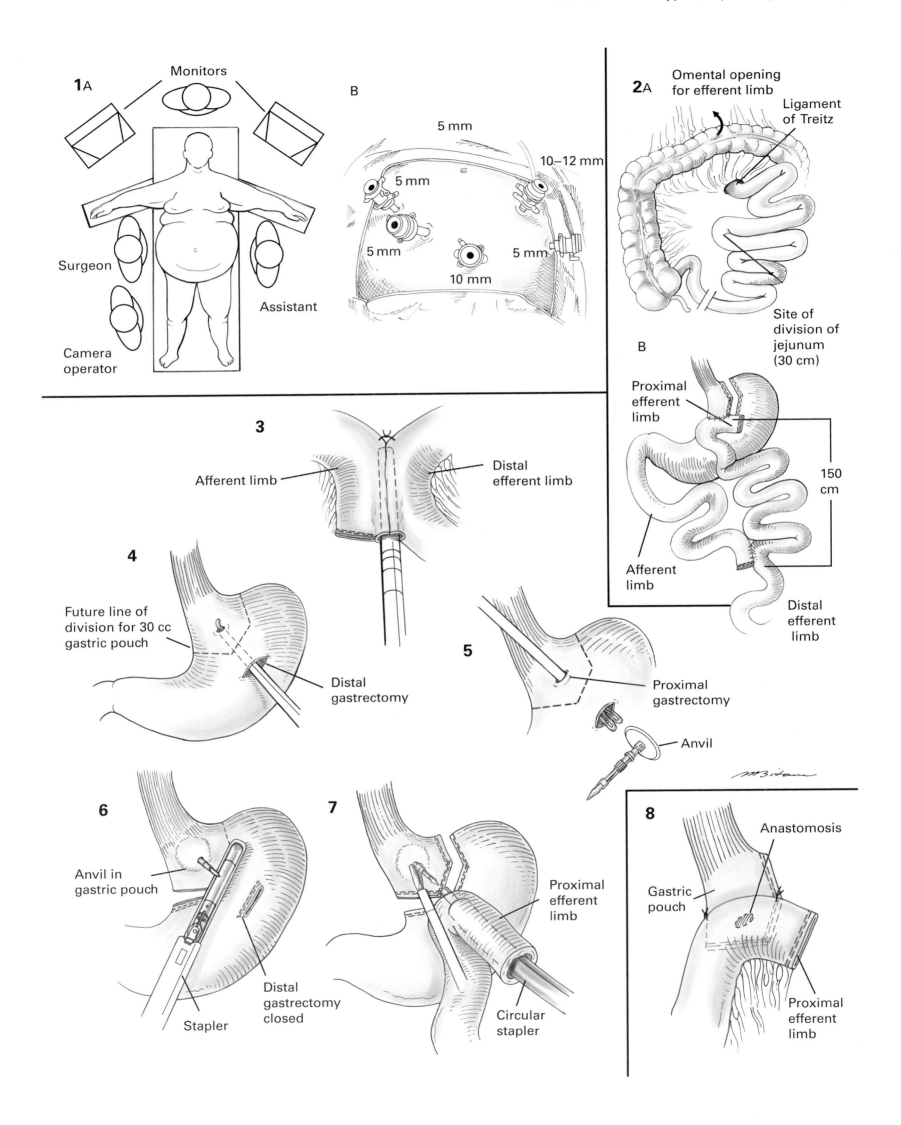

1A Monitors

Surgeon

Camera operator

Assistant

B 5 mm

5 mm

5 mm

10–12 mm

5 mm

10 mm

2A Omental opening for efferent limb

Ligament of Treitz

Site of division of jejunum (30 cm)

B Proximal efferent limb

150 cm

Afferent limb

Distal efferent limb

3 Afferent limb

Distal efferent limb

4 Future line of division for 30 cc gastric pouch

Distal gastrectomy

5 Proximal gastrectomy

Anvil

6 Anvil in gastric pouch

Distal gastrectomy closed

Stapler

7 Proximal efferent limb

Circular stapler

8 Anastomosis

Gastric pouch

Proximal efferent limb

SLEEVE GASTRECTOMY, LAPAROSCOPIC

INDICATIONS The vertical sleeve gastrectomy is an accepted primary or staged bariatric procedure with indications that follow current NIH guidelines. Body mass index (BMI) of greater than 40 kg/m², or greater than 35 kg/m² with significant comorbid conditions related to obesity, as well as, failure of conservative medical management needs to be documented. Other common requirements include medical, dietary, and psychological evaluations, and a history of past attempts at medical weight management. Informed consent should include a dietary and behavior modification educational program to ensure patients are aware of how the operation will impact their ability to eat and provide strategies for lifetime success. Sleeve gastrectomy may be chosen over other bariatric procedures for its minimal malabsorption due to normal gastrointestinal continuity, including access to the duodenum, its lower risk of marginal ulceration, and patient preference. Relative contraindications include severe gastroesophageal reflux disease.

PREOPERATIVE PREPARATION As with all morbidly obese patients comorbidities should be evaluated and optimized before surgical intervention. This may include screening for and treating obstructive sleep apnea, an appropriate cardiac and pulmonary functional evaluation, airway evaluation, and optimizing glucose control in diabetics. It is suggested that these patients have an upper endoscopy to evaluate anatomy and diagnose functional or pathologic changes before resection. All patients receive preoperative antibiotics and prophylaxis for deep vein thrombosis (DVT) per institutional guidelines. In addition, there is some evidence that having patients on a "liver shrink" (low calorie, low fat) diet preoperatively can help make the operation technically easier by decreasing the volume of the liver and improving compliance of a thick abdominal wall.

ANESTHESIA The operation is performed with general endotracheal anesthesia. Difficulties are related to morbid obesity and may include a difficult airway, difficult venous access and challenges with monitoring, and positioning the patient due to their large body habitus. Communication with anesthesia is essential to the safe performance of this operation especially related to orogastric tube management, Bougie placement, fluid management, and medications to prevent postoperative nausea and emesis. Postextubation pathways should be in place related to obstructive sleep apnea (Continuous Positive Airway Pressure-CPAP and Bilevel Continuous Airway Pressure-BiPAP use) and pain management.

POSITION The operation is typically performed with the patient supine or in modified lithotomy with a split leg table (FIGURE 1A). Morbidly obese patients should be secured well to the table to avoid movement when in steep reverse Trendelenburg, as well as, have pressure points well padded to avoid injury and risk of rhabdomyolysis. Knowledge of table capacities, foot rests, and table extenders are helpful and should be available in the operating room.

OPERATIVE PREPARATION Patients should receive preoperative antibiotics dose appropriate for their body weight per institutional guidelines, timely DVT prophylaxis and correct-sized sequential compression devices placed on their lower extremities. A urinary catheter may sometimes be placed. An orogastric tube should be placed by anesthesia before initial trocar access. Bougies, staplers, extra-long instrumentation, and energy device preferences should be available as needed.

INCISION AND EXPOSURE Typical access to the abdomen is achieved by the method the surgeon is most comfortable performing, however due to the thickness of the abdominal wall, left upper quadrant access with a Veress needle or optical viewing trocar has been shown to be safe. Trocar position is chosen to allow dissection and manipulation of both the inferior aspect of the stomach and the gastroesophageal junction at the angle of His (FIGURE 1B). The initial 5-mm trocar is placed in the abdomen around the left, midclavicular line, a hands-width below the costal margin. The abdomen is explored with a 5-mm, 30-degree laparoscope and additional 5-mm periumbilical and 5-mm left-lateral trocars are placed relative to the position of the initial trocar and distance to the stomach. A 15-mm trocar is placed to the right of the supraumbilical trocar (FIGURE 1B). As the staplers are placed through this port its position should be such that the stapler insertion can be close to parallel to the lesser curve of the stomach. A subxiphoid trocar is placed for liver retraction and a flexible liver retractor may be secured to the bed on the patient's right (FIGURE 3). The operation is best performed with the patient in some degree of reverse Trendelenburg.

DETAILS OF THE PROCEDURE A vertical sleeve gastrectomy involves a greater curve resection to fashion a longitudinal gastric tube that produces a restrictive bariatric procedure. To perform this procedure the greater curve must be dissected free of all its attachments from a point 5 cm proximal to the pylorus

to the angle of His and left crura. To begin the operation the camera is placed in the midclavicular, left upper quadrant port site and held by the assistant on the patient's left side who also uses the left-lateral port to assist. The surgeon stands on the patient's right and uses an atraumatic grasper and energy device in the 15-mm and 5-mm right-sided ports. Typical dissection begins along the greater curve near the angularis in an area where it is easier to gain access to the lesser sac. The gastroepiploic vessels are divided close to the stomach and this is continued up toward the short gastric vessels (FIGURE 2). Division of the vessels can be performed using bipolar or ultrasonic dissectors. Extra care must be taken as you approach the superior pole of the spleen where the stomach may be in close approximation to the spleen to avoid thermal injury to the stomach or cause bleeding (FIGURE 3). At this point the energy device may be moved to the left lateral most port to facilitate dissection. The dissection continues to completely mobilize the angle of His until the left crura is identified. Dissection and division of the most proximal and posterior short gastric vessel is often necessary. When this dissection is complete the hiatus should be examined for evidence of a hernia. If one is found the sac and stomach should be reduced and the crura repaired. Once proximal dissection is completed, attention is then taken distally to divide the greater curve attachments to approximately 5 cm proximal to the pylorus (FIGURE 4). Once the greater curve is completely dissected free of attachments and hemostasis is achieved, attention is taken to ensure the stomach is mobilized posteriorly. Only attachments on the most medial aspect of the posterior wall of the lesser curve should be left behind in order to allow the staplers to be safely fired and be able to divide the stomach completely.

The orogastric tube is removed and a nontapered Bougie is placed into the stomach under laparoscopic vision and directed along the lesser curve toward the pylorus below the divided attachments (FIGURE 5). Sequential firings of a stapler are used to divide the stomach along the Bougie. The initial firing begins at a point approximately 5 cm proximal to the pylorus and should be fired at angle that is close to parallel with the proximal lesser curve (FIGURE 5). With each subsequent firing, care should be taken to ensure the stapler is in close proximity to the Bougie but avoids excessive tension on the tissue. In addition, care should be taken to have nearly equal lengths of anterior and posterior stomach in the sleeve to avoid "spiraling" the sleeve, which can lead to future complications. As the division approaches the angle of His many surgeons will angle the stapler around the esophageal fat pad and preserve it. Once the greater curve is completely amputated (FIGURE 6) the stomach is removed through the 15-mm port site with or without a specimen retrieval bag.

The Bougie is removed and the sleeve should be examined intraoperatively for length and caliber, integrity of the staple line, hemostasis, and to identify areas of potential narrowing from technical errors. This may all be done with careful upper endoscopy.

Technical variations of the procedure include varying stapler sizes that best match staple height to the thickness of the tissue, adding buttress material to some or all of the stapler firings, oversewing of the staple lines, and Bougie size. Bougie size may be varied to optimize weight loss versus prevention of complications such as leaks of the staple line. Bougie sizes between 32-Fr and 36-Fr have been thought to induce the best weight loss however, sizes under 40-Fr have correlated to higher leak rates.

CLOSURE The 15- and 10-mm port sites are closed with #1 absorbable suture and is facilitated by use of a port closure device. After the fascia is closed the subcutaneous tissues are well irrigated before skin closure. The 5-mm port sites require skin closure only.

POSTOPERATIVE CARE Typical hospital stay after a vertical sleeve gastrectomy is 1 to 2 days and depends upon the patient's ability to tolerate enough liquids to maintain hydration, tolerate their medications with control of their medical problems, ambulate and not have signs or symptoms of potential complications. Orogastric tubes may be used but are not necessary. Diet is advanced to liquids on postoperative day 1 and a liquid/full liquid diet is typically continued for a month. Medication by mouth should be minimized and necessary pills that are not very small may be crushed or converted to liquid form. Nausea, reflux symptoms, and discomfort when eating can be more common after sleeve gastrectomy than other bariatric procedures and the patient should be educated and treated appropriately. Prophylactic regimens beginning in the operating room can be effective.

Centers performing bariatric procedures employ pathways for managing and monitoring sleep apnea, DVT prophylaxis, pain management, early ambulation, and complication identification. Tachycardia continues to be the most consistent sign suggestive of a complication and may include bleeding, leak, or other cardiopulmonary complications. Lifetime follow-up of these patients is recommended. ■

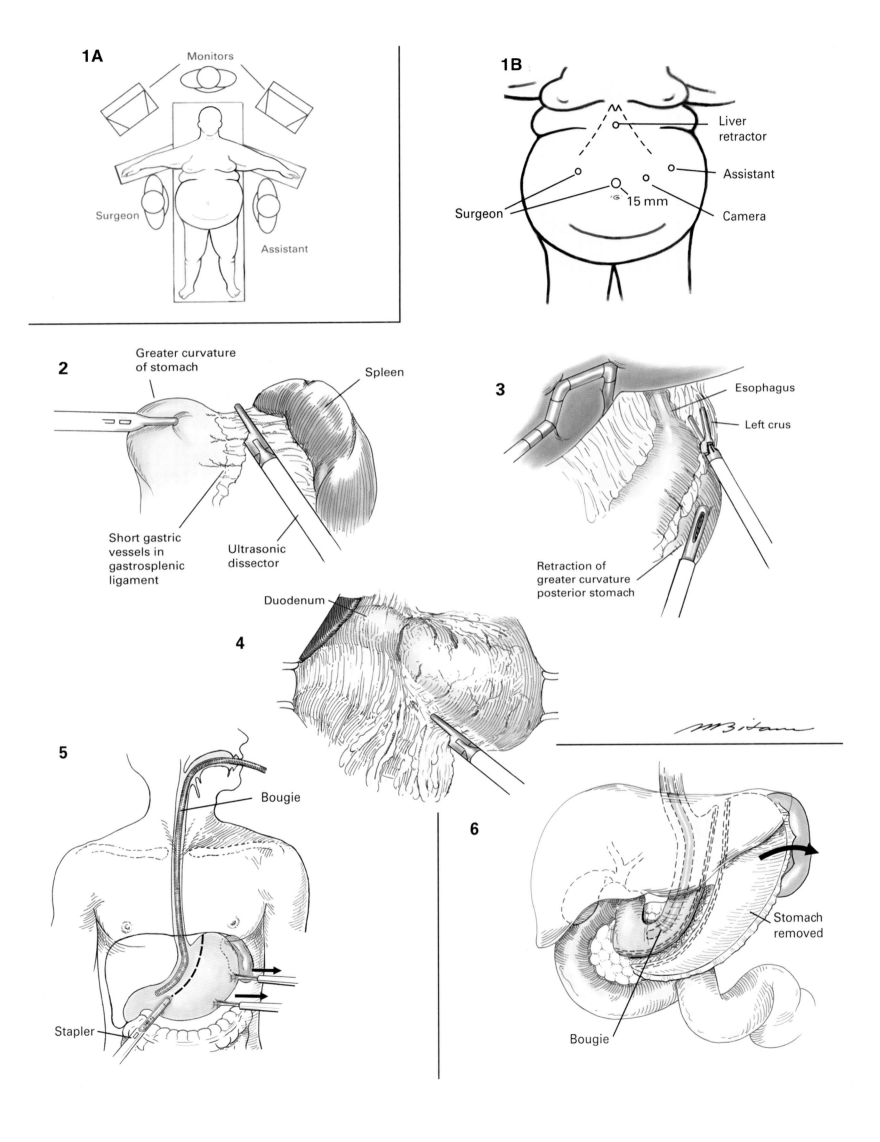

1A Monitors

Surgeon

Assistant

1B Liver retractor

Assistant

Surgeon   15 mm   Camera

2 Greater curvature of stomach

Spleen

Short gastric vessels in gastrosplenic ligament

Ultrasonic dissector

3 Esophagus

Left crus

Retraction of greater curvature posterior stomach

4 Duodenum

5 Bougie

Stapler

6 Stomach removed

Bougie

THE ADJUSTABLE GASTRIC BAND, LAPAROSCOPIC

INDICATIONS A surgeon may select the use of a gastric band to restrict the gastric size. The same selection criteria used for the Roux-en-Y gastric bypass apply.

PREOPERATIVE PREPARATION Preoperative preparation and anesthetic considerations are similar to the gastric bypass.

OPERATIVE PREPARATION Prophylactic antibiotics and venous thromboembolism prophylaxis are employed. A Foley catheter is not inserted into the bladder because of the short duration of the procedure.

POSITIONING The patient is positioned in a modified lithotomy position. The surgeon is positioned between the legs and the assistant to the patient's left. The room setup is shown in FIGURE 1.

INCISION AND DETAILS OF THE OPERATION The port placement is similar to that of a Roux-en-Y gastric bypass, with the exception of a left subcostal 15-mm port that is used to introduce the gastric band (FIGURE 2). Fewer ports may be used in some patients. The patient is placed in the reverse Trendelenburg position. The GE junction is exposed by retracting the liver proximally (FIGURE 3). Blunt dissection is used to create a retrogastric tunnel as shown in FIGURE 4. Retraction of the stomach inferiorly facilitates exposure of the greater curve side of the GE junction. The retrogastric dissection is minimal and the goal should be to create a narrow tunnel that will act to prevent slippage of the device. The tunnel is created superior to the left gastric artery. The orogastric tube placed by anesthesia is removed and a calibration balloon inserted and inflated with 15 mL of saline. The band is placed into the abdomen using an insertion device (FIGURES 5 and 6). It is placed through a 15-mm port or passed directly through the abdominal wall (FIGURE 6). An atraumatic grasper is used to advance the gastric band from the opening along the greater curvature near the angle of His to the previously made opening in the soft tissue along the lesser curvature (FIGURE 7). The band is placed around the stomach just below the intragastric balloon (FIGURE 8). The balloon is deflated and the band is buckled close (FIGURE 9). The orogastric sizing balloon is removed. The final position of the band is shown in FIGURE 9. Several interrupted nonabsorbable sutures (2-0) are used to imbricate the stomach over the band in order to prevent slippage (FIGURE 10). The distal tubing is retrieved through a left paramedian incision at the 15-mm port site (FIGURE 2). A subcutaneous pocket is made for the port used to adjust the band. The port is tacked to the anterior rectus sheath with four 0 nonabsorbable sutures (FIGURE 11).

CLOSURE Closure follows the same procedures outlined for the laparoscopic Roux-en-Y gastric bypass.

POSTOPERATIVE CARE The patient is permitted clear liquids the night of surgery and advanced to an initial diet on postoperative day 1. The patient is discharged within 23 hours of surgery if the initial diet is tolerated. A contrast study to determine band position is not necessary prior to discharge. Adjustment of the band is not performed for 6 weeks. The initial adjustment is performed under fluoroscopic guidance. ■

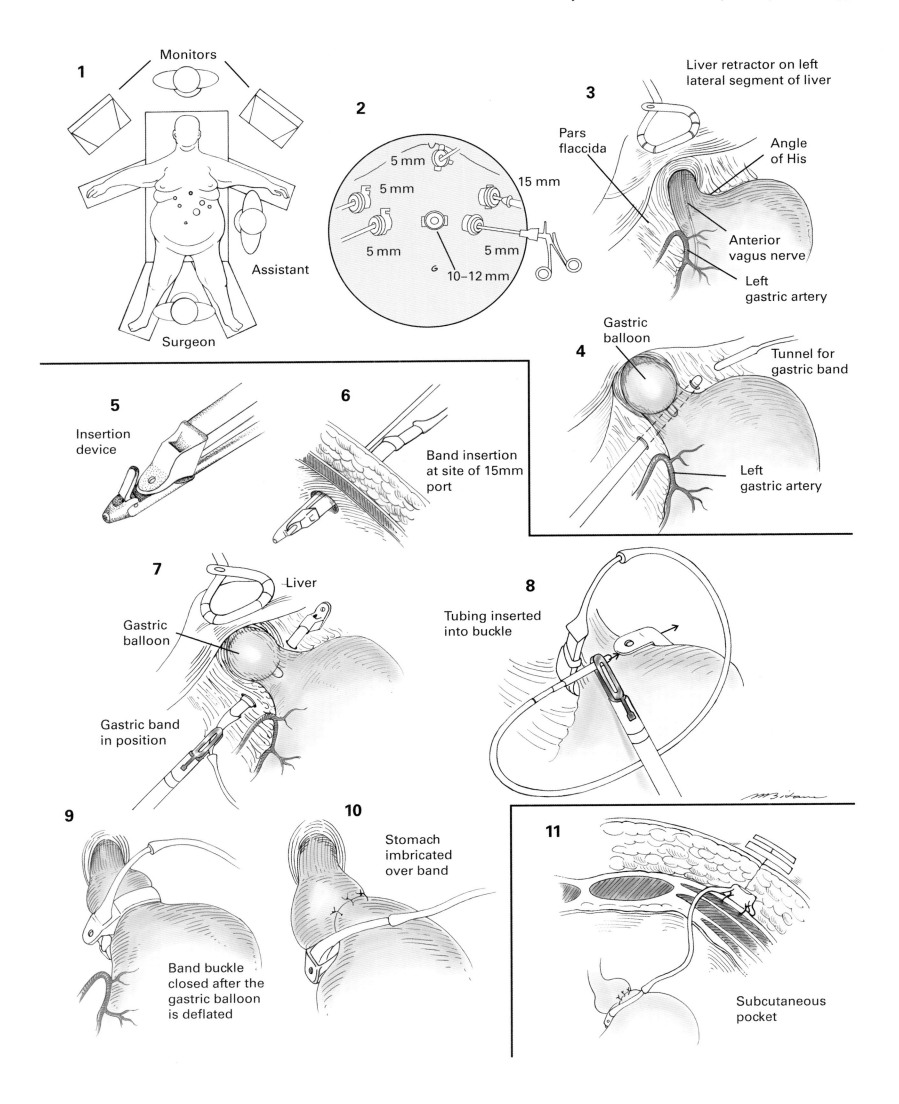

1 Monitors

Assistant

Surgeon

2 5 mm

5 mm

15 mm

5 mm

5 mm

10–12 mm

3 Liver retractor on left lateral segment of liver

Pars flaccida

Angle of His

Anterior vagus nerve

Left gastric artery

4 Gastric balloon

Tunnel for gastric band

Left gastric artery

5 Insertion device

6 Band insertion at site of 15mm port

7 Liver

Gastric balloon

Gastric band in position

8 Tubing inserted into buckle

9 Band buckle closed after the gastric balloon is deflated

10 Stomach imbricated over band

11 Subcutaneous pocket

INDICATIONS Transhiatal esophagectomy with cervical esophagogastrostomy is indicated for most conditions that require esophageal resection and reconstruction. Common indications include carcinoma of the esophagus or gastroesophageal junction, end-stage achalasia, and severe esophageal strictures refractory to endoscopic dilation. This approach may be utilized for primary resection of early stage cancers or Barrett's esophagus with multifocal high-grade dysplasia as well as following neoadjuvant chemoradiation for locally advanced cancers.

Transhiatal esophagectomy is contraindicated in patients with upper or middle third esophageal cancers with concern for tracheobronchial invasion based on imaging studies or bronchoscopy. In patients with a history of previous esophageal surgery, including fundoplication, esophagomyotomy or repair of esophageal perforation, the surgeon must be prepared to convert to a transthoracic approach as transabdominal esophageal mobilization may prove difficult or impossible in these settings. Finally, in cases where carcinoma involves the gastric cardia and may require a significant gastric resection, the colon should be evaluated preoperatively and prepared for use in esophageal reconstruction.

PREOPERATIVE PREPARATION The preoperative workup for patients with esophageal and GE junction cancers includes a thorough history and physical examination, esophagogastroduodenoscopy with biopsy for diagnosis. Esophageal nodules may be adequately staged by endoscopic mucosal resection, whereas larger tumors require endoscopic ultrasound and PET-CT imaging for complete clinical staging. Bronchoscopy should be considered for patients with squamous cell carcinomas, lesions involving the proximal third of the thoracic esophagus, and respiratory symptoms such as cough or hemoptysis.

Before proceeding with esophageal resection, the patient's medical condition and nutritional status should be considered carefully as patients with poor nutritional status and multiple comorbid medical conditions are subject to increased perioperative complications. Thorough cardiovascular and respiratory evaluations are particularly important and objective testing such as cardiac stress tests, echocardiography, and pulmonary function tests should be obtained liberally if there are concerns. Smoking cessation and a daily walking program should be strongly encouraged as these lifestyle modifications significantly reduce pulmonary complications, and enteral tube feedings via nasogastric or jejunal feeding tubes should be considered in patients with significant weight loss or other signs of severe malnutrition.

Patients should be administered a mechanical bowel preparation on the evening prior to surgery in the rare event that esophageal reconstruction with a colon interposition is necessary. Appropriate prophylactic antibiotics are administered intravenously prior to incision. Sequential compression devices and subcutaneous heparin are used for deep vein thrombosis prophylaxis.

ANESTHESIA The procedure is performed under general endotracheal anesthesia. Adequate peripheral intravenous access and a radial artery catheter are placed to allow for adequate fluid administration and blood pressure monitoring during the procedure.

POSITION The patient is placed in the supine position with the arms tucked at the sides. A nasogastric tube is placed to decompress the stomach and aid in identification of the esophagus during mediastinal mobilization. A roll is placed behind the shoulders to facilitate neck extension, and the head is turned to the right and supported on a soft head ring. The neck, anterior chest, and abdomen are prepped and draped from the mandible to pubis.

INCISION AND EXPOSURE

OVERVIEW OF THE OPERATION FIGURE 1 shows the incisions in the midline abdomen and the left cervical area. FIGURE 2 shows the relevant anatomy and arterial supply of the stomach and the anticipated line of transection form removal of the proximal stomach and esophagus.

ABDOMINAL PORTION OF THE OPERATION The initial portion of the operation is performed through a midline laparotomy extending from the xiphoid to the umbilicus. The abdomen is inspected for metastatic disease and other pathology. Suspicious lesions outside the field of resection should be biopsied and sent for frozen section analysis. A self-retaining retractor aids in exposure of the upper abdomen and mediastinum. The round and falciform ligaments are divided; and the left lobe of the liver is dissected free from its diaphragmatic attachments and retracted to the right to expose the esophageal hiatus.

DETAILS OF PROCEDURE Following the assessment of the stomach as a suitable conduit for esophageal replacement, the lesser sac is entered by incising the gastrocolic ligament at the level of the inferior pole of the spleen. The gastrocolic ligament is sequentially divided with energy (bipolar or ultrasonic), or between clamps and ligated (FIGURE 3). Care is taken to preserve the right gastroepiploic artery which is traced to its origin, and the pancreaticogastric attachments are divided using electrocautery. The gastrosplenic ligament is sequentially divided with energy (bipolar or ultrasonic), or between clamps and ligated and the posterior gastric attachments are divided to completely mobilize the gastric fundus (FIGURE 4). **CONTINUES**

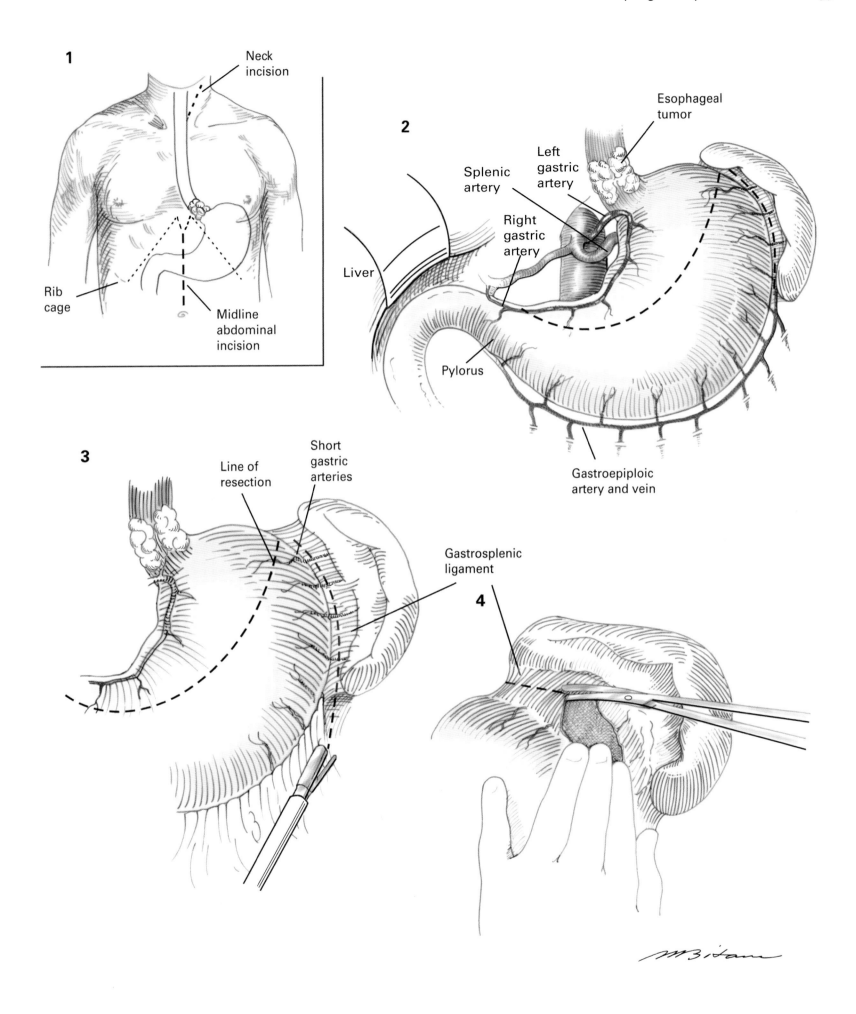

DETAILS OF PROCEDURE CONTINUED The pars flaccida of the lesser omentum is divided to expose the right crus and the phrenoesophageal ligament is divided, taking care not to injure the esophagus or GE junction (FIGURE 5). The crura are dissected and the distal esophagus is mobilized and encircled with a Penrose drain (FIGURE 6). In order to allow free movement of the pylorus to the level of the esophageal hiatus without tension, the hepatic flexure of the colon is mobilized and retracted inferiorly and the duodenum is mobilized from its retroperitoneal attachments by performing a Kocher maneuver (FIGURE 7). The dotted lines in FIGURE 7 show the course of the division of the gastrohepatic omentum and the gastrocolic omentum. The left gastric artery and a coronary vein are identified and divided near their origin using a linear cutting stapler, with care taken to maintain as much lymph node–bearing soft tissues as possible with the specimen (FIGURE 8). CONTINUES

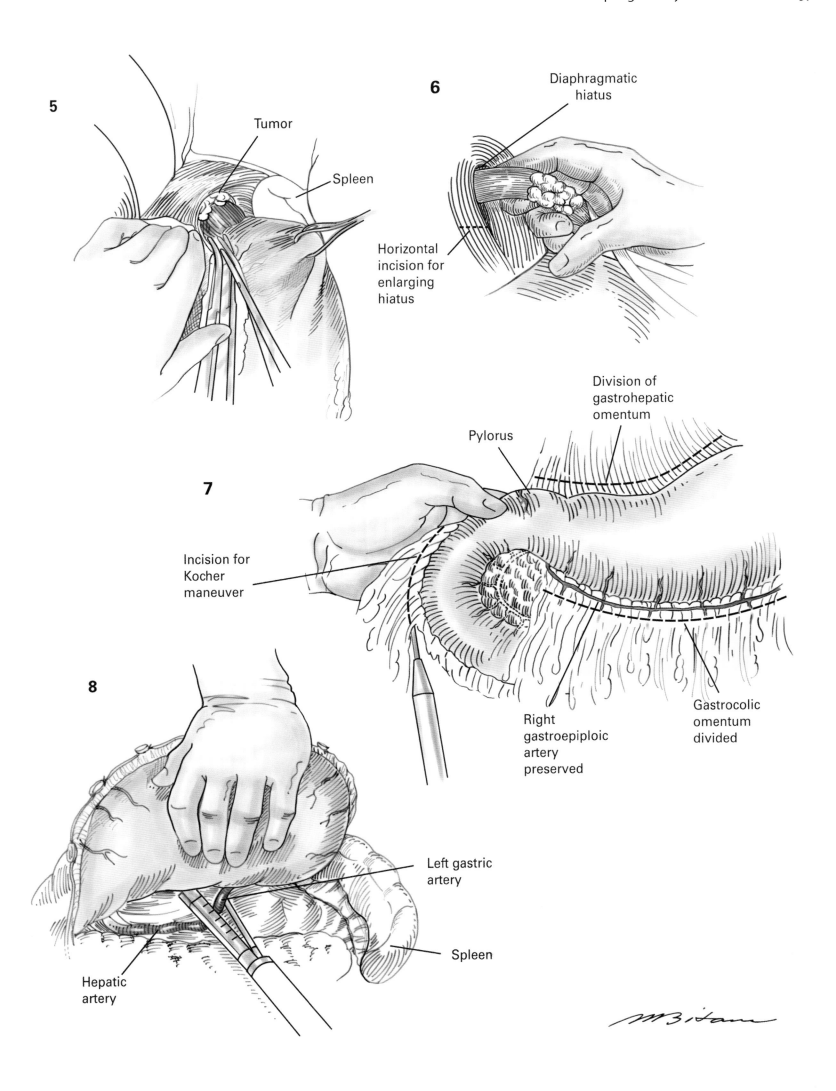

5

Tumor

Spleen

6

Diaphragmatic hiatus

Horizontal incision for enlarging hiatus

7

Division of gastrohepatic omentum

Pylorus

Incision for Kocher maneuver

Right gastroepiploic artery preserved

Gastrocolic omentum divided

8

Left gastric artery

Spleen

Hepatic artery

DETAILS OF PROCEDURE ◀ CONTINUED ▶ With the gastric mobilization, Kocher maneuver, and distal esophageal dissection complete, attention is turned to the cervical esophageal dissection. An incision is made along the anterior border of the left sternocleidomastoid muscle extending from the sternal notch to just above the cricoid cartilage (FIGURE 9). The platysma muscle and fascia along the anterior border of the sternocleidomastoid muscle are incised and the omohyoid muscle is identified and divided. The omohyoid fascia is incised and the carotid sheath is retracted laterally to allow access to the tracheoesophageal groove. The middle thyroid vein may be divided to facilitate this exposure. The prevertebral space is entered by blunt finger dissection (FIGURE 10). The anterior strap muscles are divided and the tracheoesophageal groove is dissected to allow anterior esophageal dissection. Care is taken to avoid the recurrent laryngeal nerve, but no specific attempt is made to visualize it. By careful finger dissection, the esophagus is circumferentially mobilized and encircled with a Penrose drain (FIGURE 11). Cephalad retraction of the rubber drain allows blunt dissection of the esophagus from the superior mediastinum.

Following completion of the cervical esophageal dissection, caudal traction is placed on the rubber drain around the gastroesophageal junction, and the surgeon's hand is passed into the posterior mediastinum along the prevertebral fascia, posterior to the esophagus (FIGURE 12). CONTINUES ▶

9

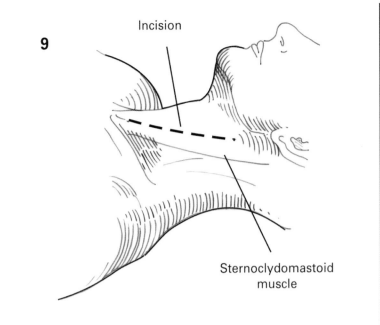

Incision

Sternoclydomastoid muscle

10

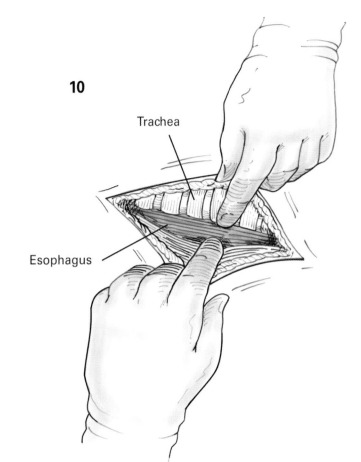

Trachea

Esophagus

11

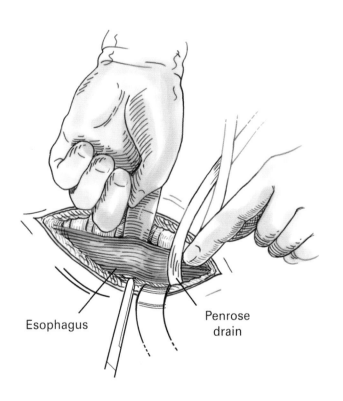

Esophagus

Penrose drain

12

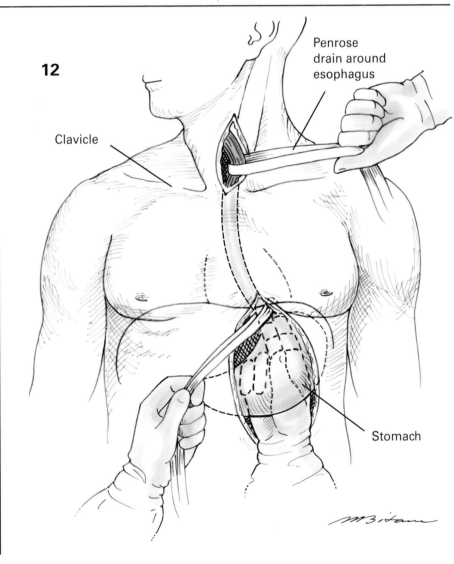

Penrose drain around esophagus

Clavicle

Stomach

DETAILS OF PROCEDURE ◄CONTINUED As the blunt dissection is extended to cephalad, a finger passed from the cervical incision can be palpated, and the posterior dissection completed (FIGURE 13). Care must be taken to closely monitor the patient's blood pressure throughout this portion of the operation. The anterior esophageal dissection is similarly performed by inserting the hand into the posterior mediastinum along the anterior surface of the esophagus with the palm facing posteriorly. Two fingers are gently advanced cephalad, with care taken to avoid injury to the pericardium or membranous trachea, until the dissection is complete in the superior mediastinum (FIGURE 14). Upon completion of the anterior and posterior dissection, cephalad retraction from the cervical incision allows blunt mobilization of the lateral attachments along the superior portion of the esophagus. Following

this, a hand is reinserted via the diaphragmatic hiatus to complete the lateral dissection by pressing the esophagus against the spine and using a posterior raking motion with the fingers.

Filmy attachments are divided bluntly, and thicker tissues and the vagal trunks are retracted toward the esophageal hiatus and divided sharply between the clips.

When the mediastinal dissection is complete, the nasogastric tube is withdrawn into the proximal esophagus and the cervical esophagus is divided using a TA stapler, with care taken to preserve adequate esophageal length to perform a tension-free anastomosis. A rubber drain is sutured to the specimen to maintain the posterior mediastinal tunnel as the esophagus is delivered into the abdomen (FIGURES 15 and 16). CONTINUES▶

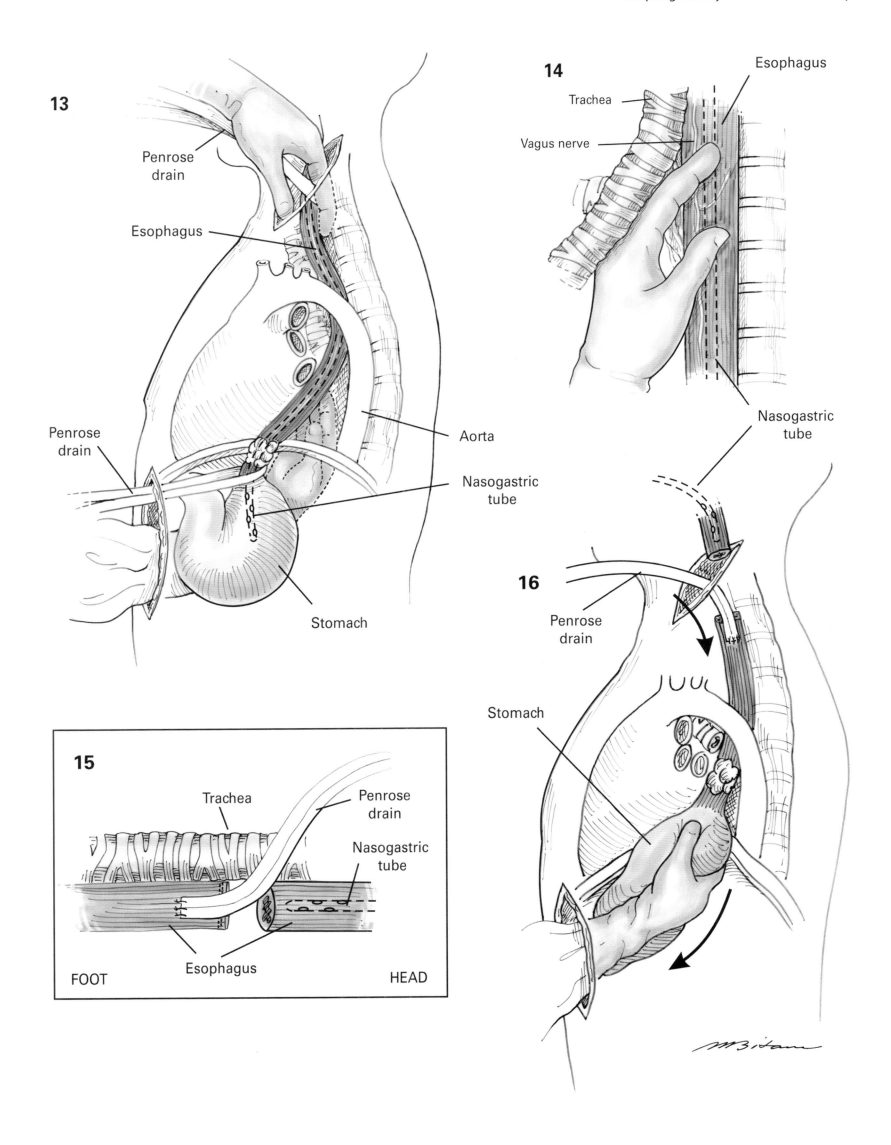

13
Penrose drain
Esophagus
Penrose drain
Aorta
Nasogastric tube
Stomach

14
Trachea
Esophagus
Vagus nerve
Nasogastric tube

15
Trachea
Penrose drain
Nasogastric tube
Esophagus
FOOT   HEAD

16
Penrose drain
Stomach

DETAILS OF PROCEDURE ◄CONTINUED Vasculature along the lesser curvature of the stomach is then divided with the linear stapling device approximately 6 cm proximal to the pylorus to mark the extent of gastric division for creation of the conduit. Branches of the right gastric artery will provide some blood flow to the distal lesser curvature and should be preserved. The stomach is divided from the fundus to the lesser curve using serial firings of the GIA 80–4.5 stapler to create a gastric tube approximately 5 cm wide (FIGURE 17). The esophagus and proximal stomach are assessed to ensure adequate margins of resection. With the gastric staple line facing the patient's right side, the stomach is sutured to the Penrose drain and pushed upward through the posterior mediastinum and grasped with surgeon's left hand or a Babcock clamp via the cervical incision (FIGURE 18). Approximately 4 to 5 cm of gastric tube are delivered into the cervical incision for creation of the anastomosis (FIGURE 19).

The cervical esophagogastrostomy may be created using a two-layer hand-sewn or linear stapled technique. A stapled cervical esophagogastrostomy is created by orienting the gastric conduit along the posterior cervical esophagus (FIGURE 20). A longitudinal gastrotomy is created and two stay sutures of 3-0 silk are placed (FIGURE 20). The esophagogastrostomy is created using a linear stapler (3.5 mm staples) (FIGURE 21). Before releasing the stapler, two 3-0 silk sutures are placed between the stomach and esophagus on each side to buttress the anastomosis. The resulting common opening is closed in two layers, with an inner layer of 3-0 running absorbable suture and an outer layer of interrupted 3-0 silk sutures. Alternatively, this can be closed with a TA stapler as shown in FIGURE 22.

The nasogastric tube is advanced past the anastomosis so that its tip is located in the distal stomach below the diaphragm. A 14-Fr feeding jejunostomy tube is then placed in a limb of proximal jejunum and brought out through a separate stab incision. We do not routinely perform a pyloroplasty due to the low incidence of delayed gastric emptying following this procedure. The abdominal and cervical incisions are closed in layers, and a Penrose drain is placed adjacent to the anastomosis and brought out through the inferior aspect of the cervical incision.

POSTOPERATIVE CARE The patient is transferred to the intensive care unit postoperatively. Early extubation is preferred, and aggressive pulmonary toilet is begun immediately. A portable chest x-ray should be obtained in order to confirm placement of life support devices and to rule out pneumo- or hemothorax. Epidural analgesia is usually not required as adequate pain control can be achieved with intermittent opioid pain medications. The patient is maintained on intravenous fluids until adequate oral or enteral nutrition is achieved, usually for several days. Intravenous beta-blockers should be administered as prophylaxis for supraventricular arrhythmias. Typically, the nasogastric tube is removed on postoperative day number three; a thick liquid diet started on day number four; and a mechanical soft diet started on day number five. An esophagram is obtained when there is clinical suspicion of possible anastomotic disruption. Jejunostomy feeds are reserved for patients who are unable to tolerate adequate oral intake due to concern for tube feeding-induced small bowel necrosis in patients who are hemodynamically and catabolically stressed. Barring complications, patients are discharged when they achieve adequate oral intake, typically within 7 to 10 days. ■

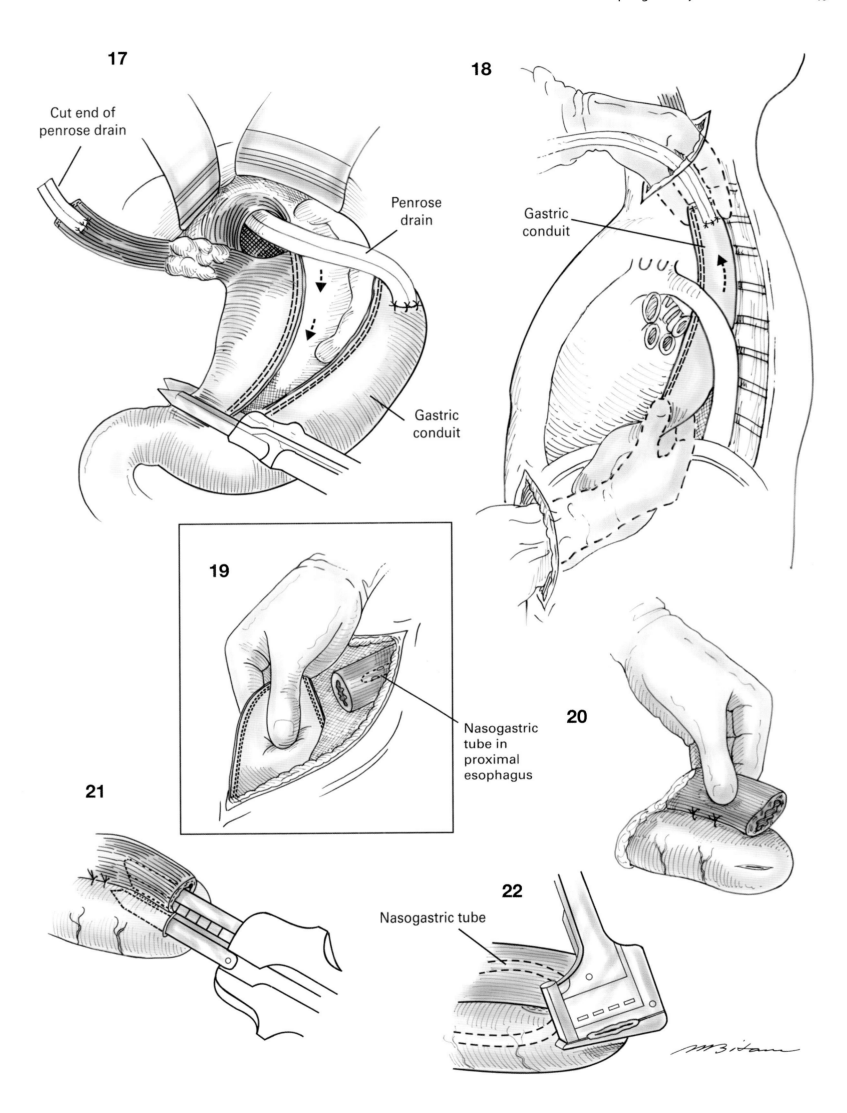

17

Cut end of penrose drain

Penrose drain

Gastric conduit

18

Gastric conduit

19

Nasogastric tube in proximal esophagus

20

21

22

Nasogastric tube

INDICATIONS Transthoracic esophagectomy is indicated for the management of surgically resectable cancers of the esophagus and gastroesophageal junction. An abdominal incision is utilized to mobilize the distal esophagus and gastroesophageal junction, including the tumor and surrounding lymph nodes. The gastric conduit is mobilized and the blood supply is based on the right gastroepiploic artery. The thoracic esophagus is then approached through a right posterolateral thoracotomy through which the specimen is resected and reconstruction is performed. Surgical resection is indicated for early staged, nonmetastatic tumors that are not amenable to endoscopic resection (T1). Surgery is also performed for nonmetastatic, intermediate staged tumors (T2–T4, N1), but usually follows a course of chemoradiation and restaging. Transthoracic esophagectomy may also be indicated for the management of benign disease such as refractory strictures, caustic injuries, or a dilated "burned esophagus" with dysphagia following treatment for achalasia.

There is some controversy regarding the optimal surgical approach for esophageal resections. Transhiatal and minimally invasive approaches have become popular due to the potential for decreased complications and data indicated equivalent outcomes. The decision to perform a transthoracic approach is made based on patient factors, surgeon preference, and experience. Potential benefits of the thoracic approach include a more thorough lymph node dissection and lower leak rates.

PREOPERATIVE PREPARATION The preoperative workup for patients with esophageal and GE junction cancers should include a thorough history and physical examination, esophagogastroduodenoscopy for diagnosis, and PET-CT imaging and endoscopic ultrasound for staging. Bronchoscopy should be considered for patients with squamous cell carcinomas, lesions involving the proximal third of the thoracic esophagus, and respiratory symptoms such as cough or hemoptysis. The patient's medical condition should be considered carefully before undertaking an esophageal resection as these procedures are extensive and patients with medical comorbidities may not tolerate them well. Thorough cardiovascular and respiratory evaluations are particularly important and objective testing such as cardiac stress tests, echocardiography, and pulmonary function tests should be obtained liberally if there are concerns. Patients should be administered a mechanical bowel preparation on the evening prior to surgery in the rare event that esophageal reconstruction with a colon interposition is necessary. Appropriate prophylactic antibiotics are administered intravenously prior to incision. Sequential compression devices and subcutaneous heparin are used for deep vein thrombosis prophylaxis.

ANESTHESIA The procedure is performed under general anesthesia. A double-lumen endobronchial tube is utilized to allow for single lung ventilation during the thoracic part of the procedure. A single lumen tube may be placed for the initial abdominal part of the procedure and then exchanged for a double-lumen tube by the anesthesia team before repositioning and performance of the thoracotomy. A nasogastric tube should be placed early during the procedure to decompress the stomach and facilitate palpation of the esophagus. This should not be secured until completion of the reconstruction as it will be repositioned several times during the procedure. A thoracic epidural may be helpful for postoperative pain control and may be associated with decreased cardiorespiratory complications.

POSITIONING The patient is initially placed in the supine position with the arms out at the sides. A bean bag should be placed under the patient, but is not deflated until repositioning after the abdominal part of the procedure has been completed. Upon completion of the abdominal part of the procedure, the patient is repositioned in the left lateral decubitus position with the right side up. An axillary roll is placed, the left arm is padded, and the right arm is placed on a padded overhead arm board and secured.

DETAILS OF PROCEDURE (abdominal portion) After general anesthesia had been induced, the abdomen is prepped and draped in standard surgical fashion. The abdomen is then entered through a midline incision extending from the xiphoid to below the umbilicus. For the abdominal portion of the procedure, please refer to Chapter 40. A 14 FR feeding jejunostomy tube is then placed in a limb of proximal jejunum in a Witzel fashion (Chapter 47, pages 160–161). Care should be taken not to compromise the lumen of the bowel. It is not necessary to routinely perform a pyloroplasty for possible delayed gastric emptying as the incidence is less than 10%. The fascia is then closed in the routine manner and the skin edges are reapproximated with staples. A dry sterile dressing is applied.

DETAILS OF PROCEDURE (thoracic portion) The patient is positioned for right thoracotomy. The right side is chosen in order to ensure adequate proximal exposure of the esophagus. The right chest is then prepped and draped in standard fashion. An occlusive drape can be useful to prevent slippage of the drapes. The chest is then entered through a standard posterolateral thoracotomy incision through the sixth intercostal space. (FIGURE 1). A rib retractor is placed and the inferior pulmonary ligament is divided using electrocautery (FIGURE 2). The esophagus is completely dissected free from its surrounding attachments, including the adjacent lymph nodes. The azygos vein is mobilized as it passes over the proximal thoracic esophagus, and is divided with the linear stapling device and secured with large hemoclips (FIGURE 3). The nasogastric tube should be withdrawn into the proximal esophagus prior to division. The proximal esophagus is stapled with a TA stapling device then divided leaving the proximal esophagus open (FIGURE 4). The gastric conduit is pulled into the chest, and the stomach is divided from the fundus to the lesser curvature using a linear stapling device (FIGURE 4). The specimen is passed off the table and sent to pathology. The gastric conduit staple line is usually oversewn using interrupted 3-0 silk sutures. Esophagogastrostomy is created in two layers using interrupted 3-0 silk sutures (FIGURE 5). The nasogastric tube should be advanced through the anastomosis prior to completion of the anterior row, and secured firmly at the nares. The conduit is secured to the chest wall laterally using interrupted 3-0 silk sutures in order to prevent torsion. Angled and straight 32-French chest tubes are placed and secured to the skin using 0 monofilament nonabsorbable sutures. The chest is then closed using looped 0 absorbable monofilament pericostal sutures. The soft tissues are closed in layers using running 0 absorbable and 2-0 absorbable sutures. The skin edges are reapproximated with staples and a dry sterile dressing is applied. Chest tubes should be connected to 20 cm H_2O pleuravac suction.

POSTOPERATIVE CARE The patient is transferred to the intensive care unit postoperatively and extubated as soon as possible. If the patient is to remain intubated because of respiratory insufficiency or other clinical issues, the double lumen endotracheal tube should be replaced with a large caliber single lumen tube. A portable chest x-ray should be obtained in order to confirm placement of life support devices and to rule out pneumo or hemothorax. The patient is maintained on intravenous fluids until adequate oral or enteral nutrition is achieved, usually for several days. Intravenous beta-blockers should be administered as prophylaxis for supraventricular arrhythmias. The nasogastric tube is removed on postoperative day number three; a clear liquid diet started on day number four; and a mechanical soft diet started on day number five. We do not usually initiate early enteral nutrition through the jejunostomy tube because of the concern for tube feeding-induced small bowel necrosis in patients who are hemodynamically and catabolically stressed. Jejunostomy feeds are reserved for patients who are unable to tolerate adequate oral intake for whatever reason. Barring any complications, patients are discharged to home once they are able to tolerate an adequate diet. Chest tubes are placed to water seal as long as there are no air leaks, and are removed after an oral diet has been established and prior to discharge. The usual hospitalization is 7 to 10 days. ■

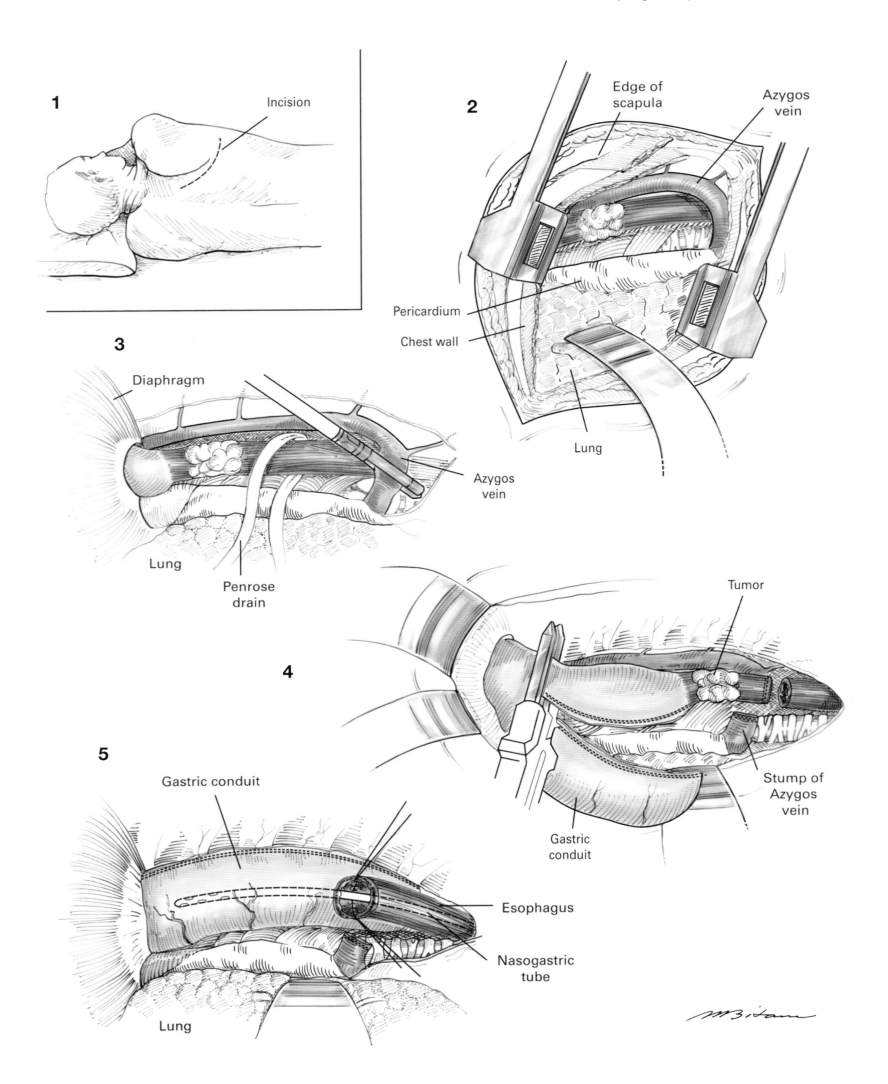

1 Incision

2 Edge of scapula — Azygos vein — Pericardium — Chest wall — Lung

3 Diaphragm — Azygos vein — Lung — Penrose drain

4 Tumor — Stump of Azygos vein — Gastric conduit

5 Gastric conduit — Esophagus — Nasogastric tube — Lung

PYLOROMYOTOMY

INDICATIONS Pyloromyotomy (Fredet–Ramstedt operation) is done in infants with congenital hypertrophic pyloric stenosis.

PREOPERATIVE CARE The diagnosis is established by the characteristic history of projectile vomiting and the physical finding of a pyloric mass or "olive" on abdominal examination. This may be confirmed by an upper gastrointestinal series but more frequently by ultrasound. The correction of dehydration and acid–base imbalance by adequate parenteral fluid therapy is as important as surgical skill in lowering the mortality rate. Although prolonged gastric intubation is to be avoided, 6 to 12 hours of preparation with intravenous hydration plus suction may be necessary to restore the baby to good physiologic condition. Oral feedings are discontinued as soon as the diagnosis is made, and an intravenous infusion is started in a scalp vein. Then 10 mL/kg of 5% glucose in normal saline is administered rapidly. This is followed by a solution of one part 5% dextrose in normal saline to one part 5% dextrose in water (one-half normal saline with 5% D/W) given at the rate of 150 mL/kg per 24 hours. The baby should be reevaluated every 8 hours with respect to state of hydration, weight, and evidence of edema. Ordinarily, this solution is continued for 8 to 16 hours. After adequate urinary output is established, potassium should be added to the intravenous solutions. In the baby who is moderately or severely dehydrated, it is wise to determine the serum electrolyte values before initiating replacement therapy and to check the values in 8 to 12 hours.

ANESTHESIA Endotracheal intubation on the conscious infant is the safest anesthetic technique, followed by general anesthesia.

POSITION A temperature-controlled blanket is placed under the infant's back to help compensate for the loss of body heat and to arch the abdomen slightly to improve the operative exposure. To prevent heat loss through the arms and legs, they are wrapped with sheet wadding, and the intravenous site is carefully protected.

OPERATIVE PREPARATION The skin is prepared in the routine manner.

INCISION AND EXPOSURE The open approach is presented. Alternatively, a laparoscopic approach may be performed. It is advisable for the general surgeon to be familiar with the open approach. A gridiron incision placed below the right costal margin, but above the inferior edge of the liver, is used. The incision is 3 cm long and extends laterally from the outer edge of the rectus muscle. The omentum or the transverse colon usually presents in the wound and is easily identified. By gentle traction on the omentum, the transverse colon is delivered and, in turn, traction on the transverse colon will deliver the greater curvature of the stomach easily into the wound. The anterior wall of the stomach is held with a moistened gauze sponge and, upward traction on the antral portion of the stomach, the pylorus is delivered into the wound.

DETAILS OF PROCEDURE The anterosuperior surface of the pylorus is not very vascular and is the region selected for the pyloromyotomy (FIGURE 2). As the pylorus is held between the surgeon's thumb and index finger, a longitudinal incision of 1 to 2 cm long is made (FIGURE 3). The incision is carried down through the serosal and muscle coats until the mucosa is exposed, but the mucosa is left intact (FIGURE 4). Great care must be taken at the duodenal end of the incision, for here the pyloric muscle ends abruptly, in contrast with the gastric end, and the mucosa of the duodenum may be perforated (see danger point) (FIGURE 1). The cut muscle is now spread apart with a straight or a half-length hemostat until the mucosa pouts up to the level of the cut serosa (FIGURES 4 and 5). Usually, hemorrhage can be controlled by applying a sponge wet with saline, and only rarely is a ligature or stitch necessary to control a bleeding vessel. The surgeon must ascertain that no perforation of the mucous membrane exists.

CLOSURE The peritoneum and transversalis fascia are closed with a running suture of 0000 chromic. The remaining fascial layers are closed with fine interrupted sutures. The skin margins are approximated with running 000000 nylon sutures or subcuticular absorbable sutures reinforced with skin-adhesive strips.

POSTOPERATIVE CARE Six hours following operation, the suction is discontinued and the nasogastric tube is removed. At this time, 15 mL of dextrose and water is offered to the infant. Following this, the infant is offered 30 mL of an evaporated milk formula every 2 hours until the morning after operation. Thereafter, the infant is fed progressively more formula on a 3-hour schedule. ■

1

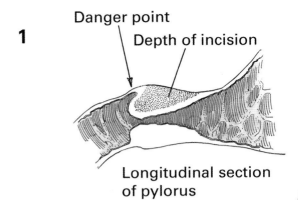

Danger point

Depth of incision

Longitudinal section
of pylorus

2

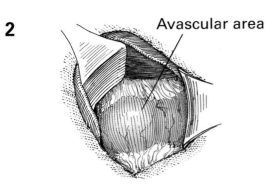

Avascular area

3

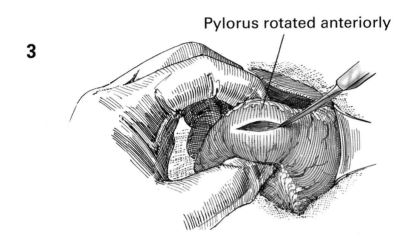

Pylorus rotated anteriorly

Incision in avascular area falls
just short of duodenal edge
of mass

4

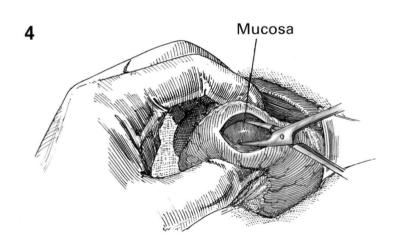

Mucosa

Spreading muscle
until mucosa bulges
to level of serosa

5

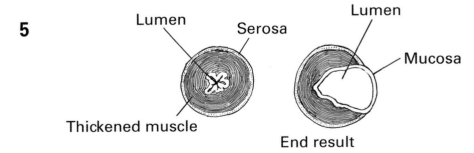

Lumen   Serosa   Lumen

Mucosa

Thickened muscle   End result

Cross section of pylorus

SECTION V
SMALL INTESTINE, COLON, AND RECTUM

INTUSSUSCEPTION AND MECKEL'S DIVERTICULECTOMY

A. INTUSSUSCEPTION

INDICATIONS Intussusception occurs most commonly in infants from the age of a few months to 2 years. Time must be taken to correct dehydration or debility by administering parenteral fluids. A stomach tube should be passed to deflate the stomach and to reduce the danger of aspirated vomitus to a minimum. If the intussusception has been of considerable duration and there is evidence of bleeding, as in the characteristic mahogany stools in infants, blood products should be administered with the operating room alerted and hydration established satisfactory for operation. The child is taken to the x-ray department, and here hydrostatic reduction by barium enema is attempted, utilizing a pressure of no more than 3 ft. As much as 1 hour may be spent in this procedure as long as manipulation of the abdomen is avoided and the exposure to fluoroscopy limited as much as possible. If the intussusception (FIGURE 1) is going to reduce, it will progressively do so. If this method fails, surgery follows immediately. If a mass lesion or cancer is suspected in an elderly patient, then a re-section should be performed rather than a manipulation.

ANESTHESIA Meperidine or morphine should be added in appropriate doses in older infants and children. Endotracheal intubation on the conscious infant is the safest anesthetic technique, followed by general anesthesia.

POSITION The patient is placed in a dorsal recumbent position. Feet and hands are held flat to the operating table by straps or pinned wrappings.

OPERATIVE PREPARATION The skin is prepared in the routine manner.

INCISION AND EXPOSURE In most instances, a transverse incision made in the right lower quadrant provides adequate exposure. The lateral third of the anterior rectus fascia and the adjacent aponeurosis of the external oblique are incised transversely. The lateral edge of the rectus muscle may then be retracted medially and the internal oblique and transversalis muscles divided in the direction of their fibers. If more exposure is required, the incision in the anterior rectus fascia may be extended, and a portion or all of the right rectus muscle may be transected.

DETAILS OF PROCEDURE The major portion of the reduction is done intra-abdominally by milking the mass back along the descending colon, transverse colon, and ascending colon. When reduction has proceeded thus far, the remainder can be delivered out of the abdominal cavity. The mass is pushed back along the descending colon by squeezing the colon distal to the intussusception (FIGURE 2). If traction is applied, it should be extremely gentle to avoid rupturing the bowel. The discolored and edematous bowel at first may not appear to be viable, but the application of warm saline solution may improve its tone and appearance. Unless the intestine is necrotic, it is better to persist in attempts at reduction than to resort to early and unnecessary resection, required in less than 5% of the cases. An etiologic factor, such as an inverted Meckel's diverticulum or intestinal polyp, is found in only 3% or 4% of childhood cases of intussusception. It is unnecessary to tack down the terminal ileum or to anchor the mesentery. Recurrences are not common, and such preventive procedures only prolong the operation. Intussusception is uncommon in adults. It may occur at any level of the small or large intestine. After the intussusception in adults has been reduced, a search should be made for the initiating cause—that is, tumors (especially intrinsic), adhesive bands, Meckel's diverticulum, and so forth. Resection is indicated if dead bowel is encountered.

CLOSURE The abdomen is closed in the routine manner. The skin margins are approximated with nylon sutures or subcuticular absorbable sutures reinforced with skin-adhesive strips.

POSTOPERATIVE CARE Nasogastric suction is continued until peristaltic activity is audible or until a stool is passed. Antibiotics and colloid replacement are not necessary in an uncomplicated intussusception but again are most valuable adjuncts in the case requiring resection. About 5 mL/kg of colloid or 5% albumin solution provides an invaluable daily supportive measure for the seriously ill child who has had resection of a gangrenous intussusception. Recurrence in the adult should suggest a cause overlooked initially but probably amenable to surgical correction, such as removal of a polyp or adhesive band.

B. MECKEL'S DIVERTICULECTOMY

INDICATIONS Excision of a Meckel's diverticulum is performed when the diverticulum is found to cause an acute abdominal condition. Frequently excision is a benign incidental procedure during a laparotomy for other causes. The majority of these diverticula cause no symptoms, but a diseased one can successfully mimic many other intestinal diseases, any of which would require exploratory laparotomy.

The presence of gastric mucosa in the diverticulum can produce ulceration with massive intestinal hemorrhage with brick-red stools, inflammation, or a free perforation with peritonitis, particularly in children. Although similar complications can occur in adults, intestinal obstruction caused by fixation of the tip of the diverticulum or a connecting band running to the umbilicus is not uncommon. The diverticulum may become inverted and form the starting point of an intussusception. Benign diverticula should be removed as incidental procedures unless contraindicated by a potentially complicating disease elsewhere in the abdomen. These congenital anomalies are remnants of the embryonic omphalomesenteric duct arising from the midgut, are found in 1% to 3% of patients, principally males, and are located usually 20 to 35 cm above the ileocecal valve. The terminal ileum should be routinely examined for a Meckel's diverticulum as part of a thorough abdominal exploration.

PREOPERATIVE PREPARATION Preoperative preparation is devoted chiefly to the restoration of blood, fluids, and electrolytes. Nasogastric suction is advisable in the presence of obstruction or peritonitis, which may require additional blood, plasma, and antibiotics.

ANESTHESIA General inhalation anesthesia is preferred; however, spinal or local anesthesia may be indicated under special circumstances.

POSITION The patient is placed in a comfortable supine position.

OPERATIVE PREPARATION The skin is prepared routinely.

INCISION AND EXPOSURE A midline incision is preferred because of its maximum flexibility. However, incidental excision of a Meckel's diverticulum may be performed through any incision that exposes it.

DETAILS OF PROCEDURE The segment of the terminal ileum involved with the Meckel's diverticulum is delivered into the wound by Babcock forceps for stabilization. The Meckel's diverticulum may be as far as 20 to 35 cm back from the level of the ileocecal valve. If a mesodiverticulum is present, it should be freed, divided between hemostats, and ligated as a mesoappendix (FIGURE 3). If the diverticulum has quite a wide neck, it may be excised either by oblique or cross clamping of the base, by wedge or V-shaped excision of the base, or by segmental resection of the involved ileum with end-to-end anastomosis (FIGURE 4). The base is double clamped with noncrushing Potts-type clamps in a direction transverse or diagonally across to the bowel. The specimen is excised with a scalpel. Traction sutures, A and B, of 00 silk are placed to approximate the serosal surface of the intestinal wall just beyond either end of the incision (FIGURE 5). When tied, these sutures, A and B, serve to stabilize the intestinal wall during the subsequent closure. Sutures of 00 silk are placed at either end of the incision, and a row of interrupted 0000 silk horizontal mattress sutures is placed beneath the clamp (FIGURE 6). The clamp is then removed, the sutures tied, and any excess intestinal wall excised. Then an inverting layer of interrupted 0000 silk horizontal mattress sutures is placed (FIGURES 6 and 7). The patency of the lumen is then tested between the surgeon's thumb and index finger. Alternatively, some surgeons prefer to amputate the diverticulum with a stapling instrument. The diverticular mesentery is divided and its vessels are ligated, as in FIGURE 3. The diverticulum is splayed transversely to the axis of the bowel using a pair of stay sutures at either side. A linear stapling device may be used, according to the surgeon's preference. After removal of the diverticulum, the transverse staple line is then inverted with a series of 000 silk mattress sutures. Again, the patency and integrity of the suture line is tested by the surgeon.

CLOSURE The usual laparotomy closure is performed.

POSTOPERATIVE CARE Postoperative care is similar to that for appendectomy or small bowel anastomosis. Fluid and electrolyte balance is maintained intravenously until intestinal motility returns. The nasogastric tube is then removed and progressive alimentation begun. Any subsiding inflammation, peritonitis, or drained abscess is treated with the appropriate systemic antibiotics plus blood and plasma replacement. The major postoperative complications are obstruction, peritonitis, and wound infection, which may require further appropriate surgical therapy. ∎

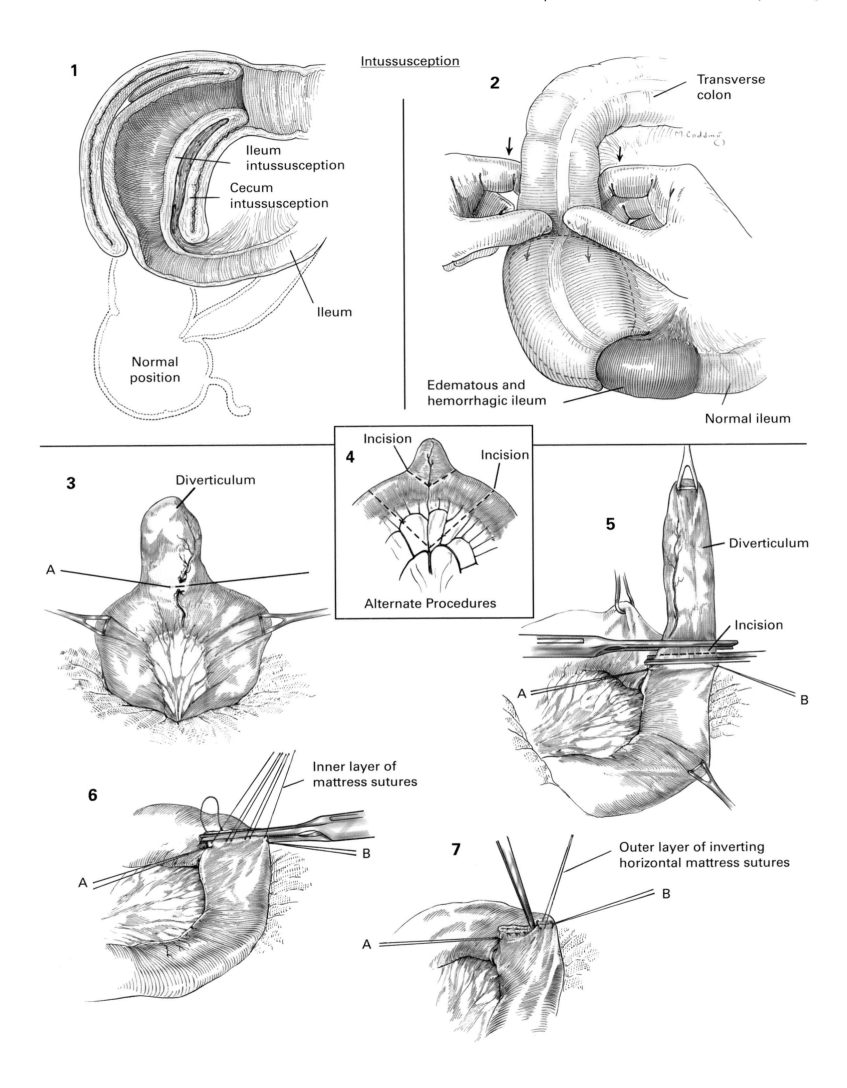

Intussusception

1

Ileum intussusception

Cecum intussusception

Ileum

Normal position

2

Transverse colon

Edematous and hemorrhagic ileum

Normal ileum

3

Diverticulum

A

4

Incision

Incision

Alternate Procedures

5

Diverticulum

Incision

A

B

6

Inner layer of mattress sutures

A

B

7

Outer layer of inverting horizontal mattress sutures

A

B

RESECTION OF SMALL INTESTINE

INDICATIONS This resection is usually an emergency procedure utilized in the presence of sudden obstruction, such as gangrenous intestine in a strangulated hernia, or from volvulus. Less frequently, it is used in mesenteric thrombosis and obstruction by tumor. Since the end-to-end anastomosis restores more accurately the natural continuity of the bowel, it is usually preferable to a lateral anastomosis; however, the surgeon should be familiar with the side-to-side anastomosis, which is favored when there is marked disparity between the sizes of the ends of bowel to be anastomosed.

PREOPERATIVE PREPARATION Since resection and anastomosis of the small intestine usually constitutes an emergency procedure, preoperative measures are necessarily limited. However, before operation is attempted, the stomach is emptied and constant gastric suction maintained. Fluid and electrolyte balance, including normal sodium, chloride, and potassium levels, should be established in accordance with the degree of fluid and electrolyte depletion and the age and cardiac status of the patient. Antibiotic therapy should be instituted if gangrenous intestine is suspected. The pulse should be slowed and a good output of urine established as evidence of adequate blood volume expansion before surgery. Constant bladder drainage may be necessary to determine accurately the urinary output in the elderly or seriously ill patient.

ANESTHESIA General anesthesia with an endotracheal tube and cuff, which permits complete sealing of the trachea, is recommended and, along with preoperative gastric decompression, is the best prophylaxis against possible aspiration pneumonia. Spinal anesthesia, either by single injection or continuous technique, may be used. However, the threat of sudden regurgitation of large volumes of upper gastrointestinal juices from the obstructed intestine must be anticipated by readily available competent suction equipment. The danger of aspiration is ever present even if an endotracheal tube is used.

POSITION The patient is placed in a comfortable supine position.

OPERATIVE PREPARATION The skin is prepared routinely.

INCISION AND EXPOSURE The incision is placed over the suspected site of the lesion. If the location of the small bowel obstruction is not known, a lower midline incision is often used, since the lower ileum is most frequently involved. The incision is made preferably above or below an old abdominal scar, if present, because the site of the obstruction will most likely be near this point, especially if the scar was tender before operation. A culture of the peritoneal fluid is taken, the amount, color, and consistency being noted. Bloody fluid indicates vascular obstruction. The dilated loops of intestine are retracted or removed carefully from the peritoneal cavity to a warm, moist surface and covered with gauze packs soaked in warm saline solution. When strangulation is present, the surgeon must determine the viability of the involved intestine by taking into consideration these factors: (1) a cadaveric odor; (2) the presence of bloody fluid indicating venous thrombosis; (3) failure of peristalsis to progress over the involved intestine; (4) loss of the normal luster and color of the serosal coat; and, most important of all; and (5) absence of arterial pulsation. What may at first appear to be nonviable intestine requiring resection will often return to viability when the cause of the obstruction has been relieved and when the bowel has been packed for a time in warm, moist gauze. There is also a prompt change in the color of viable bowel when 100% oxygen is inhaled. Infiltration of the mesentery with 1% procaine hydrochloride solution may also overcome vascular spasm and bring about arterial pulsations in questionable cases. The intra-arterial (or systemic intravenous) injection of fluorescein followed by ultraviolet lamp illumination may be used to evaluate the regional perfusion. A handheld Doppler ultrasound device in a sterile cover may also be useful in verifying the arterial supply.

In the presence of tumor, the mesentery should be explored for metastatic nodes. If there is any doubt as to the site of the obstruction, the surgeon should not hesitate to eviscerate the patient until the offending lesion is adequately exposed and to pass the bowel between the fingers, section by section, from the ligament of Treitz to the cecum. The surgeon must be certain no secondary lesion or distal cause of obstruction exists. In the presence of markedly abnormal anatomy, it may be helpful to start at the ileocecal valve and follow the decompressed bowel proximally to the point of obstruction.

DETAILS OF PROCEDURE The intestinal wall should be resected 5 to 10 cm beyond the grossly involved area, even if it means sacrificing several feet of small intestine (FIGURE 1). The bowel and mesentery are divided, preferably the mesentery first (FIGURE 2). The surgeon must be certain (1) that clamps are not applied too far downward toward the base of the mesentery, since the blood supply to a long segment of bowel may be accidentally

divided; (2) that the resection extends into the base of the mesentery only in the presence of malignant disease; and (3) that a sizable pulsating vessel is preserved to nourish the bowel adjacent to the point of resection. The bowel should be cleaned of mesentery for at least 1 cm beyond the proposed line of resection (FIGURE 2) to ensure the safe application of serosal sutures along the mesenteric border. A pair of narrow, straight clamps with fine atraumatic teeth is applied to the intestine. The clamp on the viable portion is placed obliquely, ensuring not only a better blood supply to the antimesenteric border but also a larger lumen for anastomosis (FIGURE 3). The bowel is divided on both sides of the lesion, and the retained bowel is covered with warm, moist sponges.

The color of the intestine is again observed to ensure that the blood supply to the bowel adjacent to the clamp is adequate and that there is sufficient serosa exposed at the mesenteric border for the placement of sutures. If the intestine appears bluish, or is there is no pulsation in the mesenteric vessels, the intestine is resected until the circulation is adequate.

After the bowel ends have been prepared for anastomosis and mobilized distally and proximally far enough to prevent any tension on the suture line of the anastomosis, the clamps are rotated to present the posterior serosal surfaces for approximation. Enterostomy clamps are placed along the intestine 5 to 8 cm from the crushing clamps to prevent leakage of intestinal contents after the clamps are removed. Silk mattress sutures are taken in the serosa at the mesenteric and antimesenteric borders. The mesenteric border must have been cleaned far enough so that the sutures include serosa only and no mesenteric fat. A layer of interrupted Halsted 000 silk sutures is placed in the serosa (FIGURE 4). The posterior mucosa is then closed either by a continuous lock stitch of absorbable suture or interrupted 0000 silk (FIGURE 5). The antimesenteric angle and anterior mucosa are closed by changing to a Connell inverting stitch (FIGURES 5 and 6). The anterior serosal layer is then closed with interrupted Halsted sutures of 000 silk (FIGURE 7). The mesentery is approximated with interrupted 0000 silk sutures placed to avoid injury to the vessels. Invaginating the bowel against the thumb with the finger verifies the patency of the anastomosis (FIGURE 8). Silver clips may be used to verify the site of the anastomosis in subsequent roentgen studies.

ALTERNATE METHOD The method of lateral anastomosis may be used. After the bowel is divided in accordance with the procedure explained above, the severed ends are closed with a continuous inversion suture of absorbable suture over the clamp (FIGURE 9). The wall of the intestine in inverted, and smooth serosa is approximated as the clamp is withdrawn (FIGURE 10). When the clamp is removed, the suture is pulled just tight enough to control the bleeding and occlude the lumen and is tied at the mesenteric border. The open end of the intestine may be closed by interrupted 000 silk sutures. The bowel end is closed with a serosal row of interrupted 000 silk mattress sutures that must not include fat or mesentery (FIGURE 11). In order to avoid interference with the blood supply, the final suture may pull the edge of the mesentery up to the point of closure but should not invert or include it.

Straight intestinal noncrushing clamps are applied to the intestine close to the mesenteric border and near the closed ends to avoid a blind segment beyond the anastomosis. The bowel is held in position with Allis, Babcock, or thumb forceps as the clamps are applied (FIGURE 12). The clamps are placed together, and the field is covered with fresh towels. Traction sutures are placed at either angle of the anastomosis (FIGURE 13). A row of interrupted 000 silk sutures is placed in the serosa. The bowel wall is incised with a knife on either side close to the suture line (FIGURE 13). The incision is lengthened with electrocautery until a stoma about two or three fingers wide is assured. The posterior mucosa is closed with a continuous absorbable suture lock stitch or interrupted 0000 fine silk sutures (FIGURE 14). The anterior layer of mucosa is closed with a Connell inverting stitch and the anterior serosal layer with interrupted 000 silk mattress sutures (FIGURE 15). The angles may be reinforced with several interrupted 000 silk sutures until the closed ends of intestine are securely anchored to the adjacent bowel (FIGURE 16). The mesentery is approximated using interrupted 000 silk sutures placed in such a way as to avoid major blood vessels (FIGURE 16).

CLOSURE Routine closure of the abdominal wall is performed.

POSTOPERATIVE CARE The fluid balance is established and maintained by the use of the intravenous Ringer's lactate solution. Blood transfusions may be indicated until the pulse rate returns toward normal, especially if the hematocrit is ≤30. Constant decompression by continuous gastric suction or temporary gastrostomy is maintained until normal emptying of the intestinal tract begins. ■

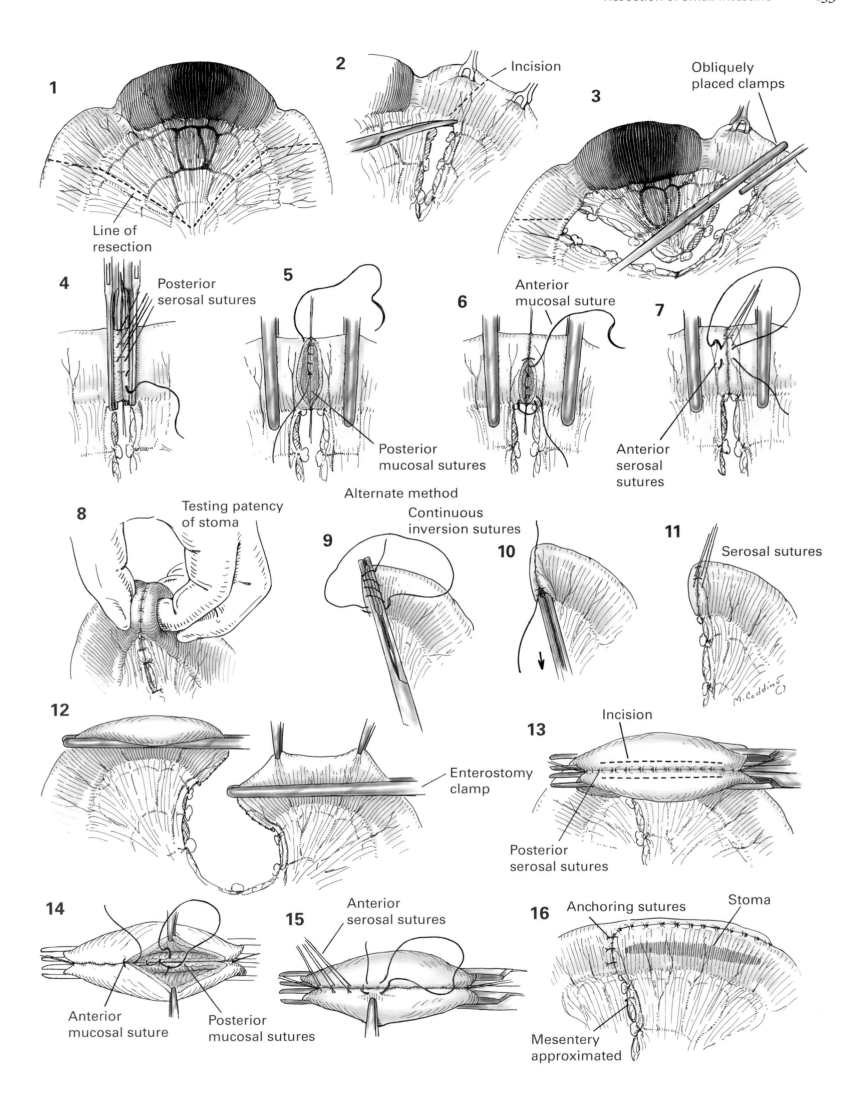

1 Line of resection

2 Incision

3 Obliquely placed clamps

4 Posterior serosal sutures

5 Posterior mucosal sutures

6 Anterior mucosal suture

7 Anterior serosal sutures

8 Testing patency of stoma

Alternate method

9 Continuous inversion sutures

10

11 Serosal sutures

M. Codding

12 Enterostomy clamp

13 Incision

Posterior serosal sutures

14 Anterior mucosal suture   Posterior mucosal sutures

15 Anterior serosal sutures

16 Anchoring sutures   Stoma

Mesentery approximated

INDICATIONS Various portions of the small intestine are resected for a variety of reasons. Emergency procedures involving interference with the blood supply by a strangulated hernia, a volvulus due to a fixed adhesion, mesenteric thrombosis, traumatic injuries, localized tumors, and regional enteritis are among the indications for small bowel resection. Occasionally it may be judicious to perform an enteroenterostomy in the presence of many adhesions or extensive regional ileitis in an effort to avoid further resection of the already shortened small bowel resulting from previous extensive resections.

PREOPERATIVE PREPARATION The indications for operation control the time allotted for fluid, electrolyte, and blood replacement (see Chapter 44). Constant gastric suction is instituted. An inlying catheter for drainage of the bladder is useful in monitoring the adequacy of urinary output in response to treatment. When the pulse is elevated and gangrenous intestine is suspected, plasma expanders or red cells may be administered. Intravenous antibiotics are given, and the patient is aggressively rehydrated using central venous pressure and urinary output as monitors.

ANESTHESIA The stomach should be on constant gastric suction, and the suction should be adequate to avoid the danger of aspiration of gastric contents. A cuffed endotracheal tube is advisable to seal off the trachea and avoid the possibility of aspiration pneumonia.

POSITION The patient is placed in a comfortable position with the operating table elevated at right angles to the working level of the surgeon. A modest reverse Trendelenburg position may be helpful in improving subsequent exposure as well as in the retraction of dilated small bowel.

OPERATIVE PREPARATION The skin is prepared in the usual manner.

INCISION AND EXPOSURE The incision is made in the general area of the suspected lesion. In the trauma patient, a long midline incision ensures adequate exposure for an extensive exploration. When an incarcerated hernia is likely to contain gangrenous intestine, some prefer to open the abdomen with an oblique incision above the groin in order to divide the viable bowel above the point of incarceration, lessening the chances of gross contamination when the hernial sac is opened. In the presence of previous scars, especially in the midline, a new incision may be judiciously made beyond the end or to one side in order to lessen the chance of injuring the underlying, probably tightly adherent small intestine.

DETAILS OF PROCEDURE A specimen of abdominal fluid is taken for culture and its color and odor evaluated as predictors of "dead intestine." The release of restrictions by adhesions or a hernia sac is the first priority in the hope that a return of adequate blood supply will follow. When the viability of the intestine is questioned, the bowel may be placed in warm, moist gauze for some minutes. Procaine may be injected carefully into the mesentery to stimulate visible arterial pulsations. Obviously gangrenous small bowel should be promptly isolated with towels in order to minimize infection. In trauma patients, the small as well as the large intestine must be thoroughly inspected for possible injury, since protruding mucosa may temporarily block contamination. Injuries to the mesentery with hematoma formation require very careful evaluation. Multiple perforations with extensive mesenteric injury may make resection of a segment of small bowel a safer procedure than an attempt at multiple repairs of a segment. The possibility of another intraluminal cause of obstruction mandates evaluation of the small intestine beyond the point of intussusception or obstruction.

OPEN-LUMEN ANASTOMOSIS OF SMALL INTESTINE Noncrushing Scudder clamps are applied proximal to the planned point of division of the small bowel as well as distal to the area to be resected. This prevents gross contamination of the obstructed bowel while controlling the blood supply. The specimen is resected (FIGURE 1) after a thin straight clamp is applied obliquely to the intestinal wall with a free mesenteric serosal border of 1 cm or more. This leaves a clear serosal area for the application of the TL60 with 4.8-mm staples.

DETAILS OF PROCEDURE The cutting linear stapler can be used to approximate the open two ends of the divided small bowel (FIGURE 2). After the bowel has been divided on the modest oblique plane with 1 cm of freed mesenteric border, the ends are aligned. This is accomplished by placing traction sutures at the mesenteric and antimesenteric borders (FIGURE 2). The antimesenteric border is approximated, and each of the cutting linear stapler forks is inserted. The bowel must be aligned evenly on the forks before the instrument is fired (FIGURE 3). The bowel walls are sewn together with the stapler and the stoma is established by the cutting knife within the cutting linear stapler (FIGURE 3A). The stapled suture line is inspected for bleeding, which, if present, is controlled with interrupted sutures.

Traction sutures (A, A′) are placed on the mesenteric border of each segment, and another is placed centrally (B) to permit traction on the end of the suture line on the antimesenteric border (FIGURE 4). The common lumen can be closed with the application of a noncutting linear stapler. The excess bowel wall beyond the suturing instrument is excised (FIGURE 5). Any bleeding points after the removal of the stapling instrument are controlled with interrupted sutures.

With time and experience, it has been found preferable to close this opening in a vertical manner from B to B′, thus approximating A to A′. This creates crossed staples only at the ends (B and B′), which are then carefully inspected for possible suture reinforcement. Again, any bleeding points are controlled with interrupted sutures. The lines of closure are carefully inspected, and the excess intestine outside of the staple lines is excised. The security of the suture line is evaluated, and the antimesenteric border can be approximated if desired with interrupted sutures for distance of the anastomosis.

The mesentery is completely approximated with interrupted sutures (FIGURE 6). The approximation may be performed before the anastomosis is created. The mesentery must be completely approximated to avoid any possibility of later internal herniation of a loop of intestine. The patency of the anastomosis is tested by palpation between the thumb and the index finger. CONTINUES ▶

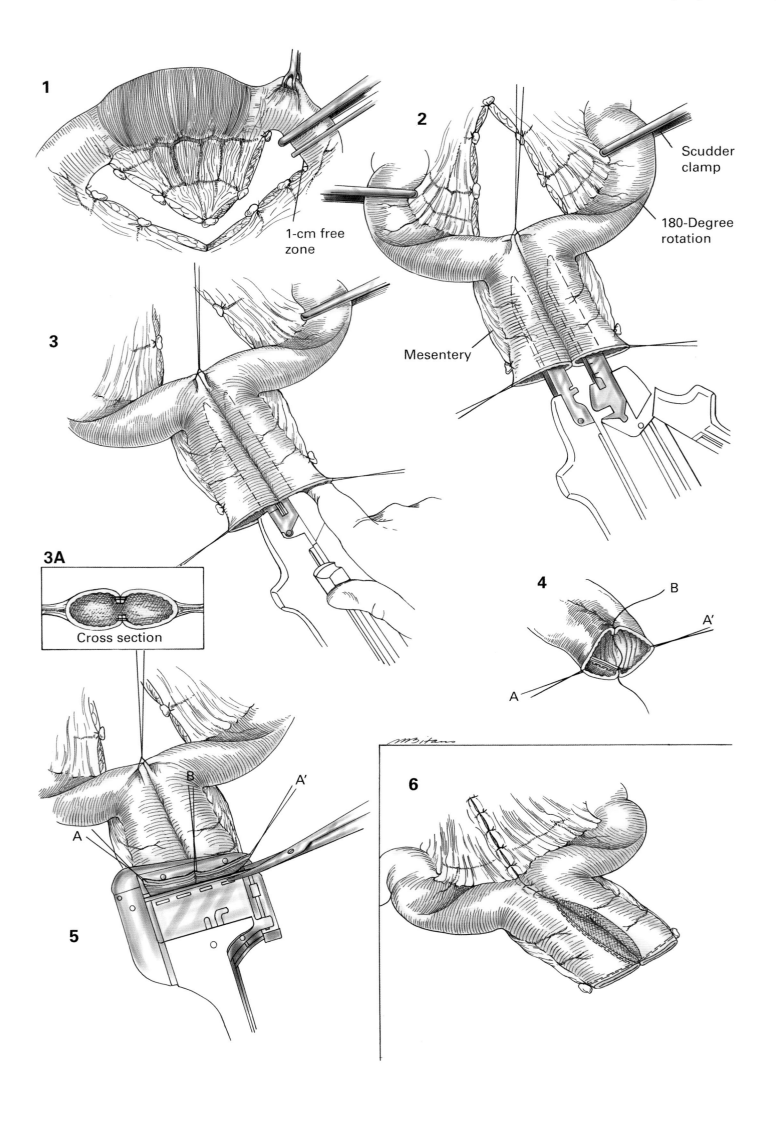

1

1-cm free zone

2

Scudder clamp

180-Degree rotation

Mesentery

3

3A

Cross section

4

B

A'

A

5

B

A'

A

6

ALTERNATIVE METHODS CONTINUED An alternative method of anastomosing the small intestine that is similar to the preceding open-lumen anastomosis may be performed after first resecting the specimen segment using the cutting linear stapler (FIGURE 7). This prevents gross contamination by closing all lumens with a row of staples. Assuming the mesenteric mobilization, ligation, and divisions have been performed, the specimen is removed. The proximal and distal limbs of remaining bowel are then rotated 180 degrees in order to align the antimesenteric borders. Traction sutures are placed near the planned staple line and approximately 6 to 8 cm distally so as to be beyond the apex of the new anastomosis. A portion of the antimesenteric border staple line is obliquely excised from each limb so as to create an opening large enough for insertion of the forks of the cutting linear stapler instrument (FIGURE 8). Both forks are inserted fully to maximize the size of the anastomotic opening. After assembling the cutting linear stapler and aligning the antimesenteric septum appropriately using the distal traction suture, the stapling instrument is discharged (FIGURE 9). The anastomosis is inspected for bleeding, which, if present, is controlled with interrupted sutures.

Traction sutures are placed at either end of the new opening, and an additional one is placed centrally, bringing together the newly created staple lines along the antimesenteric border. The three traction sutures are brought within the jaws of a noncutting linear stapler, which then closes the common opening (FIGURE 10). The excess tissue is excised above the stapling instrument and this suture line is inspected for hemostasis. The mesentery is reapproximated with interrupted sutures and the patency of the anastomosis is tested by palpation (FIGURE 11).

POSTOPERATIVE CARE See Chapter 44. ■

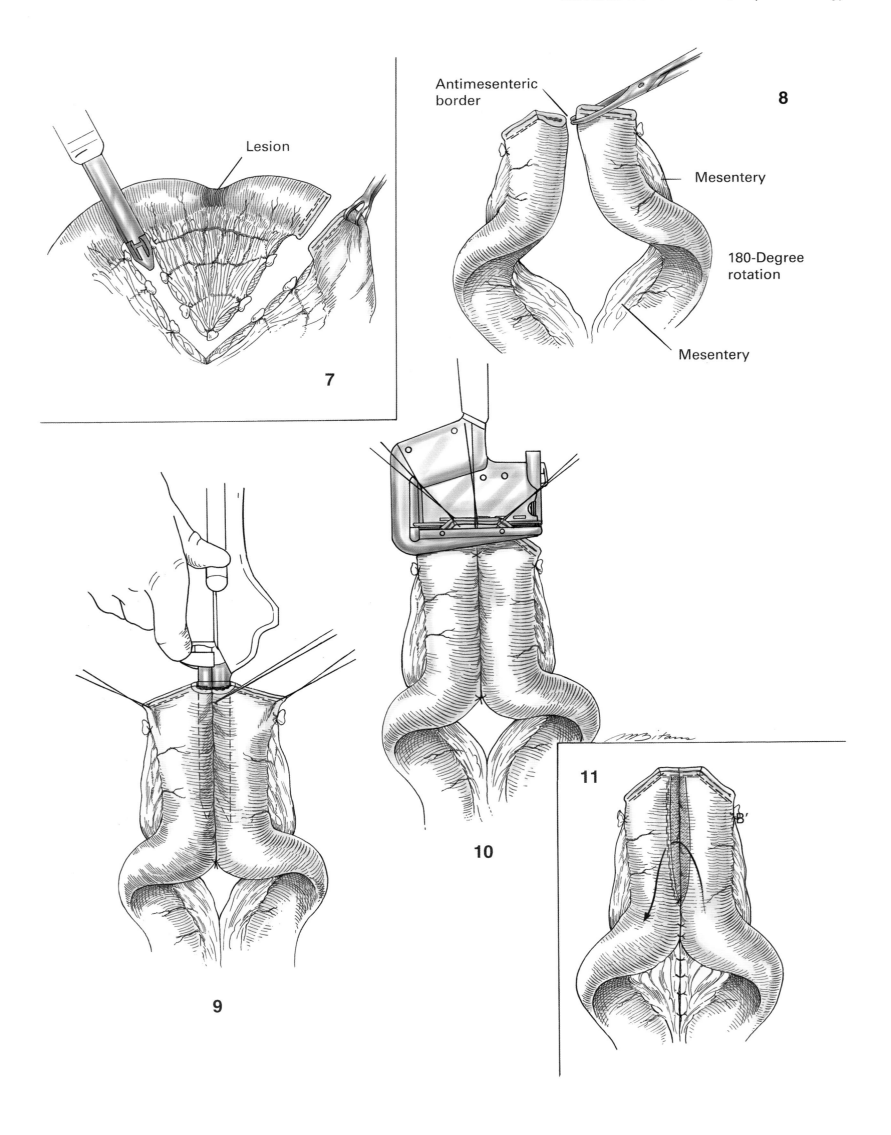

Lesion

7

Antimesenteric border

Mesentery

180-Degree rotation

Mesentery

8

9

10

11

ENTEROENTEROSTOMY, STAPLED

INDICATIONS On occasion, an enteroenterostomy may be used to bypass an obstructed segment of small intestine involved with regional ileitis, tumor, or extensive adhesions. A great difference in diameter of the intestine that enters and exits a point of obstruction may make an end-to-end anastomosis difficult. In some patients, a side-to-side anastomosis can provide relief of the obstruction with minimum risk and without sacrificing extensive segments of small intestine. In patients who have had previous small bowel resection or regional ileitis, it may be the procedure of choice rather than a radical resection leading to further nutritional problems, despite the risk of subsequent malignancy in the involved area of enteritis. The enteroenterostomy is also used to reestablish the continuity of the small intestine after a variety of Roux-en-Y procedures.

DETAILS OF PROCEDURE The two loops selected for the enteroenterostomy are grasped with Babcock forceps, and noncrushing Scudder clamps may be applied to control bleeding and limit contamination from the obstructed intestine (see FIGURE 12, Chapter 44).

Traction sutures are placed in the antimesenteric border beyond the ends of the planned anastomosis. Several additional sutures may be placed and tied to provide stabilization of the two sides in preparation for introduction of the stapler (FIGURE 1).

With the area well walled off with sterile towels, a small stab wound is made with a number 11 knife blade in the antimesenteric border of each loop. The opening is made just large enough to admit freely the fork of the cutting linear stapler instrument. After both forks have been introduced, the bowel walls are realigned before the instrument is fired. The knife in the instrument divides the septum ensuring an adequate stoma between the two rows of staples (FIGURE 2).

The cutting linear stapler instrument is removed and the staple line is inspected for potential bleeding. Additional sutures may be required to control any bleeding points. Traction sutures re-placed through the ends of both staple lines to approximate the wound edges in an everted manner while the stoma is held open (FIGURE 3). The mucosal margins may be approximated with Babcock forceps, which, along with the angle retention sutures, ensure a complete inclusion of the bowel walls within the noncutting linear stapler. The stapler is fired, and all excess bowel beyond the staples is excised by cutting along the outside surface of the stapler (FIGURE 4). The new staple suture line is inspected for hemostasis. Several additional sutures are placed to secure the angles of the anastomosis (FIGURE 5), while some prefer to place additional sutures inverting the final external staple line. The adequacy of the stoma is determined by compressing the opposing intestinal wall between the thumb and the index finger.

POSTOPERATIVE CARE Constant gastric suction is maintained. The indications for the procedure and the amount of blood loss at the time of operation dictate the need for blood replacement. The type and duration of antibiotic therapy will be related to the diagnosis and the presence of contamination at the time of operation. A careful daily check of fluid and electrolyte levels and weight is made. The input and output of the patients are evaluated daily. While oral liquids may be tolerated, the diet is restricted until bowel action has resumed. Early ambulation is encouraged and the patient is alerted to report any abdominal cramps, nausea, or vomiting. ■

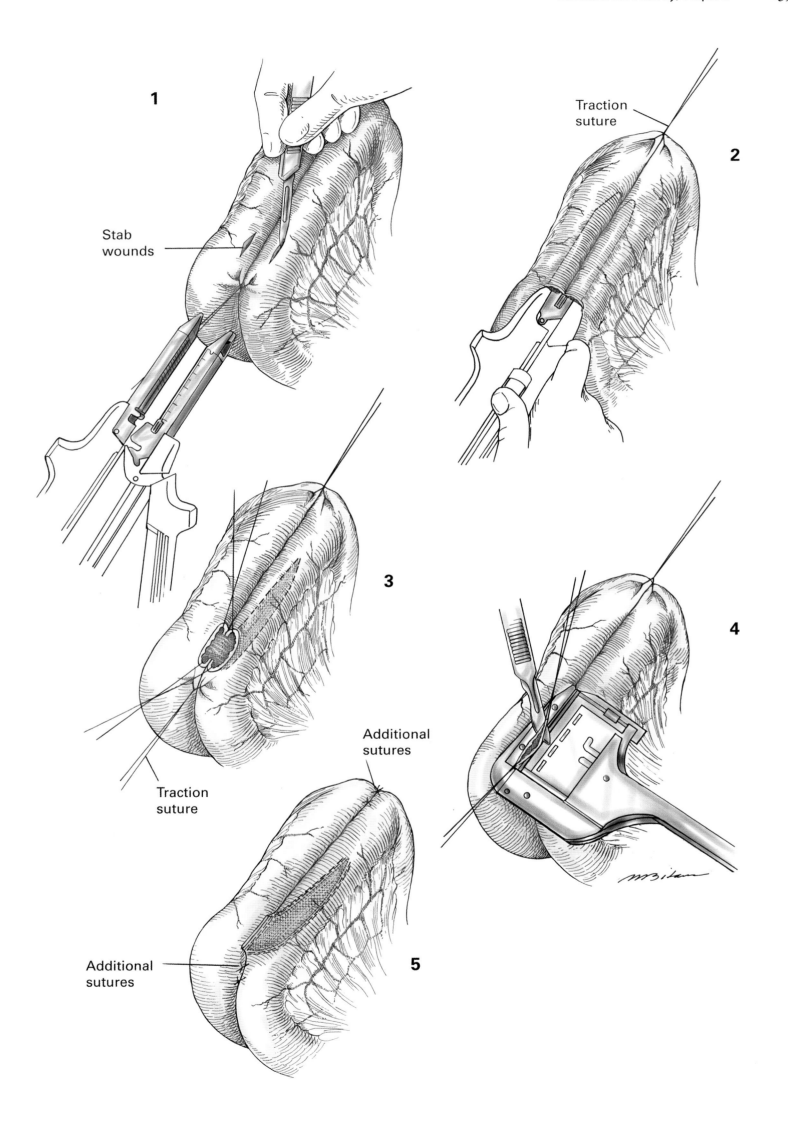

1

Stab
wounds

2

Traction
suture

3

Traction
suture

4

Additional
sutures

5

Additional
sutures

INDICATIONS Enterostomy in the high jejunum may be utilized for feeding purposes in malnourished patients, either before or after major surgical procedures. Enterostomy in the low ileum may be clinically indicated in the presence of adynamic ileus when intubation and other methods of bowel decompression have failed to relieve the obstruction or when the patient's condition will not permit the removal of the cause. Enterostomy may also be done to decompress the gastrointestinal tract proximal to the point of major resection and anastomosis or to decompress the stomach indirectly after gastric resection by directing a long tube in a retrograde fashion back into the stomach. Bile, pancreatic juice, as well as gastric juice lost from intubation or a fistula can be re-fed through the tube.

PREOPERATIVE PREPARATION The preoperative preparation is determined by the underlying conditions found preoperatively. Often an enterostomy is done in conjunction with another major surgical procedure on the gastrointestinal tract.

POSITION The patient is placed in a comfortable supine position.

OPERATIVE PREPARATION The skin is prepared routinely.

INCISION AND EXPOSURE As a rule, a midline incision is placed close to the umbilicus. If the enterostomy is performed for adynamic ileus in the presence of peritonitis, the incision should be so small that few sutures are necessary in the closure. When the procedure is part of a major intestinal resection or for feeding purposes, the enterostomy tube is brought out through a stab wound, preferably some distance away from the original incision. If the enterostomy is primarily for feeding purposes, or for draining the stomach, the incision should be made in the region of the ligament of Treitz in the left upper quadrant.

A. STAMM ENTEROSTOMY

INDICATIONS When used for feeding purposes, either preliminary, complementary, or supplementary to a major resection, a Stamm enterostomy should be made close to the ligament of Treitz in the jejunum. When intended to relieve distention in adynamic ileus, the first presenting dilated loop may be utilized.

DETAILS OF PROCEDURE In the enterostomy used as a means of feeding, a loop of jejunum close to the ligament of Treitz is delivered into the wound, and the proximal and distal ends of the bowel are identified. The bowel is stripped of its contents, and enterostomy clamps are applied. Two concentric purse-string 00 nonabsorbable sutures are taken in the submucosa of the antimesenteric surface (FIGURE 1). A small stab wound is made through the intestinal wall in the center of the inner purse-string suture (FIGURE 2), through which the catheter is slipped into the lumen of the distal portion of the intestine. The clamps are removed. The inner purse-string suture is tightened about the catheter. The outer purse-string suture is pulled snug to anchor the catheter to the intestinal wall and serves to invert a small cuff of intestine about the catheter (FIGURE 3).

CLOSURE The proximal end of the catheter is brought out through a stab wound in the abdominal wall. The intestine adjacent to the catheter is anchored to the overlying peritoneum with four fine nonabsorbable sutures (FIGURE 4). The catheter is anchored to the skin with a nonabsorbable suture (FIGURE 5).

B. WITZEL ENTEROSTOMY

INDICATIONS The Witzel enterostomy may be preferred when a long-term need for a small bowel enterostomy is clearly indicated. This procedure provides valvelike protection to the opening into the jejunum.

DETAILS OF PROCEDURE The loop of small bowel selected for the enterostomy is stripped of its contents and noncrushing clamps may be applied. A purse-string 00 nonabsorbable suture is placed opposite the mesenteric border at the planned site of entrance (FIGURE 6). A modest-sized soft catheter with several openings is then brought through the abdominal wall placed on the intestinal wall while interrupted sutures are placed about 1 cm apart, incorporating a small bite of the intestinal wall on either side of the catheter (FIGURE 7). When these sutures are tied, the catheter is buried within the wall of the small intestine for 6 to 8 cm. Following this, an incision is made into the bowel in the midportion of the purse-string suture, and the end of the catheter is inserted into the small intestine (FIGURE 8) and threaded the desired distance into the lumen, after which the purse-string suture is tied. The remaining exposed portion of the catheter and the area of the purse-string suture are further buried with three or four interrupted 00 nonabsorbable sutures (FIGURE 9). A stab wound is made in the abdominal wall and a clamp inserted as a guide to the placement of sutures between the small intestine and the peritoneum adjacent to the suture line (FIGURE 10). A broad-based attachment is desirable to avoid twisting or angulating the small intestine. After the first layer of sutures is tied, the catheter is withdrawn through the stab wound, permitting the anterior layer of sutures to be placed between the peritoneum and the small intestine, which completely seals off the area of the catheter. It is advisable to attach the small intestine to the parietes for 5 to 8 cm in order to avoid volvulus of the small intestine around a small fixed point. The intestine should be anchored to the peritoneum in the direction of peristalsis.

Alternatively, a simplified feeding enterostomy may be fashioned using an 8 or 10 French plastic or Silastic tube introduced through a needle passed through the abdominal wall some distance from the incision. The needle is tunneled intramurally through the bowel wall and the catheter directed into the bowel lumen. It is secured by one or two purse-string sutures about the entrance site. The bowel about the tubing is anchored to the perineum at its entry through the abdominal wall, and the adjacent segment of intestine is sutured to the peritoneum over approximately 10 cm (three or four sutures) to prevent rotation and possible volvulus.

CLOSURE The abdomen is closed routinely. The catheter is anchored to the skin with a suture and an additional adhesive dressing.

POSTOPERATIVE CARE When the enterostomy is performed to relieve an adynamic ileus, the catheter is attached to a drainage bottle and approximately 30 mL of sterile water or saline may be injected over 2 to 4 hours to ensure adequate drainage through the tube. If the enterostomy is used for feeding, the patient's fluid and calorie requirements can be partially met by homogenized milk and glucose in water or saline or with one of the many commercial enteral feeding mixtures. These may be started through the enterostomy tube by continuous gravity drip at the rate of 50 mL per hour. The calorie intake should be increased slowly because of the common complication of diarrhea and abdominal discomfort. Enterostomy feedings should not be continued during the night because of the possibility that distress and/or diarrhea may develop. The catheter usually is removed within 10 to 14 days unless it is required for feeding purposes, or if the obstruction has not been relieved, as proved by recurrent symptoms after clamping of the catheter. ∎

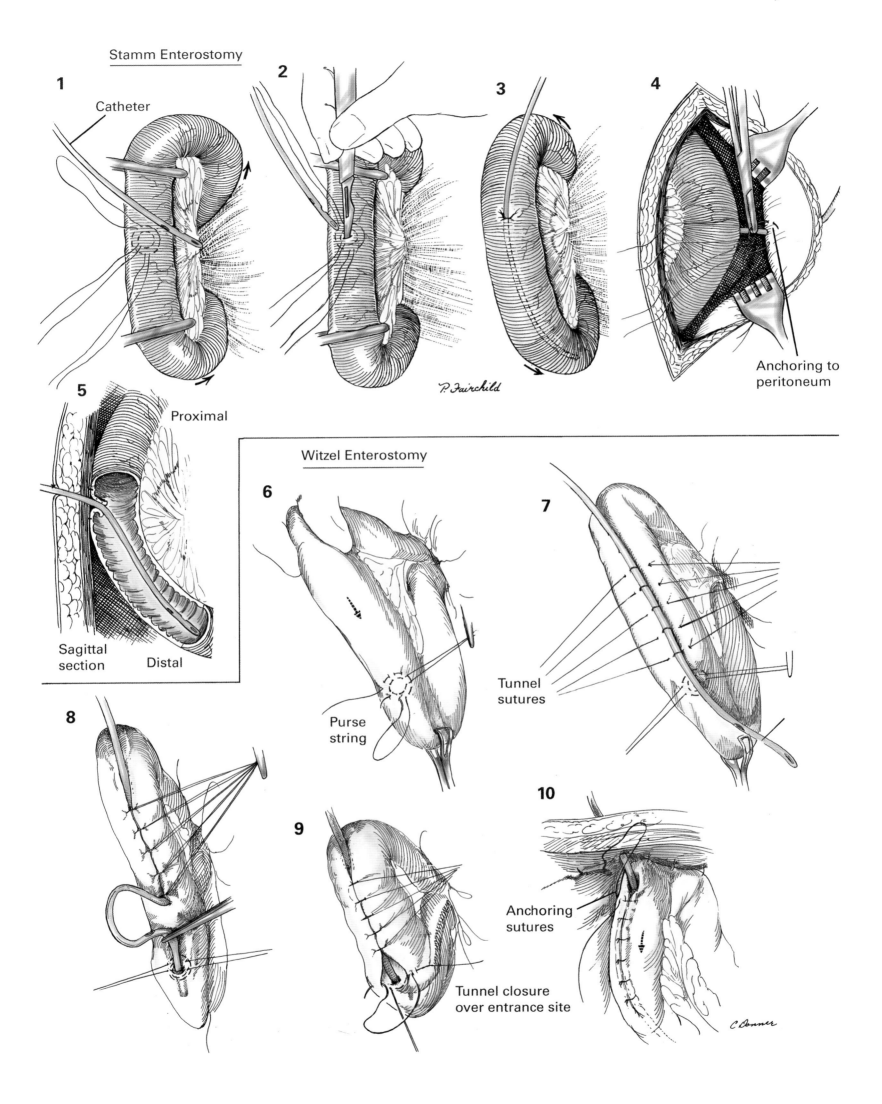

Stamm Enterostomy

1 Catheter

2 P. Fairchild

3

4 Anchoring to peritoneum

5 Proximal

Sagittal section   Distal

Witzel Enterostomy

6 Purse string

7 Tunnel sutures

8

9 Tunnel closure over entrance site

10 Anchoring sutures

C. Conner

APPENDECTOMY

INDICATIONS Acute appendicitis is a bacterial process that is usually progressive; however, many locations of the appendix allow this organ to mimic many other retrocecal, intra-abdominal, or pelvic diseases. When the diagnosis of acute appendicitis is made, prompt operation is almost always indicated. Delay for administration of parenteral fluids and antibiotics may be advisable in toxic patients, children, or elderly patients.

If the patient has a mass in the right lower quadrant when first seen, several hours of preparation may be indicated. Often a phlegmon is present and appendectomy can be accomplished. When an abscess is found, it is drained and appendectomy performed concurrently, if this can be done easily. Otherwise, the abscess is drained and an interval appendectomy is carried out at a later date.

If the diagnosis is chronic appendicitis, then other causes of pain and sources of pathology should be ruled out.

PREOPERATIVE PREPARATION The preoperative preparation is devoted chiefly to the restoration of fluid balance, especially in the very young and in aged patients. The patient should be well hydrated, as manifest by a good urine output. A nasogastric tube is passed for decompression of the stomach so as to minimize vomiting during induction of anesthesia. Antipyretic medication and external cooling may be needed since hyperpyrexia complicates general anesthesia. If peritonitis or an abscess is suspected, antibiotics are given.

ANESTHESIA Inhalation anesthesia is preferred; however, spinal anesthesia is satisfactory. Local anesthesia may be indicated in the very ill patient.

POSITION The patient is placed in a comfortable supine position.

OPERATIVE PREPARATION The skin is prepared in the usual manner.

INCISION AND EXPOSURE In no surgical procedure has the practice of standardizing the incision proved more harmful. There can be no incision that should always be utilized, since the appendix is a mobile part of the body and may be found anyplace in the right lower quadrant, in the pelvis, up under the ascending colon, and even, rarely, on the left side of the peritoneal cavity (FIGURES 1 and 3). The surgeon determines the location of the appendix, chiefly from the point of maximum tenderness by physical examination, and makes the incision best adapted for exposing this particular area. The great majority of appendices are reached satisfactorily through the right lower muscle-splitting incision, which is a variation of the original McBurney procedure (FIGURE 1, incision A). If the patient is a woman and laparoscopic evaluation is not available, many surgeons prefer a midline incision to permit exposure of the pelvis. If there is evidence of abscess formation, the incision should be made directly over the site of the abscess.

Wherever the incision is, it is deepened first to the aponeurosis of the outer layer of muscle. In the muscle-splitting incision the aponeurosis of the external oblique is split from the edge of the rectus sheath out into the flank parallel to its fibers (FIGURE 4). With the external oblique held aside by retractors, the internal oblique muscle is split parallel to its fibers up to the rectus sheath (FIGURE 5) and laterally toward the iliac crest (FIGURE 6). Sometimes the transversalis fascia and muscle are divided with the internal oblique, but a stouter structure for repair results if the transversalis fascia is opened with the peritoneum. The rectus sheath may be opened for 1 or 2 cm to give additional exposure (FIGURE 7). The peritoneum is picked up between forceps, first by the operator and then by the assistant (FIGURE 8). The operator drops the original bite, picks it up again close to the forceps of the first assistant, and compresses the peritoneum between the forceps with the handle of the scalpel to free the underlying intestine. This maneuver to safeguard the bowel is important and should always be carried out before opening the peritoneum. As soon as the peritoneum is opened (FIGURE 8), the abdominal wall structures are protected with gauze pads to minimize any potential contamination. The edges of the peritoneum are then clamped to the moist gauze sponges already surrounding the wound (FIGURE 9). Cultures are taken off the peritoneal fluid.

DETAILS OF PROCEDURE As a rule, if the cecum presents almost immediately, it is better to pull it into the wound, to hold it in a piece of moist gauze, and to deliver the appendix without feeling around blindly in the abdomen (FIGURE 10). The peritoneal attachments of the cecum may require division to facilitate the removal of the appendix. Once the appendix is delivered, its mesentery near the tip may be seized in a clamp, and the cecum may be returned to the abdominal cavity. Following this, the peritoneal cavity is walled off with moist gauze sponges (FIGURE 11). The mesentery of the appendix is divided between clamps, and the vessels are carefully ligated (FIGURES 2 and 12). It is better to apply a transfixing suture rather than a tie to the contents of the clamps, for when structures are under tension, the vessels not infrequently retract from the clamp and bleed later into the mesentery. With the vessels of the mesentery tied off, the stump of the appendix is crushed in a right-angle clamp (FIGURE 13). **CONTINUES** ▶

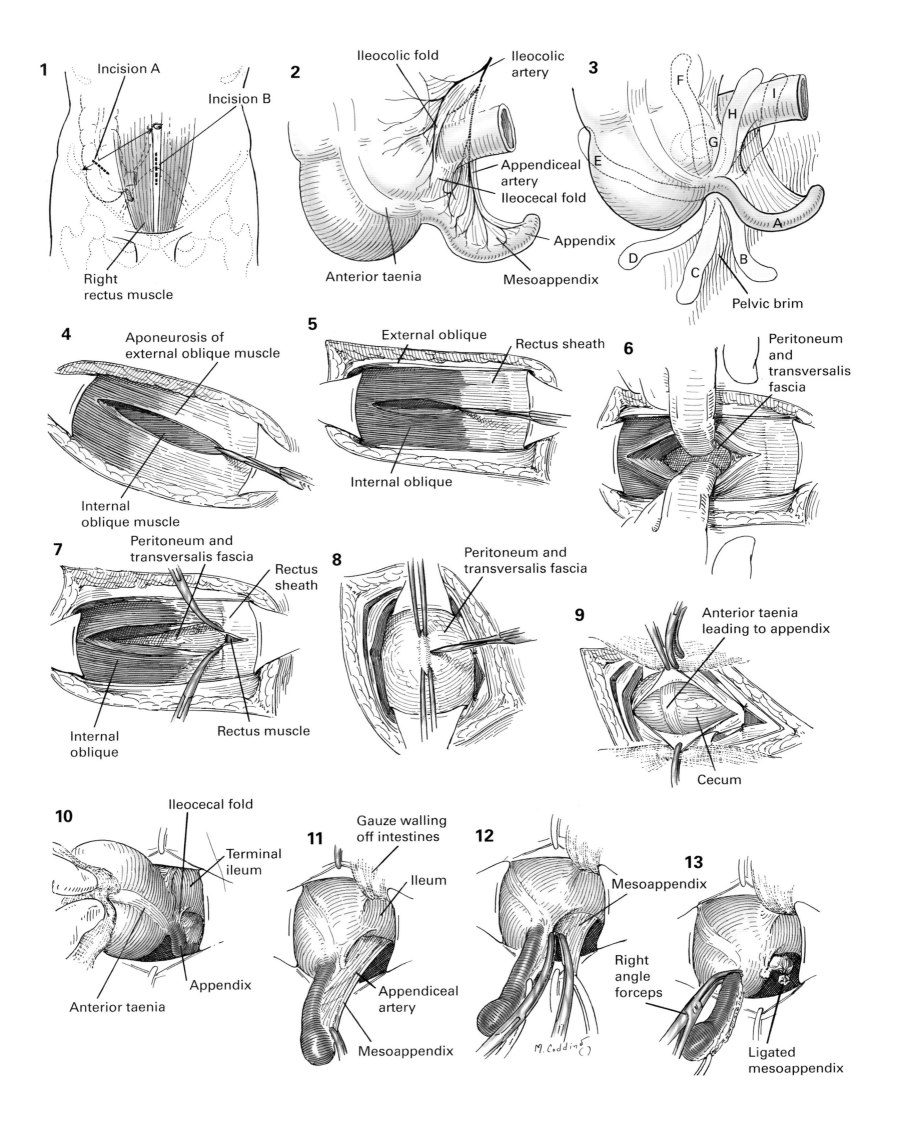

1 Incision A Incision B Right rectus muscle

2 Ileocolic fold Ileocolic artery Appendiceal artery Ileocecal fold Appendix Mesoappendix Anterior taenia

3 F H I G E A D C B Pelvic brim

4 Aponeurosis of external oblique muscle Internal oblique muscle

5 External oblique Rectus sheath Internal oblique

6 Peritoneum and transversalis fascia

7 Peritoneum and transversalis fascia Rectus sheath Internal oblique Rectus muscle

8 Peritoneum and transversalis fascia

9 Anterior taenia leading to appendix Cecum

10 Ileocecal fold Terminal ileum Anterior taenia Appendix

11 Gauze walling off intestines Ileum Appendiceal artery Mesoappendix

12 Mesoappendix Right angle forceps

13 Mesoappendix Ligated mesoappendix

M. Codding

DETALS OF PROCEDURE ◀**CONTINUED**▶ The right-angle clamp is moved 1 cm toward the tip of the appendix. Just at the proximal edge of the crushed portion, the appendix is ligated (FIGURE 14) and a straight clamp is placed on the knot. A purse-string suture is laid in the wall of the cecum at the base of the appendix, care being taken not to perforate blood vessels where the mesentery of the appendix was attached (FIGURE 15). The appendix is held upward; the cecum is walled off with moist gauze to prevent contamination; and the appendix is divided between the ligature and clamp (FIGURE 16). The suture on the base of the appendix is cut and pushed inward with the straight clamp on the ligature of the stump to invaginate the stump into the cecal wall. The jaws of the clamp are separated, and the clamp is removed as the purse-string suture is tied. The wall of the cecum may be fixed with tissue forceps to aid in inverting the appendiceal stump (FIGURE 17). The cecum then appears as shown in FIGURE 18. The area is lavaged with warm saline and the omentum is placed over the site of operation (FIGURE 19). If there has been a localized abscess or a perforation near the base, so that a secure closure of the cecum is not possible, or if hemostasis has been poor, drainage may be advisable. Drains should be soft and smooth, preferably a silastic sump drain. On no occasion should dry gauze or heavy rubber tubing be used, since these may cause bowel injury. Some surgeons do not drain the peritoneal cavity in the presence of obvious peritonitis that is not localized, relying upon peritoneal irrigation, parenteral antibiotic, and systemic antibiotic therapy to control it.

If the appendix is not obviously involved with acute inflammation, a more extensive exploration is mandatory. In the presence of peritonitis without involvement of the appendix, the possibility of a ruptured peptic ulcer or sigmoid diverticulitis must be ruled out. Acute cholecystitis, regional ileitis, and involvement of the cecum by carcinoma are not uncommon possibilities. In the female, the possibility of bleeding from a ruptured graafian follicle, ectopic pregnancy, or pelvic infection is ever present. Inspection of the pelvic organs under these circumstances cannot be omitted. On occasion a Meckel's diverticulum will be found. Closure of the abdomen, with subsequent study and adequate preparation for bowel resection at a later date, may be indicated.

CLOSURE The muscle layers are held apart while the peritoneum is closed with a running or interrupted absorbable suture (FIGURE 19). Transversalis fascia incorporated with the peritoneum offers a better foundation for the suture. Interrupted sutures are placed in the internal oblique muscle and in the small opening at the outer border of the rectus sheath (FIGURE 20). The external oblique aponeurosis is closed but not constricted with interrupted sutures (FIGURE 21). The subcutaneous tissue and skin are closed in layers. The skin may be left open for a delayed secondary closure if pus is found about the appendix.

ALTERNATIVE METHOD In some instances, in order to avoid rupturing a distended acute appendix, it is safe to ligate and divide the base of the appendix before attempting to deliver the appendix into the wound. For example, if the appendix is adherent to the lateral wall of the cecum (FIGURE 22), it is occasionally simpler to pass a curved clamp beneath the base of the appendix in order that it may be doubly clamped and ligated (FIGURE 23). Following ligation of the base of the appendix, which is often quite indurated, it is divided with a knife (FIGURE 24). The base of the appendix is then inverted with a purse-string suture (FIGURES 25 and 26). The attachments of the appendix are divided with long, curved scissors until the blood supply can be clearly identified (FIGURE 27). Curved clamps are then applied to the mesentery of the appendix, and the contents of these clamps are subsequently ligated with oo sutures (FIGURE 28).

When the appendix is not readily found, the search should follow the anterior taenia of the cecum, which will lead directly to the base of the appendix regardless of its position. When the appendix is found in the retrocecal position, it becomes necessary to incise the parietal peritoneum parallel to the lateral border of the appendix as it is seen through the peritoneum (FIGURE 29). This allows the appendix to be dissected free from its position behind the cecum and on the peritoneal covering of the iliopsoas muscle (FIGURE 30).

On occasion the cecum may be in the upper quadrant or indeed on the left side of the abdomen when failure of rotation has occurred. A liberal increase in the size of the incision and even a second incision may be, on occasion, good judgment.

POSTOPERATIVE CARE The fluid balance is maintained by the intravenous administration of Ringer's lactate. The patient is permitted to sit up for eating on the day of operation, and he may get out of bed on the first postoperative day. Sips of water may be given as soon as nausea subsides. The diet is gradually increased.

If there has been evidence of peritoneal sepsis, frequent doses of antibiotics are administered. Constant gastric suction is advisable until all evidence of peritonitis and abdominal distention has subsided. Accurate estimate of the fluid intake and output must be made.

Pelvic localization of pus is enhanced by placing the patient in a semisitting position. The patient is allowed out of bed as soon as his or her general condition warrants. Prophylaxis against deep venous thrombosis is instituted. In the presence of persistent signs of sepsis, wound infection and pelvic or subphrenic abscess should be considered. In the presence of prolonged sepsis, serial computed tomography (CT) imaging scans beginning about 7 days after surgery may reveal the causative site. ∎

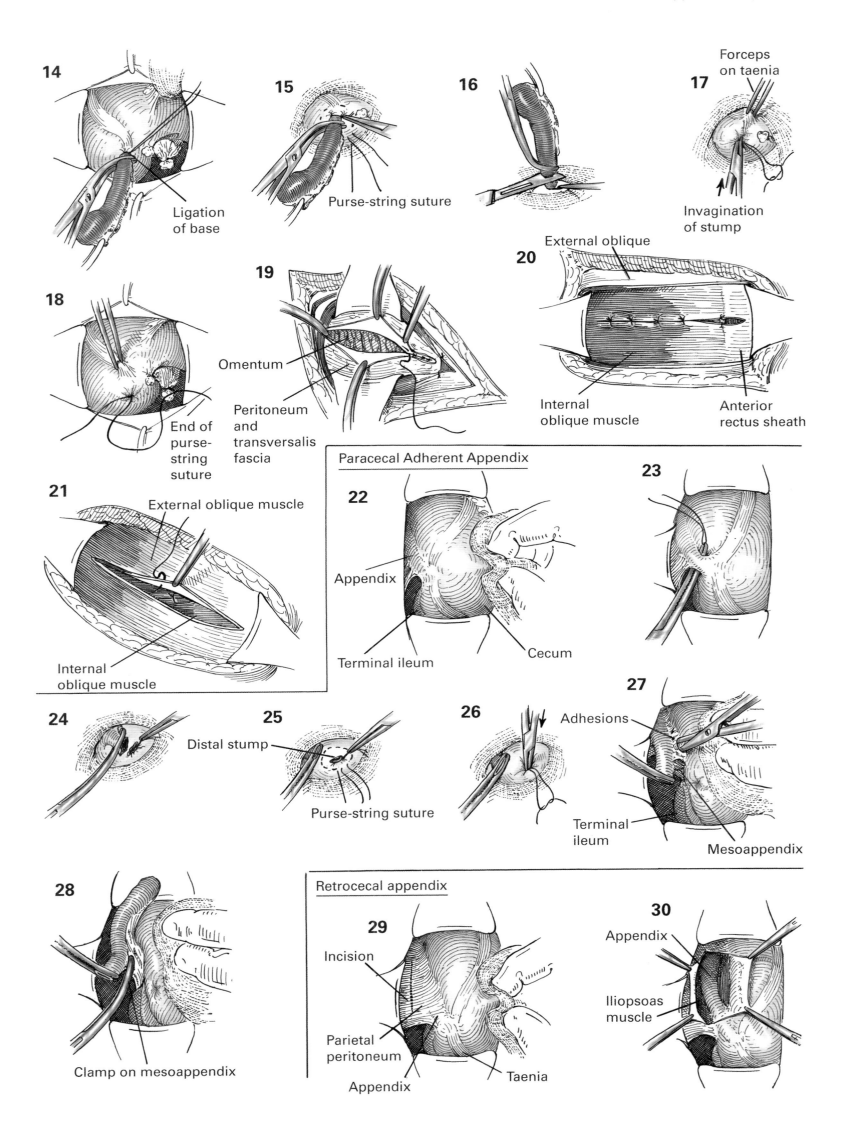

14 Ligation of base

15 Purse-string suture

16

17 Forceps on taenia / Invagination of stump

18 End of purse-string suture

19 Omentum / Peritoneum and transversalis fascia

20 External oblique / Internal oblique muscle / Anterior rectus sheath

21 External oblique muscle / Internal oblique muscle

Paracecal Adherent Appendix

22 Appendix / Terminal ileum / Cecum

23

24

25 Distal stump / Purse-string suture

26

27 Adhesions / Terminal ileum / Mesoappendix

28 Clamp on mesoappendix

Retrocecal appendix

29 Incision / Parietal peritoneum / Appendix / Taenia

30 Appendix / Iliopsoas muscle

CHAPTER 49

APPENDECTOMY, LAPAROSCOPIC

INDICATIONS Acute appendicitis is a clinical diagnosis, the accuracy of which has improved with modern diagnostic imaging techniques including CT scan of the abdomen and pelvis, which has an accuracy of 90% or more. The diagnosis is made using a combination of history, physical examination, and laboratory tests plus an elevated temperature and white blood cell count. A positive imaging study is helpful and gives reassurance about the diagnosis. In equivocal cases, serial observations and studies over time improve the accuracy of diagnosis, but at the risk of an increasing rate of perforation.

Laparoscopic appendectomy is appropriate for virtually all patients and is preferred in obese patients, who require longer open incisions with increased manipulation and the resultant increase in surgical-site infections. The laparoscopic technique is also indicated in females, especially during the reproductive years, when tubal and ovarian pathology may mimic appendicitis. Laparoscopy not only provides direct observation of the appendix but also allows evaluation of all intra-abdominal organs, especially those in the female pelvis. Laparoscopic appendectomy has been shown to be as safe as open appendectomy in the first trimester of pregnancy; however, there is always risk to the fetus with any anesthesia or operation. Later or third-trimester pregnancies as well as any process that creates intestinal distention will make entering the intraperitoneal space more difficult and leave no room for maneuvering the instruments for a safe laparoscopic operation. Finally, laparoscopic appendectomy results in less incisional pain after surgery, allows a faster return to normal function or work, and produces a better cosmetic result.

PREOPERATIVE PREPARATION As healthy youngsters and young adults constitute the most common population with appendicitis, the usual preoperative evaluation for anesthesia and surgery is performed. Intravenous fluids for hydration and preoperative antibiotics are given. Extra time may be needed in the very young or old for correction of electrolyte and fluid imbalances. Hyperpyrexia should be treated with antipyretics or even external cooling, so as to lessen the risk of general anesthesia. Additional discussion concerning preparation is contained in the discussion accompanying Chapter 48.

ANESTHESIA General anesthesia with placement of an endotracheal tube is preferred. After induction, an orogastric tube may be placed by the anesthesiologist. This tube is removed before the end of the case or is replaced with a nasogastric tube if prolonged decompression is anticipated.

POSITION The patient is placed in a supine position. The right arm may be extended for intravenous and blood pressure cuff access by the anesthesiologist while the left arm with the pulse oximeter is tucked in at the patient's side. This allows for easier movement by the surgeon and the assistant operating the videoscope. The fiber-optic light cable and gas tubing are usually placed to the head of the table; the video monitor is placed across from the operating team; and the electrocautery and suction irrigator are placed toward the foot of the table, where the scrub nurse and Mayo instrument tray are positioned.

OPERATIVE PREPARATION A Foley catheter is usually placed and the abdomen is prepped in the routine manner.

DETAILS OF PROCEDURE A typical placement for access ports is shown at the umbilicus, left lower quadrant, and lower midline (FIGURE 1). Some surgeons prefer a right upper quadrant port instead of the one in the left lower quadrant. As in most laparoscopic procedures, some form of triangulation is employed, with the longest and widest angle given to the operating ports and instruments. The videoscope port is created first. Although some use an initial inflation of the abdomen with a Veress needle (see Chapter 12), most general surgeons employ the open Hasson technique (see Chapter 11). The surgeon may enter at the superior or inferior margin of the umbilicus with either a vertical or semicircular transverse incision. After the Hasson port is placed and secured with the stay sutures, the abdomen is inflated with CO_2. The surgeon sets the maximum gas pressure ($\leq$15 mm Hg) and flow rate while he or she monitors the actual intra-abdominal pressure and the total volume of gas insufflated. The abdomen then enlarges and becomes tympanitic.

The videoscope is attached to the telescopic instrument, which may be straight (zero degree) or angled. The system is white-balanced and the focus adjusted. After the optical end of the instrument has been cleaned with antifog solution, it is introduced down the Hasson port. A careful visualization of all four quadrants of the abdomen is performed and a record is made of all normal and abnormal findings.

Under direct vision with the videoscope, two additional 5-mm ports are put into the abdomen. One is in the left lower quadrant and is placed lateral to the rectus muscle with its epigastric vessels. The light of the videoscope is used to transilluminate the abdominal wall at the proposed site so as to avoid trocar placement through vessels in the oblique muscles. The surgeon infiltrates the 5-mm site with local anesthetic. This infiltrating needle can be advanced through the abdominal wall and the videoscope will see the needle enter the anticipated site for this port. A 5-mm skin incision is made and the subcutaneous tissue dilated with a small hemostat down to the level of the fascia. The 5-mm port is placed through the abdominal wall while the surgeon views the safe entrance of the pointed trocar into the intraperitoneal space. The third port is placed through the midline linea alba in a suprapubic position so as to avoid the bladder, which has been decompressed with a Foley catheter. The strategy for a widely spread (hand's breadth) triangular pattern of port placement now becomes apparent as the three instruments compete for room to maneuver.

The patient is placed in the Trendelenburg position and the right side of the operating table may be elevated using gravity to hold the small bowel away from the right lower quadrant. If a normal appendix is found, a search for other inflammatory processes is begun. Tubo-ovarian diseases, inflammatory bowel disease, and Meckel's diverticulitis are most commonly found. Once the diagnosis of appendicitis is established, the appendix is mobilized. The appendix and its mesentery must be clearly visualized. The position of the appendix is quite variable, and it may be covered with peritoneum or even the cecum (FIGURE 2). Safe opening of any peritoneal covering or the equivalent of the lateral line of Toldt along the cecum may require placement of an additional operating port. If the surgeon cannot obtain complete visualization of the appendix, mesoappendix, and base of the cecum for a safe transection, the operation is converted to an open procedure. **CONTINUES ▶**

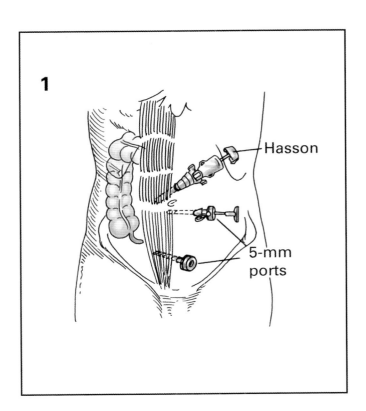

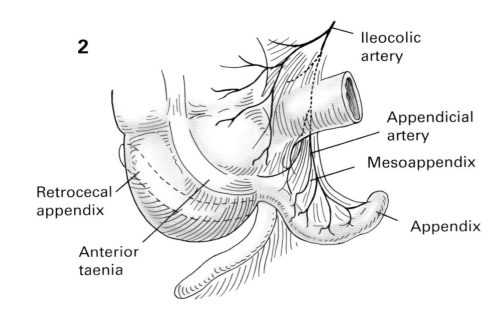

DETAILS OF PROCEDURE ◀CONTINUED▶ Laparoscopic removal begins with a splaying out of the mesoappendix using a grasping forceps upon the mesentery (FIGURE 3). The inflamed tip of the appendix is not grasped, as this could cause it to rupture. The surgeon opens through the mesentery at the base of the appendix using a dissecting instrument. If maneuvering of the appendix and its mesentery is difficult using the grasping forceps, some surgeons prefer to lasso the inflamed end of the appendix with a loop suture that is applied snugly. The cut end of this suture may be grasped more securely with the maneuvering forceps (FIGURE 4). The mesoappendix is divided (FIGURE 4) in one or more transections using an endoscopic vascular stapling instrument that is passed through the large Hasson port. This assumes that a 5-mm videoscope is available for use through the left lower quadrant port. Otherwise, the left lower quadrant port is enlarged to 10 mm, as both the videoscope and endoscopic vascular stapler require large ports. The base of the appendix is divided with the endoscopic cutting linear stapler (FIGURE 5). An important maneuver with any division using this stapler is to rotate it about 180 degrees, so as to visualize the entire length and the contents within its jaws (FIGURE 5A). This rotation should also be done during the stapling of the mesoappendix.

A small, minimally inflamed appendix can be removed safely through the shaft of a 10-mm port. Most surgeons place an enlarged or suppurative appendix into a plastic bag for removal through the abdominal wall (FIGURE 6). This lessens the chances of infection at the surgical site. The appendiceal stump and stapled mesoappendix are inspected for security and hemostasis. The area is lavaged with the suction irrigator and a regional inspection is made to verify the integrity of the cecum and small bowel.

Each of the 5-mm ports is removed under direct vision with the videoscope to make sure that there are no bleeding abdominal wall vessels.

CLOSURE The abdomen is decompressed and the Hasson port removed. Routinely, only the 10-mm port sites require fascial closure. Some surgeons tie the stay sutures together if this provides a secure closure to inspection and finger palpation. Others place new 00 delayed absorbable sutures through the fascia for its closure. Scarpa's fascia and the subcutaneous fat are not closed. The skin is approximated with fine 0000 absorbable sutures. Adhesive skin strips and small, dry sterile dressings are applied.

POSTOPERATIVE CARE The orogastric tube is removed before the patient awakens from anesthesia. The Foley catheter is discontinued as soon as the patient is alert enough to void. If a long-acting local anesthetic was used at the port sites, postoperative pain can be controlled with oral medications. There may be some transient nausea, but most patients can be weaned from intravenous fluid to simple oral intake within a day. Antibiotic therapy is often perioperative but may continue for a few days, depending on the operative findings. Most patients are discharged home within a day or two.

ALTERNATIVE METHODS There are many variations upon the technique described above. These involve the placement of the ports and the methods for transecting the appendix and mesoappendix.

Virtually all laparoscopic appendectomies begin with placement of the videoscope through an umbilical site. Insufflation using the Veress needle technique is preferred by some, although most general surgeons enter the abdomen in a more controlled, open manner using the Hasson technique. Placement of additional ports is determined by the surgeon's preference. In general, the sites should be widely spaced to avoid instrument competition. The size of the second port is a function of whether or not the surgeon has a 5-mm videoscope and whether he or she plans to use (1) the vascular stapler or (2) large ultrasonic, cautery, or laser devices for transection and hemostasis. Most of these devices currently require a 10-mm port.

Alternatively, some surgeons use metal clips for transection of the mesoappendix and a pair of absorbable loop sutures for occlusion of the stump of the appendix, whose mucosal center is cauterized. However, vascular staples are preferred by most for their security and the avoidance of unrecognized thermal damage. ■

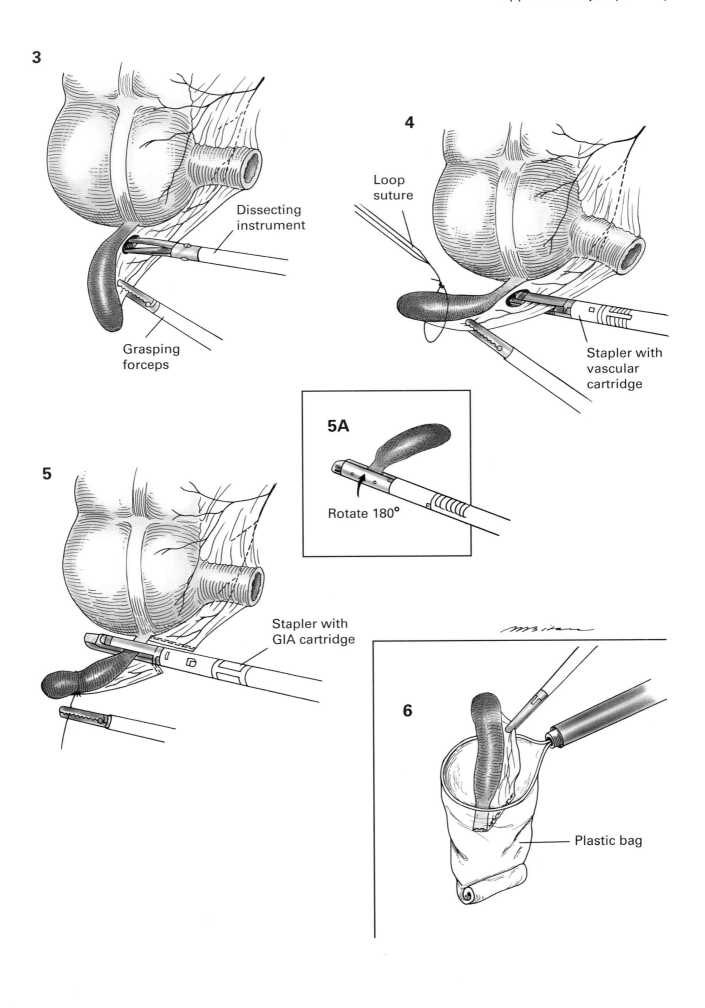

3

Dissecting instrument

Grasping forceps

4

Loop suture

Stapler with vascular cartridge

5A

Rotate 180°

5

Stapler with GIA cartridge

6

Plastic bag

CHAPTER 50 SURGICAL ANATOMY OF LARGE INTESTINE

Several important anatomic facts influence the technique of surgery in the large intestine. As a consequence of its embryologic development, the colon has two main sources of blood supply. The cecum, ascending colon, and proximal portion of the transverse colon are supplied with blood from the superior mesenteric artery, while the distal transverse colon, splenic flexure, descending colon, sigmoid, and upper rectum are supplied by branches of the inferior mesenteric artery (see FIGURE 1).

Advantage may be taken of the free anastomotic blood supply along the medial border of the bowel by dividing either the inferior mesenteric artery or the middle colic artery and by depending upon the collateral circulation through the marginal artery of Drummond to maintain the viability of a long segment of intestine. The peritoneal reflection on the lateral aspect of the colon is practically bloodless, except at the flexures or in the presence of ulcerative colitis or portal hypertension, and may be completely incised without causing bleeding or jeopardizing the viability of the bowel. When the lateral peritoneum is divided and the greater omentum freed from the transverse colon, extensive mobilization is possible, including derotation of the cecum into the right or left upper quadrant. Care should be taken to avoid undue traction on the splenic flexure lest attachments to the capsule of the spleen be torn and troublesome bleeding occur. In the presence of malignancy of the transverse colon, the omentum is usually resected adjacent to the blood supply of the greater curvature of the stomach.

After the colon has been freed from its attachments to the peritoneum of the abdominal wall, the flexures, and the greater omentum, it can be drawn toward the midline through the surgical incision limited only by the length of its mesentery. This mobility of the colon renders the blood supply more accessible and often permits a procedure to be performed outside the peritoneal cavity. The most mobile part of the large bowel is the sigmoid, because it normally possesses a long mesentery, whereas the descending colon and right half of the colon are fixed to the lateral abdominal wall.

The lymphatic distribution of the large bowel conforms to the vascular supply. Knowledge of this is of great surgical importance, especially in the treatment of malignant neoplasm, because an adequate extirpation of potentially involved lymph nodes requires the sacrifice of a much larger portion of the blood supply than would at first seem essential. The lymphatic spread of carcinoma of the large intestine along the major vascular supply has been responsible for the development of classic resections. Local "sleeve" resection for malignancy may be indicated in the presence of metastasis or because of the patient's poor general condition.

When a curative resection is planned, the tumor and adjacent bowel must be sufficiently mobilized to permit removal of the immediate lymphatic drainage area.

Basically, the resections of the colon should include either the lymphatic drainage area of the superior mesenteric vessels or that of the inferior mesenteric vessels. While this would approach the ideal, experience has shown that approximately four types of resections are commonly performed: right colectomy, left colectomy, anterior resection of the rectosigmoid, and abdominoperineal resection. For years lesions of the cecum, ascending colon, and hepatic flexure have been resected by a right colectomy with ligation of the ileocolic, right colic, and all or part of the middle colic vessels (A). Lesions in the cecal area may be associated with involved lymph glands along the ileocolic vessels. As a result, a segment of the terminal ileum is commonly resected along with the right colon. Lesions in the region of the splenic flexure are in the one area where left colectomy by a sleeve resection may be performed. Extensive resections can be carried out with good assurance of an adequate blood supply, since the marginal vessels are divided nearer their points of origin. In addition to the marginal vessels, the left colic artery near its point of origin and the inferior mesenteric vein are ligated even before manipulation of the tumor is carried out to minimize the venous spread of cancer cells. End-to-end anastomosis without tension can be accomplished by freeing the right colon of its peritoneal attachments and derotating the cecum back to its embryologic position on the left side. The blood supply is sustained through the middle colic vessels and the sigmoidal vessels. Although the veins tend to parallel the arteries, this is not the case with the inferior mesenteric vein. This vein courses to the left before it dips beneath the body of the pancreas to join the splenic vein (B).

Lesions of the lower descending colon, sigmoid, and rectosigmoid may be removed by an anterior resection. The inferior mesenteric artery is ligated at its point of origin from the aorta (C) or just distal to the origin of the left colic artery. The upper segment for anastomosis will receive its blood supply through the marginal arteries of Drummond from the middle colic artery. The viability of the rectosigmoid is more uncertain following the ligation of the inferior mesenteric artery. Accordingly, the resection is carried low enough to ensure a good blood supply from the middle and inferior hemorrhoidal vessels. This level is usually so low that the anastomosis must be carried out in the pelvis anterior to the sacrum. Here again the principle of mobilizing the flexures as well as the right colon may be required to ensure an anastomosis without tension.

The most extensive resection involves lesions of the low rectosigmoid, rectum, and anus. High ligation of the inferior mesenteric vessels and ligation of the middle and inferior hemorrhoidal vessels, along with wide excision of the rectum and anus, are required. Since the lymphatic drainage to the anus and lower rectum may drain laterally even to the inguinal region, wide lateral excision of low-lying rectal and anal neoplasms is mandatory.

Since bowel anastomosis must be performed in the absence of tension, it is imperative that considerable mobilization of the colon, especially of the splenic flexure, be carried out if continuity is to be restored following extensive resection of the left colon. The presence of pulsating vessels adjacent to the mesenteric margin, which has been cleared preparatory to the anastomosis, should be assured. Injection of 1% procaine into the adjacent mesentery will sometimes enhance arterial pulsation. Occasionally, pulsations are not apparent since the middle colic artery is compressed as a result of the small bowels being introduced into a plastic bag and displaced to the right and outside of the abdominal wall. A sterile Doppler probe may be used to verify the adequacy of the blood supply.

The large intestine bears an important relation to a number of vital structures. Thus, in operations on the right half of the colon, the right ureter and its accompanying vessels are encountered behind the mesocolon. The duodenum lies posterior to the mesentery of the hepatic flexure and is always exposed in mobilizing this portion of the bowel. The spleen is easily injured in mobilizing the splenic flexure. The left ureter and its accompanying spermatic or ovarian vessels are always encountered in operations on the sigmoid and descending colon. In an abdominoperineal resection of the rectum, both ureters are potentially in danger of injury. The surgeon must not only be aware of these structures, but must positively identify them before dividing the vessels in the mesentery of the colon.

The anatomic arrangement of the colon that permits mobilization of low-lying segments sometimes tempts the surgeon to reconstruct the normal continuity of the fecal current without adequate extirpation of the lymphatic drainage zones. Extensive block excision of the usual lymphatic drainage areas, combined with excision of a liberal segment of normal-appearing bowel on either side of a malignant lesion, is mandatory. Primary anastomosis of the large intestine requires viable intestine, the absence of tension, especially when the bowel becomes distended postoperatively, and a bowel wall of near-normal consistency. Although the danger from sepsis has decreased substantially in recent years, the fact remains that the surgical problems concerned with the large intestine are often complex and require more seasoned judgment and experience than does almost any other field in general surgery. ■

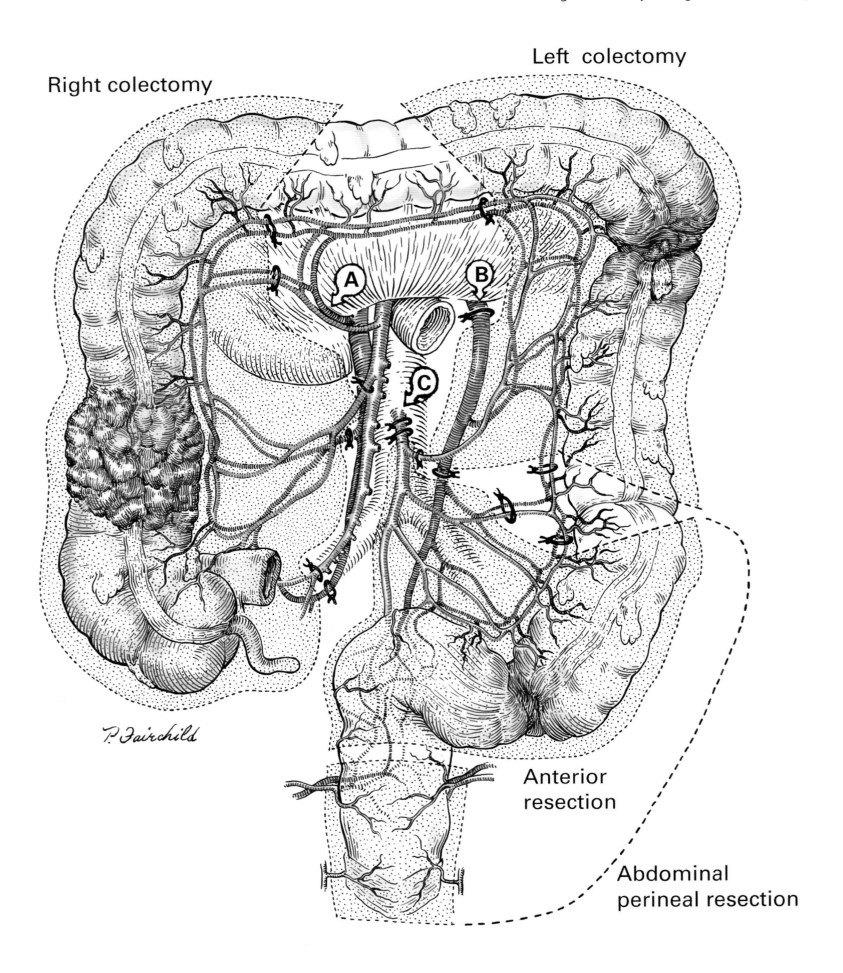

Right colectomy

Left colectomy

P. Fairchild

Anterior
resection

Abdominal
perineal resection

LOOP ILEOSTOMY

INDICATIONS A distal loop ileostomy is most commonly used for temporary diversion of the gastrointestinal contents to protect a colonic anastomosis. When it is constructed with a dominant proximal limb, this ostomy provides nearly complete diversion of succus. The loop ileostomy has replaced the traditional right transverse colon loop colostomy in many circumstances, as this loop is easier to construct and close. Additionally, the loop ileostomy has proven to be no more difficult for the patient to manage than a proximal colostomy. A loop ileostomy, however, does not decompress the colon when the ileocecal valve is intact. In those patients who require acute colon decompression, a loop colostomy will allow both colon decompression and colon preparation for a staged procedure.

PREOPERATIVE PREPARATION Most patients undergoing emergency or complex operations on the colon are counseled by the surgeon about the potential need for an ostomy. If available, an enterostomal therapist should visit the patient prior to surgery. The potential ostomy site should be marked with indelible ink (FIGURE 1). An ostomy is best placed near the lateral edge of the rectus muscle and sheath. It may be placed either above or below the umbilicus. The position chosen must take into consideration the span of the ostomy gasket, such that it has a smooth, wide surface for adherence. The costal margin, indentation of the umbilicus, uneven scars, and skin folds will not allow secure placement of the ostomy gasket. In general, the belt line should be avoided, and the patient should both stand and sit with an appliance in place during this marking. The patient should be reassured about his or her ongoing care with the enterostomal therapist. Reading material and samples are often provided. If an enterostomal therapist is unavailable, the surgeon should make every effort to educate the patient using these written and pictorial aids.

DETAILS OF PROCEDURE The anesthesia, position, and abdominal incision and exposure are determined by the colon operation being performed. When markings are made preoperatively, they should be scratched gently into the skin with an "X" prior to skin preparation. If this is not done, at the end of a long and difficult case, the inked markings will likely be gone. Upon completion of the colon anastomosis and prior to closure of the abdomen, the ostomy site is revisited. The cut edge of the abdominal wall, namely, the linea alba in the midline incision, is grasped with Kocher clamps and retracted to the central position it will occupy after closure. In patients with a thick abdominal wall, an additional clamp may be placed on the dermis to hold the abdominal wall in its usual alignment. A 3-cm circle of skin is excised and the dissection is carried down through the subcutaneous fat to the anterior fascia of the rectus muscle. A two finger–sized opening is made through the fascia. Some prefer a single slit, while others make a cruciate incision. The rectus muscle is spread or retracted medially. Care should be taken not to injure the epigastric vessels that run deeply in the center of this muscle. Another two finger–sized opening is made through the posterior sheath and peritoneum.

An appropriate segment of terminal ileum, usually about 1 ft or so proximal to the ileocecal valve, is selected. This section of small bowel must have sufficient mobility to reach through the abdominal wall without stretch or tension. It should also be proximal enough to allow side-to-side anastomosis at the time of ostomy closure. A blunt Kelly hemostat is used to create a mesenteric opening just beneath the wall of the ileum. A segment of umbilical tape or a soft rubber Penrose drain is drawn through the opening (FIGURE 2) and a seromuscular absorbable suture is placed to mark the proximal limb of the ileum. The opening in the abdominal wall is checked

again for size relative to the thickness of the ileal loop and its mesentery. In general, a two finger–sized opening is adequate. The tape and the ileal loop are brought through the abdominal wall using gentle traction with a rocking motion (FIGURE 3). The loop is oriented in a vertical manner with the active proximal limb and its marking suture placed at the cephalad or 12 o'clock position. The loop ileostomy should protrude about 5 cm above the level of the skin. A plastic ostomy rod replaces the umbilical tape or Penrose drain to prevent retraction following closure of the abdomen.

Closure of the abdomen is generally completed prior to maturing the colostomy to avoid unnecessary contamination of the abdomen with ileal contents.

The caudal or inactive side of the loop is opened transversely for two-thirds of its diameter in a position about halfway up from the skin level to that where the tape or Penrose drain penetrates the mesentery. Submucosal bleeding sites are secured with fine 0000 silk ligatures or cautery. The distal inactive stoma is matured first by placing fine 0000 absorbable sutures that traverse the entire thickness of the ileal bowel wall (FIGURE 4). This suture is completed as a transverse subcuticular bite beneath the skin edge. Three or four sutures are required for full eversion of the stoma (FIGURE 4A). To create a Brooke ileostomy the suture includes the mucosa and seromuscular layer at the open edge of the intestine and also a bite more proximal on the serosa to allow for greater eversion. The marking suture is cut or removed, and the proximal active stoma is everted. This maneuver is assisted by using the rounded, blunt end of the scalpel handle. The handle tip applies countertraction as the free mucosal edge is brought down to the skin with forceps or a similar grasping instrument (FIGURE 5). The cephalad bowel wall is then secured about its perimeter to the subcutaneous skin with interrupted fine absorbable sutures. Rods with "T" ends need not be secured. Others should be secured by placing a nonabsorbable monofilament suture at each end of the rod (FIGURE 6). In order to avoid difficulty with appliance application some surgeons prefer not to suture the rod to the skin, but to rather have the suture placed in either end of the rod and tied so as to prevent migration into the abdomen.

The viability of the stoma is rechecked and the intra-abdominal portion of the loop is examined. The loop must come up without angulation or tension, since postoperative ileus may distend the abdomen. Finally, the ileal loop opening through the abdominal wall is re-evaluated for snugness. An opening that allows passage of the loop plus one finger is recommended to minimize constriction or herniation.

CLOSURE A sterile ostomy appliance is placed after closure of the main abdominal incision.

POSTOPERATIVE CARE The ostomy is observed for viability and its output is measured. As the patient resumes oral intake, the volume of succus will increase. Careful monitoring of fluid and electrolyte balance is required, especially if an overly large (≥2 L/day) output occurs. Dietary regulation may require supplementation with antimotility drugs. The enterostomal therapist should teach the patient how to care for the stoma. Many patients will benefit from a home visit by the nurse or therapist, wherein both patient and caregiver become proficient in changing the appliance. The plastic rod is removed 3 to 5 days after surgery, after sufficient time for the serosa to be adherent to the subcutaneous fat and skin. The timing for closure of this temporary diverting loop ileostomy is determined by the healing of the colon anastomosis being protected. ■

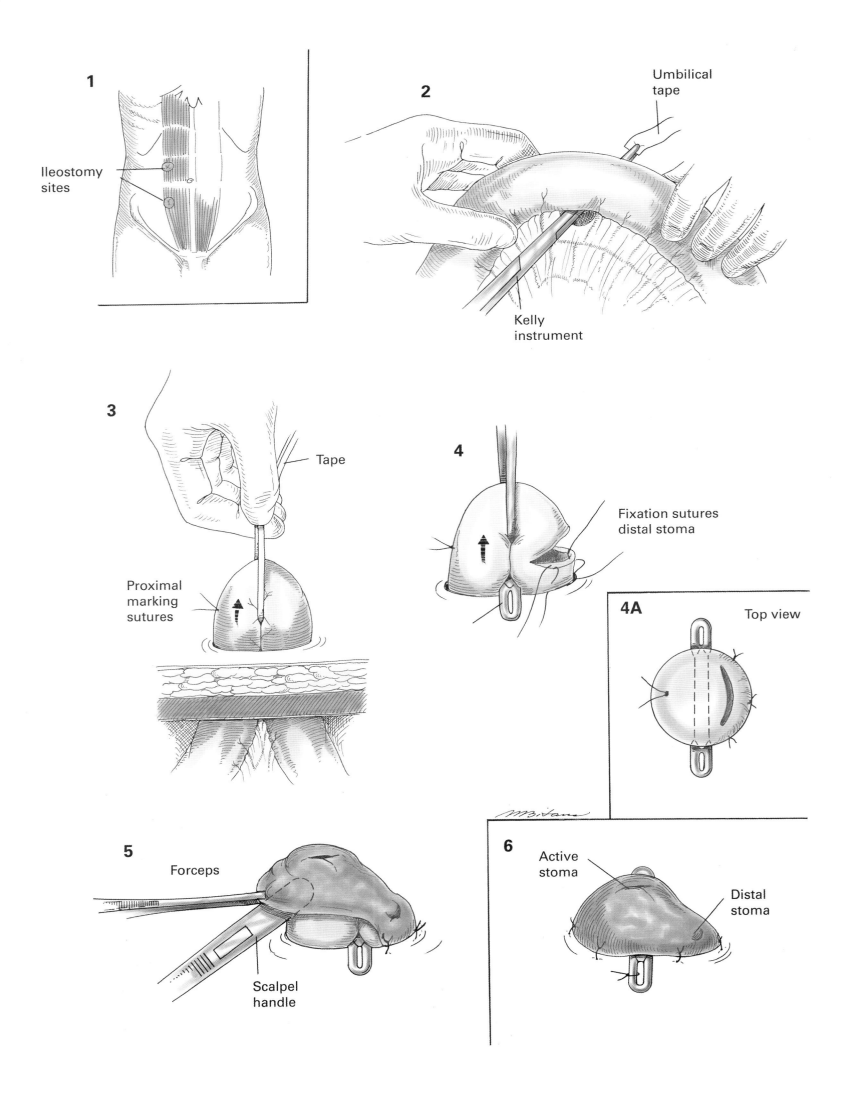

1

Ileostomy sites

2

Umbilical tape

Kelly instrument

3

Tape

Proximal marking sutures

4

Fixation sutures distal stoma

4A

Top view

5

Forceps

Scalpel handle

6

Active stoma

Distal stoma

TRANSVERSE COLOSTOMY

INDICATIONS The right transverse colostomy is preferred by many over cecostomy for decompression of the obstructed colon due to a left-side lesion. This procedure completely diverts the fecal stream and permits an efficient cleansing and preparation of the obstructed colon proximal to the lesion. When simple diversion of the fecal stream is needed as a complementary component of an elective colonic operation, the surgeon should consider placement of a proximal diverting loop ileostomy (see Chapter 51).

PREOPERATIVE PREPARATION Since this procedure is usually performed to relieve acute obstruction of the left colon, the preoperative preparation is limited to the correction of fluid and electrolyte imbalance as well as blood volume deficits. Flat and upright roentgenograms of the abdomen are made with a marker, such as a coin, on the umbilicus. An emergency water-soluble contrast enema is indicated to locate conclusively the left-sided point of obstruction. A sigmoidoscopic or colonoscopic examination may be done. Prophylactic antibiotics are administered intravenously within 1 hour of incision.

ANESTHESIA Usually, endotracheal anesthesia, which provides a cuff for secure closure of the trachea, is indicated to avoid aspiration of regurgitated gastrointestinal contents.

POSITION The patient is placed in a comfortable supine position with the proposed site for the incision presenting.

INCISION AND EXPOSURE The incision is placed in the right upper quadrant. A vertical or transverse incision can be made in a location over the distended colon as indicated from a study of the abdominal roentgenograms. Currently it is believed that the opening should be made through the rectus muscle with consideration being given for the span of the ostomy appliance gasket, which should be away from skin folds, bony prominences, or the valley of the umbilicus. Marking is further discussed in the section on loop ileostomy. The tentative site should be checked with the patient standing and sitting and taking special note of the proximity to the patient's belt line which should be avoided. The opening into the abdomen, while limited in length, must be large enough to permit easy identification and mobilization of the tightly distended transverse colon. If the bowel is tightly distended, it is essential to deflate it through a large needle or trocar, since the collapsed bowel can thus be handled more easily and safely.

DETAILS OF PROCEDURE A knuckle of transverse colon is delivered into the wound, and the omentum is retracted upward. If the intestine is tremendously distended, a large-bore needle attached to a syringe is inserted obliquely through its wall to allow gas to escape. Decompression through a small trocar attached to a suction apparatus may be indicated before the distended bowel can be safely mobilized. If necessary to avoid contamination, the small opening is closed with a purse-string suture. Under such circumstances the decompression of the bowel permits a safe delivery of a larger segment of the transverse colon through a smaller incision. The greater omentum, which is frequently more vascular than usual under these circumstances, should be dissected free of the colon that is to be used as a colostomy (FIGURE 1). All bleeding points should be ligated before replacing the omentum in the abdomen. The principle utilized is similar to that described in Chapter 27, FIGURES 1 and 2. Some surgeons prefer to pass a curved clamp through an avascular portion of the omentum and transverse mesocolon beneath the colon, following which a finger is inserted as a guide (FIGURE 2). The omentum is divided over the presenting portion of the transverse colon and reflected to either side (FIGURE 3). It may be necessary to divide several small blood vessels where the omentum is attached to the colon above the anterior taenia. After an adequate through-and-through

opening has been made beneath the transverse colon, a sterile large rubber catheter (equal to 32 French) is inserted as the finger is removed (FIGURE 4). The rubber catheter tip is cut off and one end is inserted into the other point. This joint is then secured with a nonabsorbable suture (FIGURE 5). The use of a rubber tube instead of a solid glass or plastic rod allows it to flex into an ostomy appliance. A liberal amount of transverse colon should be exteriorized to ensure a complete diversion of the fecal stream.

CLOSURE The fat tabs on the loop of bowel are now anchored to the adjacent peritoneum with fine sutures, great care being taken not to penetrate to the lumen of the bowel (FIGURE 6). The use of sutures in anchoring the intestine to the parietes is advantageous, since these will serve as a guide to the individual layers when the colostomy is closed. In the presence of great distention where the intestinal wall is quite thin, it is wiser to depend upon the fixation of the intestine by the rubber tube and postoperative inflammation, since perforation of the intestine may take place with resultant leakage and peritonitis if sutures are taken to anchor the bowel to the abdominal wall.

If a very liberal incision was necessary to deliver the dilated intestine, the peritoneal opening may be partially closed by interrupted fine sutures (FIGURE 7). The peritoneal closure should not constrict the arms of the knuckle of the intestine but should permit the introduction of the index finger directly into the peritoneal cavity about the intestine. The fascia is approximated with interrupted 00 sutures (FIGURE 7). In general, this fascial closure should allow the passage of one finger plus the loop. The subcutaneous tissue and skin are closed in a similar manner. Subcuticular interrupted absorbable sutures may be used to provide a firm closure and a wound less likely to be irritated by the subsequent constant fecal soilage. The ostomy is matured in most cases. A transverse incision is made only after the closure is complete (FIGURE 8). In some cases the bowel requires decompression with a tube secured by a purse-string suture as shown in FIGURE 9. The distal or inactive stoma is matured first by placing fine 0000 absorbable sutures that transverse the thickness of the colon bowel wall. The suture is completed as a traverse subcuticular bite beneath the skin edges (FIGURE 10). The proximal or active stoma is then matured in a similar fashion. In cases of healthy bowel, the proximal end can be made more prominent by creating the incision closer to the distal end of the exposed loop, as seen in Chapter 51. In some cases it may be preferred to delay the opening of the stoma, in which case tube drainage of the proximal limb is sometimes used.

POSTOPERATIVE CARE It is usually better judgment to open the colostomy before the initial dressings are applied rather than to delay 2 or 3 days to avoid possible infection of the wound, since the dangers of unrelieved obstruction are greater than the possible complications of wound infection.

In cases of acute obstruction, it may be desirable to continue constant gastric suction for several days. Following this, the patient is given fluids the first day and a soft diet for the next few days, progressively increasing to a high-vitamin, high-calorie, high-protein, low-residue diet. Early ambulation is permitted. Irrigations of the proximal colon may be given through the colostomy opening in preparation for secondary surgical procedures or to establish regular emptying of the colostomy if the colostomy is to be permanent. Following diversion of the fecal stream, the reaction about the obstructing tumor tends to subside and the obstruction may be relieved. Through-and-through irrigations for cleansing purposes may then be possible. Blood transfusions, high-calorie solutions, and Ringer's solution are given as required, depending on the degree of the patient's debility. Antibiotic therapy is discontinued after a few days or so unless the patient has a continuing infection. ■

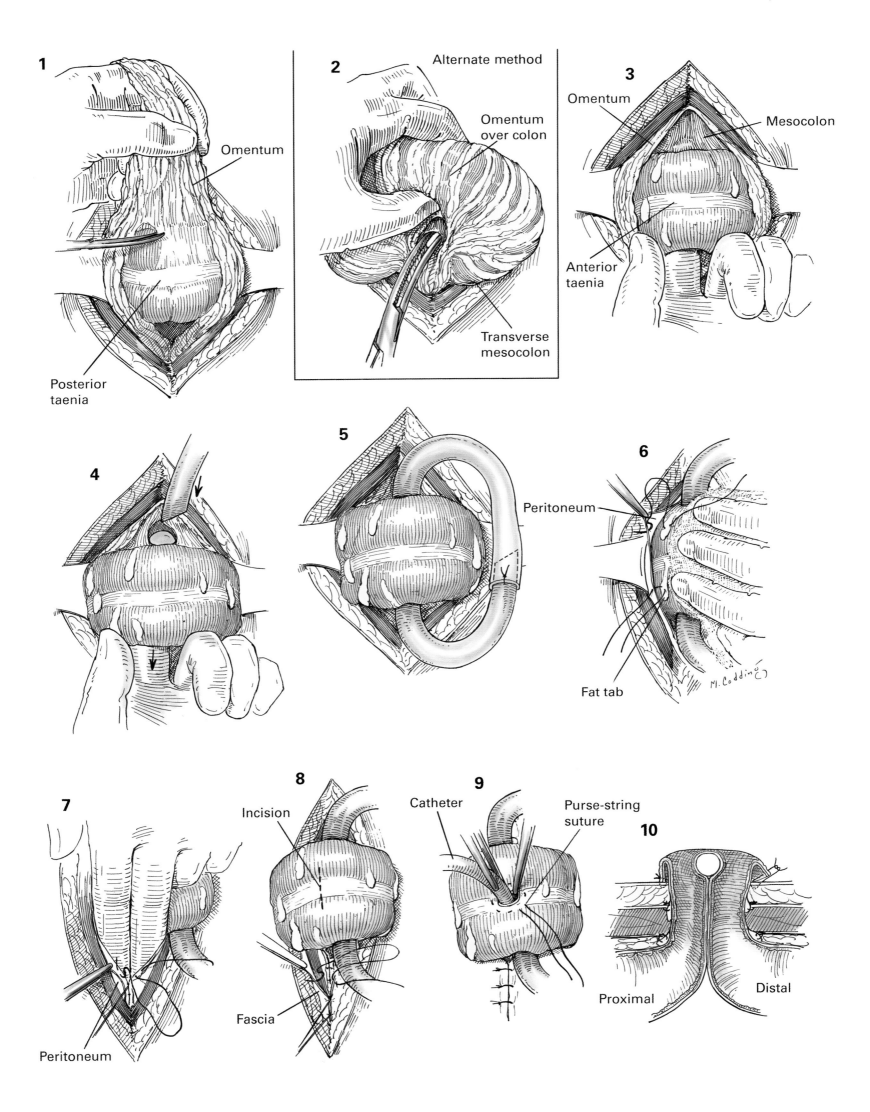

1

Omentum

Posterior
taenia

2   Alternate method

Omentum
over colon

Transverse
mesocolon

3

Omentum

Mesocolon

Anterior
taenia

4

5

Peritoneum

6

Fat tab

M. Codding

7

Peritoneum

8   Incision

Fascia

9   Catheter

Purse-string
suture

10

Proximal   Distal

CLOSURE OF COLOSTOMY

INDICATIONS In every instance an interlude that may be as long as 10 weeks should be allowed between the performance of a colostomy and its closure. This enables the patient's general condition to improve, the site of the colostomy to become walled off, local immunity to the infected contents of the intestine to develop, any infection in the wound to subside, and the wounds from technical procedures carried out on the distal colon to heal. This time may be drastically shortened if the colostomy was performed to decompress or exteriorize a traumatized normal colon. Occasionally, the colostomy partially or completely closes itself after the obstruction has been removed, which permits the fecal current to return to its normal route through the site of the anastomosis. Closure should be delayed until the edema and induration of the bowel about the colostomy opening have subsided and the intestine has resumed a normal appearance. The patency of any anastomosis of the intestine distal to the colostomy should be assured by contrast study using fluoroscopy.

A stapled anastomosis may also be created to close a loop colostomy. See Chapter 54.

PREOPERATIVE PREPARATION The patient is placed on a low-residue diet with oral antibiotics before operation, and the intestines are emptied as completely as possible. During the 24 hours preceding operation, repeated irrigations in both directions through the colostomy opening are done to empty the colon. Other preoperative preparation is in accordance with that outlined in Chapter 57.

ANESTHESIA Spinal or general anesthesia may be used.

POSITION The patient is placed in a comfortable supine position.

OPERATIVE PREPARATION Supplementary to the routine skin preparation, a sterile gauze sponge may be inserted into the colostomy opening.

INCISION AND EXPOSURE FIGURE 2 shows the cross-sectional anatomy of the colostomy. While a piece of gauze is held in the lumen of the intestine, an oval incision is made through the skin and subcutaneous tissue about the colostomy (FIGURE 1). This incision may include the original scar or, alternatively, an elliptical incision may be made that includes the entire scar and colostomy.

DETAILS OF PROCEDURE The operator's index finger is inserted into the colostomy to act as a guide to prevent incision through the intestinal wall or opening into the peritoneal cavity as the skin and subcutaneous tissue are divided by blunt and sharp dissection (FIGURES 3 and 4).

In the case of a colostomy that has been functioning for some time, the ring of scar tissue at the junction of mucous membrane and skin must be excised before proceeding with the closure (FIGURE 5). With the index finger still in the lumen of the intestine, the operator makes an incision with scissors around the margin of the mucosal reflection (FIGURE 6). This incision is carried through the seromuscular layer down to the submucosa in an effort to develop separate layers for closure (FIGURE 6).

CLOSURE With its margin held taut with forceps, the mucous membrane is closed transversely to the long axis of the bowel. A continuous fine absorbable suture is used (FIGURE 7). Following closure of the mucosa, the previously developed seromuscular layer, which has been freed of any fat, is approximated with interrupted Halsted sutures of fine silk (FIGURE 8). The wound is irrigated repeatedly, and clean towels are applied around the wound. All instruments and materials are removed, gloves are changed, and the wound is closed only with clean instruments.

The closed portion of the bowel is held to one side while the adjacent fascia is divided with curved scissors. The detachment of the fascia from the bowel is facilitated by exposure of the silk sutures previously placed for fixation of the bowel at the time of colostomy (FIGURE 9). The peritoneal cavity is not opened in this method of closure.

The patency of the bowel is tested by the surgeon's thumb and index finger. If a small opening has been accidentally made in the peritoneum, it is carefully closed with interrupted sutures. The wound is irrigated repeatedly with warm saline. The suture line is depressed with forceps, while the margins of the overlying fascia are approximated with interrupted sutures of 00 long-lasting absorbable suture (FIGURE 10). The subcutaneous tissue and skin are closed in layers in the routine manner (FIGURE 11). Some omit closure of the skin because of the possibility of infection and perform a delayed secondary closure.

ALTERNATE METHOD

INCISION AND EXPOSURE Instead of attempting to incise the ring of scar tissue at the junction of mucous membrane and the serosa of the bowel, some operators prefer to divide the full thickness of the bowel adjacent to the colostomy opening. After the bowel has been freed from the surrounding tissues, the surgeon's index finger may be inserted into the colostomy to serve as a guide while the bowel is being divided with curved scissors adjacent to the margin of the presenting mucous membrane (FIGURE 12). It may be necessary to free the intestine from the peritoneum and open into the peritoneal cavity in order to mobilize a sufficient amount of the bowel for a satisfactory closure.

DETAILS OF PROCEDURE The intestinal wall is excised until the scarred edges of bowel around the colostomy opening are completely cut away, leaving normal-appearing intestinal wall to be closed. The bowel is closed transversely to the long axis of the intestine to prevent stenosis. The bowel wall is held taut with either Allis or Babcock forceps above and below the angles of the new opening. The mucous membrane of the intestine is closed on the inner side with a continuous fine absorbable suture of the Connell type. Interrupted 0000 silk sutures on a French or straight milliner's needle are preferred by many (FIGURE 13). Interrupted mattress sutures of 00 silk or 00 absorbable synthetic sutures are placed to invert the mucosal suture line and to approximate the seromuscular layer over it (FIGURE 14).

CLOSURE The wound is irrigated with saline. All contaminated instruments, gloves, and towels are discarded, and clean materials are used if it is necessary to open the peritoneal cavity about the margin of the bowel in order to replace the closure within the peritoneal cavity (FIGURE 15). The patency of the lumen of the bowel is assured by palpation between the surgeon's thumb and index finger. If possible, the omentum is tucked over the site of the closure. The peritoneum is closed with interrupted sutures of 00 absorbable synthetic suture material, followed by a routine closure of the layers of the abdominal wall (FIGURES 16 and 17). When gross contamination has occurred, some prefer to partially approximate the subcutaneous tissue and omit skin approximation by sutures. The wound is covered with a sterile dressing.

POSTOPERATIVE CARE Parenteral fluids are administered for several days. A clear liquid diet is given for a few days, followed by a low-residue diet; a regular diet can be resumed after bowel action has started. Occasionally, a leak may occur at the closure site, but no immediate effort is made to repair the fistula (unless it is causing systemic illness or peritonitis) because closure is frequently spontaneous. Early ambulation is encouraged. ■

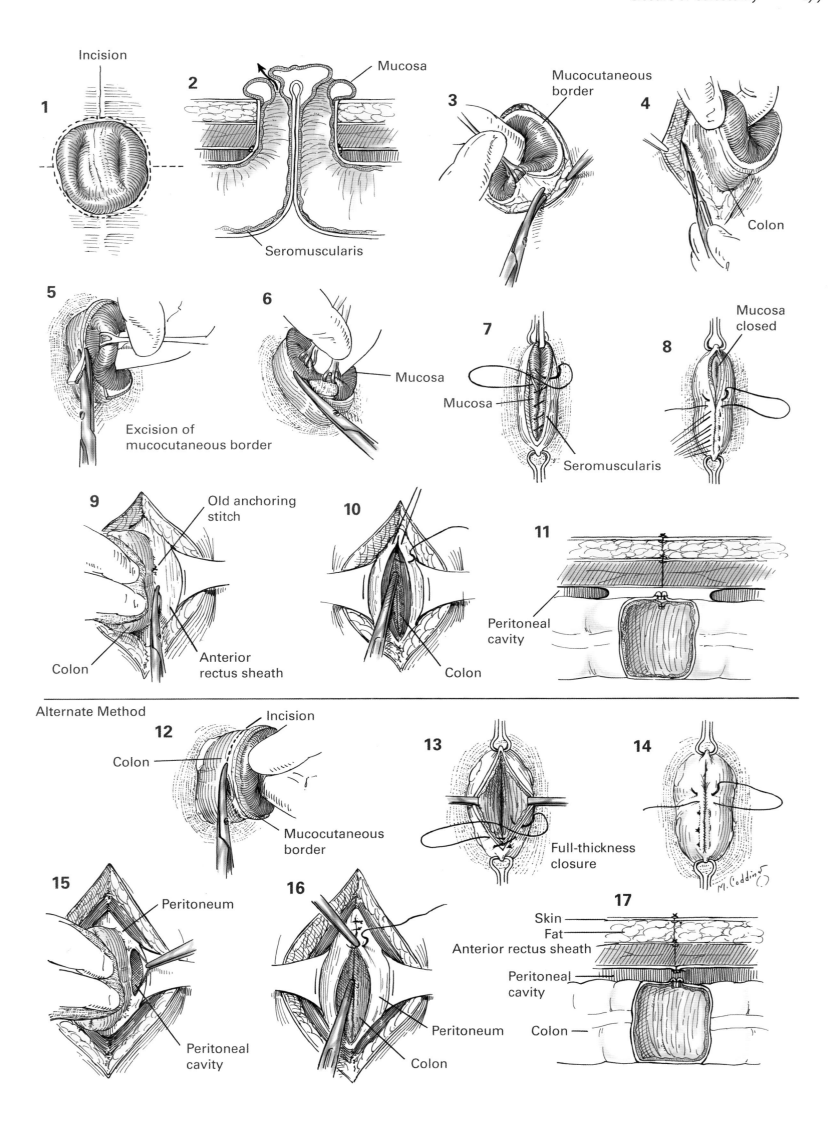

1 Incision

2 Mucosa
Seromuscularis

3 Mucocutaneous border

4 Colon

5 Excision of mucocutaneous border

6 Mucosa

7 Mucosa
Seromuscularis

8 Mucosa closed

9 Old anchoring stitch
Colon
Anterior rectus sheath

10 Colon

11 Peritoneal cavity

Alternate Method

12 Incision
Colon
Mucocutaneous border

13 Full-thickness closure

14 M. Codding

15 Peritoneum
Peritoneal cavity

16 Peritoneum
Colon

17 Skin
Fat
Anterior rectus sheath
Peritoneal cavity
Colon

COLON ANASTOMOSIS, STAPLED

ALTERNATIVE METHOD—TRIANGULATION An alternative method of open anastomosis for large intestine involves the method of triangulation using three separate staple lines. It is particularly useful in colocolostomy anastomoses as in left-sided colectomies since it does not require rotation of the mesentery. It can also be used to close a loop colostomy as an alternative to the sutured technique in Chapter 53.

DETAILS OF PROCEDURE The section of the bowel to be excised is isolated with Kocher clamps while thin straight clamps, such as Glassman clamps, are placed transversely on the colon (FIGURE 1). Several inches beyond these, noncrushing Scudder or rubber-shod clamps are applied to prevent gross contamination. The specimen is excised between the Kocher and straight clamps. The field is walled off with laparotomy pads and the clamps are opened. Obvious bleeding points are controlled with fine ligatures. The two limbs of open bowel are brought in approximation with correct mesentery-to-mesentery alignment (FIGURE 2). The mesenteric opening is closed with interrupted fine silk sutures (FIGURE 3). Anterior and posterior traction sutures (A and B) are placed halfway between the mesenteric and antimesenteric borders. The full thickness of bowel wall along the mesenteric border is aligned with several through-and-through traction sutures or a row of Allis

clamps (FIGURE 4). The noncutting linear stapler (TL 60) is positioned transversely below the Allises and traction sutures (FIGURE 5). This ensures inclusion of all bowel wall in the deep staple line. After discharging the stapling instrument, the excess tissue is cut from above the instrument jaws while preserving the traction sutures on either end (FIGURE 6).

A bisecting third traction suture (C) is placed through each stoma in a position corresponding to the apex of the antimesenteric border (FIGURE 7). The open jaws of the noncutting linear stapler (TL 60) are positioned for the second side of the triangle using traction suture (B) to elevate the end of the posterior staple line within the jaws (FIGURE 8). After discharging the staple gun, the excess tissues above the jaws are excised, leaving the apical traction suture (C) intact.

The procedure is then repeated using the two remaining traction sutures (C and A). This final limb of the triangulation must transect each of the other two staple lines (FIGURE 9). Upon its completion, the excess tissue is excised. The bowel is inspected for hemostasis and any bleeding points are secured with fine silk ligatures. Any residual mesenteric defect is closed with interrupted sutures. The anastomosis is palpated for patency (FIGURE 10) and the bowel on either side may be compressed to verify that no leak is present. ■

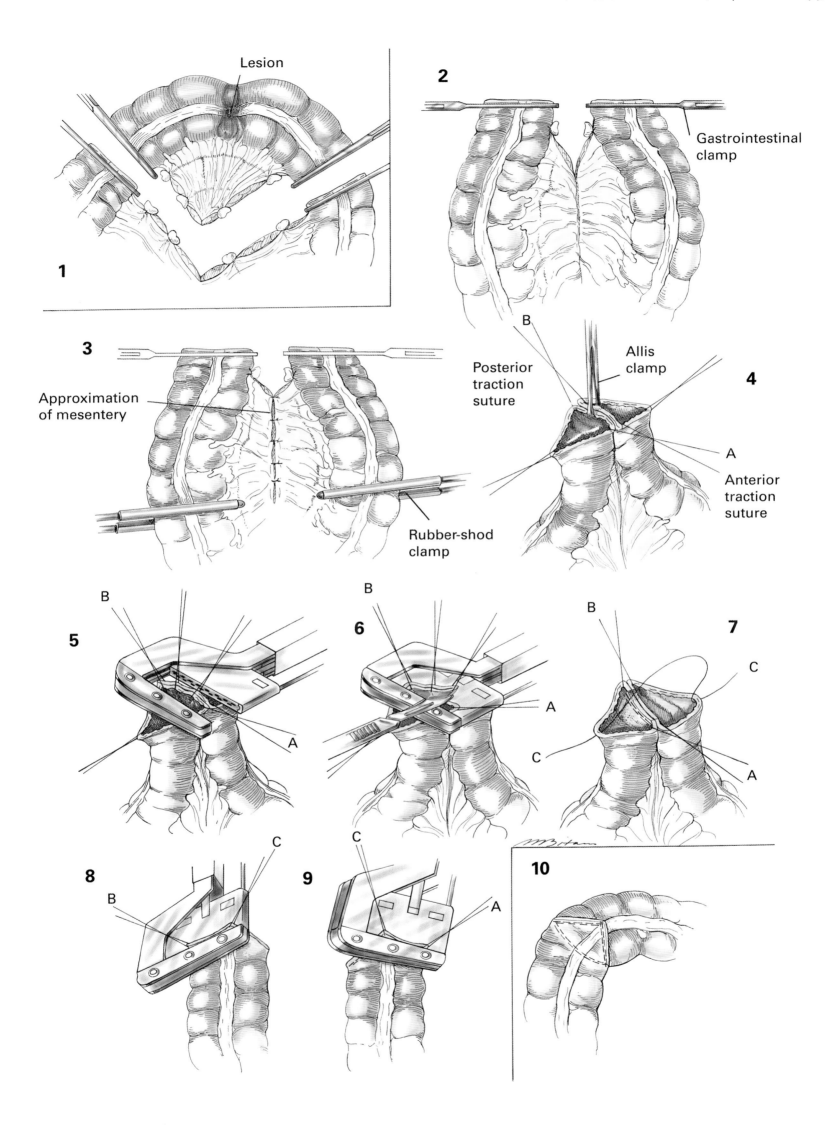

1 Lesion

2 Gastrointestinal clamp

3 Approximation of mesentery   Rubber-shod clamp

4 Posterior traction suture   Allis clamp   B   A   Anterior traction suture

5 B   A

6 B   A   C

7 B   C   A

8 B   C

9 C   A

10

INDICATIONS Resection of the right colon is commonly indicated for carcinoma, inflammatory bowel disease, and more rarely for tuberculosis or volvulus of the cecum, ascending colon, or hepatic flexure.

PREOPERATIVE PREPARATION Some tumors of the right colon present as an obstruction and may require relatively urgent operation for excessive cecal distention (≥15 cm) in the presence of a competent ileal cecal valve. Such a patient is resuscitated with correction of fluid and electrolyte imbalances. The proximal bowel is decompressed with a nasogastric tube. Once the patient's physiologic status is optimized, he or she will proceed to urgent operation, wherein a right colectomy can be performed in an unprepared bowel. The prudent surgeon should verify that there is not a second or metachronous colorectal lesion. If the right colectomy is being done in an elective setting, the entire colon should be evaluated with either colonoscopy or barium enema. Blood transfusion may be advisable, especially in older patients with cardiovascular disease, when a silent and unrecognized iron deficiency anemia has been created by a silent, longstanding neoplasm of the right colon. Any pre-existing steroid therapy is continued with intravenous replacement as the patient prepares for surgery. Perioperative systemic antibiotics are given.

ANESTHESIA Either general inhalation or spinal anesthesia is satisfactory.

POSITION The patient is placed in a comfortable supine position. The surgeon stands on the patient's right side.

OPERATIVE PREPARATION The skin is prepared in the routine manner and a sterile drape is applied.

INCISION AND EXPOSURE A liberal midline incision centered about the umbilicus is made. A transverse incision just above the level of the umbilicus also provides an excellent exposure. The lesion of the right colon is inspected and palpated to determine whether removal is possible. In the presence of malignancy, the liver is also palpated for the evidence of metastasis. If the lesion is inoperable, a side-to-side anastomosis may be performed between the terminal ileum and the transverse colon without any resection (see Chapter 46). After resection has been decided upon, the small intestines are walled off with packs and the cecum is exposed.

DETAILS OF PROCEDURE An incision is made in the peritoneal reflection close to the lateral wall of the bowel from the tip of the cecum upward to the region of the hepatic flexure (FIGURE 1). A liberal margin should be ensured in the region of the tumor. Occasionally, the full thickness of the adjacent abdominal wall may require excision to include the local spread of tumor. Since the entire hepatic flexure is usually removed as part of a right colectomy, the hepatocolic ligament, which contains some small blood vessels, must be divided and ligated, but there will be no blood vessels of importance in the peritoneal attachments along the right gutter. With the

lateral peritoneal attachment divided, the large bowel may be lifted mesially with the left hand, while the loose areolar tissue lying under it is dissected off with a moist gauze sponge over the right index finger (FIGURE 2). In elevating the right colon toward the midline, the surgeon must positively identify the right ureter and be certain that it is not injured. Care is taken also toward the top of the ascending colon and near the hepatic flexure to avoid injury to the third portion of the duodenum, which underlies the large bowel (FIGURE 3). The raw surface remaining after the intestine has been freed and brought outside the peritoneal cavity is covered with warm, moist gauze pads. The middle colic vessels are identified, along with the right-hand branches heading toward the hepatic flexure and the planned zone of transection. The mesentery of the large bowel is clamped and divided just distal to the hepatic flexure or wherever the bowel is to be resected. The right branches or all of the middle colic vessels are divided and doubly ligated. The bowel at the selected level for division is freed of all mesentery, omentum, and fat on both sides. All vessels must be carefully ligated. The right half of the greater omentum is divided near the greater curvature of the stomach and excised along with the right colon.

The terminal ileum is prepared for resection some distance away from the ileocecal valve, depending upon the amount of blood supply that must be sacrificed to ensure excision of the lymph node drainage area of the right colon. After the small intestine has been prepared at its mesenteric border, a fan-shaped excision of the mesentery to the right colon is carried out. This usually includes part of the right branches of the middle colic vessels. In the presence of malignancy, the lymph node dissection should descend as far as possible along the course of the right colic and ileocolic vessels without compromising either the middle colic vessels or the superior mesenteric vascular supply of the remaining small bowel (FIGURE 4). The blood vessels of the mesentery are doubly tied.

A straight vascular clamp, or some other type of straight clamp, is applied obliquely to the small intestine about 1 cm from the mesenteric border to ensure a serosal surface for the placement of sutures for the subsequent anastomosis. Stone, Kocher, or Pace-Potts clamps are next applied across the large intestine, which is then divided between the clamps. The intervening section of bowel, with its fan-shaped section of mesentery and nodes, is excised. The divided proximal end of the small intestine is covered with gauze moistened with saline, and closure of the stump of the large bowel is started unless an end-to-end or end-to-side anastomosis is planned. Many surgeons prefer to use stapling devices, in which case the colon and terminal small bowel are resected using a linear stapling device. The ileum and transverse colon may then be anastomosed in an antimesenteric side-to-side manner using the technique shown in Chapter 45, Resection of Small Intestine, Stapled. As staples may not be universally available, the techniques for hand-sewn anastomoses are shown in the continuing figures of Chapter 55. **CONTINUES** ▶

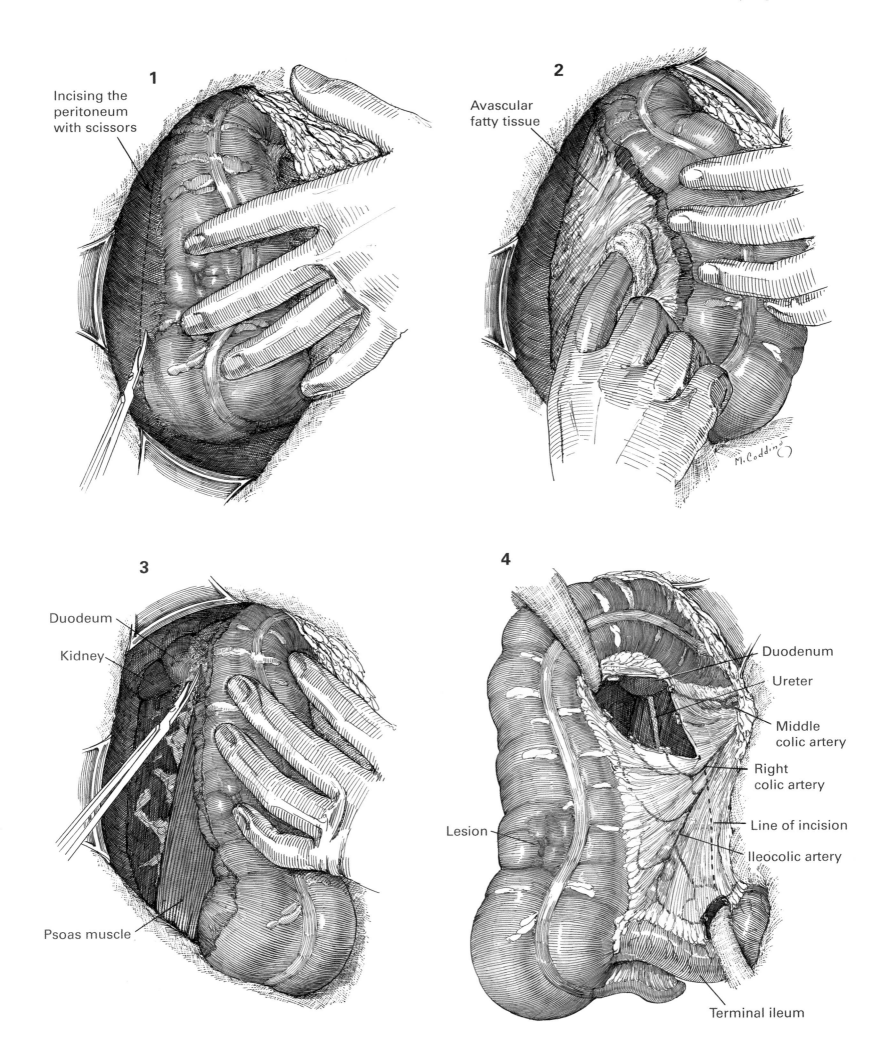

1

Incising the peritoneum with scissors

2

Avascular fatty tissue

M. Codding

3

Duodeum

Kidney

Psoas muscle

4

Duodenum

Ureter

Middle colic artery

Right colic artery

Line of incision

Ileocolic artery

Lesion

Terminal ileum

DETAILS OF PROCEDURE ◀CONTINUED▶ The end of the colon is closed by a continuous absorbable suture on an atraumatic needle and whipped loosely over a Pace-Potts or similar noncrushing clamp (FIGURE 5). Interrupted ooo silk sutures placed beneath the clamp may be used. The clamp is then opened and removed. If a continuous suture is used, it is pulled up snugly and tied. A single layer of ooo silk Halsted mattress sutures is placed about 2 or 3 cm from the original suture line; care being taken that no fat is included. As these sutures are tied, the original suture line is invaginated so that serosa meets serosa (FIGURE 6). The surgeon must determine before closing the ends of the colon whether an end-to-end, end-to-side, side-to-end, or lateral anastomosis is to be carried out (FIGURES 14, 16 to 18).

The end-to-side approximation is physiologic, simple, and safe to perform. The small intestine, still held in its clamp, is brought up adjacent to the anterior taenia of the colon (FIGURE 7). The small intestine should retain a good color and give evidence of adequate blood supply before the anastomosis is attempted. If its color indicates an inadequate blood supply, the surgeon should not hesitate to resect a sufficient length until its viability is unquestionable. Next, the omentum, if not previously excised, is retracted upward, and the anterior taenia of the transverse colon is grasped with Babcock forceps at the site chosen for anastomosis (FIGURE 7). Following this, the edge of the mesentery of the small intestine should be approximated to the edge of that of the large intestine, so that herniation of the small intestine cannot occur beneath the anastomosis into the right gutter (FIGURE 14). This opening is closed before the anastomosis is started, since on rare occasions the blood supply may be injured by the procedure and the viability of the anastomosis jeopardized. A small, straight crushing clamp is applied to the anterior taenia, including a small bite of the bowel wall (FIGURE 8). Following this, the clamps on the terminal ileum, as well as on the anterior taenia of the transverse colon, are so arranged that a serosal layer of interrupted ooo mattress or nonabsorbable synthetic sutures can be placed, anchoring the terminal ileum to the transverse colon (FIGURE 9). The two angle sutures are not cut and serve as traction sutures (FIGURE 9). An opening is made into the large intestine by excising the protruding contents of the crushing clamp that has been applied to the anterior taenia (FIGURE 10). An enterostomy clamp is then applied behind each of the crushing clamps. The crushing clamps are removed, and the terminal ileum is opened; likewise, the crushed contents of the transverse colon are separated. Sometimes it is necessary to enlarge the opening in the mucosa of the colon, since the previous excision of the contents of the crushing clamp did not provide a sufficiently large stoma for satisfactory anastomosis. The mucosa is then approximated with a continuous locked nonabsorbable suture on atraumatic needles, which is started in the midline posteriorly. The sutures, A and B, are continued as a Connell inverting suture around the angles and anteriorly to ensure inversion of the mucosa

(FIGURES 11 and 12). Interrupted fine ooo silk sutures are preferred by some for closing the mucosal layer. An anterior row of mattress sutures completes the anastomosis. Several additional mattress sutures may be placed to reinforce the angles (FIGURE 13). The patency of the stoma is tested. It should permit introduction of the index finger. If the tension is not too great, the raw surface over the iliopsoas muscle may be covered by approximating the peritoneum of the lateral abdominal wall to the mesentery.

The second method shown is a direct end-to-end anastomosis (FIGURES 15 and 16). The discrepancy in the size of the terminal ileum and the transverse colon can be overcome safely by attending to certain technical details. Added luminal circumference can be provided by exaggerating the oblique division of the terminal ileum. During the anastomosis, slightly larger bites are taken in the colonic side to compensate for the discrepancy between the two sides of the anastomosis. Following completion of the anastomosis, any remaining gap between the mesenteries is approximated. The patency of the lumen is determined by palpation.

If a side-to-end anastomosis is preferred by the surgeon, the stump of the small intestine is closed as previously described for the large intestine. The small intestine is then brought up to the open end of the large intestine (FIGURE 17), the posterior row of serosal sutures is placed, the small intestine is opened, and the continuous mucosal suture or the inverting sutures are placed as well as, finally, the anterior serosal sutures of interrupted ooo silk or nonabsorbable synthetic material. Whenever this type of procedure is carried out, care should be taken that only a very small portion of small intestine protrudes beyond the suture line, since blind ends of bowel that are in the peristaltic line form a stagnant pouch against which peristalsis tends to work, increasing the chance of eventual breakdown.

In the fourth method, the ends of the large and small intestines are closed, and a lateral anastomosis is carried out. Only a small portion of small intestine should protrude beyond the suture line. The small intestine should be anchored to the colon with interrupted sutures of silk or nonabsorbable synthetic material, including both angles of the stoma as well as the closed end of small bowel (FIGURE 18). The stapled equivalent of each of the variations can be found in earlier chapters illustrating the use of various stapling instruments in small bowel anastomoses.

CLOSURE Drains are undesirable unless gross infection has been encountered. The site of anastomosis is covered with omentum. The abdominal wall is closed in routine fashion, and a sterile dressing is applied.

POSTOPERATIVE CARE The patient should be in a comfortable position. Diarrhea or frequent bowel movements may be satisfactorily controlled by medication and diet. The need for continued steroid therapy, particularly in patients with regional ileitis, should not be overlooked in the immediate postoperative period. ■

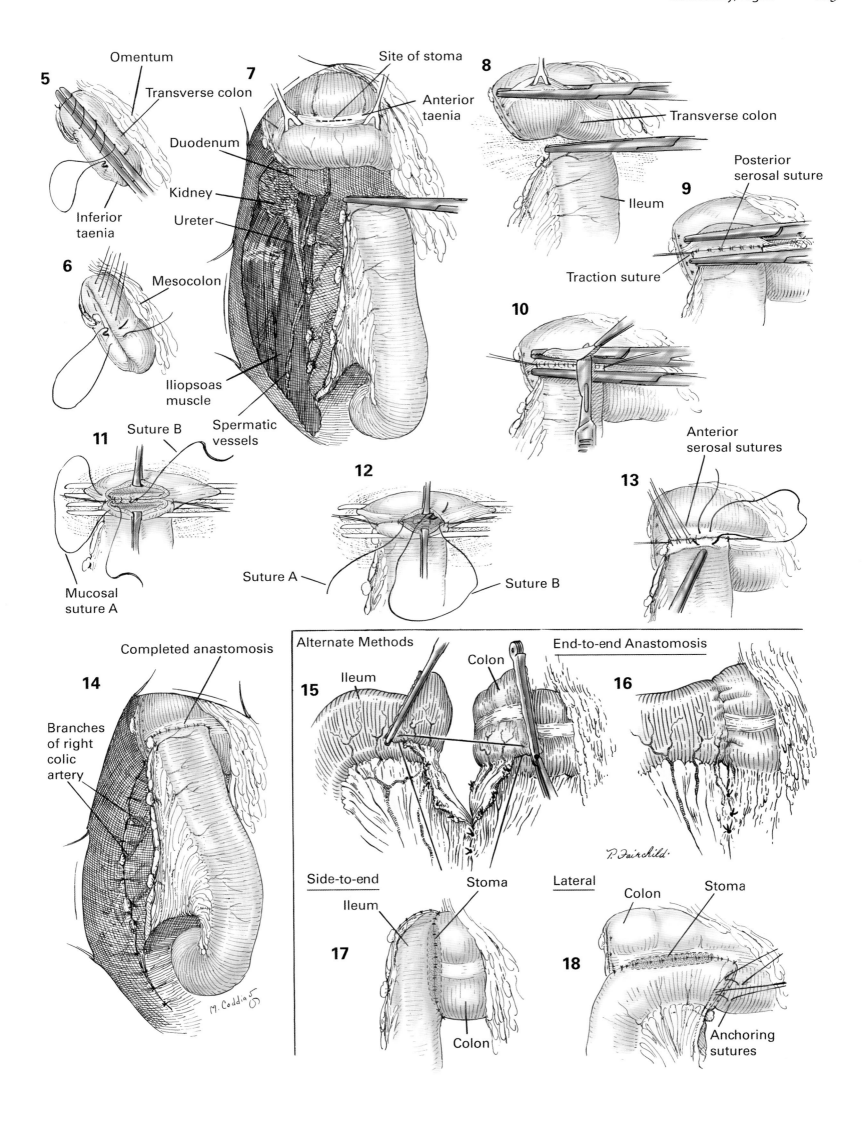

5 Omentum, Transverse colon, Inferior taenia

6 Mesocolon

7 Site of stoma, Anterior taenia, Duodenum, Kidney, Ureter, Iliopsoas muscle, Spermatic vessels

8 Transverse colon, Ileum

9 Posterior serosal suture, Traction suture

10

11 Suture B, Mucosal suture A

12 Suture A, Suture B

13 Anterior serosal sutures

14 Completed anastomosis, Branches of right colic artery

Alternate Methods   **End-to-end Anastomosis**

15 Ileum, Colon, Stoma

16

Side-to-end

17 Ileum, Stoma, Colon

Lateral

18 Colon, Stoma, Anchoring sutures

M. Coddin   P. Fairchild.

COLECTOMY, RIGHT, LAPAROSCOPIC

INDICATIONS Laparoscopic colectomy is indicated in both benign and malignant conditions as long as it is performed by qualified surgeons with appropriate resources. In general this approach is not recommended in patients with emergency conditions such as obstruction, perforation, or massive bleeding.

PREOPERATIVE PREPARATION For patients having surgery for polyps and most neoplasms, it is essential to have the lesion tattooed during colonoscopy or localized by a preoperative barium enema. Identification of the tumor during laparoscopy is usually difficult. The use of intraoperative colonoscopy is difficult during laparoscopic procedures; hence, accurate preoperative localization is necessary. If intraoperative colonoscopy is necessary, the use of CO_2 insufflation rather than air will speed the resolution of colonic distention that can greatly impede the laparoscopic approach. The patient should receive a standard mechanical bowel preparation, and prophylactic antibiotics are administered within 1 hour of the incision and are to be discontinued within 24 hours of surgery. Subcutaneous heparin is administered and sequential compression devices are placed for the prevention of venous thromboembolism.

ANESTHESIA General anesthesia is required. An orogastric or nasogastric tube is inserted.

POSITION The patient is positioned in the modified lithotomy position with the legs supported on stirrups. Padding is used to protect all pressure points. The left arm is tucked. The patient should be secured to the operating table with tape, as repositioning of the table may be needed to enhance exposure during the operation. The operating room setup is shown in FIGURE 1A. The surgeon and camera operator stand to the patient's left. The assistant stands between the patient's legs. Two video monitors are used as shown.

OPERATIVE PREPARATION The skin is prepared in the routine manner and a sterile drape is applied.

INCISION AND EXPOSURE Access to the peritoneal cavity is achieved by an open or Hasson technique. An infraumbilical incision is made and a 10- to 12-mm Hasson port inserted. The abdomen is insufflated to 15 mm Hg. A 30-degree-angled scope is employed. After the Hasson port is inserted, there are three commonly used port placements (FIGURE 1B). The first configuration, shown in FIGURE 1B, has a 10- to 12-mm trocar to the left of the midline in the left lower quadrant with a 5-mm port in the left upper quadrant and another 5-mm port the right lower quadrant if needed. Using this method, the extraction incision is made as a vertical midline either at the level of the umbilicus or in the suprapubic area. The second configuration is a 10- to 12-mm port in the left lower quadrant and 5-mm ports in the suprapubic midline and a right upper quadrant in the subcostal location in the midclavicular line. The upper 5-mm port on the right side may allow better mobilization of the hepatic flexure in some patients. With this configuration, the extraction incision is either midline as described above or in the transverse direction at the site of the 5-mm right upper quadrant port or a transverse right lower quadrant incision. The third configuration uses a hand port in the midline, a 10- to 12-mm port if the left lower quadrant, and 5-mm ports at the subxiphoid midline location and the right subcostal area. A hand port is used to extract the specimen.

DETAILS OF PROCEDURE Mobilization of the right colon is shown by a lateral to medial approach. A medial to lateral approach may be used but is not described here. In the lateral medial approach, mobilization begins at the cecum. The patient is placed in the Trendelenburg position and tilted 30 degrees to the left. The cecum is grasped with an atraumatic instrument and retracted medially and anteriorly (FIGURE 2). Using a monopolar cautery endoscissors or another energy device, an incision is made in the peritoneal reflection close to the lateral wall of the bowel at the tip of the cecum (FIGURE 2). The assistant then grasps the ascending colon and retracts it medial and cephalad, permitting the incision to be extended upward to the region of the hepatic flexure using a traction counter-traction technique (FIGURE 3). As the dissection begins, care should be taken to avoid ureteral injury. As one approaches the hepatic flexure, the duodenum may

be visualized and protected (FIGURE 3). For mobilization of the hepatic flexure, the patient should be placed in the reverse Trendelenburg position. If there is a 10- to 12-mm trocar in the right lower quadrant, repositioning the laparoscope to this sight may provide better visualization. The hepatic flexure is then retracted medially and inferiorly. An energy device is used to divide the peritoneal attachments (FIGURE 3). Care is taken to avoid injury to the underlying duodenum during hepatic flexure mobilization. For mobilization of the hepatic flexure the patient should be placed in the reverse Trendelenburg. If there is a 10- to 12-mm trocar in the right lower quadrant reposition the laparoscope to this site may provide better visualization. The hepatic flexure is then retracted medially and inferiorly. An energy device is used to divide the peritoneal attachments (FIGURE 4). Next the proximal transverse colon is mobilized by dividing the omental attachments along the line of dissection in FIGURE 2. The assistant grasps the omentum and holds this upward. The surgeon grasps the mesenteric side of the transverse colon to put tension on the omental attachments. The omental attachments are divided with ultrasonic shears or electrocautery taking care not to injure the colon. Division of the gastro colic ligament is frequently necessary to completely mobilize the hepatic flexure from the liver. The extent of omental detachment may vary depending on the location of the lesion and the degree of reach needed.

The mesentery is divided in the next series of steps. The ileocolic vessels are grasped and retracted toward the anterior abdominal wall. The peritoneum overlying the mesentery is incised at a point beneath the ileocolic vessels with electrocautery endoscissors and a window created. For malignancy, this should be near the root of the mesentery. The cecum is grasped and retracted laterally to elevate the ileocolic vessels. The vessels are skeletonized and then divided with the linear laparoscopic stapler with 2.5-mm staples or clips (FIGURE 4A and B). The dissection is carried toward the hepatic flexure and the stapling process repeated until the mesentery is divided. The dissection is continued to and including the right branch of the middle colic artery.

In FIGURE 4A, the right colic artery is being dissected. FIGURE 4B shows the ligated ileocolic artery, right colic artery, and the right branch of the middle colic. The line of resection is shown in FIGURE 5. After complete mobilization the bowel is externalized through a 6- to 10-cm incision by extending the right lower quadrant incision or the umbilical incision. A plastic wound protector is used. The terminal ileum and colon are exteriorized through this opening. The proximal and distal margins of the specimen are then divided using a linear stapler (3.5-mm staples). Larger staples may be needed depending on the thickness of the bowel wall. A side-to-side hand-sewn or stapled anastomosis may be performed. To perform a side-to-side stapled anastomosis, stay sutures are placed to secure the two antimesenteric walls of the ileum and the colon. An enterotomy for the introduction of the stapling device is created by excising a small portion of the staple lines along the ileum and transverse colon with curved Mayo scissors (FIGURE 6A). The linear stapler is then introduced and closed (FIGURE 6A). The posterior aspect of the bowel is examined to be certain that no mesentery is included in the closed stapler. Once this is ensured, the stapler is discharged and the anastomosis created. Through the enterotomies, the staple line is inspected for bleeding. Small bleeding points are sutured with 000 silk figure-of-eight sutures. The enterotomy is closed with a stapler (FIGURE 6B). The final appearance is shown in FIGURE 6B. The mesenteric defect does not require closure and the bowel returned to the peritoneal cavity.

CLOSURE The incision used to exteriorize the bowel and complete the extracorporeal anastomosis is closed with interrupted or running sutures. The port sites greater than 5 mm are closed with sutures as well.

POSTOPERATIVE CARE The orogastric or nasogastric tube is removed in the operating room. Intravenous fluids are administered and vital signs and urine output monitored every 4 hours. Prophylactic antibiotics are discontinued within 24 hours of the surgery. The bladder catheter is removed on postoperative day 1 or 2. An initial postoperative diet consisting of clear liquids is started immediately or on postoperative day 1 if there is no distention or indications of complications and this is advanced as tolerated. ■

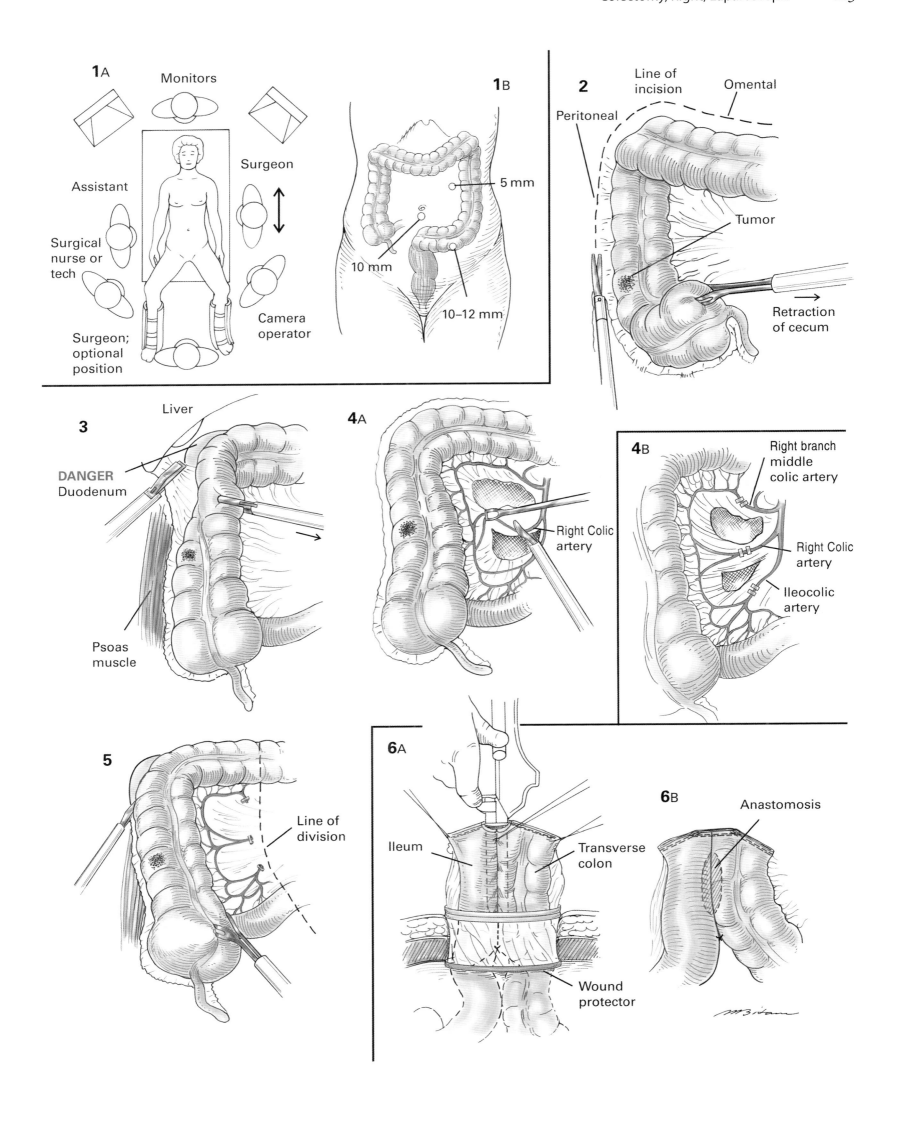

1A

Monitors

Assistant

Surgeon

Surgical nurse or tech

Surgeon; optional position

Camera operator

1B

5 mm

10 mm

10–12 mm

2

Line of incision

Peritoneal

Omental

Tumor

Retraction of cecum

3

Liver

DANGER Duodenum

Psoas muscle

4A

Right Colic artery

4B

Right branch middle colic artery

Right Colic artery

Ileocolic artery

5

Line of division

6A

Ileum

Transverse colon

Wound protector

6B

Anastomosis

COLECTOMY, LEFT, END-TO-END ANASTOMOSIS

INDICATIONS The operation is performed chiefly for tumor of the left colon or a complication of diverticulitis.

PREOPERATIVE PREPARATION Tumors of the left colon are frequently of the stenosing type. Patients with this condition often come to the surgeon with symptoms of impending intestinal obstruction.

When obstruction is not complete, the bowel can best be prepared over a period of days by oral administration of the appropriate cathartics and a clear liquid diet for the last 48 hours. The frequency with which cathartics and cleansing agents are administered will vary depending upon the amount of obstruction. The level and nature of the obstruction may be confirmed by barium enema; however, colonoscopy allows biopsy for pathologic identification, identification and removal of additional lesions such as polyps, and potential evaluation of the proximal colon. In the presence of total obstruction, a nasogastric tube is passed for decompression and the colon is emptied from below with enemas. Evaluation of the distal colon with colonoscopy is valuable. A virtual colonoscopy may be obtained with special CT imaging to evaluate the proximal colon, although it requires bowel preparation and air insufflation and not an obstruction in patients with near or complete obstruction. A baseline carcinoembryonic antigen (CEA) blood test is obtained. If this and enzymatic liver function tests are elevated, CT or imaging scans of the abdomen and liver may be obtained to evaluate metastatic spread. Perioperative antibiotics are given. A Foley catheter is inserted after induction of anesthesia.

ANESTHESIA General anesthesia is preferred.

POSITION The patient is placed in a comfortable supine position and rotated slightly toward the operator. A slight Trendelenburg position may be used, although it can rarely lead to lower extremity compartment syndrome. If the colon tumor or process is in the lower left colon or sigmoid region, most surgeons will position the patient in a modified lithotomy manner using Allen stirrups supporting the knees and ankles. This will allow for prepping and draping of the rectal region for potential passage of a circular stapling device. The legs are spread and the knees elevated sufficiently to provide this access to the rectum but not so high or wide as to interfere with the abdominal portion of the operation. If there is any doubt as to the location of the tumor, lithotomy position is recommended.

OPERATIVE PREPARATION The skin is prepared in the routine manner.

INCISION AND EXPOSURE The operator stands on the patient's left side. A liberal midline incision is made centered below the level of the umbilicus. The liver as well as other possible sites for metastasis are explored. The small intestines are then packed away medially with warm, moist packs. A pack is placed toward the pelvis and another along the lateral wall up to the spleen.

DETAILS OF PROCEDURE Precautions against possible spread of the tumor should include limited manipulation of the growth. As soon as possible, the tumor should be covered with gauze and its major blood supply clamped.

With the bowel at the point of the lesion held in the left hand, the lateral peritoneal reflection of the mesocolon is incised close to the bowel except in the region of the tumor over as wide an area as seems essential for its free mobilization (FIGURE 1). Following this, the bowel is retracted toward the midline and the mesentery is freed from the posterior abdominal wall by blunt gauze dissection. Troublesome bleeding may occur if the left spermatic or ovarian vein is torn and not ligated. The left ureter is identified because it must not be drawn up with the mesentery of the intestine and accidentally divided. A fan-shaped incision of sufficient size is made so that the entire left colic artery and vein down to their origins can be removed in order to maximize removal of regional lymph nodes (FIGURE 2). Some surgeons perform this division as soon as possible to minimize angiolymphatic spread of tumor from manipulation and traction of the specimen. In this technique, originally called "no touch," it is essential that the surgeons have already identified the left ureter as well as the inferior mesenteric and sigmoid vessels (see Chapter 7: Anatomy of the Large Intestine, Vessels 8 and 9). At least 10 cm of margin from the gross border on either side of the lesion should be allowed. The contents of the clamps applied to the mesentery are tied. The mesenteric border of the bowel at the proposed site of resection is cleared of mesenteric fat in preparation for the anastomosis (FIGURE 3).

In most patients, the splenic flexure of the colon is mobilized to avoid an anastomosis under tension. This maneuver is easier and safer to accomplish if the midline incision is extended up to the xiphoid. This technique is shown in FIGURES 15 to 17. Alternatively, the omentum may be removed in its relatively avascular junction along the left colon until the splenocolic region is reached. The descending left colon is then mobilized superiorly along the extension of the lateral line of Toldt. By approaching both ends toward the middle, the sometimes difficult splenocolic omental attachments are safely visualized and divided with minimal risk of splenic injury.

Most surgeons would currently use a stapled closure for a left hemicolectomy or sigmoidectomy, as described in Chapter 62. In either case, care must be taken to divide distally below the rectosigmoid junction both to avoid leaving sigmoid diverticula and because it allows better mobility of the rectum and easier advancement of the circular stapling device. For cases where the surgeon does not have access to staplers, the following hand-sewn method is described. Paired crushing clamps of the Stone or similar type are placed obliquely across the bowel above the lesion within 1 cm of the limits of the prepared mesentery (FIGURE 4). The field is walled off with gauze, and the bowel is divided. A pair of noncrushing clamps is then applied to the prepared area below the lesion, and the bowel is divided in a similar fashion. The ends of the large intestine are brought end to end to determine whether the anastomosis can be carried out without tension. The clamps are approximated and manipulated so that the posterior serosal surface of the intestine is presented to facilitate placement of a layer of interrupted mattress 000 silk sutures (FIGURE 5). The mesenteric border should be free of fat to achieve accurate approximation of the serosa. The sutures at the angles are not cut and are utilized for traction (FIGURE 6).

Enterostomy clamps are placed several centimeters from the crushing clamps, and the crushing clamps are removed (FIGURE 6). The portions of excessive bowel that were beyond the clamps may be excised. The field is completely walled off with moist, sterile gauze packs, and a direct open anastomosis is carried out. The mucosa is approximated with a continuous lock suture on an atraumatic needle starting in the middle of the posterior layer (FIGURE 7). At the angle, the lock suture is changed to one of the Connell type to ensure inversion of the angle and the anterior mucosa (FIGURES 8 and 9). A second continuous suture is started adjacent to the first one and is carried out in a similar fashion (FIGURE 10). After the mucosa has been accurately approximated, the two continuous sutures, A and B, are tied with the knot on the inside (FIGURE 11). A layer of interrupted 000 silk sutures or nonabsorbable sutures is utilized to approximate the anterior serosal layer. Particular attention is given to either angle to ensure accurate and secure approximation.

Alternative techniques for colon anastomoses include the use of single layer of delayed absorbable interrupted sutures with knots within the lumen and the use of stapling instruments. The latter technique is shown in Chapter 54, Colon Anastomosis, Stapled. **CONTINUES ▶**

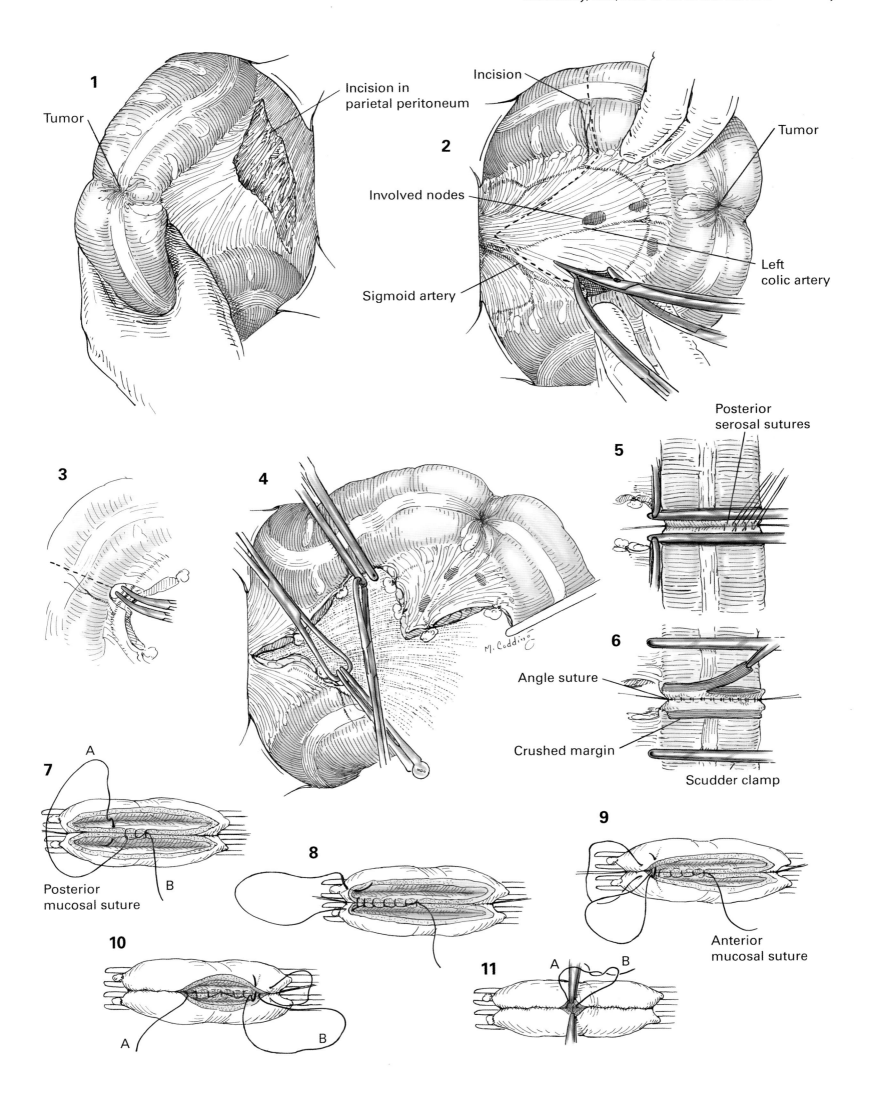

1

Tumor

Incision in parietal peritoneum

2

Incision

Tumor

Involved nodes

Sigmoid artery

Left colic artery

3

4

M. Coddine

5

Posterior serosal sutures

6

Angle suture

Crushed margin

Scudder clamp

7

A

B

Posterior mucosal suture

8

9

Anterior mucosal suture

10

A

B

11

A

B

DETAILS OF PROCEDURE ◂CONTINUED▸ Following the approximation of the mucosal layer, all contaminated instruments are discarded. The field is covered with fresh moist gauze sponges and towels. It is desirable for the members of the surgical team to change gloves. The anastomosis is further reinforced by an anterior serosal layer of interrupted ooo silk sutures (FIGURE 12). It is sometimes advisable to reinforce the mesenteric angle with one or two additional mattress sutures. Any remaining opening of the mesentery is then closed with interrupted sutures of fine silk. If there is a great deal of fat in the mesentery, which tends to hide the location of blood vessels, it is unwise to pass a needle blindly through it lest a hematoma form between the leaves of the mesentery. It is safer to grasp the peritoneal margins of the mesentery with small, pointed clamps and effect a closure by simple ligation of their contents. Finally, adequacy of the blood supply to the site of the anastomosis should be inspected. Active, pulsating vessels should be present adjacent to the anastomosis on both sides (FIGURE 13). If the blood supply appears to be interfered with and the color of the bowel is altered, it is better to resect the anastomosis rather than risk leakage and potentially fatal peritonitis. The patency of the stoma is carefully tested by compression between the thumb and the index finger (FIGURE 14). It is usually possible to obtain a two-finger stoma.

To ensure easy approximation of the open ends of the large bowel, especially if the lesion is located near the splenic flexure, it is necessary to free the intestine from adjacent structures. The abdominal incision may have to be extended up to the costal margin, since exposure of the uppermost portion of the splenic flexure may be difficult. After the relatively avascular peritoneal attachments to the descending colon have been divided, it is necessary to free the splenic flexure from the diaphragm, spleen, and stomach. The splenocolic ligament is divided between curved clamps, and the contents are ligated to avoid possible injury to the spleen, with troublesome hemorrhage (FIGURE 15). Following this, a pair of curved clamps is applied to the gastrocolic ligament for the necessary distance required to mobilize the bowel or remove sufficient intestine beyond the growth. Sometimes, in the presence of growths in this area, it is necessary to carry the division adjacent to the greater curvature of the stomach. The surgeon should not hesitate to remove a portion of the left gastroepiploic artery, if indicated, since the stomach has such a good collateral blood supply. In some instances, a true phrenocolic ligament can be developed, which must be divided to free the splenic flexure (FIGURE 16).

If it is necessary to free a portion of the transverse colon, the omentum may be freed from the bowel by incising its avascular attachments adjacent to the colon (FIGURES 15–17; see also Chapter 27). In some instances, omentum may be involved with the growth, and it may be desirable to remove all or part of it. The splenic flexure is reflected medially following the division of its attachments, and care is taken to avoid the kidney and the underlying ureter. It is usually necessary to divide a portion of the transverse mesocolon (FIGURE 18). This should be done carefully, taking into consideration possible injury to the underlying jejunum in the region of the ligament of Treitz. The large inferior mesenteric vein will also require division and double ligation as it dips down under the inferior margin of the body of the pancreas to join the splenic vein. The bowel is freed of all fatty attachments at the site selected for anastomosis. Noncrushing clamps are applied, and the bowel is divided (FIGURE 19). Arterial pulsations in the mesentery on both sides should be verified. The anastomosis is carried out as previously described. If it becomes necessary to ligate the middle colic artery, the entire transverse colon, including the hepatic and splenic flexures, may need to be resected to ensure an adequate blood supply at the site of anastomosis. In this situation the viability of the colon depends upon the right colic artery on one side and the left colic artery on the other.

CLOSURE The closure is made in the usual manner.

POSTOPERATIVE CARE The patient is encouraged to cough, sit up, and ambulate as soon as possible. The nasogastric tube provides decompression until bowel activity returns, usually on the first or second day after surgery. Oral intake of clear liquids is begun and advanced as tolerated, whereupon intravenous hydration and electrolytes are discontinued. ■

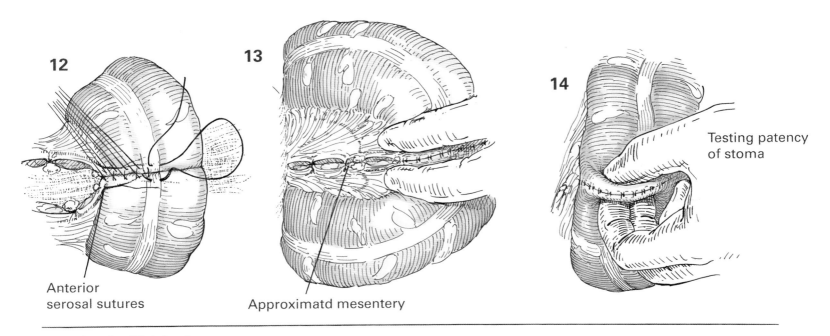

12

Anterior serosal sutures

13

Approximatd mesentery

14

Testing patency of stoma

Resection for High Lesion

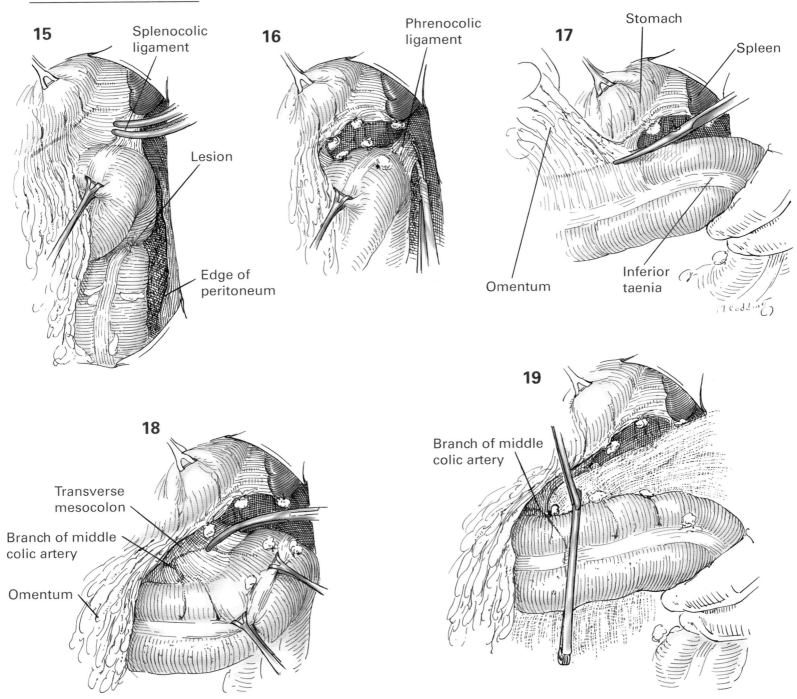

15

Splenocolic ligament

Lesion

Edge of peritoneum

16

Phrenocolic ligament

17

Stomach

Spleen

Omentum

Inferior taenia

18

Transverse mesocolon

Branch of middle colic artery

Omentum

19

Branch of middle colic artery

COLECTOMY, LEFT, LAPAROSCOPIC

INDICATIONS Laparoscopic colectomy is indicated in both benign and malignant conditions as long as it is performed by qualified surgeons with appropriate resources. In general, this approach is not recommended in patients with emergency conditions such as obstruction, perforation, or massive bleeding.

PREOPERATIVE PREPARATION For patients having surgery for polyps and occult neoplasms, it is essential to have the lesion tattooed during colonoscopy or localized by a preoperative barium enema. Identification of the tumor during laparoscopy is usually difficult. The use of intraoperative colonoscopy is difficult during laparoscopic procedures, hence accurate preoperative localization is necessary. The patient should receive a standard mechanical bowel preparation and prophylactic antibiotics are administered within 1 hour of the incision and are to be discontinued within 24 hours of surgery. Subcutaneous heparin is administered and sequential compression devices are placed for the prevention of venous thromboembolism.

INCISION AND EXPOSURE The setup is similar to the laparoscopic right colectomy. However, the surgeon and camera operator stand on the patient's right and the first assistant on the patient's left (FIGURE 1). The surgeon and camera operator may switch places during the procedure to facilitate exposure and operating angles. The surgeon moves between the legs during portions of the operation, in particular during the creation of the colorectal anastomosis. The port placement is the same as the right colectomy except that the upper abdominal 5-mm trocar is the right upper quadrant in the midclavicular line (FIGURE 2A and B). This port may facilitate mobilization of the splenic flexure (FIGURE 3). FIGURE 2B shows an alternative port placement.

DETAILS OF PROCEDURE For the initial mobilization of the sigmoid colon, the patient is rotated to the right. The sigmoid colon is grasped with an atraumatic forceps and retracted medially. The peritoneal attachments are then divided using the ultrasonic shears and blunt dissection (FIGURE 3). Care is taken to identify the ureter and avoid ureteral injury. The peritoneal attachment is divided up to the splenic flexure. This is facilitated by the first assistant or surgeon providing counter-traction of the colon. As the dissection nears the splenic flexure, it is best to stay underneath the omentum and develop a plan between the omentum and the splenic flexure (FIGURE 4). Dissection between the omentum and the spleen can lead to splenic injury. The omentum is separated for a variable distance along the transverse colon depending on the amount of colon to be removed and the amount of mobility that will be necessary to complete a tension-free anastomosis. Mobilization of the splenic flexure and the transverse colon may be facilitated by a reverse Trendelenburg position. The proximal rectum is mobilized (FIGURE 5). In FIGURE 5, the orientation of the dissection is rotated so the head is to the reader's left and the foot to the right. The line of mesenteric incision is shown. The surgeon needs to know the anticipated position of the left and right ureter. CONTINUES▶

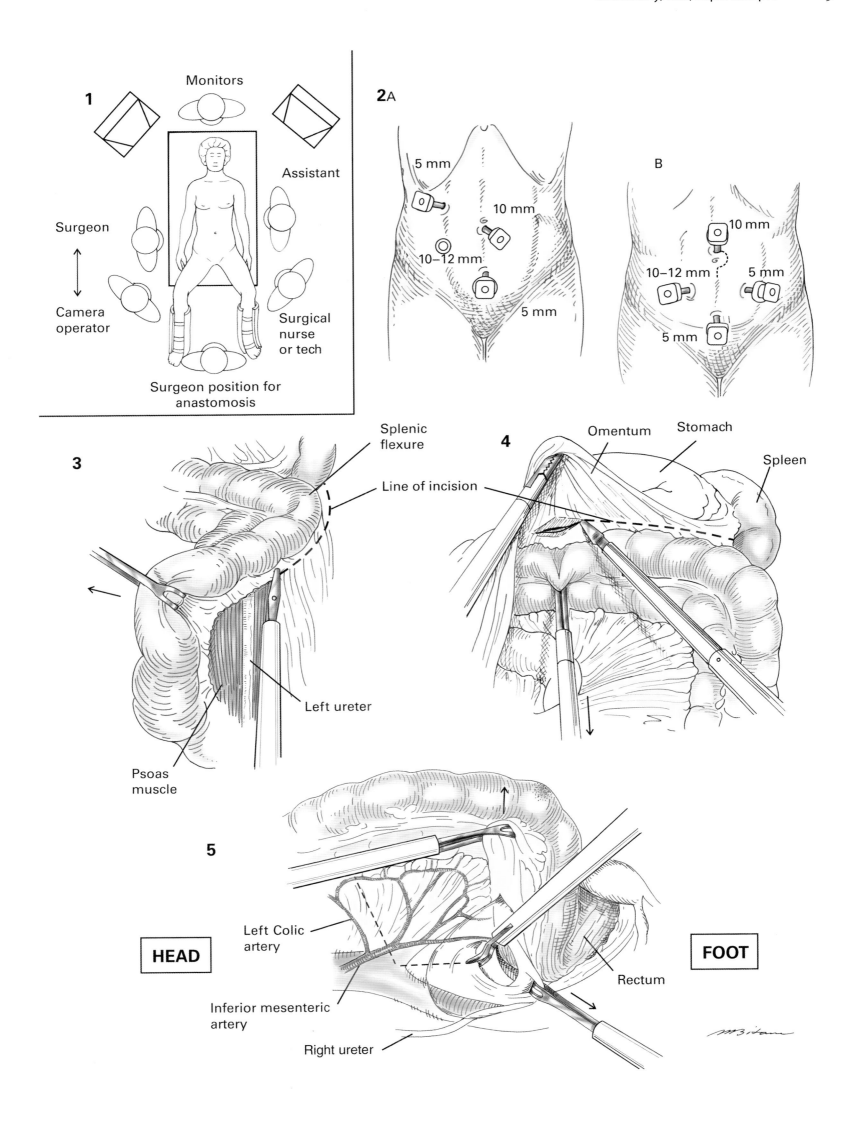

1

Monitors

Assistant

Surgeon

Camera operator

Surgical nurse or tech

Surgeon position for anastomosis

2A

5 mm

10 mm

10–12 mm

5 mm

B

10 mm

10–12 mm

5 mm

5 mm

3

Splenic flexure

Line of incision

Left ureter

Psoas muscle

4

Omentum

Stomach

Spleen

5

Left Colic artery

Inferior mesenteric artery

Right ureter

Rectum

HEAD

FOOT

DETAILS OF PROCEDURE ◀**CONTINUED** Next, control and division of the mesenteric vessels is accomplished. The mesocolon is incised. The course of the ureter should be reverified at this point. A window is made in the peritoneum near the inferior mesenteric vessels. The mesenteric vessels may be divided with linear vascular staples, individually doubly clipped or with coagulation devices designed for this purpose (FIGURE 6). FIGURE 6 shows the line of division of the mesentery. Staple application provides the most efficient method, but most costly as well. A medial to lateral dissection may be employed, reserving the mobilization of the lateral attachments and splenic flexure until the mesocolon has been divided. Once the mesentery is divided, the transverse colon is brought into the pelvis ensuring adequate mobility for a tension-free anastomosis. The distal colon/rectum is divided using a transversely placed reticulated linear stapler (FIGURE 7). This results in the distal staple line as shown in the figures labeled B. The proximal colon may be divided intracorporally with an endoscopic stapler or after the bowel is exteriorized with a linear stapler through extension of the midline or left lower quadrant trocar incisions. This results in the proximal staple line A. The umbilical incision is extended inferiorly to permit extraction of the specimen, extracorporeal division of the bowel, and preparation of the proximal colon for the anastomosis. Alternatively a left lower quadrant transverse or a Pfannenstiel incision may be made. Prior to bringing the colon through the abdominal wall, a plastic wound protector is used to prevent contamination of the subcutaneous tissue and skin. The anastomosis between A and B is created using a double-staple technique. The exteriorized proximal colon is cleaned and the staple line removed. Dilators are used to dilate the opening of the proximal colon (A).

A purse-string suture is placed in the proximal colotomy (FIGURE 8). The anvil for the circular stapler is placed in the bowel (FIGURE 9). The purse-string suture is tied and the colon returned to the peritoneal cavity. The circular stapler is inserted transanally, and the stapler spike is placed through the distal staple line or posterior to it under direct vision (B). The spike is removed with a laparoscopic forceps and removed. The end of the anvil is then inserted into the circular stapler. The stapler is closed and discharged (FIGURE 10). The stapling device is removed and the donuts are inspected for completeness. An incomplete donut indicates an incomplete suture line that will require oversewing. The abdomen is filled with saline and rigid proctoscopy with air insufflation performed in order to examine the anastomosis and to detect air leakage. If air bubbles are encountered, the anastomosis is oversewn with nonabsorbable 3-0 sutures and the air insufflation repeated to verify anastomotic integrity. The mesenteric defect does not require closure. The abdomen should be visually inspected for bleeding.

CLOSURE The incision is closed with running or interrupted absorbable sutures. No drains are used. The fasciae at all large trocar sites (>5 mm) are closed with sutures. The skin is closed with staples.

POSTOPERATIVE CARE The orogastric or nasogastric tube is removed in the postoperative care unit. Intravenous fluids are administered and urine output and vital signs monitored every 4 hours. Prophylactic antibiotics are discontinued within 24 hours of the surgery. The bladder catheter is removed on postoperative day 1 or 2. Clear liquids are started according to institutional protocol (day 0–2) and advanced as tolerated. ■

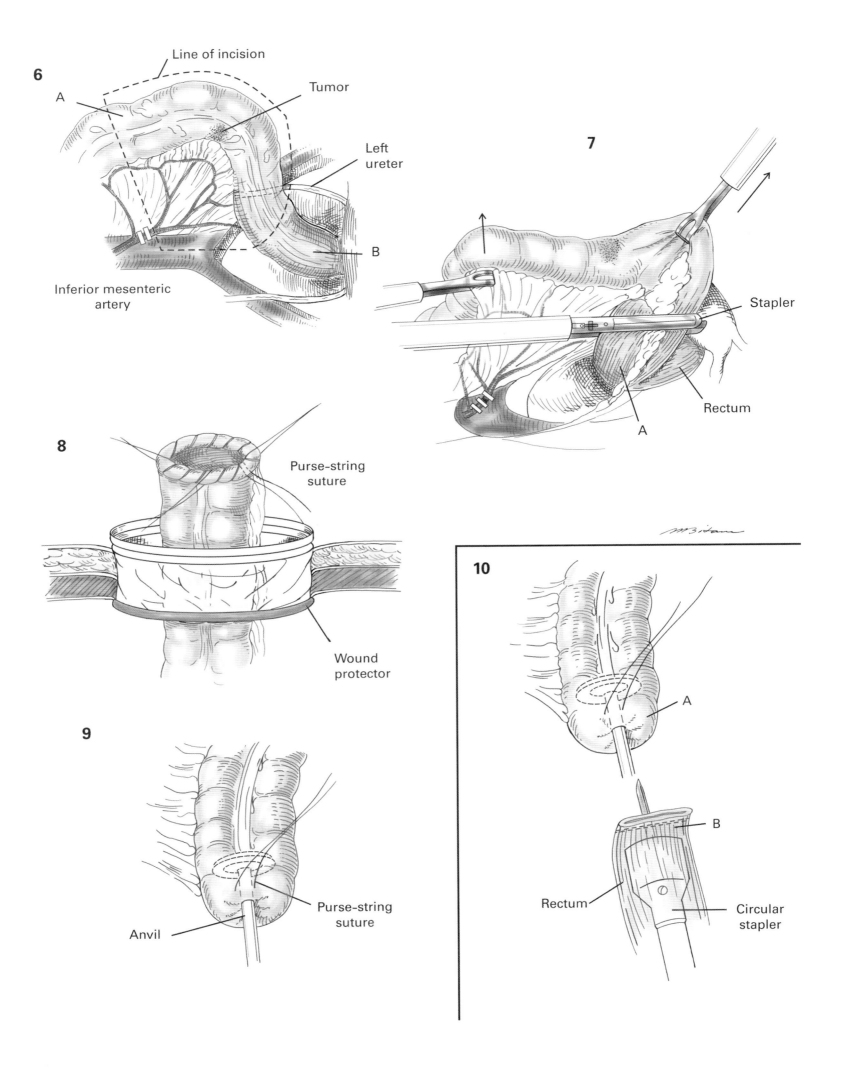

6

Line of incision

A

Tumor

Left ureter

B

Inferior mesenteric artery

7

Stapler

Rectum

A

8

Purse-string suture

Wound protector

9

Purse-string suture

Anvil

10

A

B

Rectum

Circular stapler

ABDOMINOPERINEAL RESECTION

INDICATIONS Abdominoperineal resection of the lower bowel is the operation of choice for very low rectal malignancies that involve the sphincter complex or cannot be removed with a 2-cm distal margin. In special circumstances, young patients may be candidates for a coloanal anastomosis, whereas others may be candidates for local wide excision and adjuvant treatment for low-grade superficial lesions. The surgeon must be familiar with all methods, including resection of the tumor and anastomosis of the intestine within the hollow of the sacrum.

PREOPERATIVE PREPARATION The patient's general condition must be studied and improved as much as possible, since the operation is one of the considerable magnitude. Unless there is evidence of acute or subacute obstruction, the patient is placed on a liquid diet for a day. Most patients receive a bowel preparation the afternoon or evening prior to surgery. Following complete evacuation of the colon with laxatives or purgative, appropriate nonabsorbable antibiotics may be given. Parenteral antibiotic coverage is given just prior to surgery. In the presence of low-lying tumors, it may be advisable to evaluate by cystoscopy whether or not the bladder or other portions of the genitourinary tract are involved. Basal carcinoembryonic antigen levels are determined before and after resection of the neoplasm. The extent of extramural spread or fixation to adjacent organs may be evaluated with endorectal ultrasound or MRI plus computed tomography (CT) imaging.

In males, an indwelling catheter is inserted into the bladder at the beginning of the procedure to maintain complete urinary drainage throughout the procedure and to aid in identifying the membranous urethra. Indwelling catheter drainage of the bladder in females is likewise advisable.

Currently, rectal carcinomas below the level of the peritoneal reflection in the pouch of Douglas are usually given combined radiation therapy and chemotherapy prior to surgery.

ANESTHESIA General anesthesia with endotracheal intubation and muscle relaxants is the preferred method.

ABDOMINAL RESECTION

POSITION The surgeon stands on the patient's left side. Most prefer a two-team approach with the patient in the semilithotomy position using Allen stirrups. This allows the perineal portion of the procedure to be carried out either simultaneously or after the abdominal portion without redraping, etc. A folded sheet is placed under the lower back so that the buttocks are lifted up off the bed, allowing better access to the posterior part of the perineal dissection. After an enema with a povidone–iodine solution, the anus is sutured shut at the anal verge (not distal to it) with a running-locked o silk suture. A moderate Trendelenburg position may facilitate retraction, as long as it is well tolerated by the patient.

OPERATIVE PREPARATION The lower abdomen, perineal, and rectal areas are prepared in the usual manner.

INCISION AND EXPOSURE A midline incision is made and extended to the left and above the umbilicus. A self-retaining retractor is inserted.

DETAILS OF PROCEDURE With the left hand, the surgeon thoroughly explores the abdomen from above downward, palpating first the liver to ascertain the presence or absence of metastases and then the region of the aorta and common iliac and hemorrhoidal vessels for evidence of lymph gland involvement. Finally, by palpation and inspection, the surgeon determines the extent and resectability of the growth itself (FIGURE 1). The inferior mesenteric artery and vein may be ligated distal to the origin of the left colic artery or at its point of origin from the aorta before the tumor is mobilized, but after identification of the ureters.

After the small intestine has been walled off in a plastic bag, the next procedure is the mobilization of the sigmoid, which is usually anchored in the left iliac fossa. The sigmoid is grasped and reflected medially in order that the surgeon may obtain a clear view of the fibrous bands that anchor the sigmoid to the reflection of the peritoneum of the left pelvic wall (FIGURE 2). The adjacent adhesive bands are divided with long curved scissors or electrocautery, and the peritoneal reflection is retracted laterally with forceps. Following this procedure, the sigmoid is usually mobilized easily toward the midline. The peritoneal surface on the left side of the colon is picked up with forceps and divided with long, curved, blunt-nosed Metzenbaum scissors, which are gently introduced downward beneath the peritoneum to separate the underlying structures, such as the left spermatic, or ovarian, vessels or ureter, from the peritoneum to avoid their accidental injury. The peritoneum is incised down to the cul-de-sac on the left side (FIGURE 3).

The next important step in the operation is the visualization of the left ureter throughout its course over the pelvic brim and down to the bladder. This is very important because, on the left side, the ureter may be in close proximity to the root of the mesentery of the rectosigmoid and may be included in the division of the latter structures unless it is carefully retracted to the left side of the pelvis (FIGURE 4). The ureter will respond with peristaltic waves that progress along its length after it is pinched with forceps.

The next step involves the division of the peritoneum on the right side of the rectosigmoid. The same technique that has been described for the left side may be utilized, or the surgeon may mobilize the rectosigmoid over the pelvic brim from the left side by blunt finger dissection, taking care to leave the mesorectal fat intact. The fingers of the surgeon's left hand can be passed completely behind the bowel toward the right side. With the fingers used as blunt dissectors, the right peritoneal reflection can be tented upward, separating it from the underlying structures, including the right ureter. This enables the surgeon to divide the peritoneum readily and safely with scissors or electrocautery (FIGURE 5).

TOTAL MESORECTAL EXCISION For almost 100 years, the pelvic dissections for rectal cancers requiring a low anterior or an abdominoperineal resection have been accomplished with blunt dissection. As described by the English surgeon Miles, the surgeon's hands and fingers mobilized this section of rectum. Little sharp dissection is required except for division of the lateral suspensory ligaments, as shown in previous editions of the Atlas. Known complications from this blunt dissection include hemorrhage from torn presacral veins, perforation into the rectum, and injury to the pelvic autonomic nerves. An improved dissection, the total mesorectal excision (TME), has been shown to lessen these complications and to provide a better radial margin of tumor clearance. The TME requires meticulous sharp or electrocautery dissection under direct vision. The procedure takes significantly more time to perform, but it is associated with a lessened rate of local recurrence for rectal cancers. The TME technique is widely used both with sphincter preservation in very low rectal anastomoses and with abdominoperineal resection. CONTINUES ▶

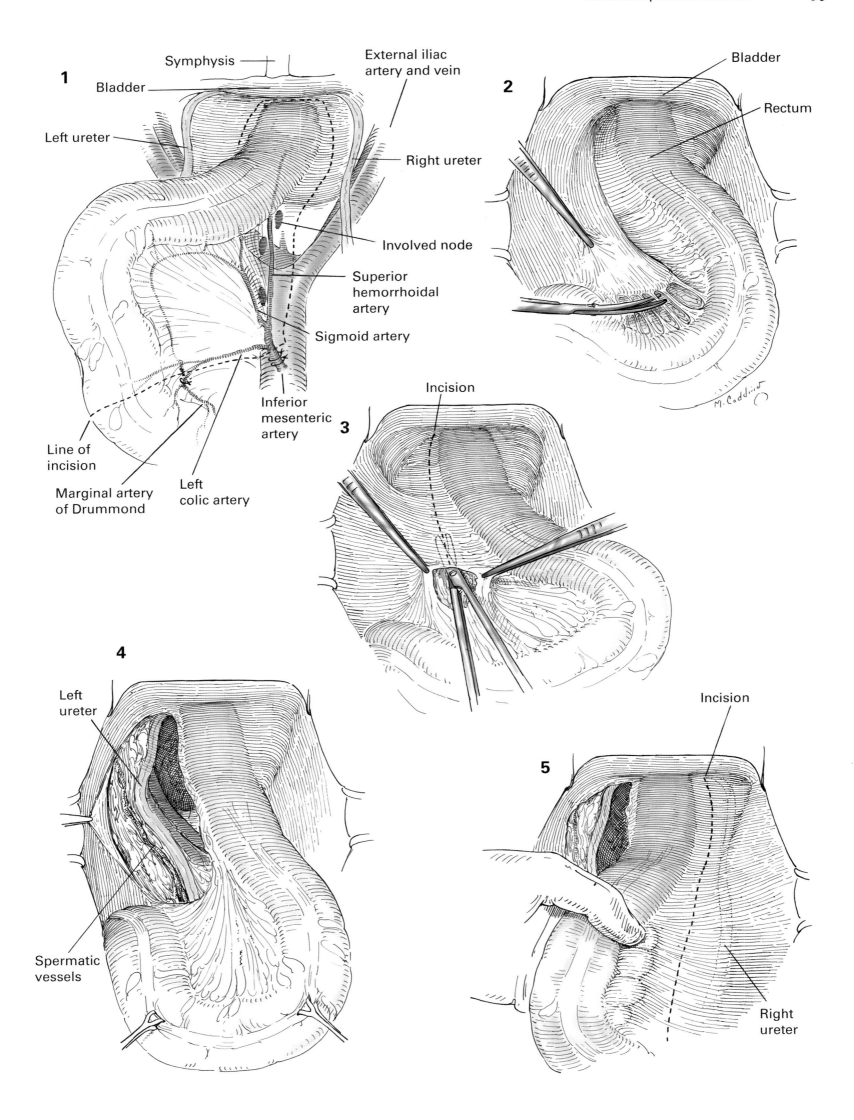

1

Symphysis

Bladder

Left ureter

External iliac
artery and vein

Right ureter

Involved node

Superior
hemorrhoidal
artery

Sigmoid artery

Inferior
mesenteric
artery

Line of
incision

Marginal artery
of Drummond

Left
colic artery

2

Bladder

Rectum

M. Coddinet

3

Incision

4

Left
ureter

Spermatic
vessels

5

Incision

Right
ureter

DETAILS OF PROCEDURE ◂CONTINUED▸ The peritoneum along the right side of the rectosigmoid junction is incised lateral to the inferior mesenteric and superior hemorrhoidal vessels (FIGURE 6). This incision extends down to the pouch of Douglas. The right ureter is identified beneath the residual peritoneum, and its course over the iliac vessels is exposed with blunt gauze dissection. The proximal bowel is retracted anteriorly and laterally. Alternatively, the proximal division of the bowel and vascular pedicles can be completed allowing the proximal end of the specimen to be moved around to aid visualization (FIGURE 13, Chapter 63). If the tumor is very large, this should be avoided at this point, as it commits one to an excision prior to complete mobilization of the tumor. The superior hypogastric nerves are visualized just below the iliac vessels and the ureters. The dissection proceeds behind the superior hemorrhoidal vessels toward the entrance of the presacral space behind the sacral promontory. Division of the retrosacral fascia or ligament just below the sacral curvature at about S2 is done sharply in the midline with scissors or electrocautery, using a long, insulated tip (FIGURE 7). The rectum is retracted anteriorly with a fiberoptic lighted deep pelvic retractor, which may be straight or curved. Under direct vision, the posterior dissection continues down to the level of the coccyx. The sacral veins are clearly visualized beneath the parietal fascia, which is kept intact, thus minimizing bleeding.

The peritoneal reflection in the pouch of Douglas is incised about 1 cm up its anterior reflection over the bladder in men (shown in this illustration) or behind the uterus in women. The bladder or uterus is retracted anteriorly using a fiberoptic lighted deep pelvic retractor. The sharp dissection proceeds anterior to Denonvilliers' fascia until the prostate and seminal vessels (FIGURE 8) or the rectovaginal septum is seen. The paths of the anterior and posterior dissections (FIGURE 9) show the close adherence to the presacral fascia posteriorly and to the actual prostate and seminal vesicles anteriorly. ◂CONTINUES▸

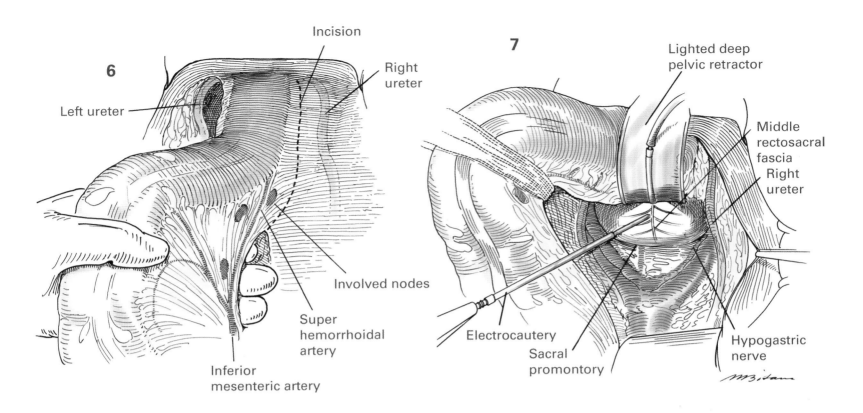

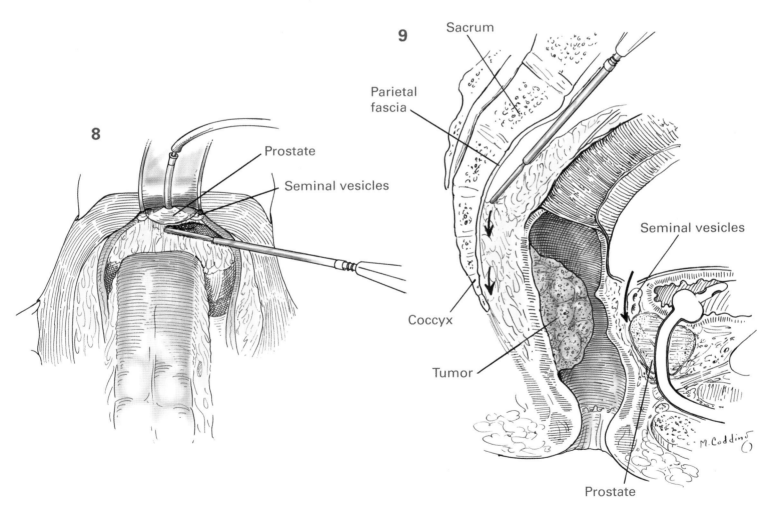

DETAILS OF PROCEDURE CONTINUED The two lateral dissections in the TME are time-consuming, as the surgeon carefully proceeds to expose the parietal fascia over the lateral pelvic wall structures. The fiberoptic lighted deep pelvic retractors are essential for clear visualization during lateral retraction of the rectum and anterior elevation of the bladder or the uterus and vagina. Better lighting may also be obtained with the use of a headlamp. The preservation of the pelvic autonomic nerve plexus and the anterior roots of sacral nerves S2, S3, and S4 is essential for anal continence and sexual function. The plexus is seen as a dense plaque of nerve tissue that comes close to the rectum at the level of the prostate or upper vagina. The TME does not encounter "lateral suspensory ligaments" but rather a fusion of the lateral mesorectum with tissue that may contain the middle hemorrhoidal arteries as the dissection heads toward the autonomic nerve plexus. This tissue is divided with electrocautery, and the middle hemorrhoidal vessels may require a ligature. The course of the ureters and the autonomic plexus is noted as the dissection is carried down to the levators (FIGURE 10).

After the rectum is mobilized, the specimen should have a wide zone of relatively smooth fat about the middle and upper rectum. In a thin patient, the pelvic nerves and autonomic nerve plexuses may just be visible beneath the parietal fascia, whereas the prostate and seminal vesicles are uncovered.

After it has been determined that the rectal tumor can be completely freed from the adjacent structures, the blood supply to the rectosigmoid is divided. The venous drainage should be ligated as early as possible to keep the vascular spread of tumor cells to a minimum. Although involved lymph nodes may not be evident in the mesentery over the bifurcation of the aorta, it is desirable to ligate the inferior mesenteric artery just distal to the origin of the left colic artery (FIGURE 11). The contents of the proximal clamps are tied, and the ligation is reinforced by a transfixing suture. Some prefer to ligate the inferior mesenteric artery as near its point of origin from the aorta as possible. Usually, this level is surprisingly near the ligament of Treitz. The blood supply to the sigmoid to be used as a colostomy is now derived from the middle artery through the marginal artery of Drummond.

Following this, the abdominal cavity and pelvis are completely walled off with gauze as a preliminary to transection with a stapling instrument that divides the bowel between double rows of staples such as a cutting linear stapler (FIGURE 12).

The redundant sigmoid, which has been retracted upward over the abdominal wall, is inspected to determine the best site (FIGURE 11) for dividing the bowel to serve as a permanent colostomy. The sigmoid is divided where it appears to be viable and will extend beyond the surface of the skin for 5 to 8 cm without being under undue tension. It is better to err in having extra colon beyond the skin margin rather than too little. Consideration must be given to the thickness of the subcutaneous tissues as well as postoperative distention in testing the length of colon mobilized for the permanent colostomy. The proximal end of the specimen is then divided at this point with a cutting linear stapler (FIGURE 13). Excessive fat tabs and thick fatty mesentery, if present, should be excised about the terminal end of the colon in anticipation of inversion of the mucosa with immediate fixation to the adjacent skin. The surgeon is now ready to begin the perineal portion of the resection. If available, a second surgical team may begin the perineal portion of the operation as the abdominal team completes the rectal mobilization.

PERINEAL RESECTION The surgeon must be satisfied with the patient's condition before proceeding with the perineal excision of the rectosigmoid. The estimated blood loss from the abdominal procedure, often more than realized unless accurately determined by the circulating nurse, should be replaced by blood transfusions, and the pulse and blood pressure should be established at a satisfactory level. Some prefer the two-team approach so that the perineal excision is carried out simultaneously with the abdominal procedure.

POSITION Historically, Miles then placed the patient on his or her left side in a modified Sims' position. Some surgeons prefer to change the patient to the lithotomy position by adjusting the stirrups to hold the legs. Some place the patient in prone-jackknife to complete the perineal resection. The change in position must be done gently and carefully; sudden shifts have been known to precipitate hypotension and shock. The pulse and blood pressure should be stabilized after the change in position before the final resection is started. Today, most surgeons prefer perform this operation as a one-stage procedure. The patient is positioned in lithotomy.

OPERATIVE PREPARATION The anus and adjacent skin surfaces are prepared with the usual skin antiseptics. The legs and buttocks are covered with sterile drapes. For a one-stage procedure, the perineum is prepped and draped as part of the initial prep. CONTINUES

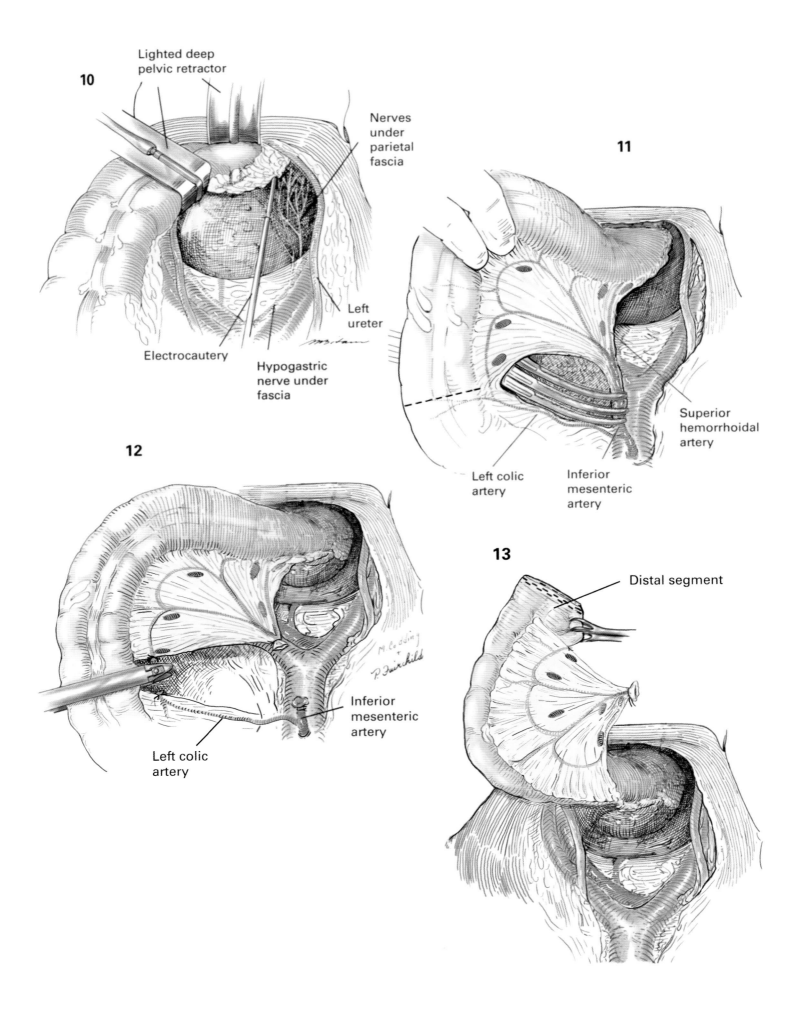

10

Lighted deep pelvic retractor

Nerves under parietal fascia

Left ureter

Electrocautery

Hypogastric nerve under fascia

11

Superior hemorrhoidal artery

Left colic artery

Inferior mesenteric artery

12

Inferior mesenteric artery

Left colic artery

13

Distal segment

INCISION AND EXPOSURE <CONTINUED> The rectum is dissected from the abdomen in to the pelvis as far as possible (FIGURE 14). This must include a wide mesenteric excision. The extent of the perineal excision is indicated in FIGURE 14. If the lesion is low and near the anus, a more radical excision is carried out. Operations for anal cancer will need to be extensive enough to excise the tumor with negative margins. If a large excision is contemplated, preoperative consultation should be made with a plastic surgeon, as myocutaneous flap reconstruction may be necessary. If the dissection has been carried down far enough from above, the perineal excision of the rectum and anus should be accomplished easily without undue loss of blood (FIGURE 14). To prevent contamination, the anus is sealed securely, either by several interrupted sutures of heavy silk or by a purse-string suture (FIGURES 15 and 16). An incision is outlined around the anus with anterior and posterior midline extensions (FIGURE 16). The skin in the region of the anal orifice is seized with several Allis forceps, and the incision is made through the skin and subcutaneous tissue at least 2 cm away from the closed anal orifice (FIGURE 17). All blood vessels are clamped and tied to prevent further loss of blood as the operation progresses (FIGURE 18). The entire dissection may be accomplished with an energy source such as electrocautery with clamps and ligatures for larger vessels .The margins of the wound are retracted laterally to assist in the exposure.

DETAILS OF PROCEDURE The posterior portion of the incision is extended backward over the coccyx, and the anus is tipped upward to enable its attachments to the coccyx to be severed more readily. After the anococcygeal raphe is severed and the presacral space is entered, the accumulated blood from above is suctioned out. The surgeon can then insert the index finger into the presacral space (FIGURE 19). The finger is swept laterally to identify the levator and muscles on either side. The levator muscle is exposed on one side and, with the finger held beneath it, is divided between paired clamps as far from the rectum as possible (FIGURE 20). Care must be taken to avoid bringing the dissection too close the rectum at this point, creating a specimen with a "waist," as this risks compromising the circumferential margin. The dissection from the perineum will meet the proximal dissection above the levators. Curved clamps should be applied to the levator ani muscles as they are divided to prevent the retraction of bleeding points. Following the ligation of all bleeding points on one side, a similar division of the levator ani muscles is carried out on the opposite side. Alternatively, the levator muscles may be transected with electrocautery, which can also control bleeding vessels. Vessels that are not easily coagulated with electrocautery should be individually secured with mattress or figure-of-eight absorbable sutures. <CONTINUES>

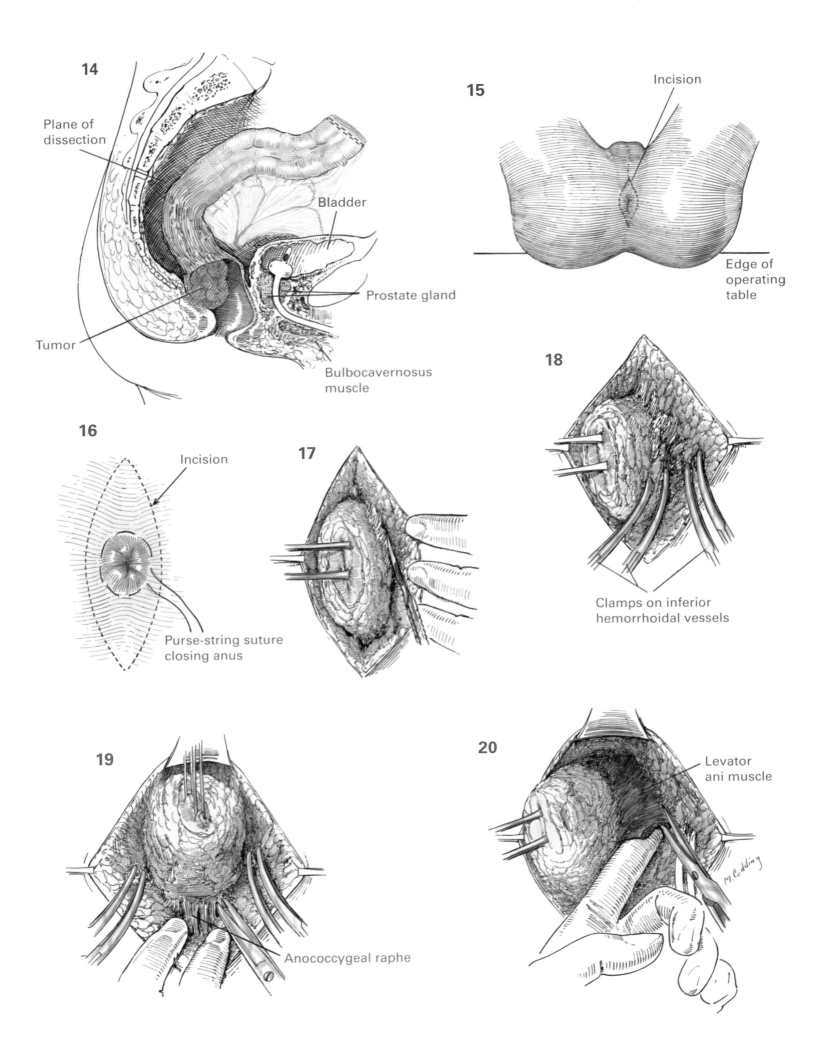

14

Plane of dissection

Tumor

Bladder

Prostate gland

Bulbocavernosus muscle

15

Incision

Edge of operating table

16

Incision

Purse-string suture closing anus

17

18

Clamps on inferior hemorrhoidal vessels

19

Anococcygeal raphe

20

Levator ani muscle

M. Codding

DETAILS OF PROCEDURE <CONTINUED> The procedure in the male is illustrated because the dissection between the rectum, membranous urethra, and prostate poses more problems than dissection in the female. Palpation of the inlying urethral catheter will facilitate the procedure by localizing the urethra and preventing accidental injury to the above-mentioned structures (FIGURE 21). The skin and subcutaneous tissue of the perineum are retracted upward, while the anus is pulled downward and backward to assist in the exposure. The rectum is pulled down, the remaining attachments of the levator ani muscles and transversus perinea are divided, and all bleeding points are ligated. In the female, the dissection between the rectum and the vagina is more easily accomplished if counter-resistance is applied to the posterior vaginal wall by the surgeon's fingers. In the presence of extensive infiltrating growths, it may be necessary to excise the perineal body as well as a portion of the posterior vaginal wall.

The upper end of the bowel segment is grasped and delivered posteriorly over the coccyx (FIGURE 22). A retractor is introduced anteriorly to assist in exposure, while any remaining anterior attachments of the rectum are divided (FIGURE 23). The large pelvic space is thoroughly inspected under direct illumination in order to clamp and ligate any active bleeding point. The cavity is packed with dry sponges until the field is free of oozing (FIGURE 24). When a two-team approach is used, irrigation may now be carried out from above.

CLOSURE It is usually possible to approximate the divided levator ani muscles in the midline (FIGURE 25). Two closed suction Silastic catheter drains are placed in the presacral space and brought out through the skin lateral in the incision and secured to the skin. The subcutaneous tissue and skin are closed with very large and widely spaced interrupted vertical mattress sutures of no. 1 nylon or silk. These are tied loosely (FIGURE 26). <CONTINUES>

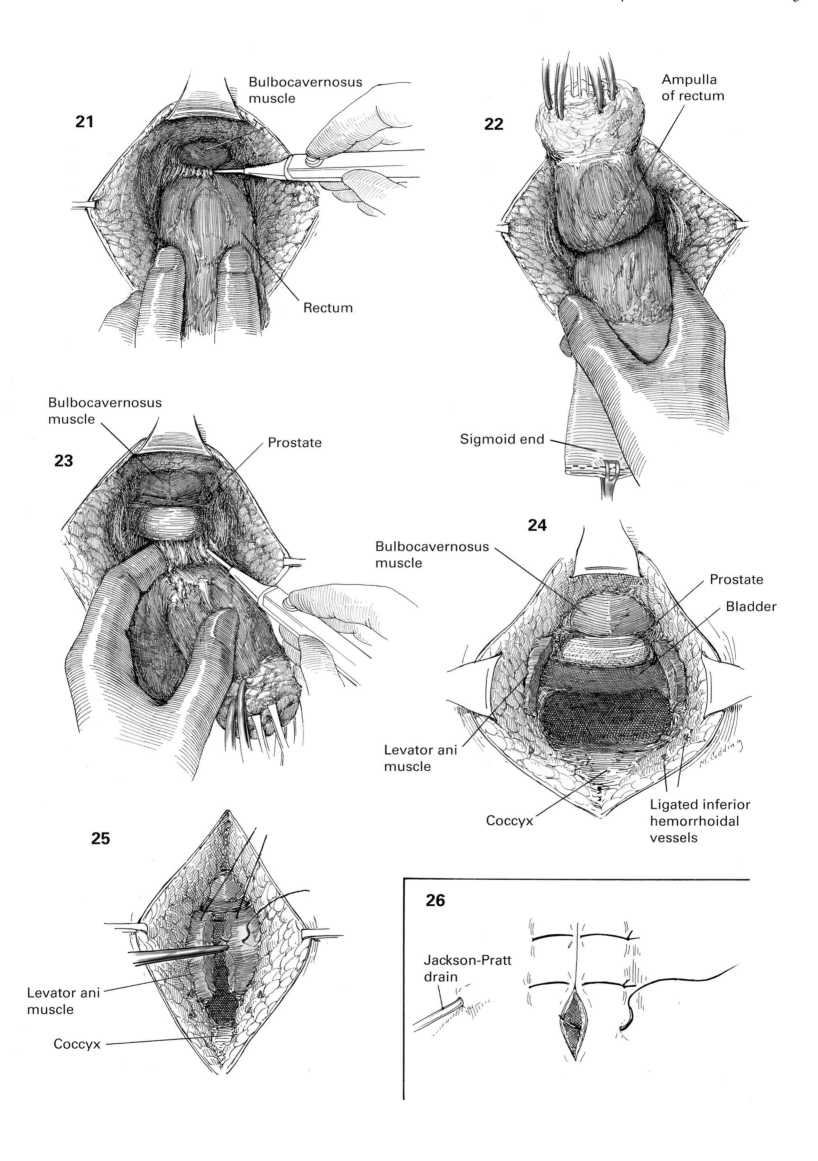

21 Bulbocavernosus muscle — Rectum

22 Ampulla of rectum — Sigmoid end

23 Bulbocavernosus muscle — Prostate

24 Bulbocavernosus muscle — Prostate — Bladder — Levator ani muscle — Coccyx — Ligated inferior hemorrhoidal vessels

25 Levator ani muscle — Coccyx

26 Jackson-Pratt drain

POSTOPERATIVE CARE CONTINUED The blood loss must be replaced during the operation and postoperatively. Intravenous Ringer's lactate solution is given and the hourly urine output monitored. With accelerated postoperative care pathways, urinary catheters are now often removed on the first postoperative day. This does not obviate the need for careful attention to voiding as described in the more traditional approach below.

The patient is traditionally maintained on constant bladder drainage for 5 to 7 days. In males the loss of bladder tone may result in one of the most distressing postoperative complications. Frequent and thorough evaluation of the patient's ability to empty the bladder is essential until good function has returned. The catheter should be clamped for several hours at a time to determine whether the patient actually has retained the sensation arising from a full bladder. In many cases, especially in males, a cystometric study should be considered before removing the catheter. The catheter should be removed early in the morning to permit all-day observations on the patient's ability to void. Overdistention should be rigorously avoided by catheterizing the patient for residual urine every 4 to 6 hours, depending upon his or her fluid intake. Diuretic liquids, such as coffee and tea, should be withheld from the evening meal in an effort to avoid overdistention of the bladder during the night. Frequent urination of small amounts indicates retention, and reinsertion of the catheter for a few days should be considered. Rigid attention to the care of the bladder with assistance from the urologic surgeon pays rich dividends in the patient's postoperative progress.

The suction catheters are removed in a few days when the drainage output has markedly decreased.

The patient is instructed in the care of a colostomy before being discharged from the hospital.

COLOSTOMY AND CLOSURE

DETAILS OF PROCEDURE After completion of the perineal resection, the pelvis is examined for bleeding and meticulous hemostasis obtained. A closed suction drain is placed and brought out through the perineum or abdominal wall. The pelvic space may be left open; some prefer to close this peritoneum. The margins of the peritoneum are mobilized in order to close the peritoneal floor securely. The peritoneum is grasped with toothed forceps and mobilized by the surgeon's hand or by blunt gauze dissection (FIGURE 27). The peritoneum in the pouch of Douglas is mobilized as widely as possible to facilitate closing the pelvic floor. The location of the ureters is reaffirmed from time to time to avoid their accidental ligation or injury. In females the uterus and adnexa may be used, if necessary, to close the new pelvic floor. At times it may be possible to close the pelvic floor in a straight line, but, more frequently, a radial type of closure is necessary to avoid undue tension on the suture line (FIGURE 28). All raw surfaces should be covered whenever possible. The omentum is placed over the peritoneal closure (FIGURE 29). Some make no attempt to close the peritoneum and rely on muscular closure.

When the patient's anatomy permits, a pedicled omental flap based on the left or right gastroepiploic artery can be created and laid into the pelvic defect. When enough omentum is available, this both fills the volume of the pelvis and covers the raw surfaces of the dissection. Some surgeons prefer to anchor the sigmoid to the lateral parietal peritoneum in order to close the left lumbar gutter and to avoid the possibility of an internal hernia. Whenever possible, these sutures should include the fat tabs or mesentery to avoid possible perforation of the bowel.

CLOSURE The omentum is returned to the region of the new pelvic floor and the table is leveled. The colostomy is created through a separate 3-cm (1¼ inch) opening selected and marked prior to surgery. In general, it is midway between the umbilicus and the left anterior superior spine (FIGURE 30). As this colostomy will be a permanent one, it is wise to choose and mark the site prior to surgery consultation with the enterostomal therapist. The adhesive ring of the colostomy bag must conform to the contour of the abdomen and must be secure when the patient is standing, bending, or sitting. After excision of the circle of skin, a two-finger-sized opening is made through the abdominal wall. The colon is grasped with Babcock forceps and brought out through the opening without undue rotation of the mesenteric blood supply. Late herniation about the colostomy can be minimized by tailoring the opening in the abdominal wall such that the colon plus one finger is a snug fit.

The abdominal wall is closed with interrupted oo silk sutures or oo synthetic absorbable sutures. Subcuticular closure of the skin should be considered since this ensures a sealed wound about an area repeatedly contaminated from the adjacent colostomy. In patients with marked obesity or cachexia, retention sutures may be utilized. The exteriorized portion of the bowel is then inspected to make certain that active pulsation is present in its blood supply. Sufficient intestine should have been provided to ensure at least 5 to 6 cm of viable bowel protruding above the skin level (FIGURE 31).

Immediate opening of the colostomy after the remainder of the wound has been covered is preferred to leaving a clamp on the exposed area completely obstructed intestine for several days. The stapled suture line is excised and the mucosa within the lumen of the bowel grasped with one or two Babcock forceps to provide fixation for the eversion of the mucosa (FIGURE 31). It may be necessary to excise several large fat tabs and additional thickened mesentery, especially in the obese patient, to facilitate the eversion of the mucosa. The mucosa is anchored to the margin of the skin with interrupted sutures or ooo synthetic absorbable sutures on a curved cutting needle (FIGURE 32). A sufficient number of sutures is taken to control bleeding as well as to seal off the subcutaneous tissue about the colostomy (FIGURE 33). The mucosa should be pink in color to ensure viability. The surgeon may insert a gloved finger into the colostomy to make certain the lumen is free and adequate without undue constriction within the abdominal wall. When the operation is complete, an ostomy appliance is applied. ■

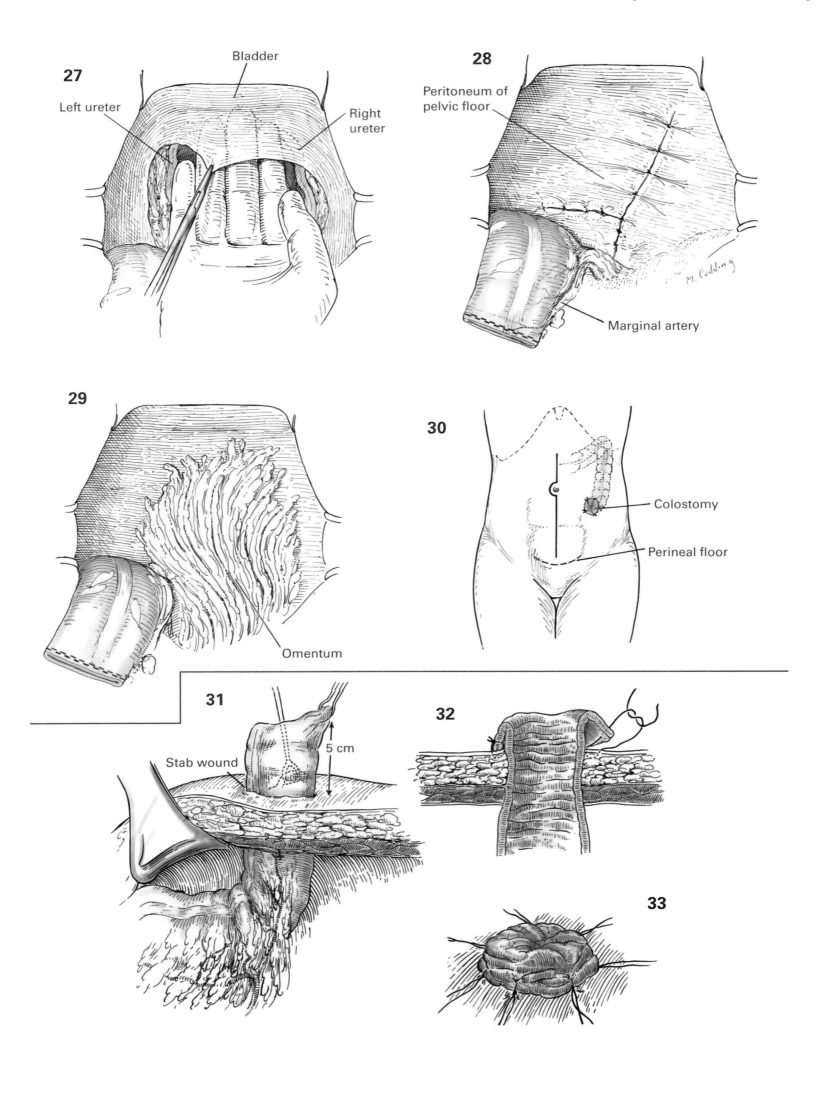

27

Bladder

Left ureter

Right ureter

28

Peritoneum of pelvic floor

M. Codding

Marginal artery

29

Omentum

30

Colostomy

Perineal floor

31

Stab wound

5 cm

32

33

TOTAL COLECTOMY AND TOTAL PROCTOCOLECTOMY

INDICATIONS The most common elective indications for total colectomy are ulcerative colitis and familial polyposis. However, sphincter-conserving procedures such as the ileoanal anastomosis (Chapter 64) should be considered in good-risk patients. In the very poor risk patient with ulcerative colitis, particularly with a complication such as a free perforation, it is judicious to perform the operation in two stages. The removal of the rectum is delayed until the patient's condition is less critical. The possibility of malignancy in patients with ulcerative colitis of many years' duration must be considered. Conservation of the anus and lower rectum by ileoproctostomy should be considered in congenital polyposis, where the polyps in the retained rectum that do not disappear spontaneously can be destroyed by repeated fulguration. Total colectomy is also performed for severe colitis of other etiologies, especially pseudomembranous colitis.

PREOPERATIVE PREPARATION Unless total colectomy is done as an emergency procedure, efforts should be made to improve the patient's nutritional status with a high-protein, high-calorie diet. Total parenteral nutrition may be used. The blood volume is restored and supplemental vitamins are provided. The surgeon must carefully evaluate the status of the steroid therapy. The patient requires special psychologic preparation for the ileostomy. This should include a visit by an enterostomal therapist who can demonstrate successful rehabilitation following this procedure. The patient should be shown the permanent type of ileostomy appliance and should be encouraged to read the literature available from an ileostomy club to prepare him or her for postoperative management. In addition, the site of the ileostomy should be selected away from bony prominences and previous scars as described in Chapter 51. A permanent type of appliance may be glued to the patient's skin for 1 to 2 days to allow him or her to move about with it in place and make any final adjustments in its eventual location. This point is marked with indelible ink to assure accurate placement of the stoma. A liquid diet is given for 1 or 2 days, followed by laxative purging the afternoon and evening prior to surgery. The male patient should be informed of the possibility of postoperative impotence, retrograde ejaculation, and difficulty in voiding. Women of child-bearing age should be counseled regarding the risk of decreased fertility after pelvic dissection.

ANESTHESIA General endotracheal anesthesia is preferred.

POSITION The patient is placed in a moderate Trendelenburg position. For total proctocolectomy, during the perineal portion of the operation, the patient may be repositioned in the lithotomy position with the thighs widely extended. Alternatively, the legs may be placed in the modified lithotomy position using the Allen stirrups for support of the feet and knees. This allows a single positioning for preparation and draping but may compromise the perineal exposure. A large rectal tube is used to lavage out the rectosigmoid with a povidone–iodine solution. This tube may be left to dependent drainage until the perineal resection begins, or the anus may be sutured closed after the enema and before skin preparation.

OPERATIVE PREPARATION The skin is prepared in the routine manner, and the ileostomy site just below the halfway mark between the right anterior iliac spine and the umbilicus is re-marked, usually by scratching the skin with the side of a hypodermic needle prior to skin preparation.

INCISION AND EXPOSURE The surgeon stands to the patient's left side. The incision must extend sufficiently high in the epigastrium to provide an easy exposure of the colonic flexures, lest undue traction of the friable bowel result in perforation and gross contamination (FIGURE 1).

After general exploration of the abdomen, the small bowel may be placed in a plastic bag. The dissection is started in the region of the tip of the cecum (FIGURE 2). The right colon is retracted medially as the peritoneum in the right lumbar gutter is incised with curved scissors (FIGURE 2). Because of the tendency to increased vascularity, it may be necessary to ligate a number of blood vessels in the free margin of the peritoneum along the right lumbar gutter.

The peritoneal attachments to the terminal ileum are divided and the cecum and terminal ileum mobilized well outside the wound (FIGURE 3). The peritoneum is tented upward before it is incised to avoid injuring the underlying right spermatic vessels and ureter. Blunt gauze dissection is utilized to push these structures away from the adjacent mesentery. The right ureter should be identified throughout its course up to the right kidney and down to the pelvic brim. Any adhesions between gallbladder, liver, and hepatic flexure are divided. During the mobilization of the ascending colon and hepatic flexure, care must be taken to identify the retroperitoneal portion of the duodenum, which may come into view rather unexpectedly. Blunt gauze is utilized to sweep away the duodenum from the overlying mesocolon. The thickened, contracted, and highly vascular greater omentum is divided between curved clamps and ligated (FIGURE 4). The greater omentum is retracted upward and the lesser omental sac entered from the right side. **CONTINUES** ▶

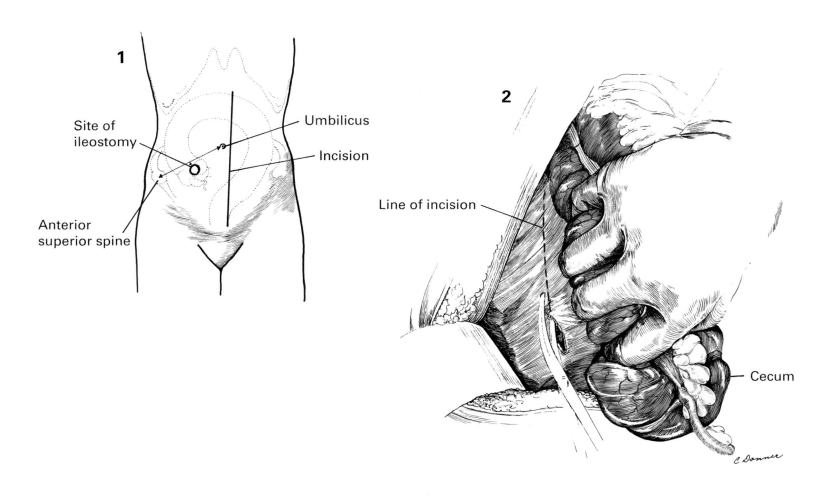

1

Site of
ileostomy

Umbilicus

Incision

Anterior
superior spine

2

Line of incision

Cecum

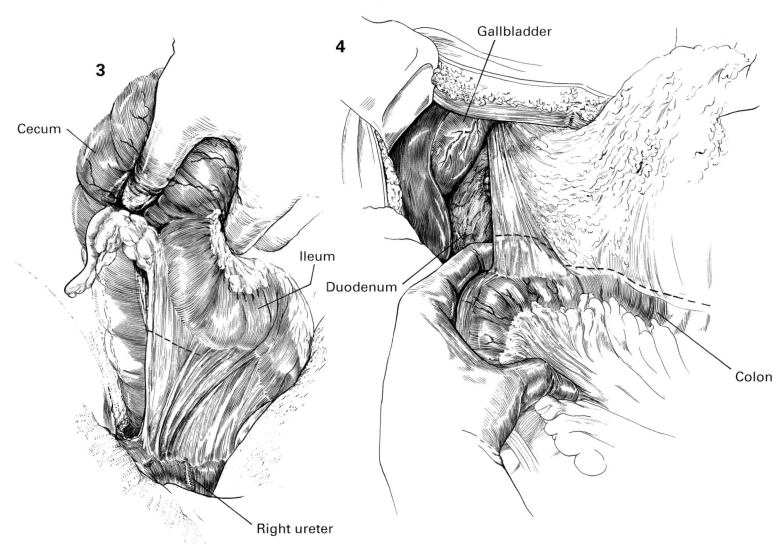

3

Cecum

Ileum

Right ureter

4

Gallbladder

Duodenum

Colon

INCISION AND EXPOSURE `CONTINUED` The thickened and vascular greater omentum is retracted upward in preparation for its separation from the transverse colon. An incision is made in the omental reflection along the superior surface of the colon (FIGURE 5). Since the omentum may be quite adherent to the colon, it may be easier to divide the gastrocolic omentum nearer the stomach than the transverse colon. This can be facilitated if the surgeon places his or her left hand, palm upward, in the lesser sac in order to better define the gastrocolic omentum. Most of the dissection can be done with electrocautery, especially if the relatively avascular plane is present where the omentum joins the transverse colon. If large vessels are encountered, paired curved clamps are applied and their contents ligated.

Special attention is required during the division of the thickened splenocolic ligament to avoid tearing the splenic capsule by undue tension (FIGURE 6). The splenocolic ligament is divided at some distance, if possible, from the inferior pole of the spleen (FIGURE 7). When the splenic flexure and descending colon have been partially freed down to the region of the sigmoid, the surgeon may wish to return to the region of the right colon and control the blood supply to the bowel before removing it in order to facilitate the eventual exposure of the pelvis for the exploration of the rectum. The mobilized right colon is drawn outside the peritoneal cavity, and the vessels in the mesentery can be identified easily (FIGURE 8). Enlarged lymph nodes often fill in the arcades about the mesenteric border. Unless malignancy has been found, the blood supply can be ligated near the bowel wall as shown in FIGURE 8. Before the blood supply is ligated, the ureter is protected posteriorly by warm, moist packs. `CONTINUES`

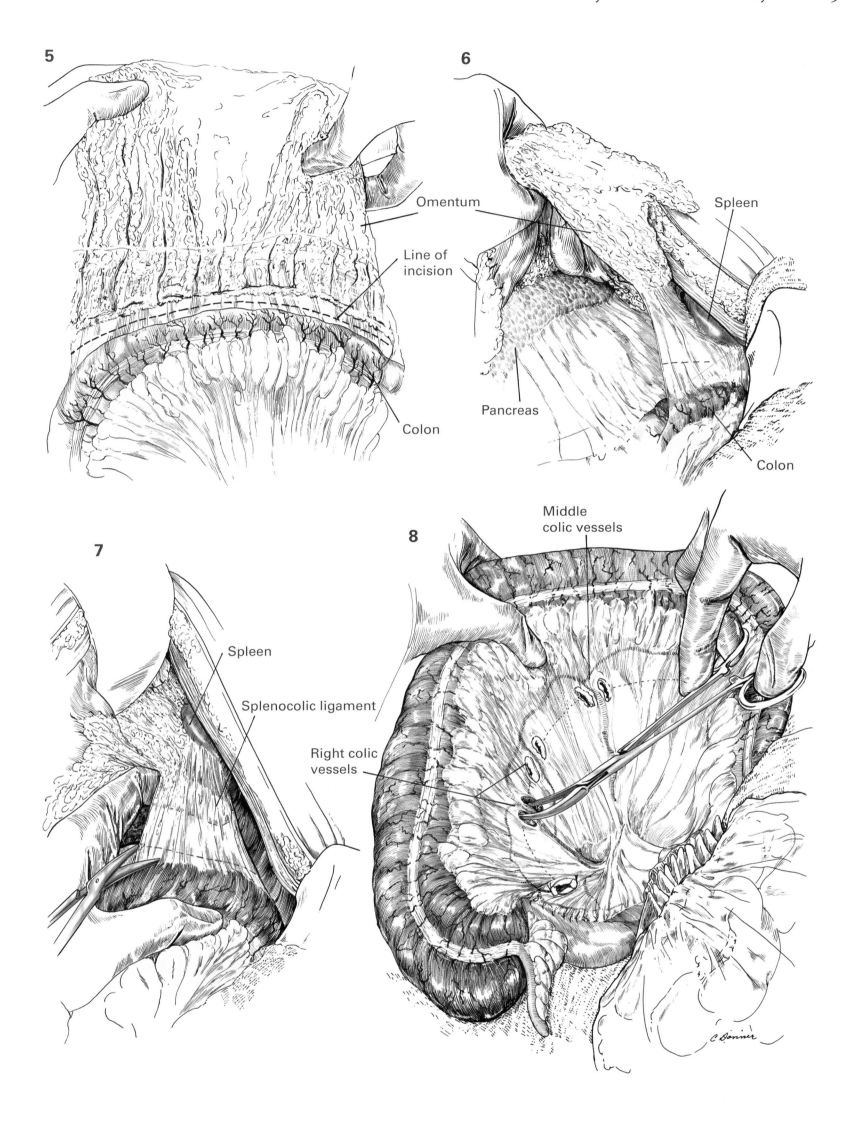

5

Omentum

Line of incision

Colon

6

Omentum

Spleen

Pancreas

Colon

7

Spleen

Splenocolic ligament

Right colic vessels

8

Middle colic vessels

INCISION AND EXPOSURE CONTINUED After the blood supply to the region of the appendix and the right colon has been divided, the terminal ileum may be further mobilized. An incision is made into the mesentery of the terminal ileum with a clear view of the ureter at all times to avoid its injury. It is often necessary to remove a portion of the terminal ileum because of its possible involvement with the inflammatory process (FIGURE 9).

Considerable time is required to separate the blood supply proximally from the site where the ileum is to be divided. Several centimeters of ileum can be denuded of blood supply in preparation for the development of an ileostomy (FIGURE 9). The blood supply to this portion of the ileum should be divided very carefully, almost one vessel at a time, maintaining the large vascular arcade at some distance from the mesenteric border. A noncrushing vascular-type clamp is applied to the ileal side and a straight Kocher clamp to the cecal side in preparation for the division of the intestine (FIGURE 10). Most commonly, however, the ileum is divided with a cutting linear stapler stapling instrument. The contents of the Kocher clamp can be ligated with heavy silk or absorbable suture to facilitate handling of the right colon (FIGURE 11).

The colon is then retracted medially, and the mesentery is divided up to the region of the middle colic vessel (FIGURE 12). Two half-length clamps should be applied proximally on the middle colic vessels because of their size and the increased vascularity in ulcerative colitis. The mesentery of the transverse colon is divided rather easily between pairs of clamps and the contents carefully ligated. This can be done at some distance from the inferior surface of the pancreas. As additional portions of colon are freed, they are incorporated in towels to avoid tearing the bowel wall and possible gross contamination. CONTINUES

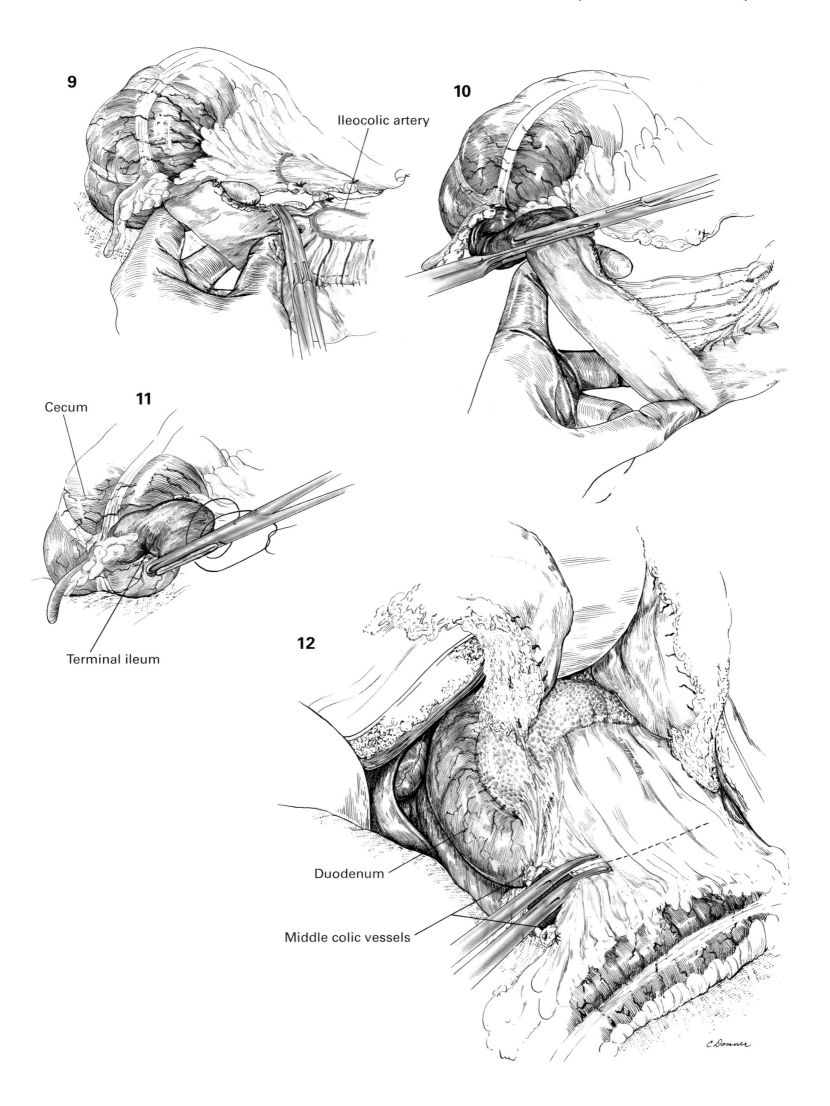

9

Ileocolic artery

10

11

Cecum

Terminal ileum

12

Duodenum

Middle colic vessels

C Donner

INCISION AND EXPOSURE ‹CONTINUED› An incision is made down the left lumbar gutter, and because the thickened and vascular peritoneum has a tendency to contract, all bleeding points should be carefully ligated (FIGURE 13). The peritoneum is lifted up until the left gonadal vessels and ureter are identified. Both should be identified throughout most of their course down over the brim of the pelvis (FIGURE 14).

In total abdominal colectomy, without planned proctectomy, the rectosigmoid junction should now be divided. The remaining vasculature to the colon can be divided close to the bowel. The superior hemorrhoidal vessels and presacral space should not be violated. When a second procedure (either ileorectal anastomosis or proctectomy and ileoanal pouch reconstruction) is contemplated, these planes should be left as virgin territory to facilitate that subsequent procedure.

TOTAL PROCTOCOLECTOMY The remaining description applies to the completion of a single-stage total proctocolectomy. As shown in FIGURE 15, the mesentery is divided adjacent to the rectosigmoid rather than up over the iliac artery bifurcation, as would be done in carcinoma. The peritoneum adjacent to the bowel is divided after identification of the ureters on either side, and the peritoneum in the pouch of Douglas between the rectum and bladder or cervix is incised. This flap is carefully elevated. This dissection along with that into the presacral space is facilitated by using lighted deep pelvic retractors, a focused headlight on the surgeon, and an extra-long insulated electrocautery tip. The dissection proceeds into the same presacral space as the mesorectal dissection, but the surgeon can stay closer to the rectum laterally and anteriorly, as this operation does not require the wide margins necessary for a malignancy. At this point, the rectum may be divided with a cutting linear stapler or endoscopic reticulating stapler or it may be transected between clamps (FIGURE 16). The distal stump is then oversewn (FIGURE 17). At this time, sharp dissection about the rectum should be carried out to free it as low as possible in order to lessen the blood loss during the subsequent perineal excision.

In the presence of multiple polyposis, a segment of rectum can be retained 5 to 8 cm above the pouch of Douglas or at a distance that can be easily reached by the sigmoidoscope for subsequent fulguration of the multiple polyps. When this is done, the terminal ileum is anastomosed to the rectal pouch in a side-to-end manner.

Absorbable sutures are used to close the peritoneal floor. The location of the ureters should be ascertained from time to time to avoid injury during the reconstruction of the pelvic floor. As in abdominoperineal resection, a pedicled omental flap can often be constructed to fill the pelvis after excision of the rectum. CONTINUES›

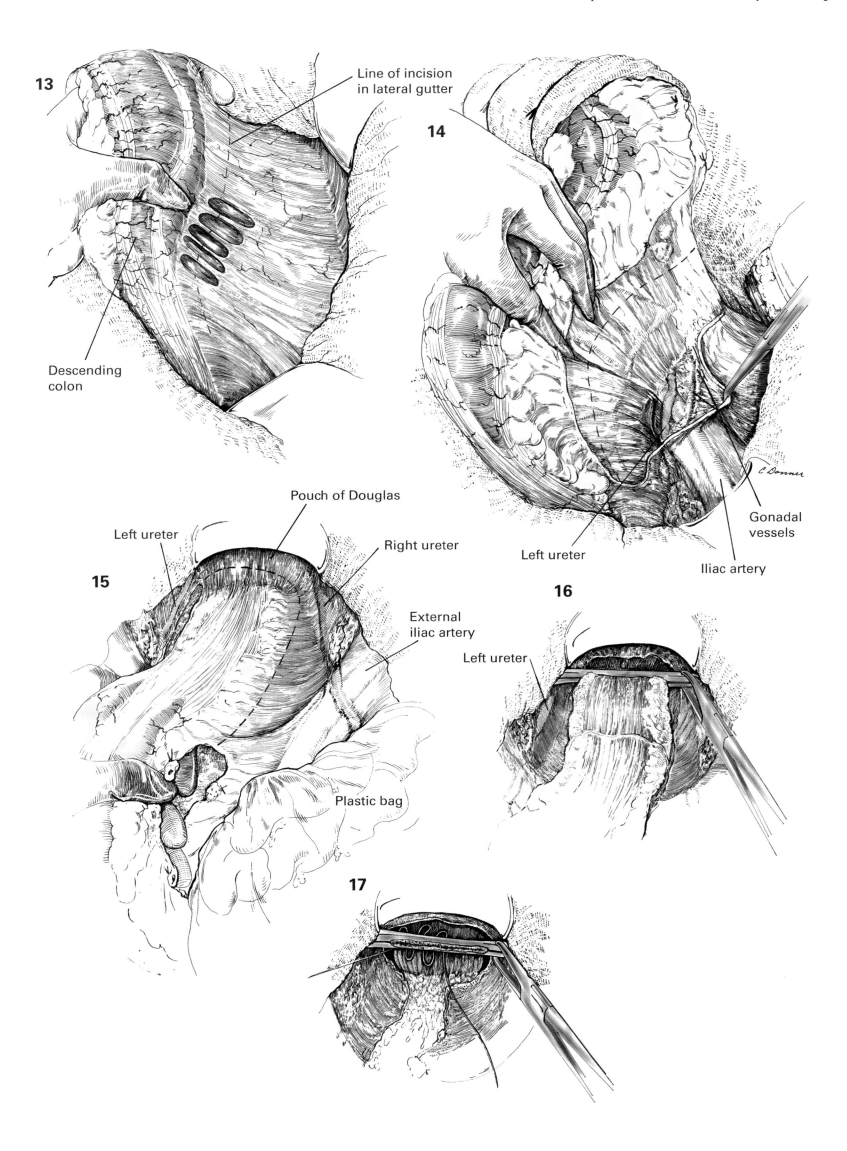

13

Line of incision in lateral gutter

Descending colon

14

Left ureter

Iliac artery

Gonadal vessels

15

Left ureter

Pouch of Douglas

Right ureter

External iliac artery

Plastic bag

16

Left ureter

17

TOTAL PROCTOCOLECTOMY `CONTINUED` After the pelvis has been reperitonealized, some of the raw surfaces in the left lumbar gutter also can be covered if the tissues are sufficiently lax (FIGURE 18). Again, the sutures should be placed so as to avoid injuring the underlying ureters and gonadal vessels. To complete the total proctocolectomy, the anus is excised as described in the perineal section of abdominoperineal resection (Chapter 59). The only exception is that it is not necessary to go wide on the levators when a simple extirpation of the sphincter muscles and bowel wall itself is carried out. The incision for the excision of the anus is shown in FIGURE 19. Primary closure with catheter suction can be used.

ILEOSTOMY The construction of the ileostomy is of major importance. The small intestine may be removed from the plastic bag and the site selected for ileostomy exposed. The location of the previously marked ileostomy site is evaluated. The midway point between the umbilicus and anterior iliac spine is again verified by a sterilized ruler. The ileostomy site is placed a little below the midway point (FIGURE 1, Chapter 60). With Kocher clamps applied to the fascial edge of the incision after removal of the self-retaining retractor, a 3-cm circle of skin is excised. After the button of skin and the underlying fat have been removed, all bleeding points are controlled. Then, while applying traction against the abdominal wall from underneath with the left hand, the surgeon makes a stellate incision through the entire thickness of the abdominal wall. Any bleeding that is encountered, especially in the rectus muscle, is clamped and ligated. An opening large enough to admit two fingers easily is usually more than sufficient.

Noncrushing vascular-type forceps are inserted through the ileostomy site and applied just proximal to the similar forceps on the terminal ileum (FIGURE 20). The original forceps are removed, and the ileum is withdrawn through the abdominal wall with the mesentery cephalad. At least 5 to 6 cm of mesentery-free ileum should be above the skin level so that an ileostomy of adequate length can be constructed. It may be necessary, especially in the obese patient, to undercut the terminal ileum under the mesenteric blood supply to attain this essential length. The viability is then reevaluated after the ileum is pulled up through the abdominal wall. The mesentery can be anchored to the abdominal wall or brought up into the subcutaneous tissue (FIGURE 21). It may be advisable to anchor the mesentery of the ileum to the parietes laterally before constructing the ileostomy because of the possibility of interfering with the blood supply to the terminal ileum. The right lumbar gutter should be closed off to avoid the potential of a postoperative internal hernia. At times it may be difficult to approximate the mesentery of the right colon and ileum to the right lumbar gutter and effect a closure (FIGURES 21 and 22). The surgeon should palpate the right gutter repeatedly and place whatever sutures are necessary to close it completely or else leave it completely open. The completed ileostomy should extend upward from the skin level at least 2.5 to 3 cm. The mucosa is anchored with interrupted fine synthetic absorbable sutures to the serosal edge of the bowel at the level of the skin and then to skin (FIGURE 22). Likewise, the mesentery may be anchored to the peritoneum, but no sutures should be taken between the seromuscular coat of the terminal ileum and the peritoneum. When the terminal ileum is divided with a cutting linear stapler, the maturation of the stoma is delayed until after closure of the abdominal wounds, the staple line is excised, and the stoma matured as described.

CLOSURE A double-looped (o or no. 1) delayed absorbable suture is used for running closure of the midline linea alba incision. In very large patients, two sutures are used that begin at either end of the incision. Interrupted fine absorbable sutures may be placed in Scarpa's fascia. The skin is closed with staples, although some prefer to use absorbable subcutaneous sutures followed by adhesive skin strips. At the end of the case, a dry sterile dressing covers the abdominal incision and an ostomy appliance is put about the ileostomy. In the presence of marked emaciation and prolonged steroid therapy, the use of retention sutures should be considered.

POSTOPERATIVE CARE Blood should be replaced as it is lost during the procedure. Additional blood or colloids may be required on the afternoon of surgery and during the early postoperative period. Constant bladder drainage is traditionally maintained for at least 4 or 5 days. Some surgeons now remove the catheter on the first postoperative day. If the patient has been on steroid therapy, this is continued during the postoperative period. A transparent temporary-type ileostomy appliance is placed over the ileostomy before moving the patient to the recovery area. This permits frequent observations of the stoma to make sure it maintains a pink and viable color. A strict intake and output chart must be maintained at all times following an ileostomy. Likewise, daily electrolyte determinations are essential because of excessive losses of electrolyte-rich fluid. Excessive amounts of fluid are occasionally lost, and large amounts of intravenous fluids, electrolytes, and colloids will be required to maintain fluid balance. The nasogastric tube is removed early and oral intake of liquids advanced as tolerated. The drains should then be removed, with serial observations as described in the discussion of abdominoperineal resection (Chapter 59). These patients require frequent and prolonged observation because of the tendency to a variety of complications ranging from abscess formation to intestinal obstruction. They should be in contact with an enterostomal therapist, who ideally may be available during office visits to the surgeon. ∎

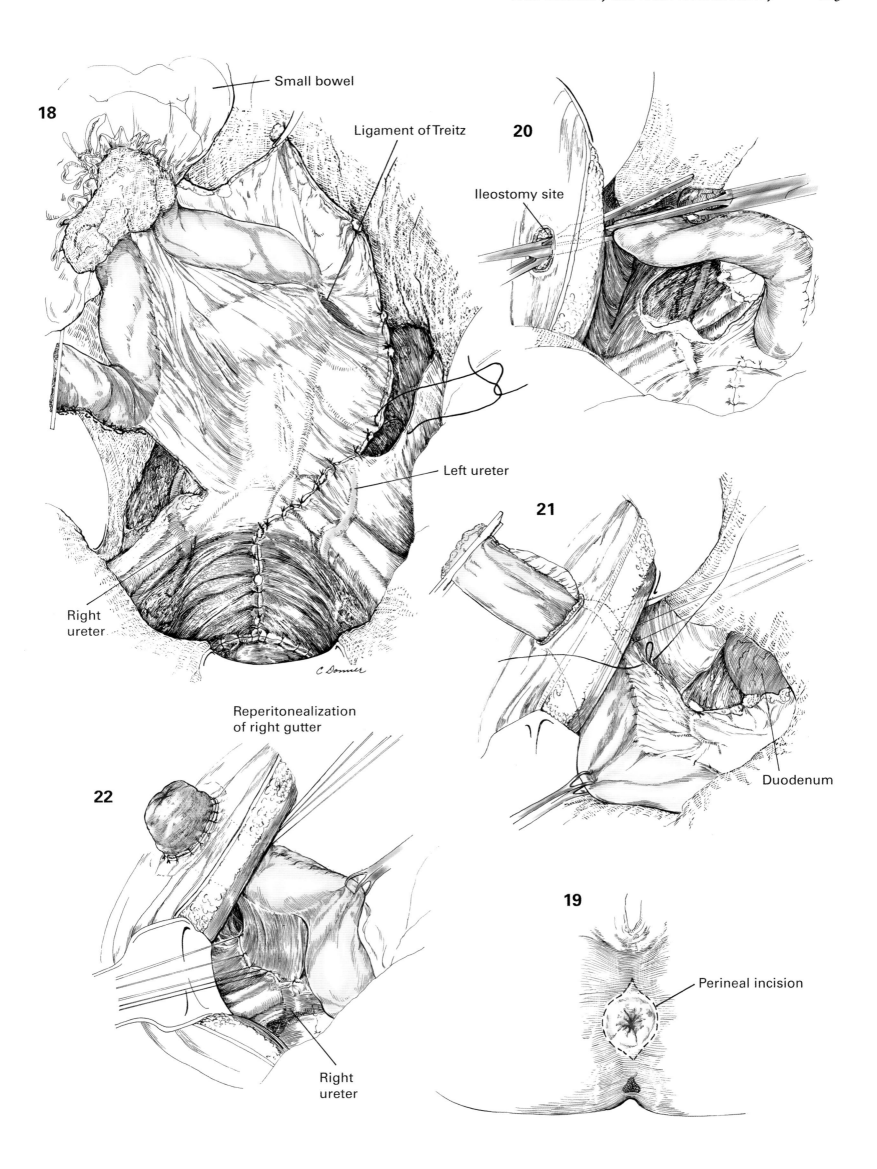

18

Small bowel

Ligament of Treitz

Left ureter

Right ureter

C. Donner

20

Ileostomy site

21

Duodenum

Reperitonealization of right gutter

22

Right ureter

19

Perineal incision

ANTERIOR RESECTION OF RECTOSIGMOID: END-TO-END ANASTOMOSIS

INDICATIONS This may be the operation of choice in selected individuals with malignant lesions in the rectosigmoid or low sigmoid area in order to re-establish the continuity of the bowel. The operation is based on the premises (**1**) that the viability of the lower rectum can be sustained from the middle or inferior hemorrhoidal vessels and (**2**) that carcinoma in this region as a rule metastasizes cephalad, only rarely metastasizing 3 to 4 cm below the primary growth. It is questionable whether an anterior resection should be advised for growths occurring within 8 cm of the pectinate line. While most patients prefer restored continuity over a permanent colostomy, there is a significant risk of postoperative bowel dysfunction (post low-anterior syndrome) that is highest in patients with preoperative dysfunction such as incontinence. The absolute indications for abdominoperineal resection are discussed in Chapter 59. The ideal situation would appear to be a small tumor located at the junction of the rectum and the sigmoid. However, there are many times when the growth can be mobilized much more than anticipated, especially when the bowel is released down to the levator muscles. The exposure is another factor that may influence the surgeon for or against a low anastomosis. A low anastomosis is much easier and safer in the female than in the male, especially if the pelvic organs of the former have been removed previously. A loop ileostomy (Chapter 51) is sometimes done at the time to divert the fecal stream temporarily from the end-to-end anastomosis or to ensure decompression of an inadequately emptied colon. A side-to-side (Baker) anastomosis should be considered when there is considerable discrepancy between the sizes of the two lumina or an excess of fat that may encroach unduly upon the lumen of an end-to-end anastomosis. Most prefer a stapling device for the anastomosis (Chapter 62).

PREOPERATIVE CARE See Chapter 62.

ANESTHESIA See Chapter 62.

POSITION The patient is placed in the Trendelenburg position. The opposite position is useful while the splenic flexure is being mobilized.

OPERATIVE PREPARATION The skin is prepared in the usual manner. A Foley catheter is inserted into the bladder.

INCISION AND EXPOSURE A midline incision is made from the symphysis to a level above and to the left of the umbilicus. The liver and the upper abdomen are carefully palpated to determine the existence of any metastases. The site of the tumor is examined with special consideration as to its size and location, the amount of dilation of the bowel proximal to the growth, and the ease of exposure. In many instances the type of resection cannot be determined until the lower segment of the bowel has been mobilized.

DETAILS OF PROCEDURE The small intestines are walled off and a self-retaining retractor is inserted into the wound. The peritoneum of the pelvic colon is freed from the region of the sigmoid downward on either side (FIGURE 3). It is important at this point to identify and isolate both ureters and the spermatic or ovarian vessels. The peritoneum is divided anterior to the rectum at the level of the base of the bladder or cervix. The growth can be further mobilized by mesorectal dissection (Chapter 59, FIGURE 8). After the peritoneal attachments have all been divided, and the rectum is freed both posteriorly and anteriorly, it is possible to bring this growth up into the wound and gain considerable distance as a result of freeing and straightening the rectum (FIGURES 1 and 2). The blood supply to the distal segment from the inferior hemorrhoidal vessels is adequate, should the middle hemorrhoidal vessels be ligated to ensure additional mobilization. The inferior mesenteric artery is ligated at the level of the superior hemorrhoidal vessels or as it arises from the aorta (FIGURE 3) and the inferior mesenteric vein is divided. This provides maximum lymphatic lymph node removal and gives additional mobility to the descending colon. The blood supply to the colon must now come from the middle colic artery through the marginal vessels of Drummond (FIGURE 3).

The bowel should be prepared for division at least 5 cm below the gross lower limits of the growth to assure removal of all adjacent lymph nodes. A Stone or a Pace-Potts anastomosis clamp is applied across the previously prepared site of division of the bowel, and a long, right-angle clamp may be

utilized for the proximal clamp (FIGURE 4). The bowel is divided between the clamps. The bowel containing the growth is then brought outside the wound, and clamps are applied to the previously prepared site well above the lesion (FIGURE 5). The surgeon must now determine that the upper segment of the bowel is sufficiently mobile to be brought down for anastomosis without tension. In order to accomplish this, it may be necessary to divide the lateral peritoneal attachment of the left colon up to and including the splenic flexure. Unless the sigmoid is very redundant, the left half of the transverse colon along with the splenic flexure must be mobilized. The midline incision is extended at this point to ensure a good exposure, since undue traction on the colon may tear the capsule of the spleen. The splenic flexure is also mobilized, as in Chapter 57. The lesser sac is entered after the splenic attachments to the colon have been divided. The greater omentum is freed from the transverse colon as shown in Chapter 27, FIGURE 1. Extra mobility and length of bowel are provided until repeated trials clearly demonstrate that the proximal segment will easily reach the site of anastomosis. The adequacy of the blood supply should be determined even when the bowel is extended down into the pelvis preliminary to the anastomosis.

The serosa along the mesenteric border of the upper segment should be cleared of fat for at least 1 cm proximal to the Pace-Potts clamps (FIGURE 5). Likewise, the margins and especially the posterior wall of the lower segment must be cleared of fat adjacent to the Pace-Potts clamp (FIGURE 5). Careful dissection with repeated application of small clamps may be necessary to accomplish a clean serosal boundary of 1 cm adjacent to the clamp in preparation for a safe anastomosis. Following this, the two ends of the clamps are approximated and then manipulated so that a posterior serosal layer of 000 silk can be placed easily (FIGURE 6). The ends of these sutures are cut, except those at either angle, which are retained for traction. As a preliminary to removing the clamp, the field is walled off with gauze, and an enterostomy clamp is gently applied to the upper segment to prevent gross soiling (FIGURE 6). The crushed contents of the clamps may be excised. The lower clamp is then removed, and the crushed margin of bowel is excised and opened (FIGURE 7). Suction is instituted to avoid any gross contamination of the field. Fine silk sutures may be inserted for traction in the midportion of the lower opening and at either angle. These traction sutures tend to facilitate the anastomosis (see Chapter 63, FIGURES 16 and 17). The posterior mucosal layer is approximated with several Babcock forceps, and the mucosa is approximated with interrupted 000 silk sutures. The anterior mucosal surface is closed with interrupted 000 silk sutures of the Connell type, with the knot on the outside. The mucosa may be closed with a continuous 000 synthetic absorbable suture (FIGURE 8) rather than interrupted silk sutures. Following this, the anterior serosal layer is carefully placed, using interrupted Halsted sutures of fine 000 silk (FIGURE 9). The peritoneum is anchored adjacent to the suture line. The patency of the anastomosis, as well as the lack of tension on the suture line, should be tested. The peritoneal floor is closed with interrupted absorbable sutures (FIGURE 10). The raw surfaces are covered by approximating the mesenteric margin of the sigmoid to the right peritoneal margin (FIGURE 10). The sigmoid is loosely attached to the left pelvic wall by anchoring the fat pads, not bowel wall, to the left peritoneal margin to prevent subsequent tension on the anastomosis as well as to cover the raw surfaces. A transverse colostomy or diverting loop ileostomy (Chapter 51) should be considered if there is any suspicion regarding the technical perfection of the anastomosis. A drain may be inserted into the left side of the pelvis and brought out at the lower angle of the wound. Some operators prefer to have a rectal tube in place, which can be guided up beyond the anastomosis to assist in decompressing the bowel during the early postoperative period. The rectal tube is anchored in position by a silk suture placed at the anal margin. Some prefer to use a surgical stapling instrument for the anastomosis. See Chapter 62.

CLOSURE Closure is performed in a routine manner.

POSTOPERATIVE CARE The rectal tube is left in place for a few days and enemas should be avoided. The patient is gradually allowed to resume a full diet. Mineral oil may be given. If a proximal diverting loop ileostomy is used, the patency of the anastomosis should be tested by contrast fluoroscopy before closure is affected several weeks after surgery. See postoperative care, Chapter 62, for general postoperative care. ■

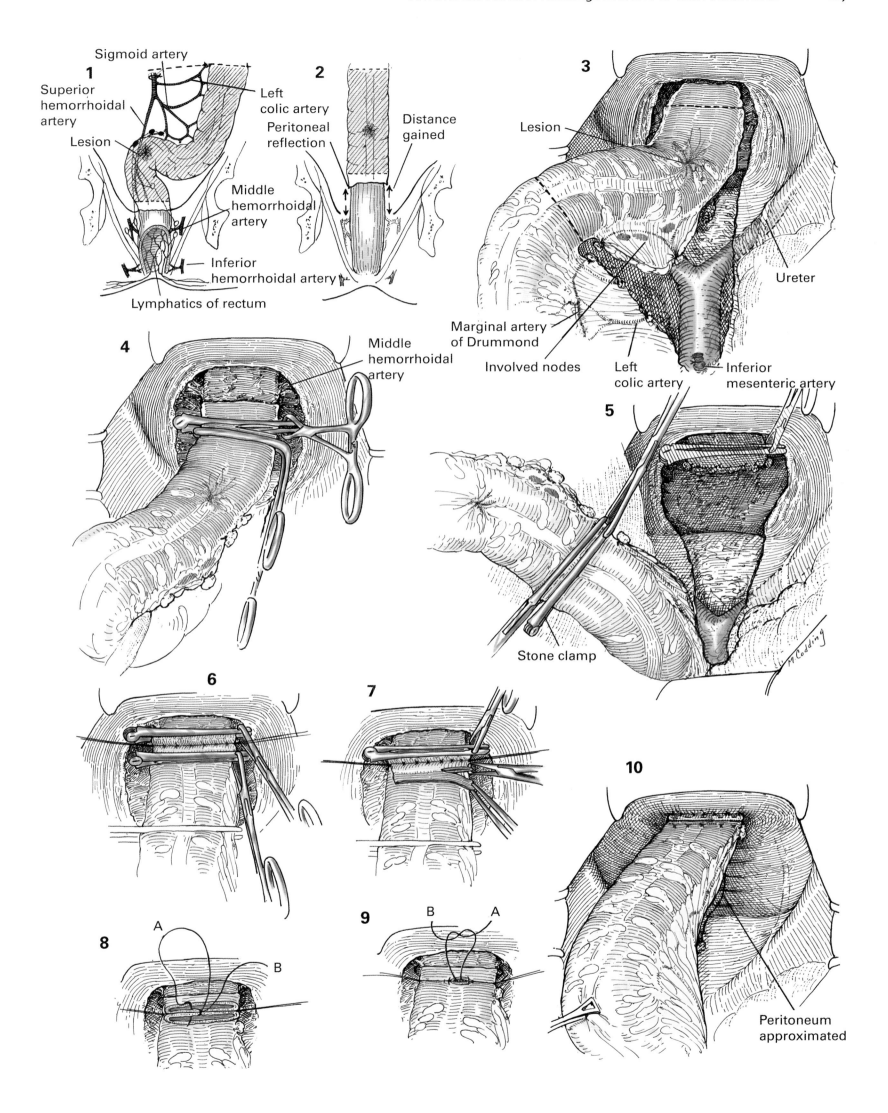

1
Sigmoid artery
Superior hemorrhoidal artery
Left colic artery
Peritoneal reflection
Lesion
Middle hemorrhoidal artery
Inferior hemorrhoidal artery
Lymphatics of rectum

2
Distance gained

3
Lesion
Ureter
Marginal artery of Drummond
Involved nodes
Left colic artery
Inferior mesenteric artery

4
Middle hemorrhoidal artery

5
Stone clamp

6

7

8
A
B

9
B   A

10
Peritoneum approximated

ANTERIOR RESECTION, STAPLED

INDICATIONS The stapler offers certain advantages in the performance of a low anterior resection, provided the surgeon is thoroughly familiar with the technique. Those favoring this method of approximating the sigmoid to a short rectal stump emphasize the ease of the anastomosis, especially in the narrow pelvis of the male. The time required for the operation may be shortened and the indications for a temporary proximal diverting loop ostomy decreased. Use of the stapler does not alter the principles of adequate resection of tumors at approximately 8 cm or less from the anus. This is because anastomoses lower than 3 cm from the anus may be associated with incontinence and because a distal margin of 2 to 3 cm below the cancer is recommended to minimize the rate of local anastomotic recurrence. The success of a properly performed anastomosis depends on an adequate blood supply to the residual bowel segments, which can be brought together easily without tension. Cancers below the peritoneal reflection in the pouch of Douglas should be evaluated with endorectal ultrasound for their staging and spread. Preoperative radiation therapy and chemotherapy should be considered for these lesions.

PREOPERATIVE PREPARATION An empty colon results from 1 day of liquid diet. The usual bowel preparation is given the day prior to surgery, while parenteral antibiotics are administered just prior to the start of the procedure. Since the stapler is to be introduced through the anus, it is mandatory that the lower colon and rectum be carefully emptied and cleansed just before the procedure is started. A large mushroom catheter is commonly introduced into the rectum for a saline irrigation until clear. Several ounces of a mild antiseptic solution such as 10% povidone-iodine can be instilled at the time the procedure is started. An inlying bladder catheter is essential for good exposure.

ANESTHESIA General endotracheal anesthesia is satisfactory.

POSITION The patient is placed in a semi lithotomy position using Allen stirrups and in a modest Trendelenburg position to enhance exposure of the deep pelvis and permit the introduction of the stapling instrument via the anus.

OPERATIVE PREPARATION Not only the abdominal wall from the xiphoid to the pubis, but the skin over the perineum, groin, and especially the anal region are prepared since the instrument will be introduced through the anus.

INCISION AND EXPOSURE A long midline incision is made starting just above the symphysis and extending to the umbilicus and around it on the left side to provide easy access to the splenic flexure (FIGURE 1). The liver is palpated for possible metastasis, and the location and mobility of the growth as well as the presence or absence of metastatic lymph nodes are verified by palpation. The small intestine may be placed in a plastic Lahey bag to which some saline solution is added. The mobility of the transverse and descending colon is evaluated with special reference to the adequate exposure of the splenic flexure. Undue traction on the omentum or colon in the region of the spleen may result in troublesome bleeding from a tear in the splenic capsule, hence many surgeons routinely mobilize the splenic flexure.

DETAILS OF PROCEDURE The indications for an anterior resection are reconfirmed, and the sigmoid and transverse colon are mobilized using the same incision and exposure techniques as in Chapter 61 (FIGURES 2 and 3). A high ligation of the inferior mesenteric lymphovascular pedicle is carried out following exposure and clear identification of the left gonadal vein and ureter. The sigmoid artery is ligated near the inferior mesenteric artery with preservation of the arcade between the ascending and descending branches of the left colic artery. The mesentery of the left colon is divided over to the junction of the sigmoid and descending colon (FIGURE 2).

Two methods of stapled closure are presented.

METHOD 1—RECTAL STAPLING A point on the sigmoid is selected for division, and the mesenteric border is meticulously cleared for a distance of approximately 2 cm (FIGURE 3). Active pulsations must be present in the mesentery, and the cleared area must be free of diverticuli. A total meso-rectal excision (Chapter 59) is carried out to at least 2 cm, preferably 5 cm, below the tumor. A linear stapler is fired across the rectum at that level (FIGURE 4) and the mesorectum is divided. Some staplers close both sides while cutting between the staple lines, while others fire only one line of staples and hence require a clamp on the proximal ("specimen") side. The rectosigmoid specimen is then lifted out of the pelvis. CONTINUES ▶

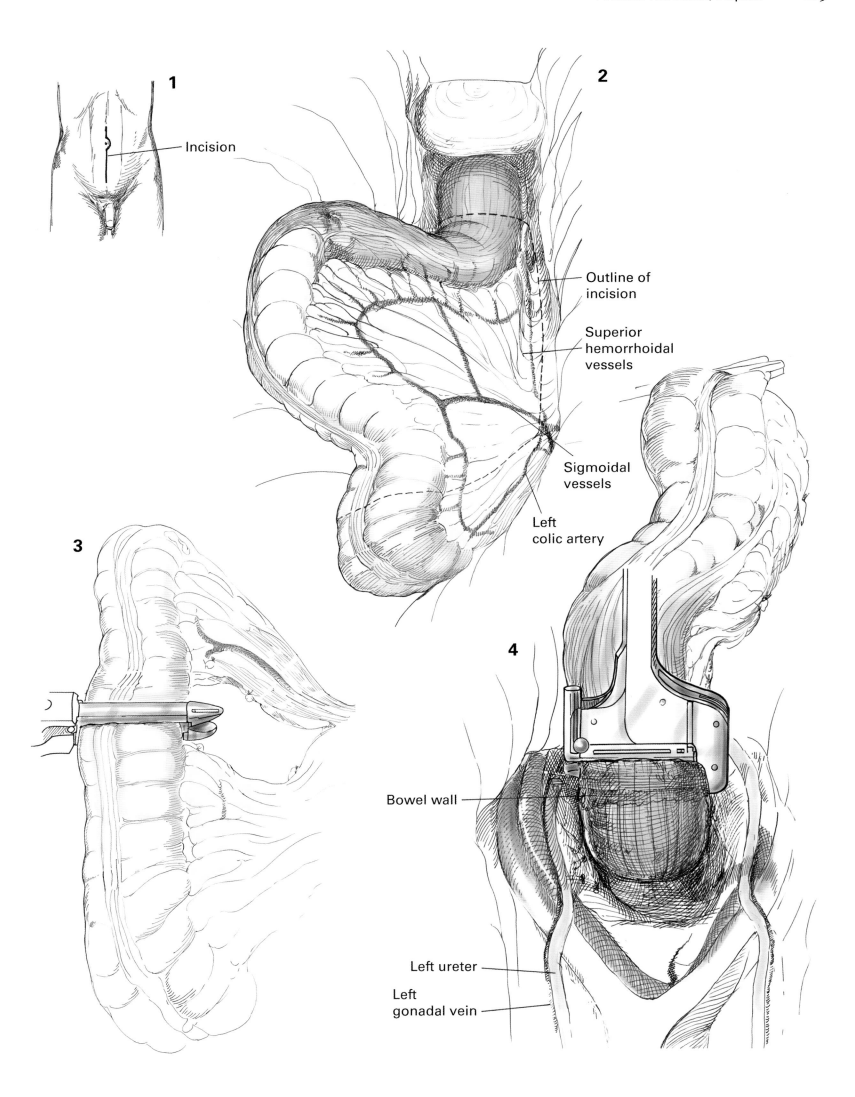

1

Incision

2

Outline of incision

Superior hemorrhoidal vessels

Sigmoidal vessels

Left colic artery

3

4

Bowel wall

Left ureter

Left gonadal vein

METHOD 1—RECTAL STAPLING ◄CONTINUED► The end of the sigmoid is then opened. If there is doubt as to the size of stapler needed, retraction stay sutures are placed and circular stapler sizers can be passed into the sigmoid to determine the largest size that fits easily (FIGURE 5). A circumferential purse string of oo polypropylene suture is placed (FIGURE 6). The open end of the sigmoid is gently manipulated over the end of the anvil, and the suture is securely tied (FIGURE 7). The assistant gently dilates the anus and inserts the curved stapler of appropriate diameter (FIGURE 8). The surgeon assists from above in the passage of the instrument as the spike advances through the rectum, usually just posterior to the stapled stump so as to avoid overlap with this staple line (FIGURE 9). Alternatively the spike may be advanced just anterior or posterior to the rectal staple line. In this case the staple line will be included in the donut.

The adequacy of the previously placed purse-string suture is carefully determined. The completeness of the mucosal closure is rechecked to be certain there is no gap between the shafts of the purse-string closure. Bulky puckering of excess tissue must be avoided, lest failure to compress the tissues adequately will lead to failure of the anastomosis. As the assistant closes the instrument from below (FIGURE 8), the surgeon from above, prevents fatty tissues or the posterior wall of the vagina from being trapped between the bowel ends. The assistant verifies that the stapler is tightened to the correct thickness for the height of its staples as shown by a color-bar indicator in the handle of the stapler. The trigger is released and the handles squeezed to fire and create the anastomosis.

After firing the stapler, the manufacturer's routine for releasing the instrument is followed carefully to avoid the possibility of disrupting the line of staples during its removal (FIGURE 10). Additional interrupted sutures may be placed around the anastomosis, and all raw surfaces in the pelvis are reperitonealized where possible.

Before closure of the abdomen, the "doughnuts" created by the instrument must be carefully inspected for 360-degree continuity (FIGURE 11). A gap indicates a possible leak which will require additional external interrupted sutures. The integrity of the anastomosis is confirmed by filling the pelvis with sterile saline, and air is injected through a catheter or proctoscope in the rectum. The appearance of air bubbles identifies the presence of a leak that must be repaired by interrupted sutures. If there is any doubt concerning the security of the final anastomosis, a temporary proximal diverting loop ileostomy (Chapter 51) should be considered.

Most surgeons prefer temporary drainage of the presacral space with closed suction silastic drains. The drains are left in place for a few days until the fluid becomes more serous and smaller in volume. If large volumes of rather clear fluid are noted, then a urea or creatinine content should be checked and the bladder and ureters evaluated.

METHOD 2—RECTAL PURSE-STRING A point on the sigmoid is selected for division, and the mesenteric border is meticulously cleared for a distance of approximately 2 cm. Active pulsations must be present in the mesentery. The cleared area must be free of diverticuli. The purse-string clamp is applied obliquely to the bowel so as to preserve the 2-cm cleared bowel proximally. This is necessary as the 2-cm zone will be enclosed within the stapler anvil and will become the upper "doughnut." If the wall is not carefully cleaned of fat, or if too thick, a turn-in is created with a purse-string suture that is placed freehand, the entire circumference of the bowel may not be brought inside the instrument. This will result in an incompetent anastomosis and leak. Accordingly the placement of the purse-string sutures and the examination of the upper and lower "doughnut" rings for intact purse-string sutures with 360 degrees of full-thickness bowel wall turn-in are most important steps with these instruments. A oo polypropylene suture on a long, straight Keith needle is passed through the special openings in the purse-string clamp, and a purse-string suture results. A straight Kocher clamp is applied on the colon distal to the purse-string clamp and the bowel is divided in between. The rectosigmoid is retracted forward toward the symphysis as the peritoneum is incised and the rectal segment mobilized from the presacral space using mesorectal dissection (Chapter 59). The posterior rectal wall is cleared of fat until at least 2 cm of only the bowel wall is exposed approximately 5 cm or more distal to the tumor. In the male and very obese patient, it is difficult to properly place the purse-string clamp and even more difficult to insert the Keith needle to complete the purse-string anastomosis. Under such circumstances, a noncrushing vascular clamp is placed across the area cleared for the anastomosis similar to that shown in FIGURES 4 and 5 on Chapter 61. A Kocher clamp secures the proximal specimen and the bowel is divided. The end of the sigmoid should be brought down to the divided end of the rectum to verify once again the adequacy of mobilization in order to avoid any chance of tension on the suture line of staples. Additional mobility may be gained by ligating and dividing the inferior mesenteric vein just below the inferior margin of the pancreas. The decision now must be made whether to perform an open sutures anastomosis as shown in FIGURES 8 and 9 on Chapter 61 or to use the transrectal circular stapler after placing the rectal stump purse-string suture by hand in a very low anastomosis. In these cases some surgeons prefer to place the purse-string suture in the very short rectal stump from below using an anal speculum. More frequently, it is technically easier to maintain compression of the rectal wall with a right angle vascular clamp while a purse-string suture is placed in the protruding mucosa. Absorbable traction sutures can be placed to serve as stay sutures, while the purse-string suture of oo polypropylene sutures includes both in the muscular and mucosal layers. Also this suture must be placed close to the cut edge so as to ensure a snug approximation of the entire bowel wall about the stapling instrument when it is tied. Circular stapler sizing instruments are passed into the open proximal bowel lumen and into the rectum to define the largest-diameter stapler possible. The assistant gently dilates the anus and inserts the circular stapler from below. The remainder of the procedure is same as described in METHOD 1.

CLOSURE Routine procedures are followed.

POSTOPERATIVE CARE Some postoperative rectal bleeding may occur but usually stops spontaneously. The diet is slowly resumed after the patient passes flatus. Some prefer to insert a catheter in the anus beyond the anastomosis for the venting of gas and anchor the catheter with a silk suture to the perianal skin. The Foley catheter is removed after 5 days with careful observation of the volume and patterns of voiding, or earlier, depending on institutional protocol. The patients may complain of increased frequency and urgency that may persist for several months. A tight anastomosis may require eventual gentle dilations. ■

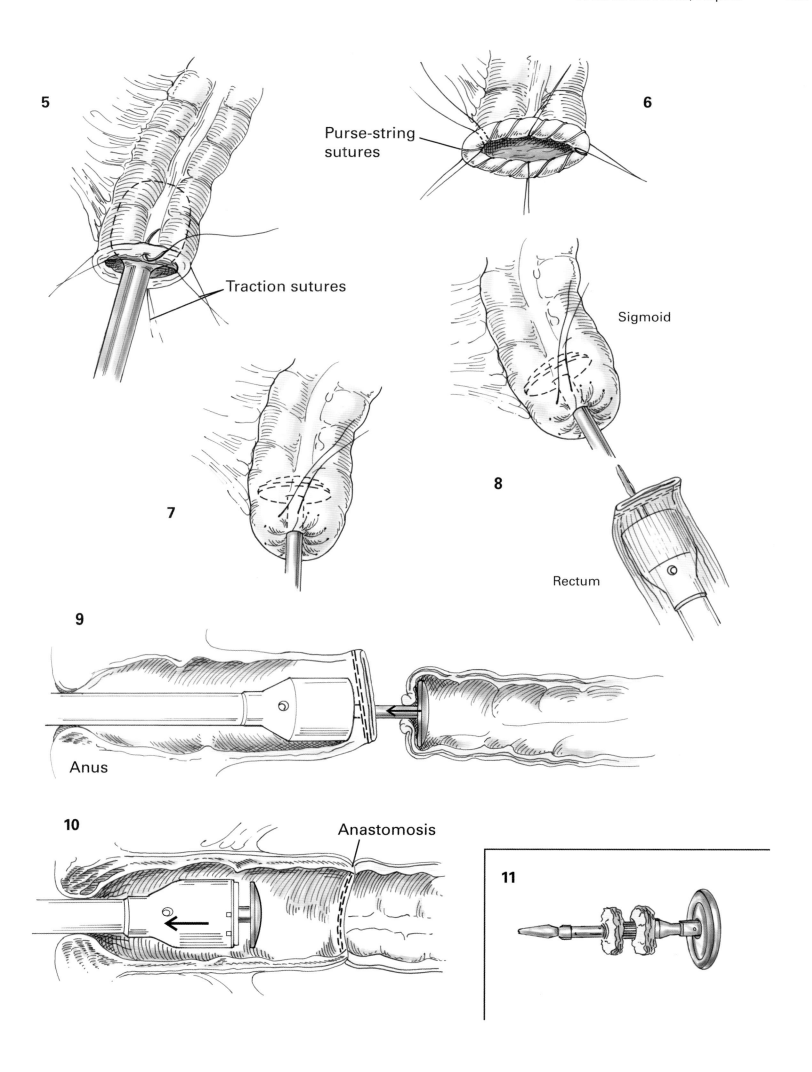

5

6 Purse-string sutures

Traction sutures

7

8 Sigmoid

Rectum

9 Anus

10 Anastomosis

11

CHAPTER 63

ANTERIOR RESECTION OF RECTOSIGMOID: SIDE-TO-END ANASTOMOSIS (BAKER)

INDICATIONS The low-lying lesions of the rectum and rectosigmoid may be resected and bowel continuity established anterior to the sacrum in a variety of ways. Although the end-to-end anastomosis (Chapter 61) can be used, side-to-end anastomosis is advantageous in cases with considerable discrepancy in size between the resected bowel and the rectal stump, particularly in obese patients. When the lesion is so low that abdominoperineal resection, with sacrifice of the rectum, ordinarily would be indicated, and in the presence of distant metastases, or when the patient refuses to give permission for a permanent colostomy, bowel continuity can be established by a very low side-to-end anastomosis. This approach may occasionally be needed in colostomy (Hartmann's) closure, and a similar ileorectal anastomosis can be used in closing an ileostomy (e.g., after total colectomy for pseudomembranous colitis).

The principles of cancer surgery should be observed, including en bloc excision of the lymphatic drainage area and early ligation of the inferior mesenteric vessels near the point of origin (FIGURES 1 and 2). The blood supply to the sigmoid will be sustained through the marginal artery of Drummond via the middle colic artery arising from the superior mesenteric artery. At least 2 cm and preferably 5 cm of the bowel should be resected below the malignant tumor to assure removal of all adjacent lymph nodes. The continuity can be reestablished after the descending colon, the splenic flexure, and the left portion of the transverse colon are mobilized (FIGURE 3).

The entire right colon can be freed from its lateral peritoneal attachments and rotated to its embryologic position on the left side of the abdomen, if more mobility is desired.

The advantages of the side-to-end anastomosis include assurance of a larger and more secure anastomosis than may be possible by the end-to-end method.

PREOPERATIVE PREPARATION After the lesion has been proved to be malignant by microscopic examination, and polyps or secondary lesions ruled out by appropriate colonoscopic and barium studies of the colon, the patient is shifted to a clear liquid diet for a day or so before surgery. A preliminary computed tomography scan with IV contrast may reveal distant spread and locate the courses of the ureters. For cancers below the peritoneal reflection, an endorectal ultrasound study will aid in the staging of the extent of disease. Appropriate tumors should be evaluated for radiation therapy and chemotherapy prior to operation. The rectum is irrigated with saline or a povidone-iodine solution. The tube is left in place for rectal decompression. An indwelling urethral catheter ensures a collapsed bladder, providing better exposure of deep pelvic structures. Systemic antibiotics are given.

ANESTHESIA General endotracheal anesthesia is satisfactory. Spinal anesthesia may be used.

POSITION The patient is placed near the left side of the table and so immobilized that the Trendelenburg position can be assumed during the final anastomosis without difficulty.

OPERATIVE PREPARATION The skin is prepared from the symphysis up to the epigastrium. If a stapled anastomosis is planned, Allen stirrups are used to create a modified lithotomy position allowing concurrent preparation and draping for later access to the rectum. The perineum and rectum are prepared and included in the draping if stapling is planned.

INCISION AND EXPOSURE A midline incision is made, starting just above the symphysis and extending down to the umbilicus and around it on the left side. The height to which the incision is carried in the epigastrium depends on the location of the splenic flexure. Because it will be necessary to detach the splenic flexure, easy exposure of this area must be provided. Undue tension of the left half of the colon and splenic flexure will tear the splenic capsule, causing blood loss and risking splenectomy.

After the abdomen is opened, a self-retaining retractor is inserted, and the liver is palpated for evidence of metastasis. Palpation should be carried out well over the top of both lobes of the liver as well as on the undersurface. Likewise, lymph nodes along the course of the inferior mesenteric artery and at the bifurcation of the aorta are inspected for evidence of involvement. The position and fixation of the tumor are ascertained by palpation. In the presence of metastasis to the liver or seeding throughout the general peritoneal cavity, a sleeve type of segmental resection is indicated. When a palliative resection is carried out, wide dissection of the inferior mesenteric blood supply up to the point of origin in the region of the ligament of Treitz is not necessary.

DETAILS OF PROCEDURE After it has been decided that the lesion is resectable, that an anterior resection is warranted, and that adequate bowel can be resected distal to the tumor, the small intestines are walled off and the transverse colon and splenic flexure are mobilized (FIGURE 4).

While the omentum is held upward, sharp dissection is used to divide the attachment of the omentum to the transverse colon. A few blood vessels may need to be ligated during this procedure. Opening into the lesser sac above the transverse colon ensures an easier and safer separation of the omentum from the splenic flexure of the colon, particularly in the obese patient. Again, great care must be exercised as the splenocolic ligament is divided in order to avoid tearing the splenic capsule. Clamps should be applied in this area so that the contents of the splenocolic ligament can be carefully divided and ligated (FIGURE 5). **CONTINUES** ▶

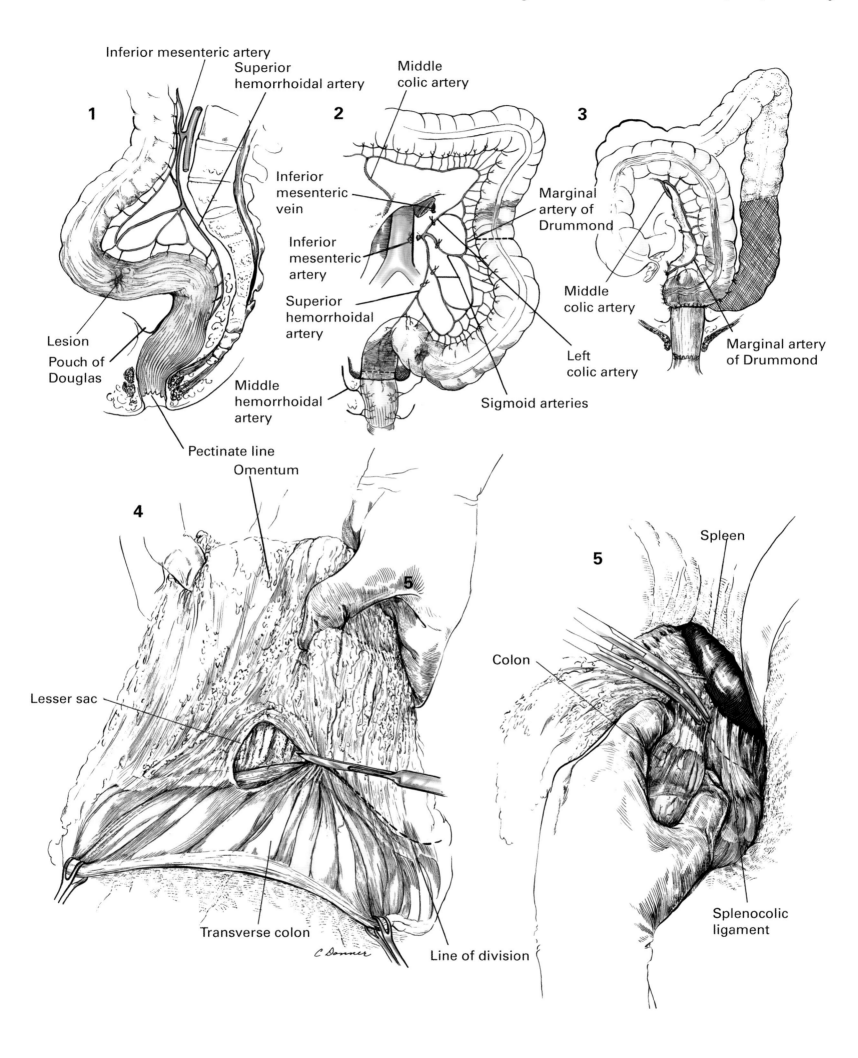

1

Inferior mesenteric artery
Superior hemorrhoidal artery
Lesion
Pouch of Douglas
Middle hemorrhoidal artery
Pectinate line

2

Middle colic artery
Inferior mesenteric vein
Inferior mesenteric artery
Superior hemorrhoidal artery
Sigmoid arteries
Left colic artery

3

Marginal artery of Drummond
Middle colic artery
Marginal artery of Drummond

4

Omentum
Lesser sac
Transverse colon
Line of division

5

Spleen
Colon
Splenocolic ligament

C Donner

DETAILS OF PROCEDURE ◀CONTINUED The peritoneum over the region of the left kidney is divided as gentle traction is maintained downward and medially on the splenic flexure of the colon. There is a tendency to grasp the colon and to encircle it completely with the fingers. This tends to puncture the thinned out mesentery. Rents can be avoided if a gauze pack is used to gently sweep the splenic flexure downward and medially (FIGURE 6). Usually, it is unnecessary to divide and ligate any vessels during this procedure. The peritoneum in the left lumbar gutter is divided, and the entire descending colon is swept medially.

The rectosigmoid is freed from the hollow of the sacrum as shown in Chapter 59. The sigmoid is first separated from any attachments to the iliac fossa on the left side, and the left gonadal vessels and the ureter are identified throughout their course in the field of operation (FIGURE 7). Often, especially in the female, a very low-lying lesion can be mobilized and lifted up well into the wound.

After the bowel has been freed from the hollow of the sacrum, the fingers of the left hand should separate the right ureter from the overlying peritoneum by blunt dissection (FIGURE 8). The peritoneum is incised some distance from the tumor, and the rectum is freed further down to the region of the levator muscles using the mesorectal dissection (Chapter 59). Division of the middle hemorrhoidal vessels with the suspensory ligaments may be necessary to ensure the needed length of bowel to be resected below the tumor. The surgeon should not hesitate to divide the peritoneal attachments in the region of the pouch of Douglas, to free the rectum from the prostate gland in the male and from the posterior wall of the vagina in the female. The inferior mesenteric artery is freed from the underlying aorta to near its point of origin (FIGURE 9). Three curved clamps are applied to the inferior mesenteric artery, and the vessel is divided and ligated with oo silk. The inferior mesenteric vein should be ligated at this time, before the tumor has been palpated and compressed due to the manipulation required during resection. CONTINUES▶

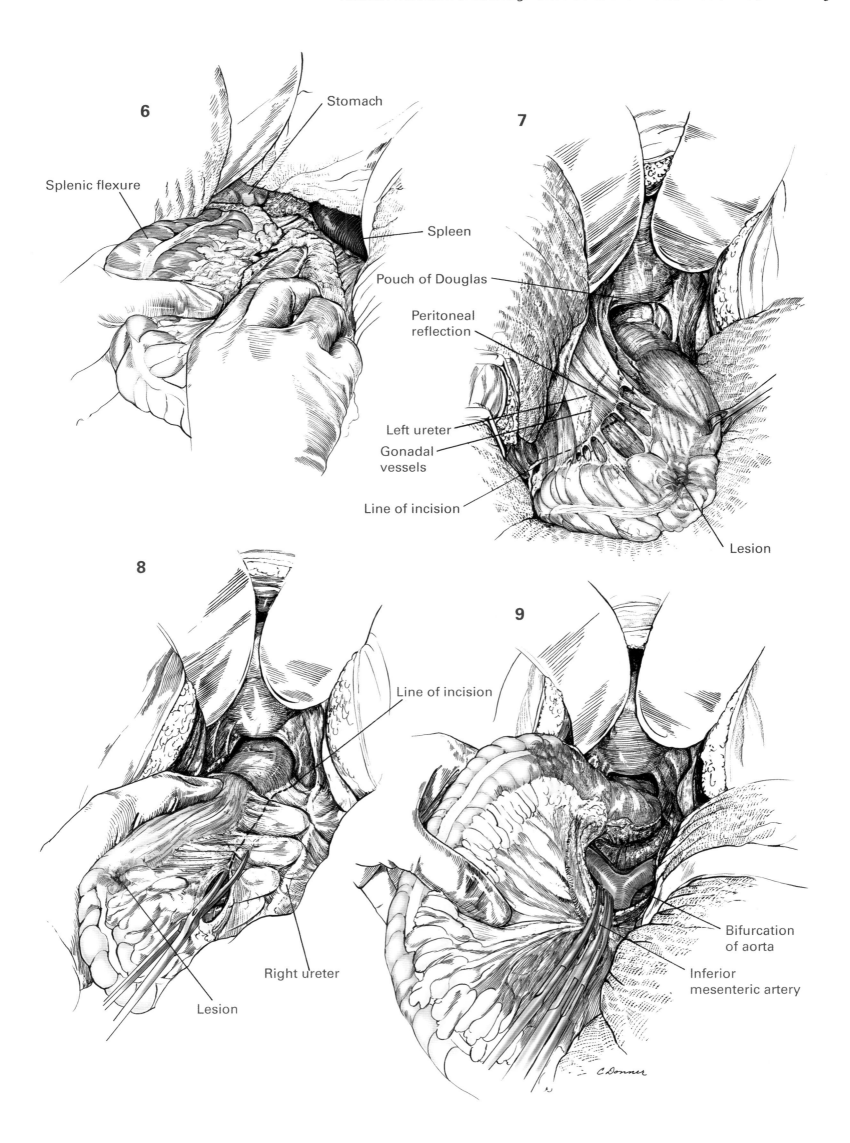

6

Stomach

Splenic flexure

Spleen

7

Pouch of Douglas

Peritoneal
reflection

Left ureter

Gonadal
vessels

Line of incision

Lesion

8

Line of incision

Right ureter

Lesion

9

Bifurcation
of aorta

Inferior
mesenteric artery

DETAILS OF PROCEDURE ◀CONTINUED After the mesenteric vessels have been ligated and the rectum has been mobilized adequately, a Pace-Potts noncrushing clamp is applied across the bowel at least 5 cm to 10 cm below the tumor (FIGURE 10A). The position of both ureters should once again be identified before the clamp is applied. A straight clamp is applied 1 cm proximal to the noncrushing clamp, and the bowel is divided (FIGURE 10B). As soon as possible the specimen is wrapped in a large pack held in place by encircling ties (FIGURE 11).

It is reassuring for the surgeon, especially in obese patients, to see active pulsations at the anastomotic site, and the surgeon should take the time to free the mobilized colon and to loosen any tension on the middle colic vessels. Procaine, 1%, can be injected into the mesentery to strengthen pulsations in elderly patients or in the presence of large fat deposits in the mesentery (FIGURE 11). The Doppler apparatus may be used to verify the adequacy of the blood supply. The small bowel should be returned to the abdomen from the plastic bag, since the base of the mesentery of the small intestine can compress the middle colic vessels, particularly if the small intestine is placed on the abdominal wall above and to the right of the umbilicus (FIGURE 12). The blood supply improves as the colon resection nears the middle colic vessels, since the descending colon is now dependent upon the marginal vessels of Drummond arising from the middle colic vessels (FIGURE 12). The entire transverse colon as well as the right colon may be mobilized by detaching the omentum and the peritoneal attachments as indicated by the dotted line (FIGURE 12).

The mesentery is divided up to the bowel wall (FIGURE 13) where active pulsations have been identified. The mesentery to the sigmoid is further mobilized and divided until a sufficient amount of bowel has been isolated proximal to the lesion.

The remaining colon must be sufficiently mobilized then to reach the rectal stump loosely and without tension. Extra mobility is mandatory, since postoperative distention of the bowel and subsequent tension on the suture line must be anticipated.

A decision is made for an end-to-end anastomosis with or without a stapling instrument or a side-to-end anastomosis. The adequacy of the exposure, the amount of omental fat, and finally, the discrepancy between the sizes of the upper and lower lumens may influence the final technical approach. CONTINUES▶

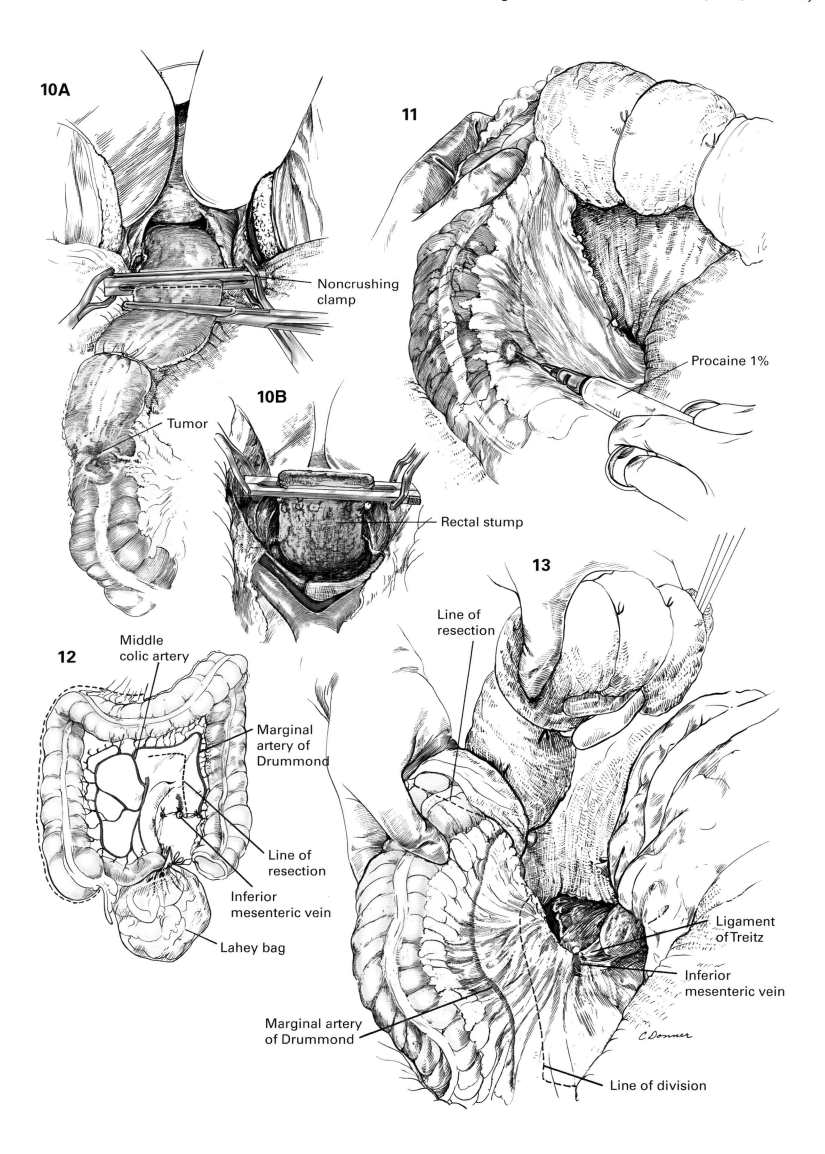

10A

Noncrushing clamp

10B

Tumor

Rectal stump

11

Procaine 1%

12

Middle colic artery

Marginal artery of Drummond

Line of resection

Inferior mesenteric vein

Lahey bag

13

Line of resection

Ligament of Treitz

Inferior mesenteric vein

Marginal artery of Drummond

Line of division

C. Donner

DETAILS OF PROCEDURE ◄CONTINUED► The bowel is divided obliquely after the mesentery has been cleared off to about 1 cm from the clamp (FIGURE 14). The mobility of this segment of bowel is tested by bringing it down to the region of the rectal stump to be absolutely certain that side-to-end anastomosis can be carried out without tension. If the initial segment is too tight, additional transverse colon may be mobilized. The hepatic flexure can be freed as well as the entire right colon. Any attachments constricting the mesentery of the descending colon can be divided. The presence of active arterial pulsations should be determined while the closed end of the colon is held deep in the pelvis. The end of the bowel is closed using a running absorbable suture followed by 000 interrupted silk Halsted mattress sutures. Alternatively, a stapled closure and division with a cutting linear stapler can be used. Some surgeons oversew this staple line with interrupted 000 silks for better security and inversion.

The *taenia* adjacent to the mesentery along the inferior surface of the mobilized segment is grasped with Babcock forceps, and traction sutures (**A** and **B**) are placed at either end of the proposed opening (FIGURE 15). These sutures keep the inferior *taenia* under traction during the subsequent placement of the posterior serosal row of interrupted 00 silk sutures (FIGURE 16). The traction suture (**B**) should be within 2 cm of the closed end of the bowel, since it is undesirable to leave a long blind stump of colon beyond the site of the anastomosis. After this, the Pace-Potts clamp is removed. The margins of the rectal stump are protected by gauze pads to avoid gross spilling and contamination. It is advisable to excise the edge of the rectal stump if it has been damaged by the clamp. The color of the mucosa and viability of the rectal stump should be rechecked. Any bleeding points on the edge of the rectal stump are grasped and ligated with 0000 absorbable sutures. It has been found useful for exposure to insert a traction suture (**C**) in the midportion of the anterior wall of the rectum (FIGURE 17). This keeps the bowel under modest traction and aids in subsequent placement of mucosal sutures. A noncrushing clamp may be applied across the colon to avoid the possibility of gross contamination. An incision is made between the traction sutures (**A** and **B**) along the *taenia*, and the lumen of the proximal bowel is opened (FIGURE 15). All contamination is removed in both angles of the openings. The same type of traction suture (**C**) can be placed in the midportion of the wall of the sigmoid. Interrupted 000 silks are placed full thickness through the posterior edges of both the descending colon and rectal stump (FIGURE 16). The knots are tied within the lumen and then cut. This layer provides absolute full thickness control for the posterior suture row. A double-ended running 00 absorbable suture is tied in the posterior midline. This proceeds laterally as a running, locking, and continuous suture until each suture line reaches the corner. A Connell inverting suture is then used as the closure proceeds from both corners to the midline. Thereafter, an interrupted row of 00 nonabsorbable sutures are placed in a submucosal mattress manner for inversion and security of the completed anterior anastomosis (FIGURE 18).

This provides a large stoma. The patency of the stoma is determined by palpation and the integrity of the anastomosis can be checked by filling the pelvis with saline and then insufflating the rectum with air using an Asepto syringe. The appearance of air bubbles signals the needs to reevaluate the suture line or even in the entire anastomosis.

After completing the anastomosis, the surgeon should recheck the adequacy of the distal blood supply and be certain that the proximal colon is not under tension. The hollow of the sacrum is irrigated with saline and the placement of a closed-system Silastic catheter in this region is optional.

To release tension from the suture line as the bowel becomes dilated in the early postoperative period, it is useful to anchor some fat pads to the peritoneal reflection in the iliac fossa. This seals off entrance into the pelvis as it anchors the bowel in this area. Likewise, the free medial edge of the mesentery should be approximated to the right peritoneal margin in order to cover all raw surfaces. As this peritoneum is closed, the course and location of both ureters must be identified repeatedly to avoid including them in a suture.

ALTERNATE STAPLED TECHNIQUE The Baker's side-to-end anastomosis as illustrated is a very safe approach when the surgeon must perform a hand-sewn anterior or low anterior resection. Most surgeons, however, have access to and proficiency with stapling instruments. In these circumstances, the proximal descending colon is transected with a cutting linear stapler while the rectal stump is divided between a pair of suture lines created with a noncutting linear stapler stapling device (FIGURE 19). The rectum is divided between the staple lines and the specimen removed. The staple line of the proximal colon is partially resected along the antimesenteric border so as to create an opening that allows passage of a circular stapler anvil, whose shaft will exit through the *taenia*, approximately 5 cm proximal to this opening. A purse string is then applied about the anvil shaft and tied in a snug manner (FIGURE 20). The open cut end of the proximal colon is closed with the noncutting linear stapler. The main circular stapler instrument is passed, with its disposable trocar retracted within, until it reaches the staple line of the rectal stump. Under direct vision, the surgeon guides the circular stapler trocar out through the posterior rectal bowel wall about 0.5 cm behind the suture line. A purse string is carefully placed about the penetrating trocar. The trocar is removed and the anvil inserted into the circular stapler instrument within the rectum. The rectal purse string is tightened and both purse strings are inspected. The two segments of bowel are carefully brought together and the instrument is fired. The firing and release require adherence to the manufacturer's instructions to verify correct tightness or compression of the tissue before firing and the correct amount of loosening for the cap to tilt before careful removal. The surgeon verifies the presence of two intact tissue rings (donuts) containing the purse strings of both the proximal and distal colon walls. After inspection of the anastomosis, the air bubble test described above is most useful, as the surgeon cannot always see fully around the anastomosis. An advantage of bringing the circular stapler stapler trocar out posterior to the rectal stump staple line is that it places the junction of the two staple lines (corners) somewhat anteriorly, where they may be most easily reinforced with interrupted 000 nonabsorbable mattress sutures.

CLOSURE The routine closure is performed.

POSTOPERATIVE CARE The Foley catheter is removed in 1 to 5 days, depending upon how much bladder and presacral dissection was performed. Careful observation of the voiding pattern, volumes, and residual volumes determines successful recovery. The initial liquid diet is advanced as tolerated. The presacral drain is monitored for output and blood content. It is usually removed in a few days unless a urine leak is suspected on the basis of a large output of clear fluid with an elevated urea content. ■

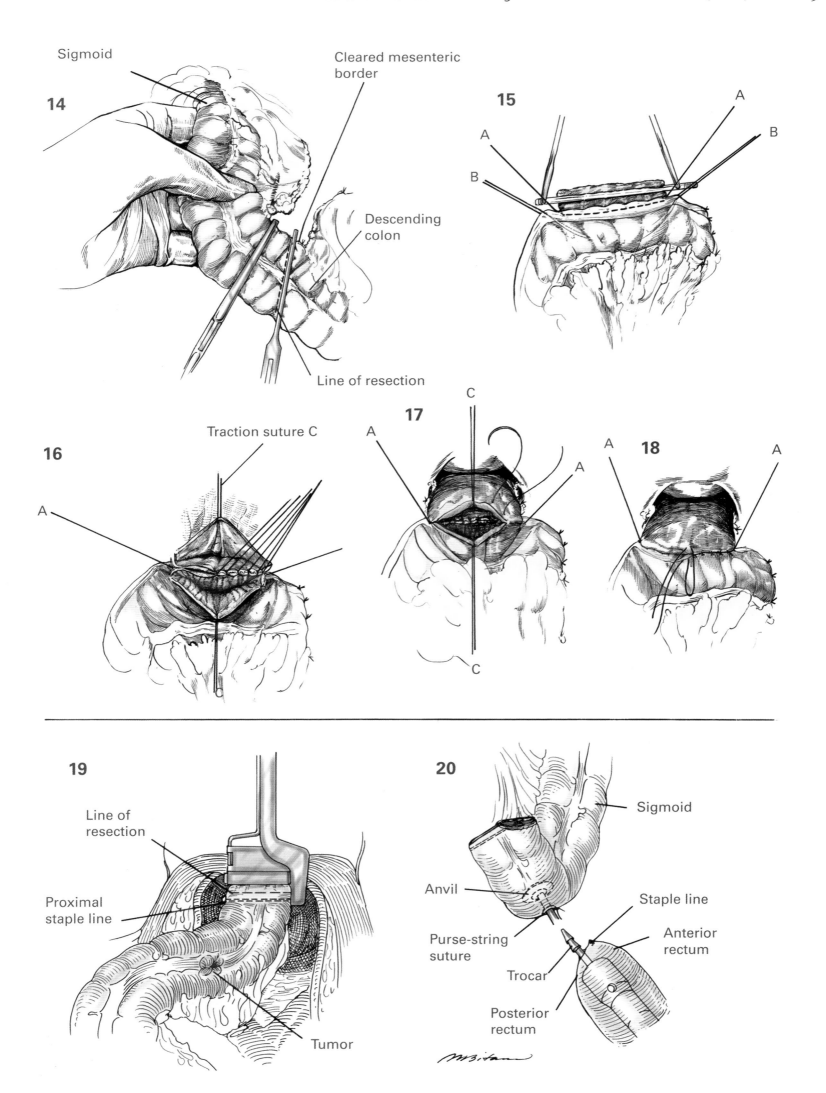

14

Sigmoid

Cleared mesenteric border

Descending colon

Line of resection

15

A

A

B

B

16

Traction suture C

A

17

A

A

C

C

18

A

A

19

Line of resection

Proximal staple line

Tumor

20

Sigmoid

Anvil

Purse-string suture

Trocar

Posterior rectum

Staple line

Anterior rectum

CHAPTER 64 ILEOANAL ANASTOMOSIS

INDICATIONS A permanent ileostomy following removal of the colon can be avoided in selected patients by removing all diseased colon and rectum down to the top of the columns of Morgagni or the pectinate line, followed by construction of an ileal reservoir, with anastomosis of the anal canal (FIGURE 1). Patients with ulcerative colitis (UC) and polyposis are candidates for this procedure, but those with Crohn's disease are generally not, because of the potential for involvement of the small intestine. The patient must have an adequate anal sphincter by digital examination or, better yet, by manometry. The rectum should be free of ulcerations, abscesses, stricture, fissures, or fistulae. This is especially important in patients with UC. This procedure can be considered in patients who are strongly opposed to an ileostomy and who are available for prolonged close follow-up. The patient should thoroughly understand the uncertainties of postoperative anal control and the need to have patience during the early months after the operation. The procedure is not recommended for frail, elderly patients and those who have fecal incontinence. Obesity may make it impossible to perform the anal pouch anastomosis. In patients with familial adenomatous polyposis (FAP) desmoid tumors involving the small bowel mesentery can make it difficult to obtain adequate length to reach the anus with the pouch. All patients should realize that a permanent ileostomy can sometimes be required due to factors not known until the procedure is underway.

Various surgical procedures have been used in an effort to improve long-term anal continence. It is questionable whether any procedure currently used is always completely successful, and the patient should be informed of this uncertainty. Increasing experience suggests the use of some type of anal pull-through procedure has a reasonable chance of providing more comfort than the terminal ileostomy or the ileal abdominal pouch.

A prolonged period of preoperative hyperalimentation or nonalimentation with catabolism may be avoided by a staged procedure, especially in the presence of toxic megacolon, poor general condition, or rectal disease. A permanent ileostomy is performed with subtotal colectomy, leaving the rectum in place, and the superior hemorrhoidal vessels undivided. This also offers the chance to review the pathology of the colon to further exclude Crohn's disease. After several months, an ileoanal anastomosis is considered and a diverting ileostomy is created at the time of the pouch. After a suitable recovery the temporary ileostomy is closed making this a three-stage procedure. Various pouches have been advocated. They include the J pouch (FIGURE 2A), the three loop S pouch (FIGURE 2B), the lateral isoperistaltic ileal reservoir (FIGURE 2C), and the four-loop W reservoir (FIGURE 2D).

PREOPERATIVE PREPARATION Documentation of the pathologic process involved is done with biopsies taken from the anal canal as well as the rectum or colon. The stomach and duodenum are inspected by gastroduodenoscopy. Patients with polyposis and UC patients with high-grade dysplasia should be informed of the potential for malignancy. It is important to have medical and surgical agreement that surgical removal of the entire colon is in the best long-term interest of the patient. Time is usually required for the patient to accept the recommendation and the patient can benefit from talking with another patient who has undergone this procedure. The patient's medications, including steroid therapy for UC, must be considered, and steroid therapy continued. Intravenous antibiotics are given before operation, and any major blood volume deficit is corrected. Patients receive a clear liquid diet for a day or two and an oral bowel preparation the day before.

In severe cases, some prefer a 6-week period of intense medication to keep the colon at rest permitting the inflammatory reaction to subside. Such patients may be placed on total parenteral alimentation, systemic steroids and steroid enemas, and systemic antibiotics when UC is present. The rectal mucosa is evaluated by sigmoidoscopic examination immediately prior to the operation. A large rectal tube is placed for irrigation with saline and povidone-iodine antiseptic solution.

Preoperative consultation with an enterostomal therapy nurse can help with the patient's understanding of the diverting and possibly permanent ileostomy as well as help to position the stoma appropriately. Excellent patient-oriented literature is also available from professional and patient support groups, which may aid the patient's understanding of both the procedure and its wide variety of possible complications.

Men should be counseled regarding the risk of impotence and retrograde ejaculation due to the pelvic dissection, and women should be counseled regarding the risk of decreased fertility due to scarring in the pelvis.

ANESTHESIA General endotracheal anesthesia is preferred.

POSITION The patient is placed in the modified lithotomy position using Allen stirrups. This allows the abdominal as well as perineal dissections to be performed without repositioning of the patient.

OPERATIVE PREPARATION The rectum is given a very limited low-pressure irrigation, and the perianal skin and buttocks are given the routine skin preparation. Constant bladder drainage is instituted and a nasogastric tube is inserted. The pubis and abdominal skin are also prepared in the routine fashion, and sterile drapes are applied.

INCISION AND EXPOSURE A lower midline incision that extends to the left of the umbilicus is made, and the abdomen is explored. Particular attention is given to the entire small intestine to make certain there is no evidence of Crohn's disease, which would contraindicate the operation. The involvement of the colon with inflammation or polyposis is evaluated. In the presence of polyposis, the possibility of encountering an unsuspected site of malignancy or metastases to the liver is ever present. If there is any question of Crohn's colitis, the colon is resected and sent to the pathologist for gross and microscopic verification.

DETAILS OF PROCEDURE The colon may be constricted, friable, and quite vascular, with firm attachments to the omentum. Gentle traction is applied to avoid tearing the friable bowel with resulting gross contamination. The mesentery of the colon can be divided and blood vessels ligated relatively near the bowel wall, except in diffuse polyposis, where there is always a possibility of metastases to regional lymph nodes. It is judicious to have the pathologist evaluate the entire specimen as soon as possible.

Before proceeding with the removal of the mucosa from the lower segment and before constructing the ileal reservoir, it is essential that sufficient ileum has been mobilized to construct the pouch. Approximately 50 cm of terminal ileum is required for the construction of the ileal reservoir. Such mobilization is accomplished by dividing the ileocolic vessels and the mesentery down to near the arcade of vessels at the very end of the ileum, but none of the latter is ligated (FIGURE 3). It may be necessary to evaluate the mobility of the small bowel all the way up to the ligament of Treitz with division of any bands that tend to limit the mobility of the small intestine (FIGURE 4). Incisions within the posterior peritoneum may be worthwhile to provide added mobility. Some divide the last ileal arcade (FIGURE 4). The adequacy of the blood supply involved should be evaluated frequently to be certain a vigorous blood supply is sustained to the end of the mobilized ileal terminal. The end of the proposed pouch should reach at least to the pubis, and preferably to the edge of the Bookwalter ring being used for retraction.

The dissection below the rectosigmoid junction is carried out close to the bowel wall to avoid damage to the presacral and parasympathetic nerves. The rectal stump is washed out with povidone-iodine, and the bowel divided at the anorectal junction. This leaves a stump about 3 to 4 cm in length (FIGURE 5). Some prefer to have a longer rectal anal stump, which requires resection of the rectal mucosa from above rather than entirely through the anus. Others use a stapling instrument for closure of the rectal stump. **CONTINUES ▶**

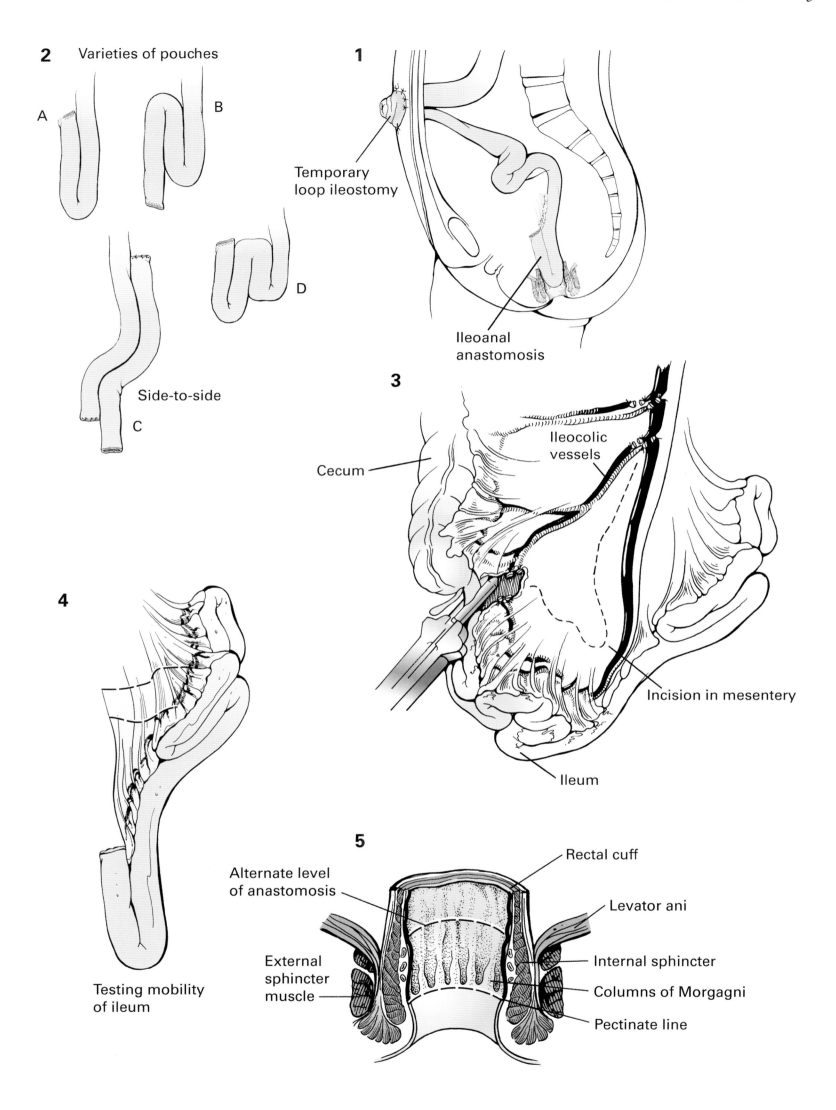

2 Varieties of pouches

A

B

D

Side-to-side

C

1

Temporary loop ileostomy

Ileoanal anastomosis

3

Ileocolic vessels

Cecum

Incision in mesentery

Ileum

4

Testing mobility of ileum

5

Alternate level of anastomosis

External sphincter muscle

Rectal cuff

Levator ani

Internal sphincter

Columns of Morgagni

Pectinate line

DETAILS OF PROCEDURE ◀CONTINUED▶ Many surgeons advocate leaving about 2 cm of mucosa above the columns. Recurrence of inflammatory bowel disease and malignant degeneration are possible and careful follow-up is essential. In general, avoidance of rectal dilatation or eversion of the stump plus a high level of anastomosis results in better fecal continence. In patients with high-grade dysplasia in the rectum, a traditional mucosectomy may be a better option, as it removes all the mucosa. If this technique is done, a hand-sewn ileoanal anastomosis would be required. The J pouch is constructed by rotating the terminal ileum clockwise to create a "J" shape (as seen from anteriorly) 15 cm long. The anterior ends are held by semicircular 000 silk sutures (FIGURE 6). The length is then checked as described above to ensure it will reach the pelvis. The distal antimesenteric end of the pouch is opened with electrocautery. A linear stapler is then inserted and fired, creating a pouch from the two limbs (FIGURE 7). Multiple firings are used to complete the full length of the pouch (to reach the upper end, the distal end is telescoped onto the stapler). A 2-0 Prolene suture is then used to create a "whip-stitch" purse-string suture around the opening in the tip of the pouch. An anvil of the circular stapler is then inserted and the purse-string tied around it (FIGURE 8). The anvil must sit so that the antimesenteric aspect of the ileum is draped across it. The circular stapling instrument is then inserted gently into the rectum by an assistant. It is advanced up to the level of the stapled rectal stump. The sharp spike then pierces through the stump just posterior to the staple line and it is approximated with the anvil (FIGURE 9). The device is then closed and fired, taking care not to include adjacent structures such as the vagina. Naive or too-vigorous insertion of the circular stapler instrument will rip through the very short rectal stump and make the procedure much more difficult. FIGURE 10 demonstrates the completed J pouch with ileorectal stump anastomosis.

If the rectal mucosa is severely diseased, then a complete mucosal proctectomy may be indicated. The mucosa is excised from the dentate line up to include the 3 or 4 cm of mucosa in the rectal stump. Some prefer to outline the dentate line with electrocoagulation followed by the submucosal injection of 1:300,000 adrenaline solution (FIGURE 11). This tends to elevate the mucosa and facilitate the dissection in a more bloodless field. All mucosa must be completely removed. This dissection is often the most time-consuming part of the technical procedure and must be done with the greatest care (FIGURE 12). The underlying muscle and nerves must not be injured. A dry field is essential.

Some prefer to grasp the stump with a Babcock forceps in the anus and everted out the anus (FIGURE 13). This facilitates the removal of the mucosa under direct vision but may result in poor fecal continence (FIGURE 14).

Others prefer to divide the mucosa at the top of the columns of Morgagni (FIGURE 5, page 231). This avoids telescoping the rectal stump and lessens the possibility of nerve injury where the patient may not be able to differentiate stool from flatus postoperatively.

If a mucosal proctectomy is performed, then a hand-sewn ileoanal anastomosis must be completed. This is demonstrated on page 235 in this chapter.
◀CONTINUES▶

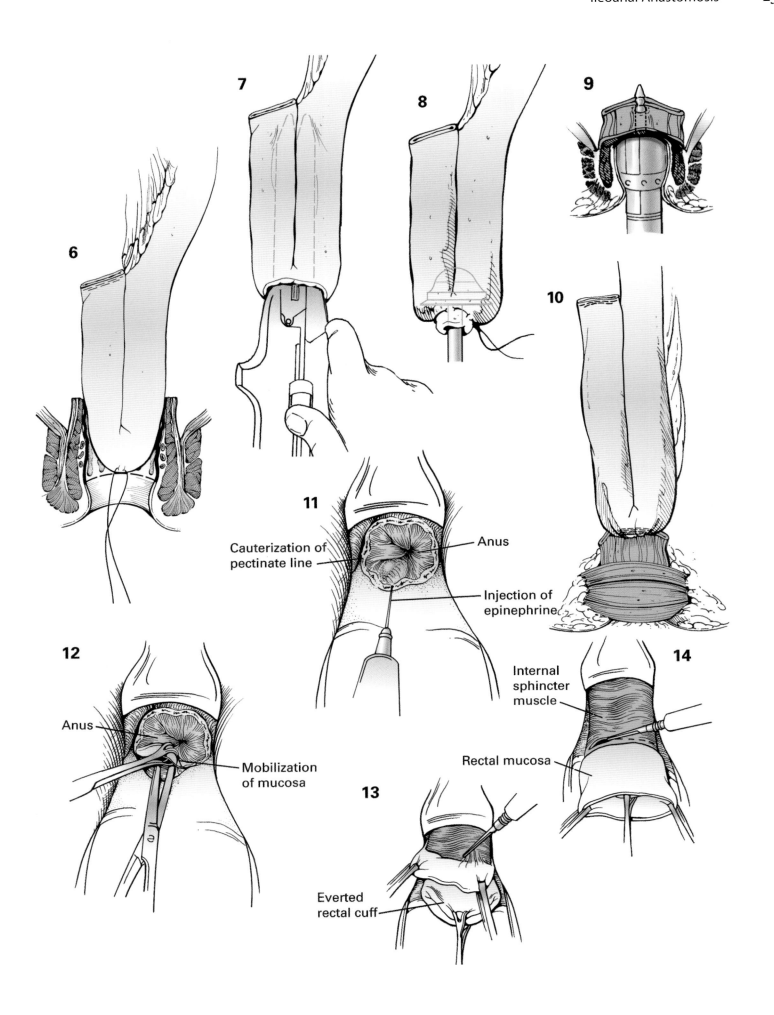

6

7

8

9

10

11

Cauterization of pectinate line

Anus

Injection of epinephrine

12

Anus

Mobilization of mucosa

13

Everted rectal cuff

14

Internal sphincter muscle

Rectal mucosa

DETAILS OF PROCEDURE ◀CONTINUED The adequacy of the blood supply to the reservoir is again double-checked. Two interrupted sutures with needles attached (FIGURE 15) are anchored on each side of the two-finger opening in the reservoir. These sutures are passed by the surgeon down through the anus, and the reservoir is placed in the proper position from above.

The two sutures on each side are then anchored to either side of the opening at the level of the dentate line (FIGURE 16). An additional suture is placed in the midline anteriorly and posteriorly. Eight or ten additional sutures may be required to ensure an accurate anastomosis. These sutures include the full thickness of the ileal wall, as well as a portion of the internal sphincter (FIGURE 17).

Any openings in the mesentery are closed with interrupted sutures to avoid intestinal hernia. The pelvic peritoneum is closed about the pouch to avoid twisting or displacement. A suture may be placed to anchor the pouch to each side of the muscular rectal cuff to secure the pouch in position and lessen the possible tension on the suture in the dentate line anastomosis. Some prefer to insert a rubber drain between the wall of the pouch and the rectal cuff. The rubber tissue drain is brought out anteriorly.

While it is tempting to avoid an ileostomy, fewer postoperative complications result if a complete diversion of the fecal stream is accomplished by ileostomy. The defunctioning ileostomy is performed through a small opening in the left lower quadrant about 40 cm from the pouch (FIGURE 18). It is advisable to ensure complete diversion of the fecal stream (FIGURE 19) by intussuscepting up the proximal limb or stoma over the rod (see also Chapter 51).

POSTOPERATIVE CARE Steroid therapy is gradually decreased until it can be omitted completely. The bladder catheter is removed after testing for sensation after a few days. The diet is slowly increased, but may need to be adjusted or limited depending upon the incidence of diarrhea.

Incidental obstruction, pelvic sepsis, and local problems around the ileostomy are occasional complications after the operation. Before closure, the integrity of the pouch and the anal anastomosis is evaluated by radiographic procedures with water-soluble contrast. Direct evaluation of the anastomosis for patency is also necessary. Frequently it strictures or develops a web across it requiring examination with sedation in the GI laboratory. Pouchoscopy can also be performed at this time. If no problems exist, the ileostomy is closed within 4 months.

The major consideration involves the degree of anal continence that has been achieved. Patience is required during the first year, as the capacity of the pouch increases and sphincter control gradually improves. The control of diarrhea during the day and soiling at night are of major concern and may require adjustment in bulk and type of food, as well as special medication. The number of daily stools varies, with an average of six per day and one or two per night. Patients with polyposis usually have fewer bowel movements per day than patients with UC.

A troublesome complication is a poorly defined syndrome known as pouchitis. The stools are increased in frequency with malaise, fever, and bloody stools, along with abdominal cramps. This complication is far more common in patients with UC than in those with multiple polyposis. Specific medication and dietary adjustments are indicated. This procedure is believed to be associated with chronic residual stasis. Intestinal obstruction may occur in 10% more of the patients.

Patients with this operation require frequent, long-term follow-up evaluations. ■

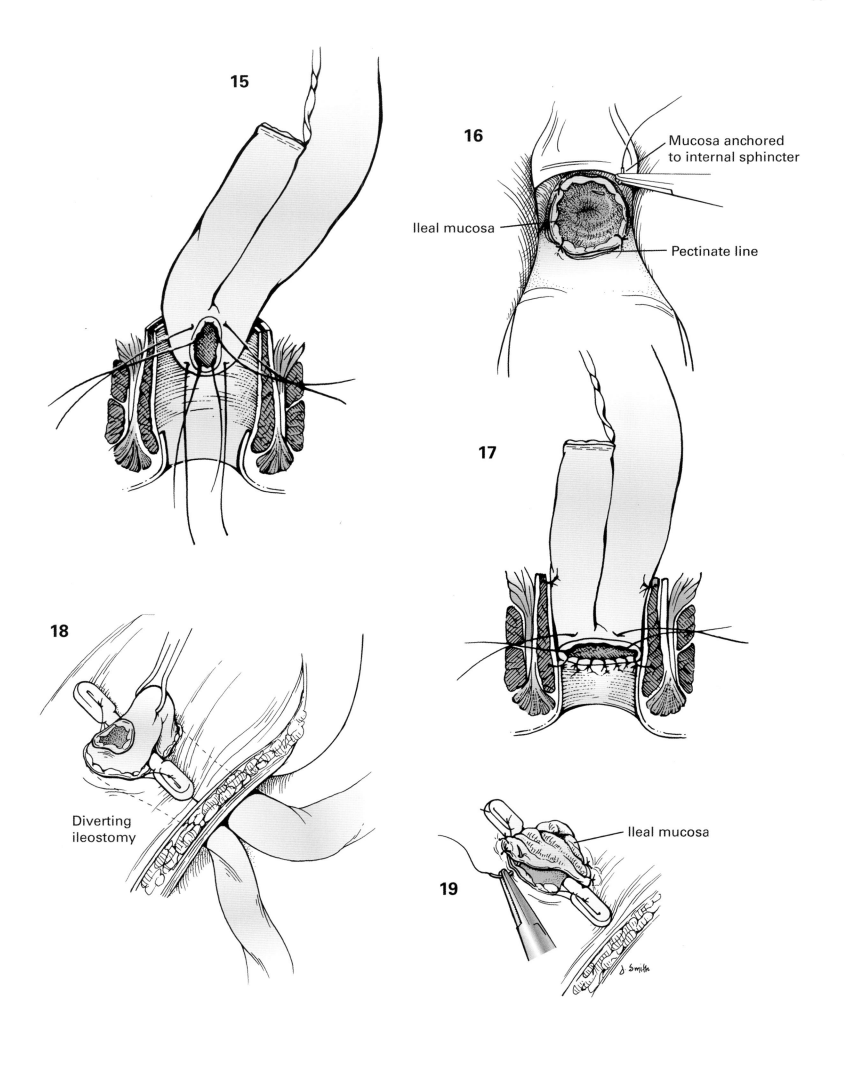

15

16

Mucosa anchored
to internal sphincter

Ileal mucosa

Pectinate line

17

18

Diverting
ileostomy

19

Ileal mucosa

J. Smith

CHAPTER 65

RECTAL PROLAPSE, PERINEAL REPAIR

INDICATIONS Operative correction of complete rectal prolapse in children is rarely indicated. However, in adults (especially in older groups) effective operative repair is worthwhile. Relatively commonly, rectal prolapse is found to be associated with or related to neurologic and psychiatric disorders as well as degenerative arteriosclerotic diseases. True prolapse of the rectum involves a herniation of the pouch of Douglas through the dilated and incompetent sphincter muscles. To correct this defect, the hernial pouch must be eliminated and the weakened pelvic floor strengthened. Obliteration of the pouch of Douglas and fixation of the rectum can be accomplished by the perineal, abdominal, or combined approach.

True prolapse of the rectum starts as an internal intussusception at the level of the levator muscles anteriorly. The rectum slides from this weak point through the anal canal. A true prolapse can be identified by circular rings of the prolapsed rectum as all layers of the bowel are present. In a first-degree prolapse, only the mucosa of the bowel is prolapsed, which is usually identified by three radial folds rather than circumferential folds. Rectal prolapse, if allowed to persist, can result in dilatation and incompetent anal sphincters. Prolapse is often present in elderly women who have perineal descent and weakness of the pelvis floor muscles. Perineal descent may often be associated with either a retocele or a cystocele. There is often an antecedent history of multiple pregnancies and pelvis surgery including hysterectomy. Operative correction by the perineal approach is usually reserved for individuals who are elderly and would otherwise be unable to tolerate a sigmoid colectomy and rectopexy, which is the ideal repair for this problem.

PREOPERATIVE PREPARATION Colonoscopy or a barium enema and sigmoidoscopic examination are essential. The use of a low-residue diet, cathartics, and enemas is necessary to obtain a clean and empty large bowel. The prolapse is reduced and reduction sustained by the application of a T-binder to minimize the associated edema and encourage the healing of any superficial ulcerations. The procedure requires a complete bowel prep including both mechanical cleansing and oral and preoperative intravenous antibiotics.

ANESTHESIA General or spinal anesthesia is satisfactory; however, general is usually preferred.

POSITION The patient is placed in a lithotomy position with the legs widely separated. The table is in a slight Trendelenburg position to decrease the venous ooze and enhance the anatomic dissection.

OPERATIVE PREPARATION The prolapse is reduced and the rectum irrigated with sterile saline. The skin about the perineum is cleansed in a routine manner. The area may be dried and a plastic drape used if desired. The bladder is catheterized, and the catheter left in place.

INCISION AND EXPOSURE The prolapse tends to present without difficulty (FIGURE 1), and Babcock or Allis forceps are applied for traction purposes to determine the extent of the prolapse. The relationship of the prolapse to the pouch of Douglas and the sphincter muscles of the anus is shown in FIGURE 2. The protruding mass is palpated to make certain the small intestine is not entrapped in the hernia sac anteriorly. Absorbable 000 sutures are placed in midline (FIGURE 3A) anteriorly, posteriorly, and at the halfway point on either side (FIGURE 3B and B₁) near the anal margin, not only to serve as a retractor but for subsequent landmarks at the completion of the procedure. The identification of the pectinate line is important, since the incision through the presenting rectal mucosa will be made 3 mm proximal to this anatomic landmark. This minimal amount of mucosa is adequate for the final anastomosis and is short enough to prevent postoperative protrusion. A sharp knife or electrocautery can be used (FIGURE 3). This area tends to be quite vascular, and meticulous hemostasis by electrocoagulation or individual ligation is essential (FIGURE 4). The incision through the outer sleeve should divide the full thickness of bowel wall, including mucosa as well as the muscularis. The pouch of Douglas is not entered. The dissection is facilitated if the surgeon inserts his index finger in a developed cleavage plane between the two layers of prolapsed bowel wall (FIGURE 5). **CONTINUES** ▶

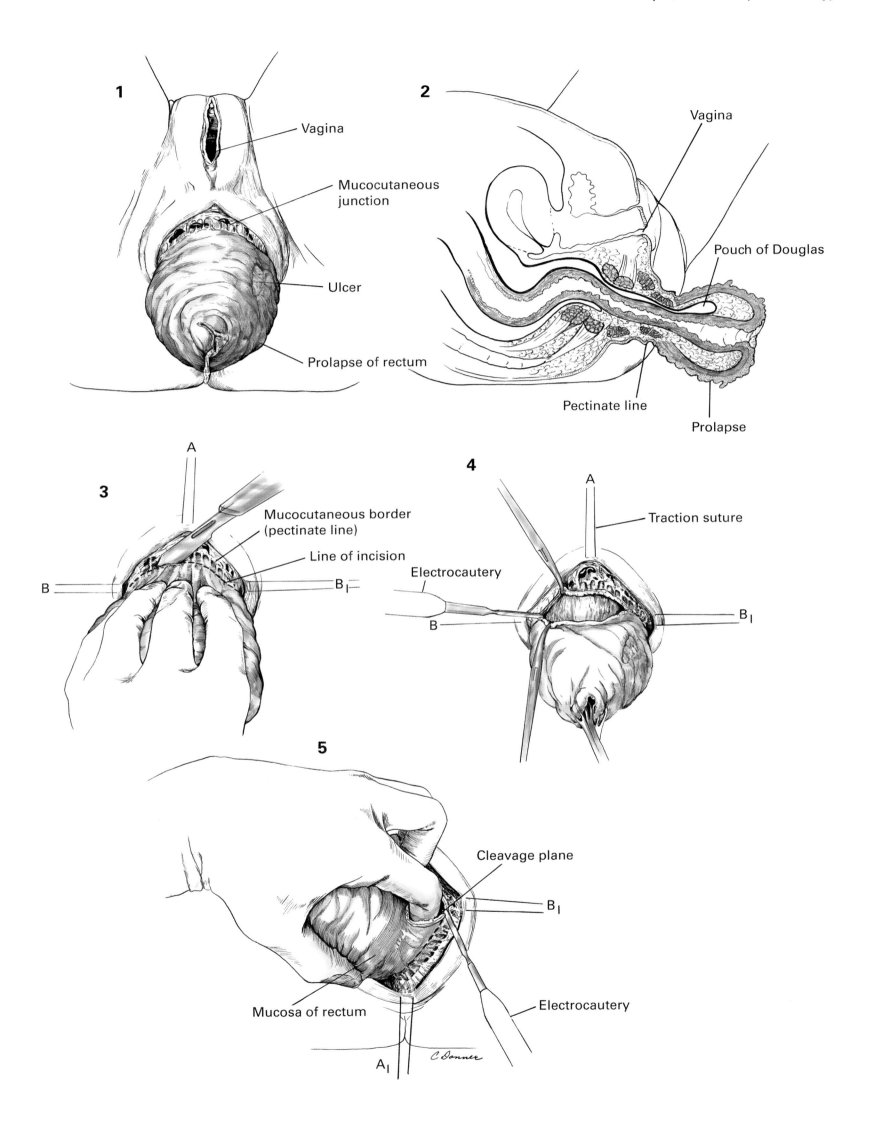

1

Vagina

Mucocutaneous junction

Ulcer

Prolapse of rectum

2

Vagina

Pouch of Douglas

Pectinate line

Prolapse

3

A

Mucocutaneous border (pectinate line)

Line of incision

B

B₁

4

A

Traction suture

Electrocautery

B

B₁

5

Cleavage plane

B₁

Mucosa of rectum

Electrocautery

A₁

C Donner

INCISION AND EXPOSURE ◀CONTINUED▶ After the mucosa and muscularis of the protruding segment have been completely divided, traction is maintained downward on the cuff of incised mucosa and muscularis (FIGURE 6). Any attachments between the bowel wall and the underlying segment are divided with the electrocoagulant unit or sharp knife, and all bleeding points are controlled. This cuff is pulled off easily and results in a segment twice as long as the original protrusion (FIGURE 7). The bowel wall is not amputated at this time, but downward traction is maintained as an attempt is made to identify the prolapsed pouch of Douglas (FIGURE 7). The resection may be started in the midline anteriorly and continued upward through the fat until the glistening wall of the peritoneum is identified. The peritoneum is gently opened (FIGURE 8), and the pouch of Douglas is explored with the examining finger. Any attachments between the small bowel or adnexa in the female should be separated to ensure freeing of as much of the pouch of Douglas as possible and to permit mobilization of the redundant rectosigmoid into the wound.

After the peritoneum is opened, the presenting intestine lying on the posterior side of the sliding hernia is grasped with forceps to determine how much mobile large intestine will require amputation to correct the tendency toward recurrent prolapse. The peritoneal opening should be extended laterally to either side. The blood supply, surrounded by a thick layer of fatty tissue, is usually identified posteriorly and on the right side of the presenting intestines (FIGURE 9). Half-length forceps and the surgeon's index finger are used as blunt dissectors until the mesentery to this segment of the bowel has been separated without injuring the bowel wall itself. At least three half-length clamps are applied to ensure a safe double ligation with o absorbable suture (FIGURE 10). The most proximal one of these sutures should be of the transfixing type, since the tissues are under some tension, and bleeding may develop unless the contents of these clamps are tied securely. No effort should be made to strip the bowel from the mesentery; however, it may be necessary to reapply clamps from either side, as well as in the midline posteriorly, until all the redundant large intestine has been pulled freely into the wound.

After the blood supply has been ligated and as much of the intestines as necessary mobilized into the wound, the pouch of Douglas can be closed in several ways. If the opening is rather large and the prolapse has included a segment of the large intestine well above the base of the pouch of Douglas, an inverted T-type closure of the peritoneum can be carried out (FIGURE 11). The peritoneum is closed in the midline anteriorly with interrupted or continuous oo absorbable suture.

The closure approximates the peritoneum around the bowel wall, and the continuous suture is tied. A suture starting at this point, including a bite of the peritoneum as well as of the bowel wall, continues around to the right side until it is anchored in the region of the ligated mesentery blood supply (FIGURE 11). The attachment of the peritoneum is made secure in a similar manner on the left side. This accounts for the so-called inverted-T closure of the peritoneum. CONTINUES▶

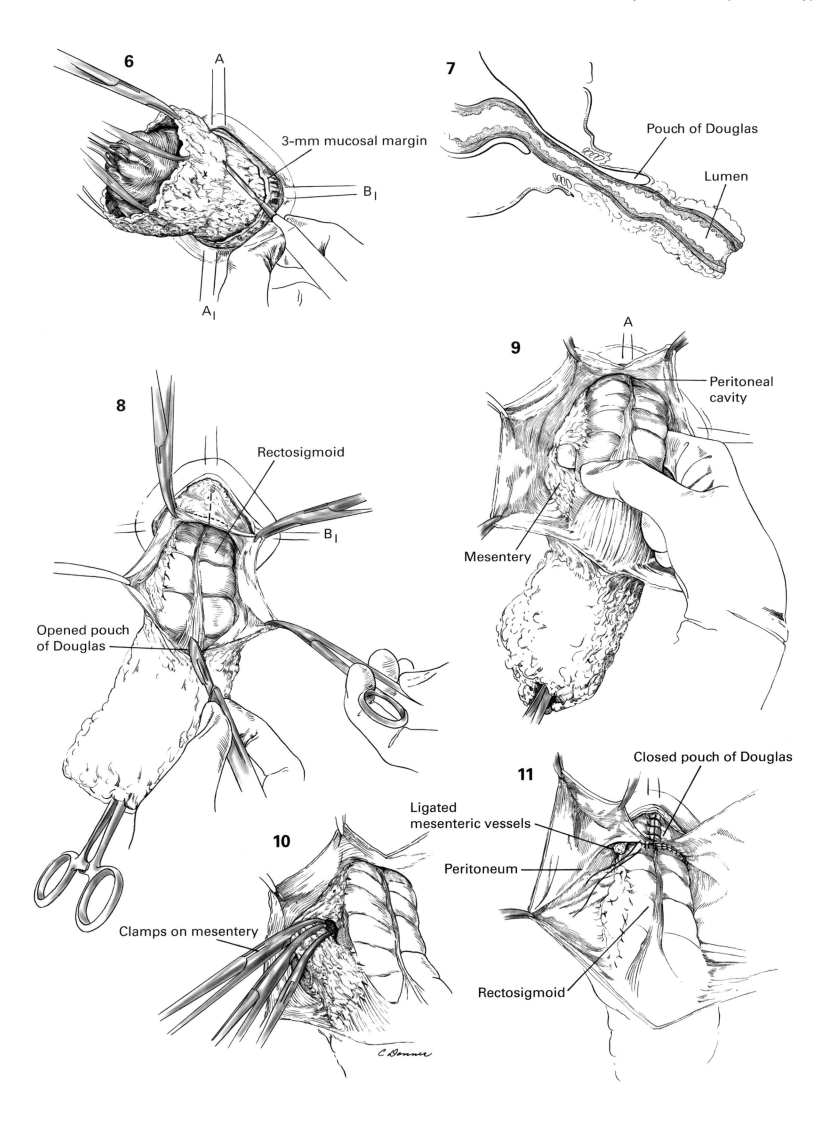

6

A

3-mm mucosal margin

B₁

A₁

7

Pouch of Douglas

Lumen

8

Rectosigmoid

B₁

Opened pouch
of Douglas

9

Peritoneal
cavity

Mesentery

10

Clamps on mesentery

11

Ligated
mesenteric vessels

Closed pouch of Douglas

Peritoneum

Rectosigmoid

C. Donner

INCISION AND EXPOSURE CONTINUED In some instances, especially when the prolapse is not particularly marked, the pouch of Douglas may be developed from the anterior rectal wall similar to a direct hernial sac (FIGURE 12). The peritoneum is then carefully incised and the margins held apart by traction with two or three forceps (FIGURE 13). The surgeon's index finger should be inserted to ascertain that the pouch of Douglas is free from attachments to either the small bowel or the adnexa in the female. It may be necessary to enlarge such an opening and insert a small retractor to accomplish this with good visualization. The pouch of Douglas should be closed as high as possible with a purse-string oo absorbable suture (FIGURE 14). Considerable time may be required to make certain that the pouch of Douglas has been obliterated as high as possible. If the obliteration cannot be done satisfactorily, it may be judicious to obliterate the pouch of Douglas by a transabdominal approach as part of a plan for a second-stage or a two-stage procedure. After the peritoneum has been closed, the redundant peritoneum is amputated, and additional sutures are taken to control bleeding and reinforce the pouch of Douglas (FIGURE 15).

The next step involves identification of the levator muscles, since the reinforcement of the pelvic floor is essential to prevent recurrence. The procedure to be followed is not unlike the approximation of the levator muscles in the performance of a posterior perineorrhaphy. A small narrow retractor can be inserted anteriorly as the surgeon inserts the index and middle fingers of the left hand to better define the levator ani muscles on the left side. An Allis or Babcock clamp grasps the levator muscles to better define their margins, and a deep oo absorbable suture is inserted (FIGURE 16). The first suture can be applied at either the top or the bottom of the proposed closure, depending on which is easier. In FIGURE 17, the first suture shown is placed in the bottom of the approximation, and a right-angle clamp depresses the bowel wall to provide a snug approximation by the levators. An additional three or four sutures are required to approximate the levators farther up in the midline (FIGURE 18).

Only after the levators are approximated should the prolapsed bowel be prepared for amputation. It is essential that the normal anatomic position of the bowel be retained. For this reason it has been found judicious to split the anterior as well as the posterior wall of the prolapsed large intestine almost up to the region where the bowel will be divided. This should be done carefully so that sufficient bowel is available for approximation to the pectinate line, yet a sufficient amount is removed to prevent recurrence (FIGURE 18). After the bowel has been divided, the surgeon should insert a finger into the lumen of the bowel to again check snugness of the approximation of the levator muscles. Enough room should be available to admit the index and middle fingers easily. If the approximation of the levators seems to be too snug and the blood supply to the bowel compromised, one of the sutures may be removed, or, if too large, an additional approximation of the levators should be considered.

Before the bowel wall is divided up as high as eventually required, the midline anteriorly should be tested for length. The bowel wall is divided up to a point where a retraction suture can be placed in the midline approximating the mucosa with the pectinate line without tension (FIGURE 19). A quadrant of the mucosa is then divided, and the mucosa is approximated to the pectinate line with either the continuous lock or interrupted oo absorbable sutures. The mucosa can be approximated more accurately if a planned quadrant anatomic fixation is carried out as shown in FIGURES 19 and 20. The importance of the traction sutures in the midline and at the halfway point on either side readily becomes apparent as the satisfactory approximation of the mucosa to the pectinate line is finally accomplished (FIGURE 20). There should be an easy approximation of the mucosa to the pectinate line, and it should have a nice pink color. The sutures should not be tied so tight as to produce bleaching of the mucosa. After completion of the procedure, the surgeon should introduce a well-lubricated finger carefully through the anastomosis to make certain of its patency as well as its adequacy (FIGURE 21). No drainage is indicated.

POSTOPERATIVE CARE Fluid balance is maintained by intravenous administration of water, glucose, and electrolytes. A liquid diet is gradually progressed to a low-residue diet. Mineral oil in doses of 1 oz two times per day is given. Digital examination is delayed unless undue distress develops about the site of operation. The possibility of development of a perirectal abscess, which may require incision and drainage, is an ever-present threat. ■

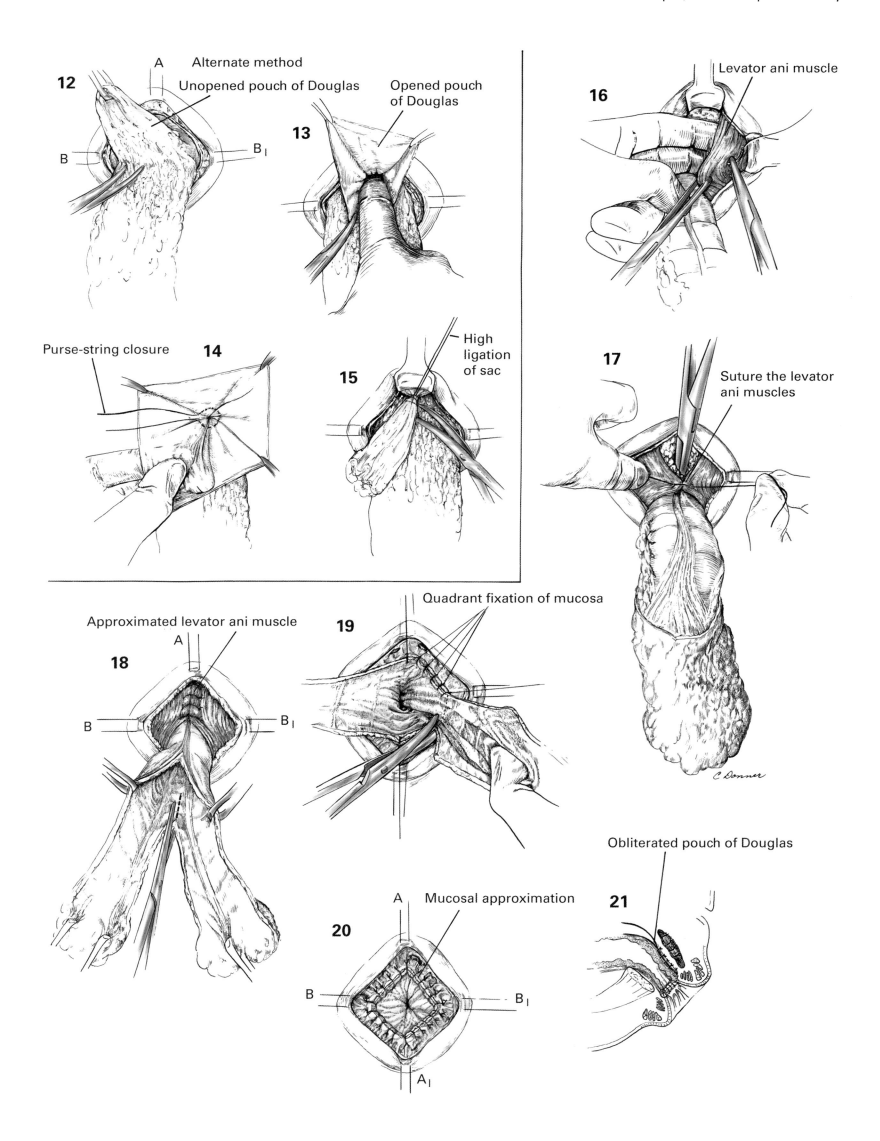

12 Alternate method
A
Unopened pouch of Douglas
B
B₁

13 Opened pouch of Douglas

Purse-string closure   **14**

15 High ligation of sac

16 Levator ani muscle

17 Suture the levator ani muscles

Approximated levator ani muscle
18
A
B
B₁

19 Quadrant fixation of mucosa

20 Mucosal approximation
A
B
B₁
A₁

21 Obliterated pouch of Douglas

C. Donner

RUBBER BANDING AND EXCISION OF HEMORRHOIDS

A. RUBBER BANDING OF HEMORRHOIDS

INDICATIONS This is an office procedure generally reserved for grade 1 or 2 hemorrhoids with minimal symptoms. The anatomy of internal and external hemorrhoids is shown in FIGURE 1.

PREPARATION Fleets enema. No anesthetic is necessary.

POSITION The patient is usually placed in a standard kneeling position on a Ritter table, although this may also be done in the left lateral position.

DETAILS OF PROCEDURE The hemorrhoidal bander is prepared with two rubber bands loaded. After digital examination, a Hirschman anoscope is inserted in the anal canal, the obturator removed, and the internal hemorrhoids are evaluated. After evaluation, which includes inspection of the internal hemorrhoids in their cardinal positions (right anterior, right posterior, and lateral), a decision is made as to which hemorrhoid is the most suitable for banding. This is usually the largest hemorrhoid. The Hirschman anoscope is positioned over the target hemorrhoid to allow prolapsed into the anoscope. Care must be taken to ensure that the site of the banding (all of the tissue encompassed by the band) is above the dentate line. An Allis clamp is first placed through the Hirschman anoscope to test the area (FIGURE 2A). The hemorrhoid in question is grabbed with the Allis clamp. If the patient has significant discomfort, the clamp is too far distal and needs to be moved more proximal. Once the correct position of the clamp is determined, the bander is placed through the Hirschman anoscope, and the hemorrhoid is prolapsed with the Allis clamp into the bander (FIGURE 2B). If there is no discomfort, the bander is fired, and the band is placed on the hemorrhoid. The instruments are then removed.

If the patient has significant, sharp pain immediately after placement of the band, it should be removed. This is done by incising the band with the tip of an 11-blade scalpel or with suture-removal scissors.

It is generally unsafe to place more than one or two bands at any one sitting. If more than two hemorrhoids are banded, they should be done at two or more office visits over the course of a couple of months. It is not unusual for the symptoms to improve after a single banding. Banding the largest hemorrhoid involved will sometimes resolve the patient's symptoms for a significant period of time.

POSTOPERATIVE CARE The patient will usually report some bleeding when the hemorrhoid sloughs in 4 to 7 days, which is entirely normal. However, the patient should be instructed to call immediately if he or she develops urinary retention or fever, as these may be early indications of pelvic sepsis. The procedure may be repeated in 6 weeks if symptoms have failed to completely resolve.

B. EXCISION OF HEMORRHOIDS

INDICATIONS Hemorrhoidectomy is usually an elective procedure performed in good-risk patients with persistent symptoms referable to proven hemorrhoids. Bleeding, protrusion, pain, pruritus, and infection are the more common indications when palliative medical measures have failed. Large external skin tags may require removal because of local pruritus. In the female, a pelvic examination is made to eliminate tumor or pregnancy as the etiology. In the male, the status of the prostate gland must be thoroughly evaluated. In older patients, a thorough colonoscopy or sigmoidoscopy and barium enema are mandatory. The presence of a serious systemic disease, such as cirrhosis of the liver, or a probable short life expectancy from advanced age or any other cause should be a general contraindication to operation unless anal symptoms are marked.

Simple internal hemorrhoids that prolapse may be treated by rubber banding using the technique shown in FIGURE 2A, B and C. Larger hemorrhoids may require excision as the first procedure, or if hemorrhoidal banding has failed.

PREPARATION A thorough cleaning enema is given the night before or early in the morning of operation, preferably several hours before operation, since residual enema fluid is more disturbing than the presence of a small amount of dry fecal material.

ANESTHESIA Spinal, epidural, or local anesthesia is satisfactory. If an inhalation anesthesia is given, it should be remembered that dilatation of the anus stimulates the respiratory centers. Spinal anesthesia must be used with caution because it may so completely relax the anal sphincter such that it cannot be properly identified by palpation.

POSITION The positioning of the patient depends on the type of anesthesia used. With spinal anesthesia, the prone jackknife position affords the surgeon the best exposure. If general anesthesia is used, an exaggerated dorsal lithotomy position is preferred, with the buttocks extending beyond the edge of the table and the legs held in stirrups.

OPERATIVE PREPARATION Extensive dilatation of the anus before hemorrhoidectomy is undesirable because it distorts the anatomy, making it impossible to remove all hemorrhoids at one operation without fear of stenosis. Gentle dilatation may be used if no more than three hemorrhoids are removed at one time.

DETAILS OF PROCEDURE Anoscopy is done, and any associated pathology is identified so that hypertrophied papillae or deep crypts may be removed.

The anal canal may be gently dilated to about two fingers' width to permit adequate exposure. A suitable self-retaining retractor is inserted into the canal, and further inspection is made. A gauze sponge is introduced into the rectum, and the retractor is withdrawn (FIGURE 3). The surgeon makes gentle traction on the sponge, reproducing, in effect, the passage of a bolus through the canal. As the sponge is withdrawn, the prolapsing hemorrhoids may be identified and are picked up with hemorrhoid clamps (FIGURE 4). Clamps are placed on all the prolapsing hemorrhoids and left in place as markers during the operation. Opposite the hemorrhoid a straight hemostatic forceps is placed on the anal verge, which is the external boundary of the anal canal. The hemorrhoid is placed under tension by simultaneous traction on the forceps and the hemorrhoid clamp (FIGURE 5). A triangular incision is made from the anal verge to the pectinate line (FIGURE 6). By traction on the two clamps and careful blunt and sharp dissection with the scalpel, it is possible to dissect off the triangular area of skin and the hemorrhoidal tissue from the outer edge of the external sphincter muscle. Many small fibrous bands will be found running upward into the hemorrhoidal mass. These represent the continuation downward of the longitudinal muscle and may be divided with impunity (FIGURE 7). Dissection is carried to the outer edge of the external sphincter. The anal skin must be divided to and slightly beyond the pectinate line. There now remain mucosa and the deep veins entering the hemorrhoidal mass. The tissue is secured with a straight clamp and a transfixing suture is placed at the apex of the hemorrhoidal mass (FIGURE 8). The hemorrhoidal tissue is removed with a knife, and an over-and-over continuous suture is made in the mucosa (FIGURE 9). The clamp is removed and a continuous suture approximates the mucosa, including the two edges of the pectinate line. As the suture is continued externally, small bites are taken in the external sphincter muscle (FIGURE 10). The deep portion of the skin is closed by a subcutaneous approximation (FIGURE 11), and the skin edges are left open to provide for better drainage and prevent postoperative edema (FIGURE 12). **CONTINUES** ▶

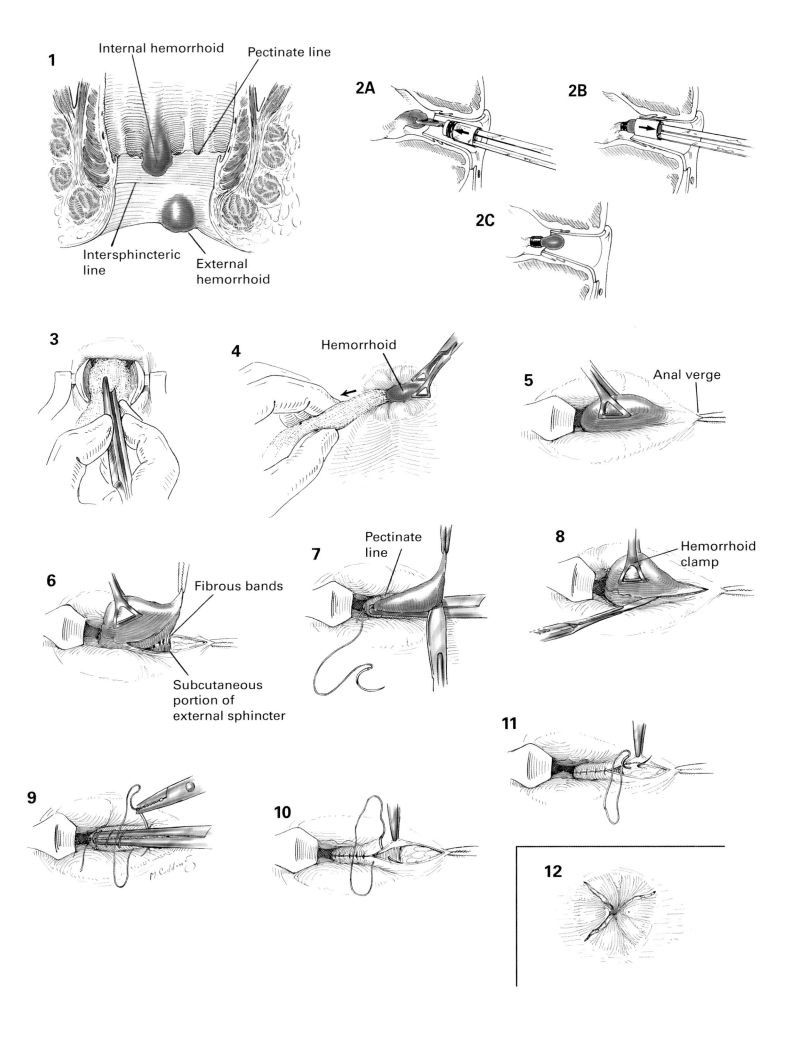

1

Internal hemorrhoid   Pectinate line

Intersphincteric line   External hemorrhoid

2A

2B

2C

3

4   Hemorrhoid

5   Anal verge

6   Fibrous bands

Subcutaneous portion of external sphincter

7   Pectinate line

8   Hemorrhoid clamp

9

10

11

12

DETAILS OF PROCEDURE <small>CONTINUED</small> Each hemorrhoidal mass is similarly removed. All possible mucosal tissue must be preserved to prevent stenosis. However, relatively large areas of skin may be safely removed in the triangular incision.

With extensive hemorrhoids it may be necessary to excise one-half of the mucosa of the entire canal in this fashion. The triangular incision may extend from the anal verge and reach the pectinate anteriorly and posteriorly. The mucosa is divided horizontally, taking small bites of tissue in a series of hemostats (FIGURE 13). This mucosal flap is sutured into the external sphincter horizontally to prevent stenosis (FIGURE 14). All redundant incisional skin margins should be excised to minimize the subsequent development of potentially damaging perianal skin tags.

POSTOPERATIVE CARE A sterile protective dressing is applied to the anus. Petrolatum may be applied locally. The diet is restricted for the first 2 or 3 days, but by the third day the patient may be allowed a full diet. Mineral oil (30 mL) is given. The patient is encouraged to have a bowel movement and usually will do so by the third day. Local application of heat is useful in alleviating discomfort. The patient may take sitz baths as desired. Weekly anal dilatation may rarely be needed postoperatively until healing is complete.

C. TREATMENT OF THROMBOSED HEMORRHOIDS

INDICATIONS Thrombosed hemorrhoids usually occur from straining or significant downward pressure. Often, individuals who have done heavy lifting or women late in their pregnancy may experience thromboses. These patients usually complain of significant pain. Diagnosis is made by inspection. The thrombosed hemorrhoid will generally be located in either the right lateral or the left lateral position. Depending upon the size of the hemorrhoid, removal might be accomplished successfully in the office. If the thrombosed hemorrhoid has been present for more than a few days, it may be unnecessary to do anything, as these will usually resolve with time. Occasionally, thrombosed hemorrhoids will present with extrusion of the clot and possible contamination, and in cases such as this, they should be removed.

PROCEDURE Once the decision is made to remove the thrombosed hemorrhoid in the office, the patient should be placed on the Ritter examination table in the standard kneeling position. With an assistant, hold the buttock apart to expose the anal canal and the thrombosed hemorrhoid. The area is first painted with betadine, and then injected with 2 to 3 mL of 1.0% xylocaine with epinephrine. This will provide both good analgesia and allow the patient comfort on the way home. The hemorrhoid is then grasped with a small hemostat and using dissecting scissors, excised using an elliptical incision (FIGURE 15). It is important to excise, and not to simply incise, the hemorrhoid as much as possible, to prevent further clot accumulation. This may be facilitated by using a small curette (FIGURE 16). The open wound is not closed. It is treated with silver nitrate and a pressure dressing placed. The patient is instructed to keep the dressing on until the next morning or bowel movement and to begin sitz baths the next day. ∎

Treatment of extensive hemorrhoidal mass

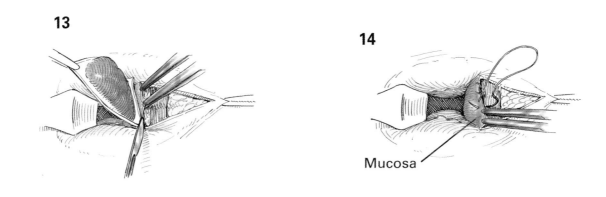

13

14

Mucosa

Treatment of thrombosed external hemorrhoid

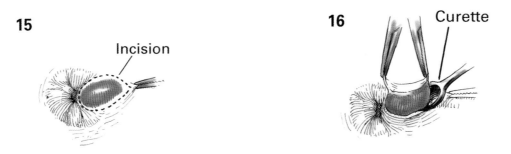

15

Incision

16

Curette

PERIRECTAL ABSCESS, FISTULA-IN-ANO, AND ANAL FISSURE

INDICATIONS The anatomy of the anal region is shown in FIGURE 1. Abscesses around the anal canal arise from infection of the anal crypt of Morgagni (FIGURE 2) and can be either superficial perianal abscesses (80%) or deeper ischiorectal abscesses (20%) (FIGURE 3). A perianal abscess is found adjacent to the anal canal, either on the right or left side, anterior or posterior. The patient usually complains of pain that may be, but not always, associated with a fever. The diagnosis is made by inspection of the perianal area, which will reveal a red, angry, and often fluctuant abscess. A digital examination should not be done due to the painful nature of the problem. FIGURE 3 shows the location of perianal and perirectal abscesses. Abscesses are classified according to the spaces they invade. Most superficial perianal abscesses can be drained safely in the office and do not require operative drainage. The most difficult to treat are those that track proximally or circumferentially within the intersphincteric plane or within the ischiorectal fossa or postanal space. Examination under anesthesia may be required to determine the location and extent of the abscess. An ischiorectal abscess, however, is large, involves either the right or the left ischiorectal space or the deep postanal space, and requires operative drainage.

PREPARATION For office drainage, the patient should be placed in the standard kneeling position on a Ritter table. For operative drainage, a prone, jackknife position is best. If done in the operating room, a general or spinal anesthetic is desirable.

OFFICE PROCEDURE For a perianal abscess, the skin over the abscess is numbed with ethylene chloride. Injection of the site with Xylocaine is excessively painful and unnecessary. Once the area is sufficiently numbed, a stab incision is made over the abscess to drain pus. This should be sufficiently large to allow adequate drainage. There is no need to excessively probe this abscess. The incision should be made as close to the anal canal as possible so that if a fistula-in-ano does develop, the fistula tract will be as short as possible.

A. OPERATIVE DRAINAGE OF ISCHIORECTAL ABSCESS

INDICATIONS Ischiorectal abscesses are drained immediately. Careful palpation often shows evidence of fluctuation not seen in the perianal tissue. Operation is not delayed until fluctuation is obvious, because a perirectal abscess may rupture through the levator muscle into the retroperitoneal tissue.

PREOPERATIVE PREPARATION No special preoperative preparation is required. Antibiotic therapy is given.

ANESTHESIA General anesthesia with endotracheal intubation may be used; however, regional anesthesia, either spinal or epidural, is satisfactory.

POSITION The prone or jackknife position is preferred for drainage.

INCISION AND EXPOSURE The common locations of ischiorectal abscesses are shown in FIGURE 3. Abscesses may be located extraperitoneally above the levator ani muscle. Careful rectal and sigmoidoscopic examination should be performed to detect associated pathologic processes after the patient has been anesthetized. An incision is made at the maximum point of tenderness (FIGURE 3) and placed either parallel or radial to the anus. If the abscess lies above the levator, great care should be taken in its drainage. Supra-levator abscesses are frequently caused by an abdominal source (e.g., diverticulitis), which should be treated through the abdomen rather than turned into an extrasphincteric abscess by perianal drainage.

DETAILS OF PROCEDURE After incision and drainage, the cavity is explored with the index finger to ensure complete drainage and to ascertain that no foreign body is in the ischiorectal space. A specimen of the draining material is obtained for bacteriologic studies. Usually, there is no communication with the rectum. If the abscess is small and a clear communication with the rectum is identified, the tract may be excised. The outer opening must be sufficiently large, for the common error is to drain a large cavity through a comparatively small incision, resulting in the development of a chronic abscess.

CLOSURE The cavity is lightly packed with a gauze tape.

POSTOPERATIVE CARE Moist compresses and sitz baths reduce inflammation and promote rapid healing. Postoperative dressings to ensure healing from the bottom are as important as the operation. An ischiorectal abscess is prone to result in an anal fistula; however, in about half of the cases, there will be primary healing with proper postoperative care. It is helpful to discuss the possibility of fistula formation with the patient preoperatively lest they feel that the fistula is a failure of the drainage procedure.

B. FISTULOTOMY

INDICATIONS The majority of anal fistulae result from infection arising in a crypt, extending into the perianal musculature, and then rupturing either into the ischiorectal fossa or superficial perirectal tissues. Operative obliteration of the fistula is always indicated if the patient's general condition is good.

ANATOMIC CONSIDERATIONS Treatment of anal fistulae presupposes a knowledge of anal anatomy, particularly of the sphincter muscles and their relation to the anal crypts. A study of FIGURE 1 will clarify several important points. As shown in FIGURE 1, the external sphincter muscle can be divided into three portions: the subcutaneous, superficial, and deep portions. The subcutaneous portion lies just beneath the skin and below the lower edge of the internal sphincter (FIGURE 1). The superficial and deep portions surround the deeper part of the internal sphincter and continue upward to join with the levator muscle (FIGURE 1). The levator ani surrounds the anal canal laterally and posteriorly, but it is absent anteriorly (FIGURE 1). The longitudinal muscle of the anus is the continuation downward of the longitudinal muscle of the large bowel (FIGURE 1). The internal sphincter muscle is a bulbous thickening of the circular muscle coat of the large bowel. The superficial external sphincter is palpated as a band surrounding the anal canal just beneath the skin (FIGURE 1). Just above it is felt a slight depression, the intersphincteric line, and the slight swelling above this point is the lower edge of the internal sphincter (FIGURE 1). If the finger is introduced into the canal and hooked around the entire anorectal ring anteriorly, it contacts the deep portion of the external sphincter, the levator being absent in this location (FIGURE 1). As the finger is rotated posteriorly, in contact with the midline of the canal laterally, a distinct thickening is felt as the levator ani (FIGURE 1) joins the canal, and posteriorly the anal canal feels thicker than it does anteriorly. Incontinence will not occur if any portion of the external sphincter or levator muscle remains intact.

Most fistulae arise in the anal glands at the base of the crypts of Morgagni; therefore, the abscess usually lies within the substance of the internal sphincter (FIGURE 2). It extravasates through the muscle, tending to follow the tissue planes created by the fibromuscular septa of the longitudinal muscle. Fistulae rarely arise from perforations of the anal canal associated with foreign bodies or abscesses, as in tuberculosis or ulcerative colitis. The internal opening may be above the pectinate line and may traverse the entire sphincter or portions of the levator (FIGURE 4). It may be necessary to operate in stages or to use the seton technique (Chapter 68) to avoid incontinence.

Fistulae-in-ano usually follow Salmon–Goodsall's rule. If located anteriorly, there is a radial tract (FIGURE 5A); if posterior, there is a curved track (FIGURE 5B–D). Simple anal fistulae (FIGURE 5A) follow a direct route in the anus. Complicated fistulae (FIGURE 5B and C) follow a more devious route, often horseshoe in shape and with numerous openings. Most complicated fistulous tracts open into the posterior half of the anus. Should the fistula have multiple sinuses, the main exit will usually be posterior, even though one opening is anterior to the dashed line (FIGURE 5); a single fistulous opening anterior to the dashed line usually extends directly into the anterior half of the anus (FIGURE 5A) (Goodsall's rule). **CONTINUES ▶**

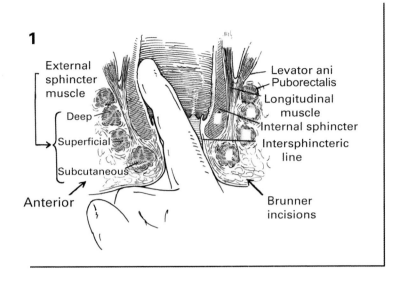

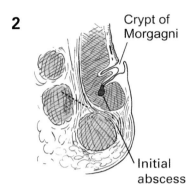

Types of Ischiorectal Abscess

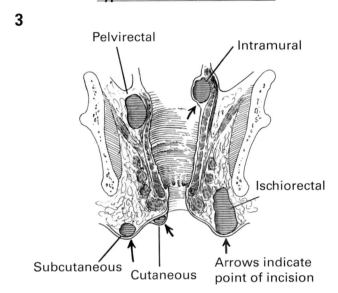

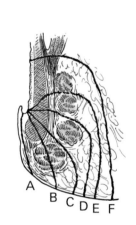

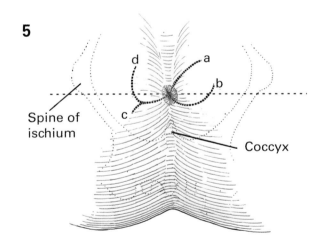

PREOPERATIVE PREPARATION ◀CONTINUED Local abscesses are drained if there is pocketing or cellulitis. If there is no severe local inflammation, a cleaning enema is given the night before operation. No cathartic is necessary.

ANESTHESIA Inhalation anesthesia is the procedure of choice when dealing with a complicated fistula. Spinal anesthesia is satisfactory for simple fistulae and may be used for more complicated fistulae; however, it provides such complete relaxation of the musculature that palpation and recognition of the divisions of the external sphincter and levator are sometimes impossible.

POSITION (See Chapter 66.)

1. TREATMENT OF SIMPLE FISTULAE

DETAILS OF PROCEDURE The anal canal may be dilated just enough to permit introduction of a self-retaining retractor. The pectinate line is directly visualized, and anal crypts that may reveal the internal opening are inspected. Gentle probing of suspected crypts may reveal an unusually deep crypt, which, from the position of its external opening, can be recognized as the source of the fistula (FIGURE 6). If a normal pectinate line is found, with shallow crypts or no crypts at all, it is likely to be a local perianal abscess with no direct communication with the anal canal. Some surgeons prefer to inject hydrogen peroxide into the external opening to trace the fistulous tract to its inner opening.

After the internal opening of a simple fistula has been identified, a probe is introduced into the external opening and gently passed down the tract into the internal opening (FIGURE 7). Care is taken to avoid creation of a false passage. The incision is made on the probe, and the tract is laid open (FIGURE 8). It is not necessary to excise the fistula. The tract should lie open as shown in FIGURE 9. In a simple superficial fistula, the entire tract may be stabilized with a probe as it is excised with scissors with electrocautery.

2. TREATMENT OF COMPLICATED FISTULAE

DETAILS OF PROCEDURE For complex fistulae such as a horseshoe fistula with an external opening anterior to the midanal line and an internal opening in the posterior midline, extensive incisions are avoided. The main posterior tract is identified with a probe (FIGURE 10). A short posterior portion of the tract is unroofed and the involved crypt excised (FIGURE 11). The anterior tracts are curetted and drained via soft rubber (Penrose) drains through secondary incisions along the tracts (FIGURE 12). The posterior tract is marsupialized (FIGURE 13). CONTINUES▶

<u>Treatment of Simple Fistula Type A</u>

6

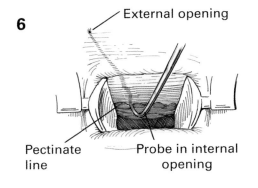

External opening

Pectinate line

Probe in internal opening

7

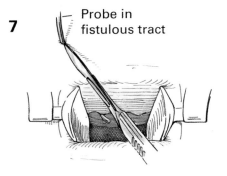

Probe in fistulous tract

8

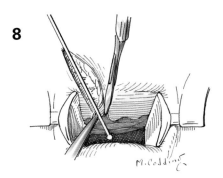

9

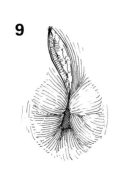

<u>Treatment of Complicated Fistula</u>

10

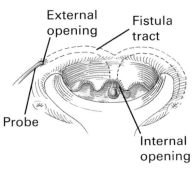

External opening

Fistula tract

Probe

Internal opening

11

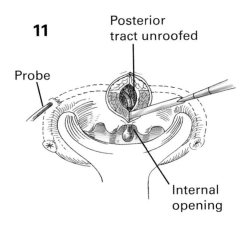

Posterior tract unroofed

Probe

Internal opening

12

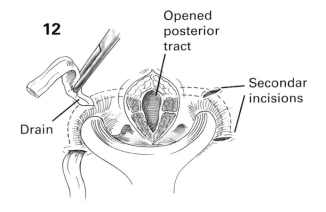

Opened posterior tract

Secondar incisions

Drain

13

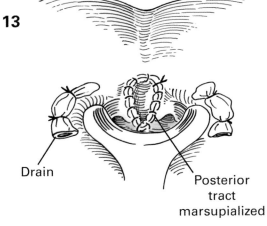

Drain

Posterior tract marsupialized

A. SETON PLACEMENT `CONTINUED`

DETAILS OF PROCEDURE If a large transsphincteric fistula involving a significant amount of external sphincter muscle is present, a seton should be placed. The probe is first passed from the external opening to the internal opening, and a 0 silk suture is tied around the groove in the probe (FIGURE 14). The probe with the suture is then pulled back through the fistula track, and the 0 silk suture is tied tightly around the muscle. All fat and skin are removed leaving the seton compressing sphincter muscle only. Silk is an irritant, and with time the silk will cut through the sphincter muscle. However, the fistulotomy will be performed incrementally giving time for the sphincter to heal. The fistula is slowly drawn out by the seton. This protects against incontinence, by preventing the sphincter muscle from separating, as would happen during a fistulotomy. A non-cutting seton using a vessel loop is indicated in chronic perianal disease.

POSTOPERATIVE CARE The patient may be out of bed as soon as the anesthesia has worn off. The patient is allowed a light diet, and there is no attempt to restrain bowel movements. Stool softeners are prescribed. Sitz baths may be started on the second day following operation. Patients may be discharged the day of surgery and are seen within 1 week.

B. ENDORECTAL ADVANCEMENT FLAP

An alternative therapy for a complex fistula is an endorectal advancement flap (FIGURE 15). A flap with mucosa and submucosa is created to include the internal opening (FIGURE 16). The dissection is carried far enough proximal until the flap can be advanced distally without tension. The internal opening is excised, and then the flap is matured to the intersphincteric groove (FIGURE 17). The external sphincter may be plicated to close the fistula opening and then the flap is sutured to the intersphincteric groove with interrupted absorbable sutures (FIGURE 17). This effectively treats a complex fistula-in-ano with minimal risk of injury to the sphincter muscles.

C. ANAL FISSURE

INDICATIONS Fissure in ano is a common painful condition that can be found in children and adults alike. These wounds usually heal spontaneously in children but may require operative correction in adults. It is usually caused by constipation or a large traumatic bowel movement, and it is almost always located posterior. The fissure, which runs between the dentate line and anal verge, if deep enough exposes the internal sphincter muscle. This causes considerable spasm and pain. Chronic fissures may be associated with a hypertrophied anal papilla and a skin tag. Over a period of time, the internal sphincter muscle hypertrophies, becoming more effective in keeping the wound open, and preventing spontaneous closure of the fissure. Topical salves and fiber are usually effective early on. Once the wound becomes chronic, surgical repair is usually necessary.

PREOPERATIVE PREPARATION No preoperative preparation is necessary. The cleaning enema, which is such an excruciating procedure to the patient, is omitted.

ANESTHESIA Spinal, epidural, or local anesthesia is satisfactory.

OPERATIVE PREPARATION The field is prepared with local antiseptic solution. No attempt is made to dilate the canal and irrigate the rectum.

DETAILS OF PROCEDURE The patient is placed in the position as shown and prepped and draped in the usual fashion. The prone jackknife position may be used. A Hill-Ferguson retractor is placed in the anal canal, and the anal canal is inspected. The fissure is usually posterior and may be associated with a right posterior hemorrhoid (FIGURE 18). The fissure and the hemorrhoid, if necessary (FIGURE 19), are excised and the anal mucosa and anoderm closed with a running 2-0 chromic suture (FIGURE 20). A lateral internal sphincterotomy is performed to reduce sphincter spasm. A separate incision is then made in the left lateral position, again excising the hemorrhoid in that location if necessary, to expose the hypertrophied internal sphincter muscle. A partial lateral internal sphincterotomy is done in this position. This wound is closed with a running 2-0 chromic stitch.

The procedure may be done as a closed technique. With the finger in the anal canal, an 11-blade is inserted into the intersphincteric plane staying below the dentate line (FIGURE 21). The blade is then moved medially, dividing the inferior one-third to one-half of the internal sphincter (FIGURE 22).

An open technique may be done. A skin incision is made (FIGURE 23). A hypertrophied band of internal sphincter is freed and elevated (FIGURE 24). The internal sphincter is then partially divided (FIGURE 25). The wound is left open. The sphincterotomy is done in the lateral position to avoid creating a keyhole deformity, a complication of the procedure that can be challenging to correct. This procedure removes the chronic fissure in ano and releases the tension on the anal canal sufficiently enough to allow the fissure to heal.

POSTOPERATIVE CARE Patients are allowed out of bed and encouraged to move their bowels as soon as possible after operation. Sitz baths can be an effective method of pain control. The patient should be kept under weekly observation after discharge until healing is complete. ∎

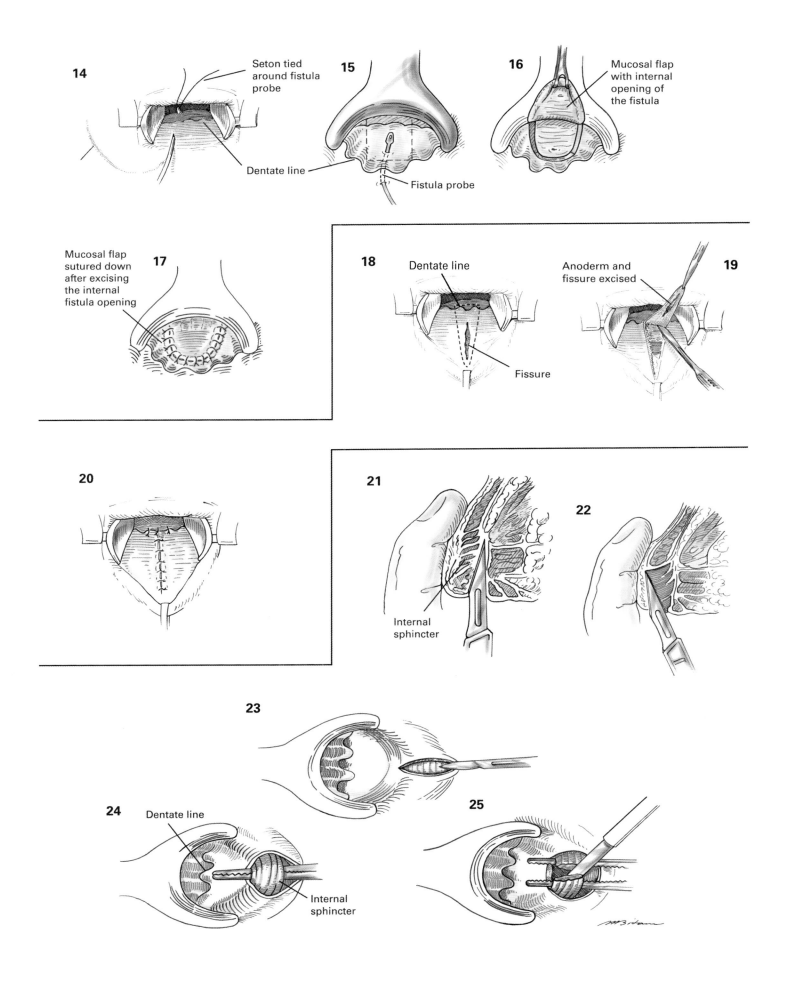

14 Seton tied around fistula probe / Dentate line

15 Dentate line / Fistula probe

16 Mucosal flap with internal opening of the fistula

17 Mucosal flap sutured down after excising the internal fistula opening

18 Dentate line / Fissure

19 Anoderm and fissure excised

20

21 Internal sphincter

22

23

24 Dentate line / Internal sphincter

25

EXCISION OF PILONIDAL SINUS

INDICATIONS Pilonidal cysts and sinuses should be completely excised or exteriorized (FIGURE 1A and B). Acutely infected sinuses should be incised and drained, followed later by complete excision after the acute infection subsides. The more limited procedure of exteriorization (marsupialization) is effective when the sinus tract is well defined (FIGURE 1B). Regardless of the various surgical approaches, such lesions may recur.

PREOPERATIVE PREPARATION In complicated sinuses with several tracts present, a dye such as methylene blue may be injected for better identification, although if a careful dissection is carried out in a bloodless field, the surgeon can identify the sinus tracts. It is important that this be done several days before the operation to avoid excessive staining of the operative area, which may occur if the injection is done at the time of operation.

ANESTHESIA Light general anesthesia is satisfactory. The patient's position requires that special care be taken to maintain an unobstructed airway. Spinal anesthesia should not be used in the presence of infection near the site of lumbar puncture.

POSITION The patient is placed on his or her abdomen with the hips elevated and the table broken in the middle (FIGURE 2).

OPERATIVE PREPARATION Two strips of adhesive tape are anchored snugly and symmetrically about 10 cm from the midline at the level of the sinus and pulled down and fastened beneath the table (FIGURE 3). This spreads the intergluteal fold for better visualization of the operative area. A routine skin preparation follows after the skin is carefully shaved.

DETAILS OF PROCEDURE An ovoid incision is made around the opening of the sinus tract off the midline about 1 cm away from either side (FIGURE 4). Firm pressure and outward pull make the skin taut and control bleeding.

An Allis forceps is placed at the upper angle of the skin to be removed, and the sinus is cut out en bloc (FIGURE 5). The subcutaneous tissue is excised downward and laterally to the fascia underneath. Great care is exercised to protect this fascia from the incision, as it offers the only defense against deeper spread of infection (FIGURE 6). Small, pointed hemostats should be used to clamp the bleeding vessels in order that the smallest amount of tissue reaction be incurred. Electrocoagulation may be used to control bleeding and to keep the amount of buried suture material to a minimum. Some prefer to avoid burying any suture material by using compression or electrocoagulation to control all the bleeding points. Extreme care should be taken in the dissection of the lower end of the incision, as many small, troublesome vessels are encountered frequently that tend to retract when divided. After careful inspection of the wound to make sure that all sinus tracts have been removed, the subcutaneous fat is undercut at its junction with the underlying fascia (FIGURE 7). This undercutting should extend only far enough to allow approximation of the edges without tension (FIGURE 8).

CLOSURE After all bleeding points are controlled, the wound should be thoroughly washed with saline. The chances for primary healing are greatly enhanced if the field is absolutely dry. If unexpected infection has been encountered, the wound should be packed open. In uncomplicated sinuses, the wound is closed after all bleeding is controlled. The closure should be off the midline. Rather than bury sutures, the skin can be closed and the dead space eliminated by a series of interrupted vertical mattress sutures (FIGURE 9). The suture is introduced 1 cm or a little more than the margins of the wound to include the full thickness of the mobilized flap of skin and subcutaneous tissue. A second bite includes the fascia in the bottom of the wound (FIGURE 9). The suture is then continued deep into the opposite flap. The suture is directed back to the original side as it passes back through the skin margins (FIGURE 10). When tied, this obliterates the dead space and accurately approximates the skin margins (FIGURE 11). The sutures should be placed at intervals of not more than 1 cm. Skin approximation must be very accurate, since even a small overlap may be surprisingly slow to heal in this area. A pressure dressing is applied with great care, and the sutures are allowed to remain in place for 10 to 14 days.

EXTERIORIZATION When the sinus appears small and in the presence of recurrence, a probe may be inserted into the sinus, and the skin and subcutaneous tissue divided (FIGURE 1A). The entire sinus, including any tributaries, must be laid wide open and all granulation tissue wiped away repeatedly with sterile gauze or a curette. The thick lining of the sinus forms the bottom of the wound. A wedge of subcutaneous tissue is excised to facilitate the sewing of the mobilized skin margins to the thick wall of the retained sinus. This ensures a cavity that can be dressed easily with a minimum of drainage as well as discomfort to the patient. The raw margins of the wound are held apart by a gauze pack until healing is complete (FIGURE 1B). This method has the advantage of being a procedure of less magnitude than complete excision. The period of hospitalization and rehabilitation is shortened and insurance against recurrence enhanced.

POSTOPERATIVE CARE Complete immobilization of the area and protection against contamination are essential. Early ambulation is advisable, but sitting upon the incision in a hard chair is not. The patient should be encouraged always to sit on a cushion or to sit to the side on one buttock or the other. The diet is restricted to clear liquids for several days, followed by a low-residue diet to decrease the chances of contamination from a bowel movement. When the sinus is packed open or exteriorized, the patient is not immobilized. Regardless of the method used, frequent and repeated dressings are indicated to avoid possible early bridging of the skin with recurrence and prolonged discomfort and disability. The importance of keeping all hair removed from the intergluteal fold until healing is complete cannot be overemphasized. Depilatory agents may be used several times per month provided that pretesting for sensitivity to the agent has been negative. ∎

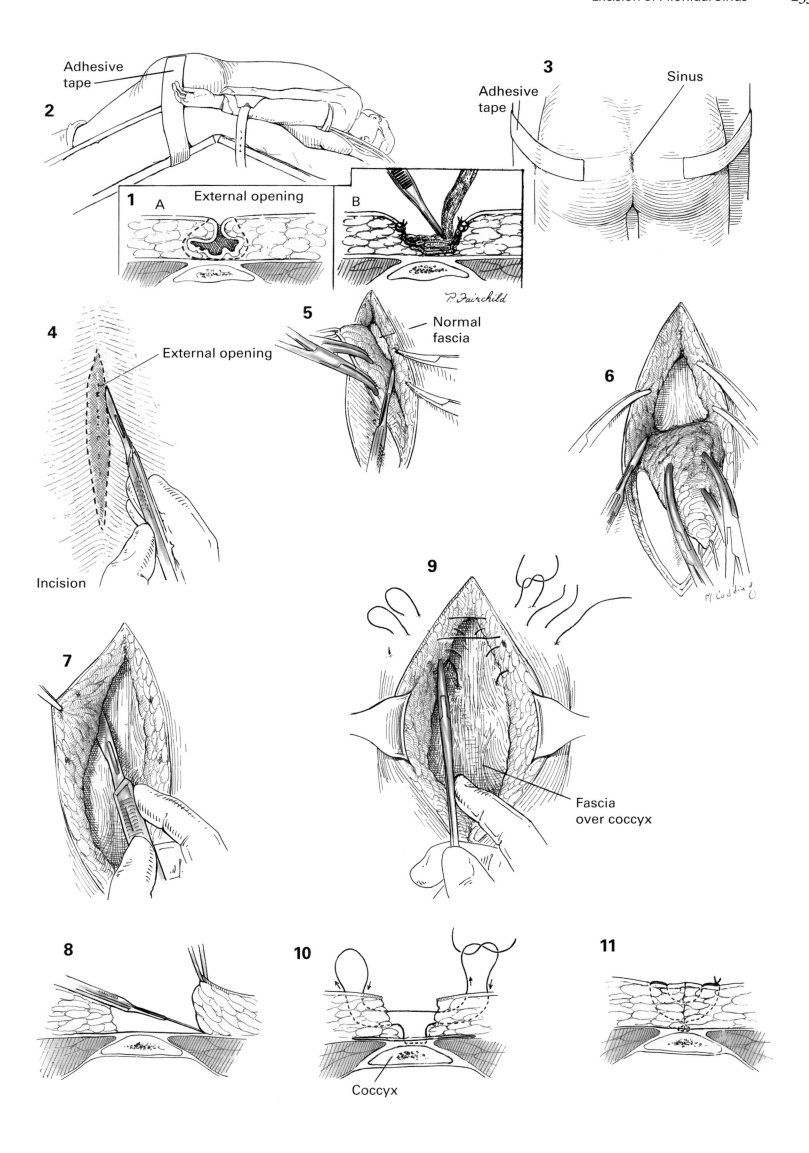

2 Adhesive tape

1 A External opening B

3 Adhesive tape Sinus

P. Fairchild

4 External opening

Incision

5 Normal fascia

6

M. Coddia...

7

9

Fascia over coccyx

8

10 Coccyx

11

GALL BLADDER, BILE DUCTS, AND LIVER

CHOLECYSTECTOMY, LAPAROSCOPIC

INDICATIONS Cholecystectomy is indicated in symptomatic patients with proven disease of the gallbladder, and the indications for laparoscopic cholecystectomy are essentially the same as those for open cholecystectomy. These include, but are not limited to, symptomatic cholelithiasis, acute calculus and acalculous cholecystitis, gallstone pancreatitis, biliary dyskinesia, and gallbladder masses and polyps that are concerning for malignancies. Cholecystectomy for mild gallstone pancreatitis should be performed during the initial admission for pancreatitis and deferred for several weeks in patients with severe pancreatitis. Contraindications include small bowel obstruction secondary to gallstone ileus, coagulopathy, and medical comorbidities prohibiting surgery. Relative contraindications are decreasing as the minimally invasive surgical experience of surgeons' increases. Factors associated with increased surgical risk include cirrhosis with portal hypertension, previous intra-abdominal surgery with adhesions, and acute gangrenous cholecystitis.

PREOPERATIVE PREPARATION Following a history and physical examination, the diagnosis of biliary disease is typically documented with ultrasound examination of the right upper quadrant. The remainder of the gastrointestinal tract may require additional studies. A chest x-ray and electrocardiogram may be performed as indicated. Routine laboratory blood tests are obtained and should include a liver function panel. Coagulation studies should be ordered if there is a concern for hepatic insufficiency or other causes of coagulopathy. The risks of laparoscopic cholecystectomy include bleeding, infection, trocar injuries to viscera or blood vessels, and bile duct injury. These should be discussed with the patient as well as the possibility of conversion to an open procedure. The management of patients with gallstones and suspected common duct stones is based on risk stratification. Preoperative endoscopic retrograde cholangiopancreatography (ERCP) with sphincterotomy and stone extraction, if necessary, is indicated in patients with jaundice and should be considered in patients with dilated bile ducts on imaging and/or elevated liver function tests.

ANESTHESIA General anesthesia with endotracheal intubation is recommended. Preoperative prophylactic antibiotics for anticipated bile pathogens are administered such that adequate tissue levels exist, although there is evidence that there may be limited benefit for low-risk patients

POSITION As laparoscopic cholecystectomy makes extensive use of supporting equipment, it is important to position this equipment such that it is easily visualized by all members of the surgical team (FIGURE 1).

The surgeon must have a clear line of sight to both the video monitor and the high flow CO_2 insufflator such that he or she can monitor both the intra-abdominal pressure and gas flow rates. In general, all members of the team are looking across the operating table at video monitors. The positions of the video monitors may require adjustment once all members step to their final positions at operation. The patient is placed supine with the arms either secured at the sides or out at right angles so as to allow maximum access to monitoring devices by the anesthesiologist at the head of the table. An orogastric tube is passed after the patient is asleep. Sequential pneumatic compression stockings should be placed for deep vein thrombosis (DVT) prophylaxis. The dispersive electrode (electrocautery grounding pad) is placed near the hip, avoiding any region where internal metal orthopedic parts or electronic devices may have been implanted. The possible need for fluoroscopic examination of the abdomen in the event that an intraoperative cholangiogram is performed should be considered when positioning the bed and patient. The legs, arms, and upper chest are covered with blankets to minimize heat loss.

OPERATIVE PREPARATION The skin of the entire abdomen and lower anterior chest is prepared in the routine manner.

INCISION AND EXPOSURE The abdomen is palpated to find the liver edge or unsuspected intra-abdominal masses. The patient is placed in a mild Trendelenburg position and an appropriate site for the creation of the pneumoperitoneum is chosen. The initial port may be placed by an open, or Hasson, technique and this is generally preferred. Alternatively, a Veress needle technique may be used. These techniques are described in Chapters 11 and 12.

DETAILS OF THE PROCEDURE Topical antifog solution is applied to the optical end of the telescope, which may be either angled (30 degrees) or flat (0 degrees) (FIGURE 2). The CO_2 source is attached to the port, and the videoscope is inserted after white-balancing and focusing the system. A general examination of the intra-abdominal organs is performed taking special note of any organ pathology or adhesions. The finding of any trocar-related injuries to intra-abdominal viscera or blood vessels requires an immediate repair using advanced laparoscopic techniques or more commonly open laparotomy.

Three additional trocar ports are placed, using direct visualization of their sites of intra-abdominal penetration. The second 10-mm trocar port is placed in the epigastrium about 1–2 cm below the xiphoid, with its intra-abdominal entrance site being just to the right of the falciform ligament (FIGURE 3). Some surgeons use a 5-mm port at this site. Two smaller 5-mm trocar ports for instruments are then placed: one in the right upper quadrant near the midclavicular line, several centimeters below the costal margin and another quite laterally at almost the level of the umbilicus. These sites may be varied according to the anatomy of the patient and the experience of the surgeon. The patient is placed in a mild (10–15 degrees) reverse Trendelenburg position with slight rotation of the patient slightly to the left (right side up) for optimal visualization of the gallbladder region.

The apex of the gallbladder fundus is grasped with a ratcheted forceps (**A**) through the lateral port. The gallbladder and liver are then lifted superiorly (FIGURE 4). This maneuver provides good exposure of the undersurface of the liver and gallbladder. Omental or other loose adhesions to the gallbladder are gently teased away by the surgeon (FIGURE 5).

The infundibulum of the gallbladder is grasped with forceps (**B**) through the middle port. Lateral traction with the middle forceps exposes the region of the cystic duct and artery. Dissecting forceps or hook cautery (**C**) are used by the surgeon through the subxiphoid port to open the peritoneum over the presumed junction of the gallbladder and cystic duct (FIGURE 6). With gentle teasing and spreading motions, the cystic duct and artery are exposed (FIGURE 6). Each structure is exposed circumferentially. If possible, both structures are dissected free and identified prior to clipping and division. To minimize bile duct injury the concept of the "critical view of safety" is helpful. In this technique, the neck of the gallbladder must be dissected off the liver bed (i.e., unfolding Calot's triangle) to achieve conclusive identification of the two structures to be divided: the cystic duct and cystic artery. In the classic view the liver is seen posterior to Calot's triangle (FIGURE 7). Division of the peritoneum to the right of the infundibulum and cystic duct can be helpful for the initial dissection and minimizes the use of blind dissection closer to the area of the common bile duct.

The window may be verified and elongated by sweeping back and forth through the space with an instrument (FIGURE 7). If the dissection is difficult because of inflammatory swelling and scarring, the surgeon should consider conversion to an open procedure. Whenever there is concern about unclear anatomy, there should be consideration for intraoperative cholangiography or conversion to an open procedure. **CONTINUES ▶**

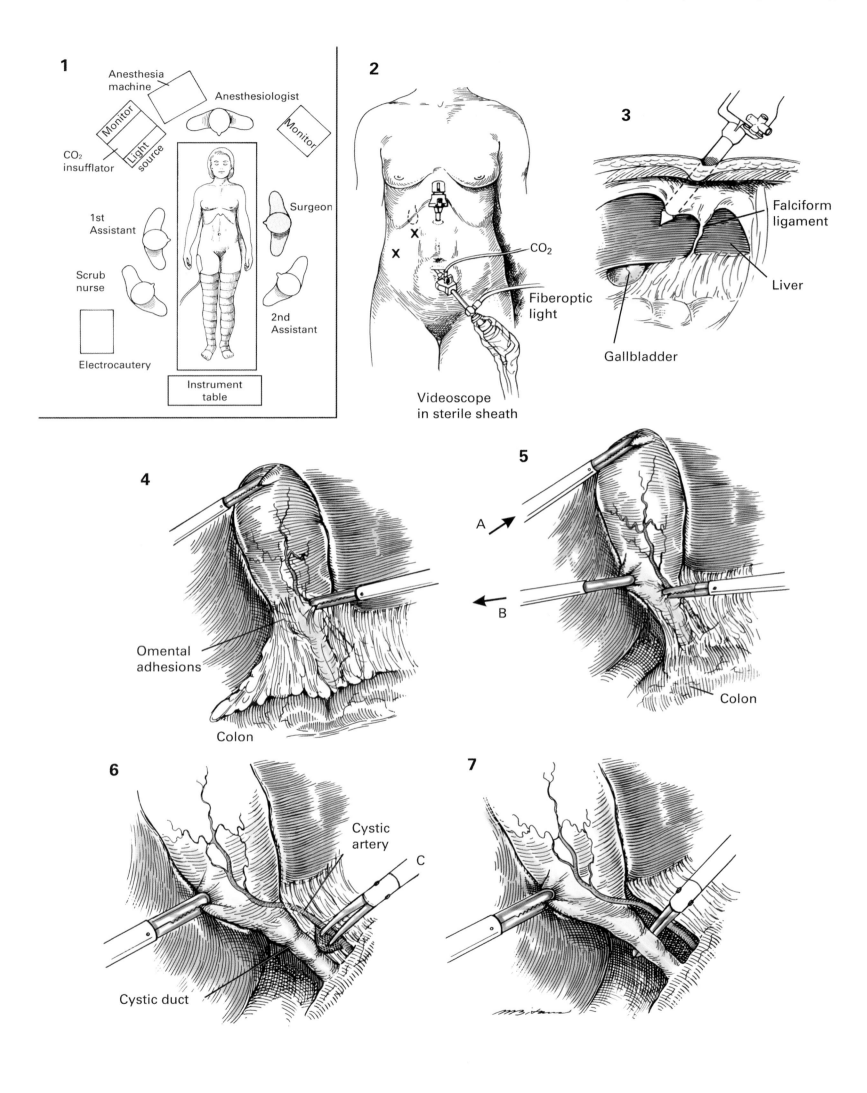

1

Anesthesia machine

Anesthesiologist

Monitor

Monitor

CO_2 insufflator

Light source

Surgeon

1st Assistant

Scrub nurse

2nd Assistant

Electrocautery

Instrument table

2

CO_2

Fiberoptic light

Videoscope in sterile sheath

3

Falciform ligament

Liver

Gallbladder

4

Omental adhesions

Colon

5

A

B

Colon

6

Cystic artery

C

Cystic duct

7

DETAILS OF THE PROCEDURE ◀CONTINUED▶ The cystic artery is cleared for a 1-cm zone and its path followed onto the surface of the gallbladder. The clear zone is then secured with metal clips both proximally and distally (FIGURE 8). The cystic artery may be divided with endoscopic scissors. The cystic duct is also cleared for about 2 cm or so such that the surgeon can clearly identify its continuity with the gallbladder and achieve the critical view of safety. A metal clip is applied as high as possible on the cystic duct where it begins to dilate and form the gallbladder. (FIGURE 9) If no cholangiogram is to be performed, then two clips are placed on the proximal cystic duct and the duct is divided. If a cholangiogram is to be performed, the surgeon should be certain that all the equipment is available. This includes a catheter of choice, two syringes (one for saline and one for contrast), a stopcock for the syringes, and extension tubing. All of the air must be emptied from the tubing prior to performing the cholangiogram. In preparation for insertion of the cholangiogram catheter, the cystic duct is opened and bile is noted (FIGURE 10). If necessary, the opening may be dilated with the scissor tips. The cholangiogram catheter of choice is passed through the middle port or through a 14-guage angiocath inserted into the abdominal wall between the midclavicular trocar and that in the anterior axillary line. The duct is cannulated and the catheter secured (FIGURE 10). Some catheters are secured within a winged clamp, whereas others rely on an inflated intraluminal Fogarty-like balloon. A simple straight plastic catheter such as a 4 French ureteral catheter may be secured with a gently applied metal clip over the lower cystic duct containing the catheter. This should be snug enough to prevent leakage but loose enough to avoid crimping the catheter and preventing dye injection. In preparation for the cholangiogram, the videoscope and metal instruments are removed. The radiolucent ports are aligned in a vertical axis so as to minimize their appearance on the x-ray. The field is covered with a sterile towel and the x-ray equipment positioned. Simple dye injections under fluoroscopy are performed. The principal ducts are visualized in order to ensure anatomic integrity, the absence of ductal stones, and flow into the duodenum. Upon completion of a satisfactory cholangiogram, the lower cystic duct is doubly clipped and the cystic duct divided with endoscopic scissors (FIGURE 11). In the event that an abnormal or confusing cholangiogram is obtained, the surgeon should convert to an open procedure with full anatomic verification. If choledocholithiasis is identified, the surgeon may choose to perform laparoscopic common bile duct exploration or to complete the cholecystectomy and plan for a postoperative ERCP.

The cystic duct–gallbladder junction is grasped with forceps through the middle port and the gallbladder is removed from its bed beginning inferiorly and carrying the dissection up the gallbladder fossa. Most surgeons score the lateral peritoneum for a centimeter or so with electrocautery (FIGURE 12) and then elevate the gallbladder from the liver bed. Appropriate traction, often to the sides, is required to provide exposure of the zone of dissection with an electrocautery instrument between the gallbladder and its bed (FIGURE 13). Vigorous traction with the forceps or dissection into the gallbladder wall may produce an opening with spillage of bile and stones. Such openings should be secured if possible using forceps, metal clips, or a suture loop, which is first placed over the forceps and then closed like a lasso over the hole and the adjacent gallbladder wall that is tented up by the forceps. CONTINUES▶

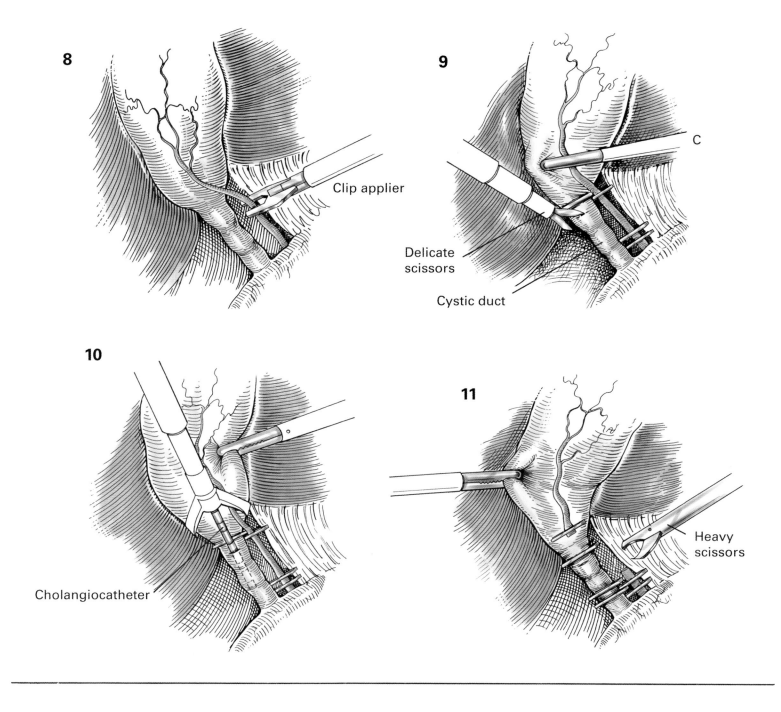

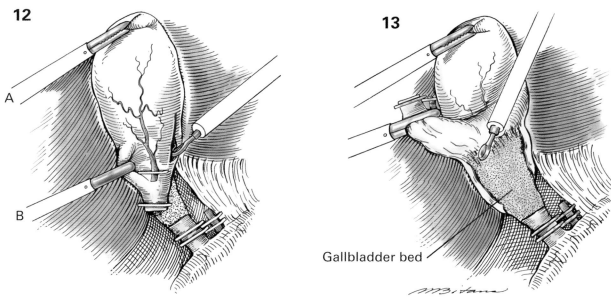

DETAILS OF THE PROCEDURE ◄CONTINUED As the dissection proceeds well up the gallbladder bed, it may be necessary for the first assistant to actively position and reposition the two forceps on the gallbladder so as to provide good exposure for the surgeon. When the dissection is almost complete and traction on the gallbladder still allows superior displacement of the liver with a clear view of the gallbladder bed and operative site, the surgeon should reinspect the clips on the cystic duct and artery for their security and the liver bed for any bleeding sites. The region is irrigated with saline (FIGURE 14) and the diluted bile and blood are aspirated from the lateral gutter just over the edge of the liver. The final peritoneal attachments of the gallbladder are divided from the liver and the gallbladder is positioned above the liver, which has now fallen back inferiorly to its normal position.

The videoscope is removed from the umbilical port and inserted in the epigastric one. If a 5-mm port was used at the subxiphoid site in order to reduce the incidence of incisional hernia, then a 5-mm laparoscope is substituted for the 10-mm scope. Consideration should be given to contain the gallbladder in a laparoscopic retrieval bag prior to removal, especially if there is a concern for malignancy, infection, or if spillage has occurred. A grasping forceps is passed through the umbilical port so as to pick up the end of the specimen in the region of the cystic duct or the specimen retrieval bag (FIGURE 15). This exchange may be somewhat disorienting to the surgeon and first assistant as left and right are now reversed in a mirror-image manner on the monitor screens. If the gallbladder stones are small, one is usually able to withdraw the gallbladder, forceps, and umbilical port back out to the level of the skin where the gallbladder is grasped with a Kelly clamp (FIGURE 16). Bile and small stones may be easily aspirated whereupon the gallbladder will exit easily through the umbilical site under direct vision of the videoscope in the epigastric port. Extraction of large stones or many medium-sized stones may require crushing prior to extraction (FIGURE 17) or require that the linea alba opening be enlarged. After extraction, the umbilical site is temporarily occluded with the assistant's gloved finger so as to maintain the pneumoperitoneum. Alternatively, the gallbladder may be removed through the 10-mm subxiphoid port.

After removal of the gallbladder and final inspection of the abdomen, all ports are removed and the sites closely inspected for bleeding. The videoscope is removed and the pneumoperitoneum is evacuated so as to lessen postoperative discomfort. Placement of peritoneal drains may be considered if there was considerable inflammation, bleeding, a wide cystic duct, or common bile ducts stones identified on intraoperative cholangiography.

CLOSURE The operative sites may be infiltrated with a long-acting local anesthetic (bupivacaine) (FIGURE 18), and the fascia at the 10-mm port sites is sutured with one or two absorbable size 0 sutures (FIGURE 19). The skin is approximated with absorbable subcuticular sutures. Adhesive skin strips and dry sterile dressings are applied.

POSTOPERATIVE CARE The orogastric tube is removed in the operating room prior to emergence from general anesthesia. Pain at the operative site is usually well controlled with oral medications. Although patients have some transient nausea, most are able to take oral liquids soon after surgery and may be discharged to home on the day of surgery. Follow-up by the surgeon is important, as biliary injuries are often occult and delayed in presentation. Prolonged or new, unexpected pain should be evaluated with physical examination, laboratory tests, and appropriate imaging studies. ∎

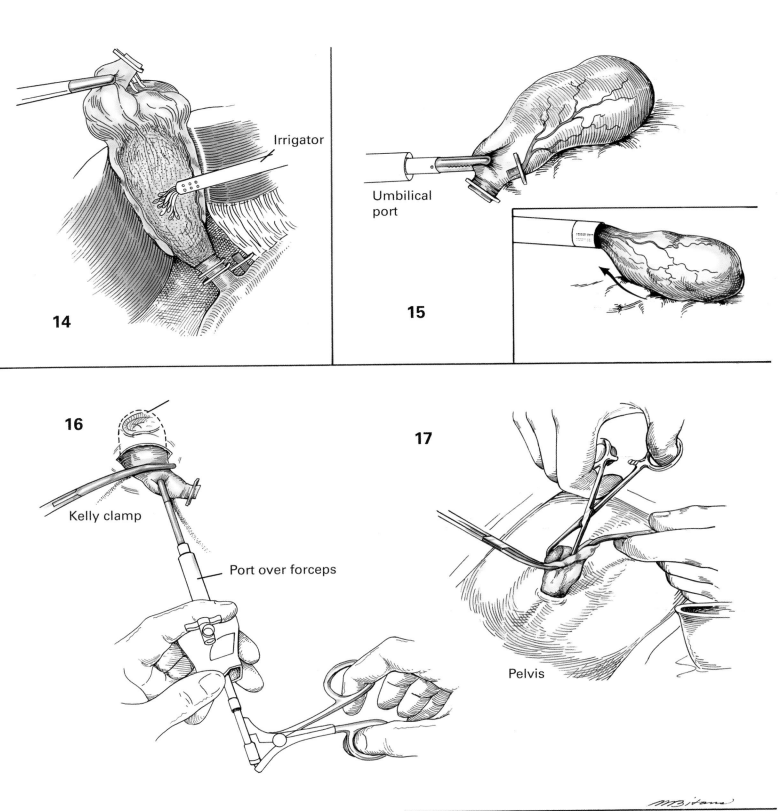

14

Irrigator

15

Umbilical port

16

Kelly clamp

Port over forceps

17

Pelvis

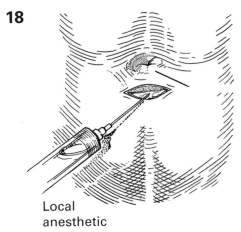

18

Local anesthetic

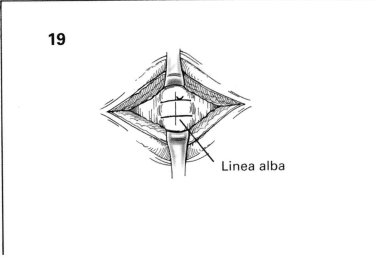

19

Linea alba

CHAPTER 70

CHOLECYSTECTOMY, OPEN RETROGRADE TECHNIQUE

INDICATIONS Cholecystectomy is indicated in patients with proven diseases of the gallbladder that produce symptoms. The incidental finding of gallstones by imaging studies, or a history of vague indigestion, is insufficient evidence for operation in itself and does not justify the risk involved, particularly in the elderly. Today, most patients have laparoscopic removal of their gallbladder. The procedure described here is called "open" and is most commonly performed at a conversion to open when the initial laparoscopic approach encounters complex technical events (swollen, gangrenous gallbladder, confusing anatomy, or abnormal cholangiograms, etc.) or major complications (ductal, blood vessel, or bowel injury) that are best treated with open exposure. Although open cholecystectomy is no longer the primary operation of choice, its mastery is essential for surgeons who perform laparoscopic cholecystectomy. A safe surgeon knows when it is appropriate to convert to an open operation, and does risk endangering the safety of the patient in order to complete the procedure laparoscopically at all costs.

PREOPERATIVE PREPARATION Following a history and physical examination, the diagnosis of biliary disease is typically documented with ultrasound examination of the right upper quadrant. The remainder of the gastrointestinal tract may require additional studies. A chest x-ray and electrocardiogram may be performed as indicated. Routine laboratory blood tests are obtained and should include a liver function panel. Coagulation studies should be ordered if there is a concern for hepatic insufficiency or other causes of coagulopathy. The risks of cholecystectomy include bleeding, infection, visceral injuries, and bile duct injury.

ANESTHESIA General anesthesia with endotracheal intubation is recommended. Deep anesthesia is avoided by the use of a suitable muscle relaxant. In those patients suffering from extensive liver damage, barbiturates as well as other anesthetic agents suspected of hepatotoxicity should be avoided. In elderly or debilitated patients, local infiltration anesthesia is satisfactory, although some type of analgesia is usually necessary as a supplement at certain stages of the procedure.

POSITION The proper position of the patient on the operating table is essential to secure sufficient exposure (FIGURE 1). Arrangements should be made for an operative cholangiogram in the event that one is necessary. A fluoroscopic C-arm requires sufficient space to be centered under the patient to ensure coverage of the liver, duodenum, and head of the pancreas. The exposure can be enhanced by tilting the table until the body as a whole is in a semi-erect position. The weight of the liver then tends to lower the gallbladder below the costal margin. Retraction is also aided in this position, because the intestines have a tendency to fall away from the site of operation.

OPERATIVE PREPARATION The skin is prepared in the routine manner. Patients are administered appropriate prophylactic antibiotics prior to the time of incision. The use of prophylactic antibiotics appears to be more efficacious in patients undergoing open cholecystectomy as compared to laparoscopic surgery, particularly for low-risk patients.

INCISION AND EXPOSURE Two incisions are commonly used: the vertical high midline and the oblique subcostal (FIGURE 2). A midline incision is used if other pathology, such as hiatus hernia or duodenal ulcer, requires surgical consideration. Benefits of the subcostal incision include good exposure, minimal early postoperative wound discomfort, and decreased risk of incisional hernia. The choice of incision is based on surgeon preference and experience. After the incision is made, the details of the procedure are identical, irrespective of the type of incision employed.

DETAILS OF PROCEDURE After the peritoneal cavity has been opened, the gloved hand, moistened with warm saline solution, is used to explore the abdominal cavity, unless there is an acute suppurative infection involving the gallbladder. The stomach and duodenum are inspected and palpated. A general abdominal exploration is performed. The surgeon next passes the right hand up over the dome of the liver, allowing air between the diaphragm and liver to aid in displacing the liver downward (FIGURE 3).

An external ring self-retaining retractor with adjustable retracting blades (such as a Bookwalter type) may be used advantageously. A half-length clamp is applied to the falciform ligament and another to the fundus of the gallbladder (FIGURE 4). Most surgeons prefer to divide the falciform ligament between half-length clamps, and both ends should be ligated; otherwise, active arterial bleeding will result. Downward traction is maintained by the clamps on the fundus of the gallbladder and on the round ligament. This traction is exaggerated with each inspiration as the liver is projected downward (FIGURE 4). After the liver has been pulled downward as far as easy traction allows, the half-length clamps are pulled toward the costal margin to present the undersurfaces of the liver and gallbladder (FIGURE 5). An assistant then holds these clamps while the surgeon prepares to wall off the field. If the gallbladder is acutely inflamed and distended, it is desirable to aspirate some of the contents through a trocar before the half-length clamp is applied to the fundus; otherwise, small stones may be forced into the cystic and common ducts. Adhesions between the undersurface of the gallbladder and adjacent structures are frequently found, drawing the duodenum or transverse colon up into the region of the ampulla. Adequate exposure is maintained by the assistant, who exerts downward traction with a warm, moist sponge. The adhesions are divided with curved scissors or electrical energy until an avascular cleavage plane can be developed adjacent to the wall of the gallbladder (FIGURE 6). After the initial incision is made, it is usually possible to brush these adhesions away with gauze sponges held in thumb forceps (FIGURE 7). Once the gallbladder is freed of its adhesions, it can be lifted upward to afford better exposure. In order that the adjacent structures may be packed away with moist gauze pads, the surgeon inserts the left hand into the wound, palm down, to direct the gauze pads downward. The pads are introduced with long, smooth forceps. The stomach and transverse colon are packed away, and a final gauze pack is inserted into the region of the foramen of Winslow (FIGURE 8). The gauze pads are held in position either with a retractor or by the left hand of the first assistant, who, with fingers slightly flexed and spread apart, maintains moderate downward and slightly outward pressure, better defining the region of the gastrohepatic ligament. **CONTINUES ▶**

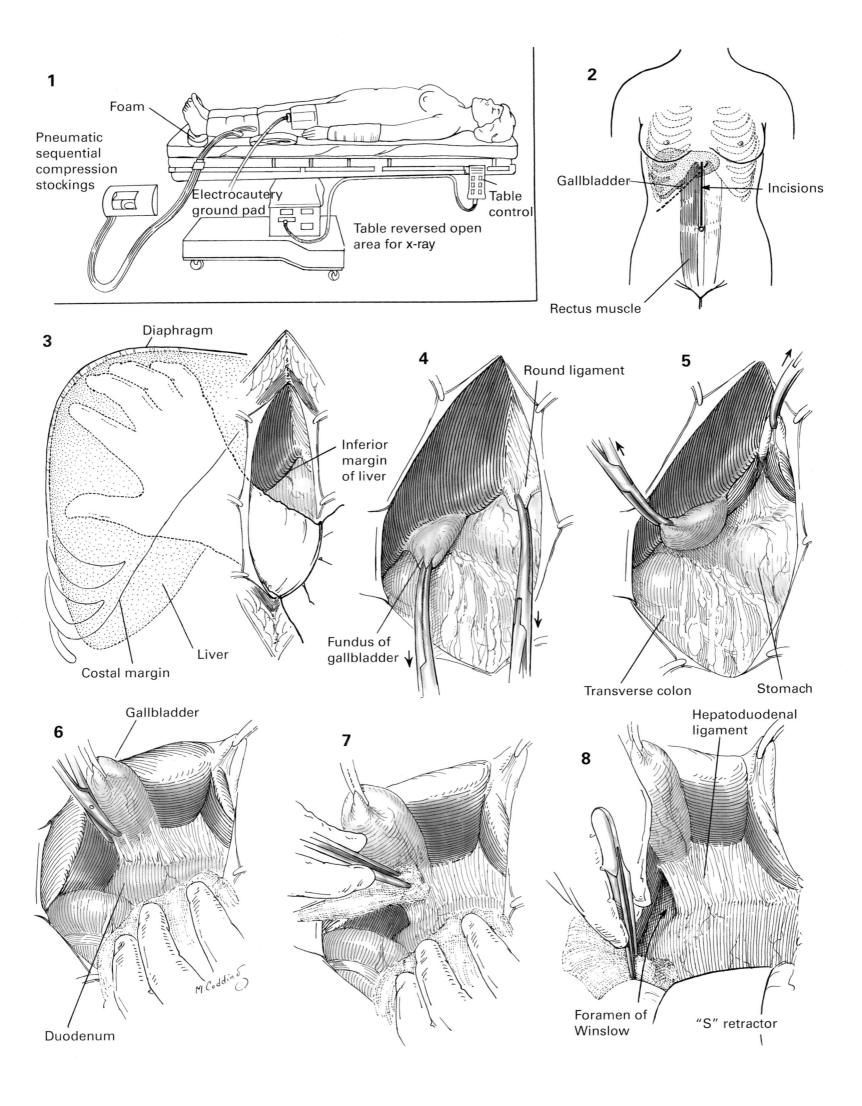

1

Pneumatic sequential compression stockings

Foam

Electrocautery ground pad

Table reversed open area for x-ray

Table control

2

Gallbladder

Incisions

Rectus muscle

3

Diaphragm

Inferior margin of liver

Costal margin

Liver

4

Round ligament

Fundus of gallbladder

5

Transverse colon

Stomach

6

Gallbladder

Duodenum

M Codding

7

8

Hepatoduodenal ligament

Foramen of Winslow

"S" retractor

DETAILS OF PROCEDURE **CONTINUED** After the field has been adequately walled off, the surgeon introduces the left index finger into the foramen of Winslow and, with finger and thumb, thoroughly palpates the region for evidence of calculi in the common duct as well as for thickening of the head of the pancreas. A half-length clamp, with the concavity turned upward, is used to grasp the undersurface of the gallbladder to attain traction toward the operator (FIGURE 9). The early application of clamps in the region of the neck of the gallbladder is one of the frequent causes of accidental injury to the common duct. This is especially true when the gallbladder is acutely distended, because the neck of the gallbladder may run parallel to the common duct for a considerable distance. If the clamp is applied blindly where the neck of the gallbladder passes into the cystic duct, part or all of the common duct may be accidentally included in it (FIGURE 10). For this reason it is always advisable to apply the half-length clamp well up on the undersurface of the gallbladder before any attempt is made to visualize the region of the neck of the gallbladder. The enucleation of the gallbladder is started by dividing the peritoneum on the inferior aspect of the gallbladder and extending it downward to the region of the neck. The peritoneum usually is divided with electrocautery or long Metzenbaum dissecting scissors. The incision is carefully extended downward toward hepatoduodenal ligament (FIGURES 11 and 12). By means of blunt gauze dissection, the region of the neck is freed down to the region of the cystic duct (FIGURE 13). After the neck of the gallbladder has been clearly defined, the clamp on the undersurface of the gallbladder is reapplied lower to the region of the infundibulum or neck.

With traction maintained on the infundibulum, the cystic duct is defined by means of blunt dissection (FIGURE 13). A long right-angle clamp is then passed behind the cystic duct. The jaws of the clamp are separated cautiously as counter-pressure is placed on the upper side of the lower end of the gallbladder by the surgeon's index finger. Slowly and with great care, the cystic duct is isolated from the common duct (FIGURE 14). The cystic artery is likewise isolated with a long right-angle clamp. If the upward traction on the gallbladder is marked, and the common duct is quite flexible, it is not uncommon to have it angulate sharply upward, giving the appearance of a prolonged cystic duct. Under such circumstances, injury to the common duct or its division may result when the right-angle clamp is applied to what is thought to be the cystic duct (FIGURE 15 and inset). Such a disaster may occur when the exposure appears too easy in a thin patient because of the extreme laxity of the common duct.

After the cystic duct has been isolated, it is thoroughly palpated to ascertain that no calculi have been forced into it or the common duct by the application of clamps, and that none will be overlooked in the stump of the cystic duct. The size of the cystic duct is carefully noted before the right-angle clamp is applied. Intraoperative cholangiography may be performed routinely or selectively and is performed through the cystic duct after it has been divided. Because it is more difficult to divide the cystic duct between two closely applied right-angle clamps, a curved half-length clamp is placed adjacent to the initial right-angle clamp. The curvature of the half-length clamp makes it ideally suited for directing the scissors downward during the division of the cystic duct (FIGURE 16). Whenever possible, unless occluded by severe inflammation, the cystic duct and cystic artery are isolated separately to permit individual ligation. Under no circumstances should a right-angle clamp be applied to the presumed region of the cystic duct in the hope that both the cystic artery and duct be included in one mass ligature. It is surprising how much additional cystic duct can often be developed by maintaining traction on the duct as blunt gauze dissection is carried out. After the cholangiogram, the cystic duct is ligated with a transfixing suture (FIGURE 17) or ligature, being sure not to encroach on the common duct. In general, the free length beyond the tie should approximate the diameter of the duct or vessel. It may be helpful to reinforce suture ligatures with metal hemoclips. **CONTINUES**

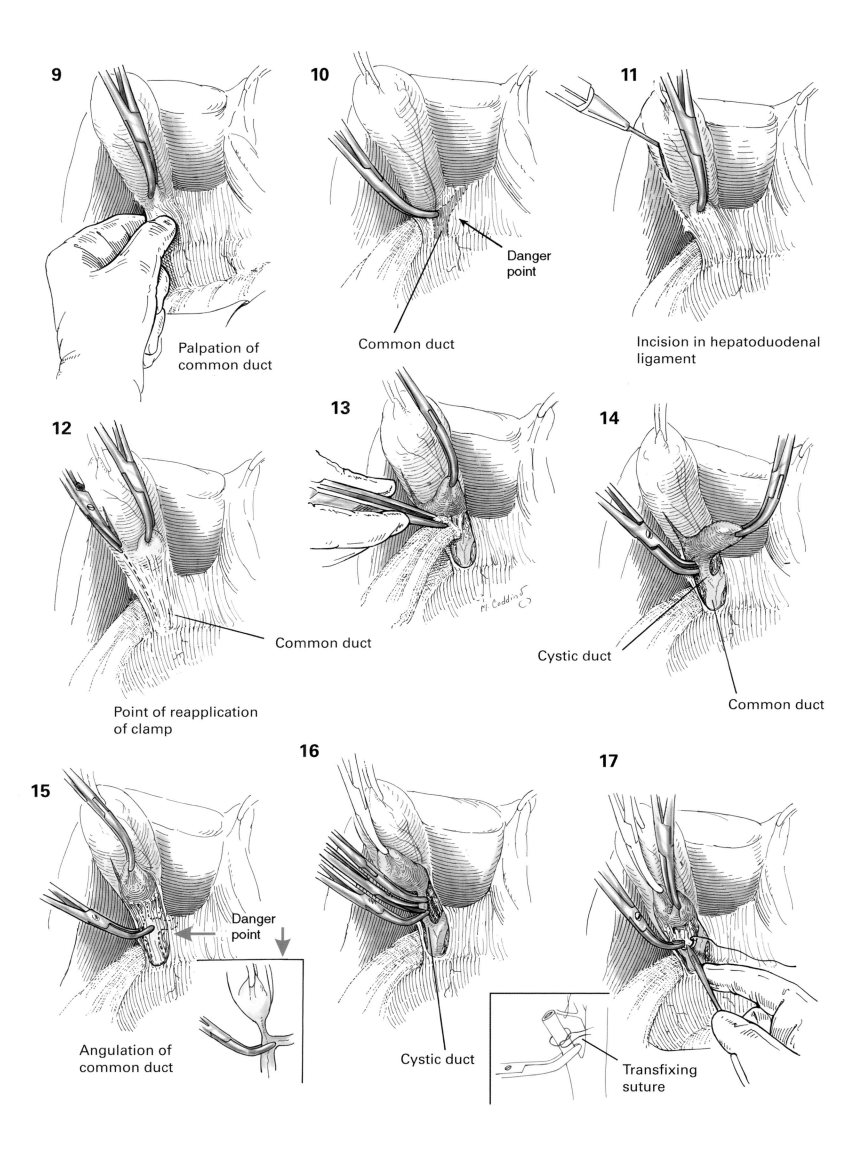

9

Palpation of
common duct

10

Danger
point

Common duct

11

Incision in hepatoduodenal
ligament

12

Common duct

Point of reapplication
of clamp

13

14

Cystic duct

Common duct

15

Danger
point

Angulation of
common duct

16

Cystic duct

17

Transfixing
suture

DETAILS OF PROCEDURE ◄CONTINUED If the cystic artery was not divided before the cystic duct, it is now carefully isolated by a right-angle clamp similar to those used in isolating the cystic duct (FIGURE 18). The cystic artery should be isolated as far away from the region of the hepatic duct as possible. A clamp is never applied blindly to this region, lest the hepatic artery lie in an anomalous location and be clamped and divided (FIGURE 19). Anomalies of the blood supply in this region are so common that this possibility must be considered in every case. The cystic artery is divided between clamps similar to those utilized in the division of the cystic duct (FIGURE 20). The cystic artery should be tied as soon as it has been divided to avoid possible difficulties while the gallbladder is being removed (FIGURE 21). Again, the use of reinforcing metal hemoclips may be useful. If desired, the ligation of the cystic duct can be delayed until after the cystic artery has been ligated. Some prefer to ligate the cystic artery routinely and leave the cystic duct intact until the gallbladder is completely freed from the liver bed. This approach minimizes possible injury to the ductal system as complete exposure is obtained before the cystic duct is divided. If the clamp or tie on the cystic artery slips off, resulting in vigorous bleeding, the hepatic artery may be compressed in the gastrohepatic ligament (Pringle maneuver) by the thumb and index finger of the left hand, temporarily controlling the bleeding (FIGURE 22). The field can be dried with suction by the assistant, and, as the surgeon releases compression of the hepatic artery, a hemostat may be applied safely and exactly to the bleeding point. The stumps of the cystic artery and cystic duct are each inspected thoroughly and, before the operation proceeds, the common duct is again visualized to make certain that it is not angulated or otherwise disturbed. Blind clamping in a bloody field is all too frequently responsible for injury to the ducts, producing the complication of stricture. Classic anatomic relationships in this area should never be taken for granted, since normal variations are more common in this critical zone than anywhere else in the body.

After the cystic duct and artery have been tied, removal of the gallbladder is begun. The incision, initially made on the inferior surface of the gallbladder about 1 cm from the liver edge, is extended upward around the fundus (FIGURE 23). With the left hand, the surgeon holds the clamps that have been applied to the gallbladder and, using electrocautery, divides the loose areolar tissue between the gallbladder and the liver. This allows the gallbladder to be dissected from its bed without dividing any sizable vessels. An operative cholangiogram (FIGURE 24) may be performed to identify common bile duct stones or confirm the biliary anatomy. Syringes of saline-diluted contrast media should be connected by a three-way adapter in a closed system to avoid the introduction of air into the ducts. The cholangiogram catheter is filled with saline and it is introduced a short distance into the cystic duct. The tube is secured in the cystic duct with a tie or clip. All gauze packs, clamps, and retractors are removed as the table is returned to a level position by the anesthesiologist. Five milliliters diluted water-soluble of contrast media are injected under fluoroscopic visualization. Limited amounts of a dilute solution prevent the obliteration of any small calculi within the ducts. A second injection of 15 to 20 mL is made to outline the ductal system completely and to ensure patency of the ampulla of Vater. The tube should be displaced laterally and the duodenum gently pushed to the right to ensure a clear image without interference from the skeletal system or the tube filled with contrast media. If no further studies are warranted, the tube is removed and the cystic duct is ligated. If the cystic duct cannot be used for the cholangiogram, a fine gauge needle, such as a butterfly, can be inserted into the common duct (FIGURE 25). The metal needle may be bent anteriorly as shown in the lateral view inset to facilitate its placement. The puncture site in the common duct is oversewn with a 0000 absorbable suture and some surgeons place a closed suction Silastic suction drain (Jackson–Pratt) in Morrison's pouch. A common bile duct exploration should be performed in all patients found to have choledocholithiasis on intraoperative cholangiography at the time of open cholecystectomy.

The portal vessel area and the gallbladder bed are inspected for hemostasis. Culture of the gallbladder bile is performed in cases where there is a concern for infection.

CLOSURE For a right subcostal incision, the fascia is closed in two layers using running, slowly absorbable, monofilament suture. The skin may be sutured or clipped closed. Most surgeons do not use drains when the field is dry and there is no evidence of leakage from accessory ducts.

POSTOPERATIVE CARE A nasogastric tube may be beneficial for a day or two if significant infection, ileus, or debility is present. Perioperative antibiotics should be discontinued within 24 hours unless the patient has an infection that requires treatment. Coughing and ambulation are encouraged immediately. The diet is advanced to as tolerated, and intravenous fluids are continued until the patient is tolerating adequate oral intake. ■

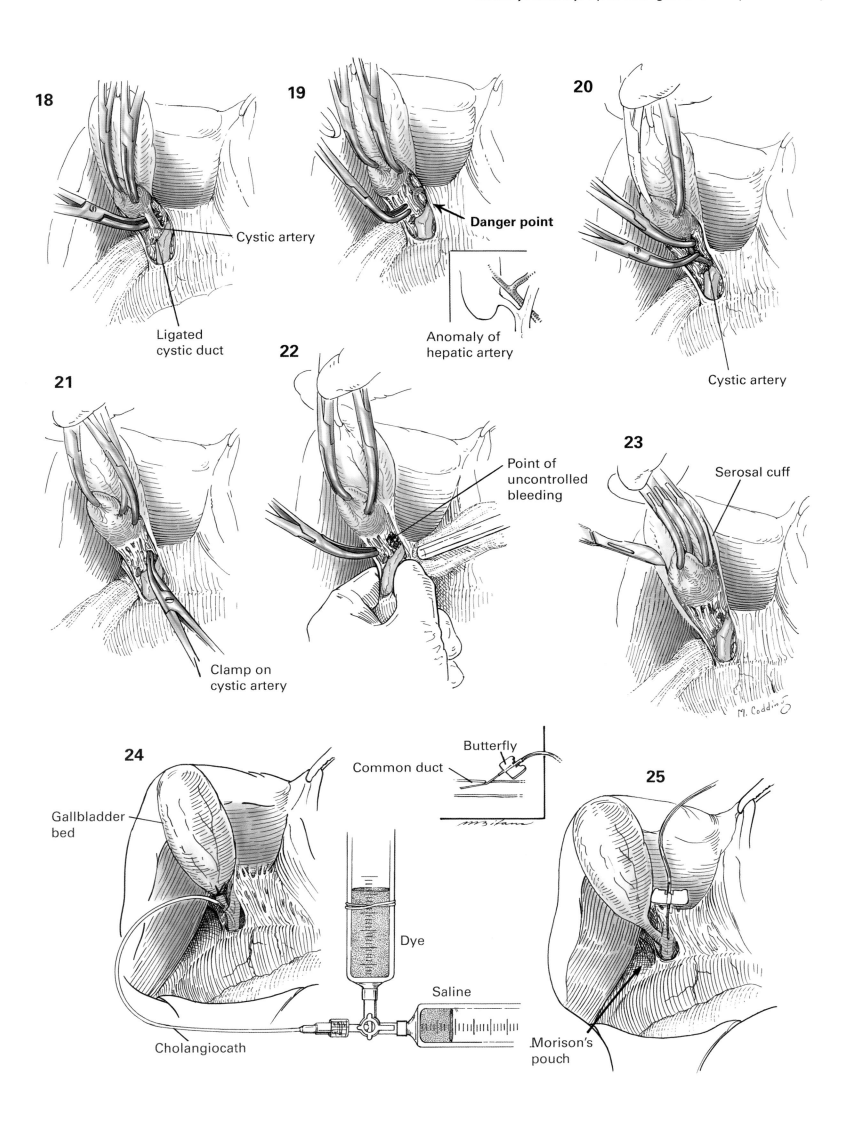

18

Cystic artery

Ligated
cystic duct

19

Danger point

Anomaly of
hepatic artery

20

Cystic artery

21

Clamp on
cystic artery

22

Point of
uncontrolled
bleeding

23

Serosal cuff

M. Codding

24

Gallbladder
bed

Cholangiocath

Butterfly

Common duct

Dye

Saline

25

Morison's
pouch

INDICATIONS Common bile duct exploration should be performed in all patients with common bile duct stones who have either failed, or are not candidates for, endoscopic therapy and who do not have medical conditions that prohibit surgical intervention. Alternative therapies, such as extracorporeal shockwave lithotripsy and dissolving solutions, are not widely available and have limited efficacy. Percutaneous transhepatic cholangiography (PTHC), electrohydraulic lithotripsy, and laser lithotripsy may be useful in a small number of selected patients who are not candidates for surgery or endoscopic therapy. Laparoscopic common bile duct exploration, open common bile duct exploration, and postoperative ERCP with stone removal are all options for the treatment of common bile duct stones identified by intraoperative cholangiography and decision making should be guided by patient-specific considerations, training and experience of the surgeon, and available endoscopic expertise.

Open common bile duct exploration remains an important technique and should be part of every gastrointestinal surgeon's armamentarium for treating hepatobiliary diseases. Open common bile duct exploration may be performed in patients requiring open cholecystectomy, for patients who have failed or suffered complications from laparoscopic common bile duct exploration, and in circumstances where necessary equipment, experience, and/or resources are limited. FIGURE 1 depicts schematically the more common locations of calculi.

PREOPERATIVE PREPARATION In the past, significant time was spent improving hepatic function, as it was believed that anesthesia and surgery were very hazardous in the presence of significant jaundice. Obviously, any coagulopathy must be corrected with vitamin K and blood products, while antibiotics should be given for sepsis or cholangitis. PTHC with retrograde catheter placement for decompression has been largely replaced by endoscopic retrograde cholangiopancreatography (ERCP) with sphincterotomy. This allows stone extraction or stent placement to relieve the obstruction. Appropriate preoperative studies should be obtained (labs, chest x-ray, EKG) as indicated. The patient should be well hydrated and any electrolyte imbalances corrected.

ANESTHESIA General anesthesia with endotracheal intubation is recommended. Anesthetic agents suspected of hepatotoxicity should be avoided. Blood is promptly replaced as it is lost so as to avoid the development of hypotension.

OPERATIVE PREPARATION The skin is prepared in the routine manner. Patients are administered appropriate prophylactic antibiotics prior to the time of incision.

INCISION AND EXPOSURE The abdomen is most commonly opened through a right upper quadrant subcostal incision, although a midline approach is acceptable as well. The use of self-retaining retractors greatly facilitates visualization. The proximal cystic duct should be ligated to prevent gallstones from migrating from the gallbladder into the cystic duct and common bile duct. The liver should be retracted superiorly, the duodenum retracted inferiorly, and the stomach retracted to the left.

DETAILS OF PROCEDURE Dissection is carried out on the anterolateral common bile duct. The peritoneum overlying the common bile duct in the hepatoduodenal ligament is incised distal to the cystic duct (FIGURE 2). Aspiration of the common duct for bile may be performed in order to confirm the anatomy and to prevent inadvertent vascular injury (FIGURE 3). 4-0 monofilament, absorbable stay sutures are placed on the common bile duct just above the level of the duodenum and the duct is opened longitudinally with a scalpel, preserving the lateral blood supply (FIGURE 4). Traction on these sutures can facilitate visualization of the duct contents and instrumentation of the duct (FIGURE 5). The choledochotomy can then be extended with Potts scissors to a length of approximately 1.5 cm. Stones can initially be extracted using a stone scoop or forceps gently inserted into the common bile duct. If this is not possible, balloon extraction can be performed with biliary Fogarty catheters, clearing the proximal duct before the distal duct. These catheters are less traumatic than metal forceps and may be preferred. Saline irrigation can facilitate the removal of fragmented debris by flushing (FIGURES 6 and 7). Choledochoscopy with wire basket retrieval can be employed in the unlikely event that balloon extraction is unsuccessful. A 14-F or larger T-tube should be placed and secured using interrupted 4-0 monofilament, absorbable sutures (FIGURES 8 and 9). The suture line is tested by injecting saline through the T-tube (FIGURE 10). Completion T-tube cholangiography should always be performed prior to closure in order to confirm duct clearance and to rule out bile leaks. Transduodenal sphincteroplasty or choledochoduodenostomy may be performed for distally impacted stones and failures of open common bile duct exploration (CBDE). In the postoperative period a retained stone may be amendable to percutaneous extraction through a mature T-tube tract.

CLOSURE The closure of the gallbladder bed may be accomplished as shown (FIGURE 11) but is usually unnecessary. A closed-system suction catheter made of Silastic is introduced down past the foramen of Winslow into Morison's pouch (FIGURE 11). The catheter and drain are brought out through a stab wound at a level that avoids acute angulation of either the drain or the T-tube (see Chapter 72, FIGURE 9). The catheter is attached to the skin of the abdomen with a skin suture and adhesive tape. The abdomen is closed in a routine manner.

POSTOPERATIVE CARE If the bile loss is excessive, sodium lactate or bicarbonate should be added to compensate for the excessive sodium loss. The fluid balance is maintained by daily administration of approximately 2,000 to 3,000 mL of Ringer's lactate solution. The T-tube catheter is connected to a drainage bag, and the amount of drainage over a 24-hour period is recorded. In the presence of jaundice or a bleeding tendency, blood products and vitamin K are given. The patient is ambulated and returned to oral intake as tolerated. In the absence of cholangitis antibiotics are discontinued within 24 hours. The T-tube should be clamped prior to discharge as long as there are no signs of cholangitis or bile leakage. Patients should be instructed to flush the catheter with 10 mL of sterile saline one to two times a day. The closed suction drain is removed in two to five days unless there is excessive bile drainage. The common duct catheter can be removed in 28 days provided a T-tube cholangiogram shows a normal ductal system and no retained stones. ■

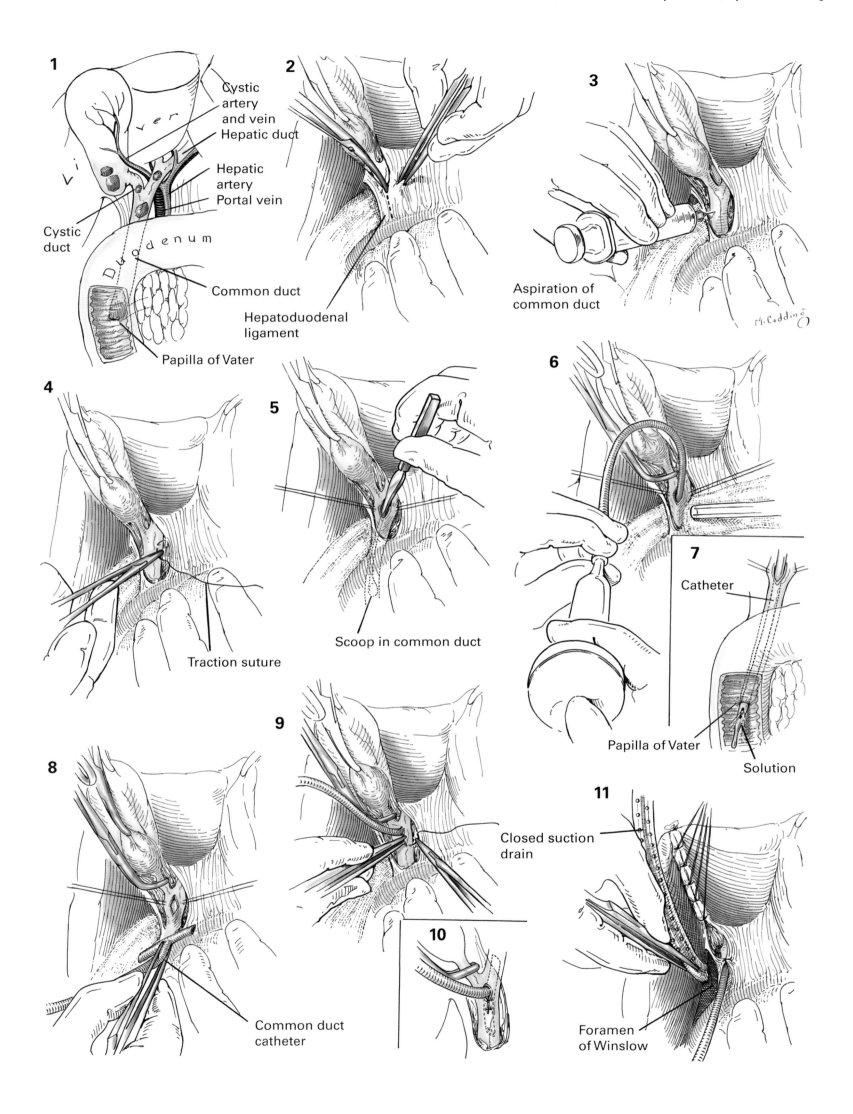

1

Cystic
artery
and vein
Hepatic duct

Hepatic
artery
Portal vein

Cystic
duct

Common duct

Hepatoduodenal
ligament

Papilla of Vater

2

3

Aspiration of
common duct

4

Traction suture

5

Scoop in common duct

6

7

Catheter

Papilla of Vater

Solution

8

9

Closed suction
drain

Common duct
catheter

10

11

Foramen
of Winslow

CHAPTER 72

COMMON BILE DUCT EXPLORATION, TRANSDUODENAL TECHNIQUE

DETAILS OF THE PROCEDURE Sometimes it is impossible to dislodge a stone impacted in the ampulla of Vater by careful and repeated manipulation, and a more radical procedure is necessary. Under such circumstances the duodenum is mobilized by the Kocher maneuver, and the common duct is exposed throughout its course down to the duodenal wall. An incision is made in the lateral part of the peritoneal attachment of the duodenum, making it possible to mobilize the second portion of the duodenum (FIGURE 1). After the peritoneal attachment has been incised, blunt gauze dissection is used to sweep the duodenum medially. Occasionally, this will expose the retroduodenal portion of the common duct and will allow more direct palpation (FIGURE 2). A blunt metal probe is introduced downward to the point of the obstruction, and the location of the stone is more accurately determined by palpation. A scoop is passed down to the region of the ampulla of the common bile duct, and its course is directed carefully with the index finger and thumb of the surgeon's left hand (FIGURE 3). With the tissues being held firmly by the thumb and index finger, it is usually possible to break up the impacted calculus with the scoop. Should this prove unsuccessful, it is necessary to open the anterior duodenal wall and to expose Vater's papilla (FIGURE 4).

Since opening the duodenum tends to increase the risk of complications, it should not be considered until all indirect methods have been tried. In fact, many surgeons will proceed directly to choledochoduoenostomy (Chapter 73), particularly in cases where there is a dilated common bile duct.

By exerting gentle pressure on a uterine sound or a biliary Fogarty inserted in to the common duct, the surgeon can determine the exact location of the papilla by palpation over the anterior wall of the duodenum. With the duodenal wall held taut in Babcock forceps or by silk sutures, an incision 3 to 4 cm long is made over this area, parallel to the long axis of the bowel. A transverse duodenotomy is also acceptable if the location of the ampulla has been identified adequately and transverse closure of defect results in less narrowing and deformity of the duodenum. The field must be completely walled off by gauze sponges, and constant suction must be maintained to avoid contamination by bile and pancreatic juice. Small gauze sponges are then introduced upward and downward within the lumen of the duodenum to prevent further soiling. Long silk sutures are attached to each of these gauze sponges to ensure their subsequent removal (FIGURE 5). Even at this point the calculus may be dislodged by direct palpation. If this is still impossible, the probe is reintroduced and directed firmly against the region of the papilla to determine the direction of the duct, so that a small incision may be made directly parallel to it (FIGURE 5). This incision enlarges the papilla so that a calculus can either be expressed or be removed with fenestrated stone forceps (FIGURE 6). Following this, the patency of the common duct is ascertained by introducing a small and soft red rubber catheter (8 French) into the opening of the common duct and downward through the papilla (FIGURE 7). Any bleeding points from the incision into the papilla are controlled by fine 0000 interrupted absorbable sutures (FIGURE 8). The pancreatic duct must not be occluded by these sutures. No effort is made to reconstruct the papilla to its natural size, the opening being allowed to remain enlarged as a result of the incision. A sphincterotomy or sphincteroplasty can be performed through this exposure. These procedures involve the pancreatic duct as well as the common duct.

The small gauze sponges that plug the duodenum are withdrawn, and the intestine is closed. The bowel is closed in the opposite direction from that in which the incision was made. This avoids constricting the lumen of the bowel (FIGURE 9). The duodenal wall is sutured with interrupted 3-0 silk sutures, starting at the angle adjacent to one of the Babcock clamps. The serosa may be reinforced with a layer of interrupted Halsted mattress sutures of 00 silk (FIGURE 10). This closure must be watertight and secure to avoid the complication of duodenal fistula. A T-tube catheter is introduced into the common duct, and the duodenum is distended with normal saline to make certain that there is no leakage. A No. 14-French T-tube is then directed into the initial opening of the common duct, and the technique from this point on is observed as described in Chapter 71, FIGURES 9, 10 and 11. A closed-system suction catheter made of Silastic is inserted down past the foramen of Winslow into Morrison's pouch in all cases and remains there until there is no danger of duodenal fistula. It is advisable to bring the common-duct catheter and the drain out through a stab wound lateral to the incision (FIGURE 11). It is safest to avoid clamping the common-duct catheter, permitting it to drain into a sterile gauze sponge until it is attached to a drainage plastic bag. The bile is cultured for bacterial content and antimicrobial sensitivities.

CLOSURE The abdomen is closed in the routine manner (see Chapter 10, pages 34–39).

POSTOPERATIVE CARE If the bile loss is excessive, sodium lactate or bicarbonate should be added to compensate for the excessive sodium loss. The fluid balance is maintained by daily administration of approximately 2,000 to 3,000 mL of Ringer's lactate solution. The T-tube catheter is connected to a drainage bag, and the amount of drainage over a 24-hour period is recorded. In the presence of jaundice with a bleeding tendency, blood products, and vitamin K are given. The patient is ambulated and returned to oral intake as tolerated. Antibiotics are discontinued within 24 hours. The T-tube should be clamped prior to discharge as long as there are no signs of cholangitis or bile leakage. Patients should be instructed to flush the catheter with 10 mL of sterile saline one to two times a day. The Silastic drain is removed in 2 to 5 days unless there is excessive bile drainage. The common duct catheter can be removed in 10 to 14 days after a T-tube cholangiogram shows a normal ductal system, but we prefer to leave them in place for four weeks. ■

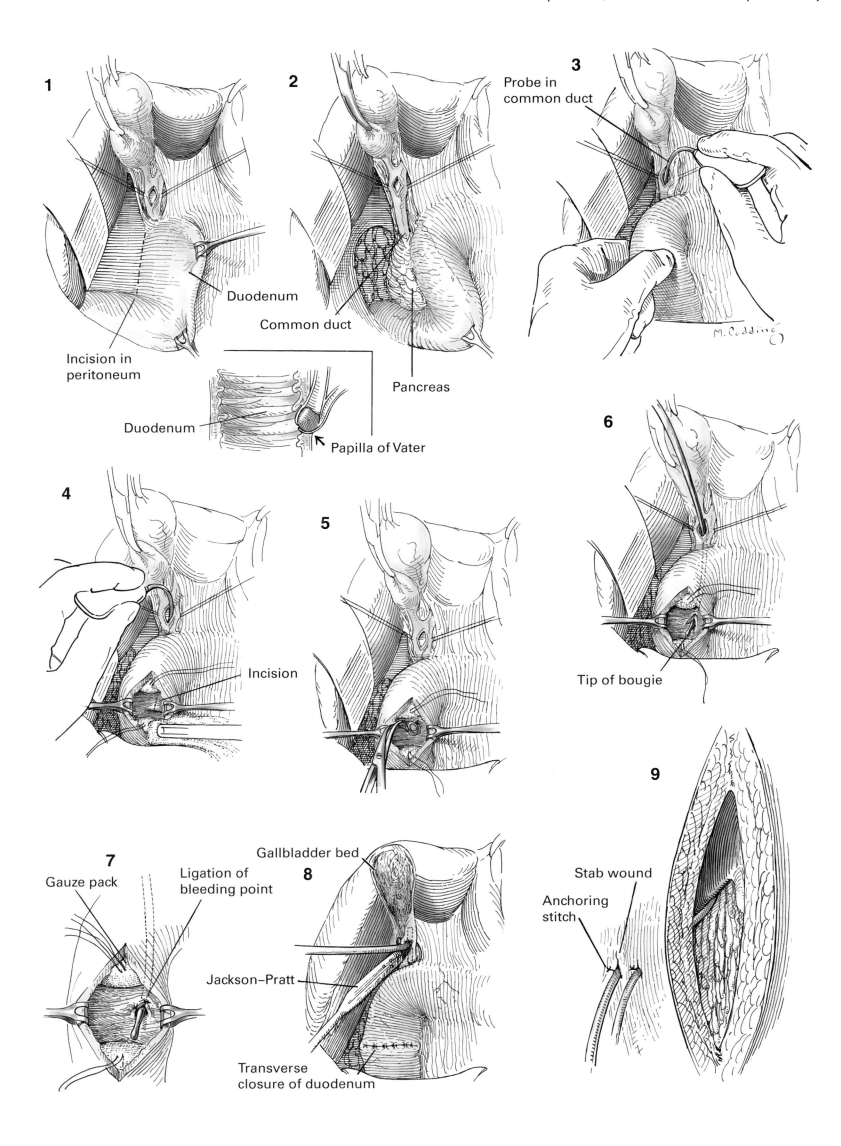

1

Incision in
peritoneum

Duodenum

2

Common duct

Pancreas

Duodenum

Papilla of Vater

3

Probe in
common duct

M. Codding

4

5

Incision

6

Tip of bougie

7

Gauze pack

Ligation of
bleeding point

8

Gallblader bed

Jackson–Pratt

Transverse
closure of duodenum

9

Stab wound

Anchoring
stitch

CHAPTER 73

CHOLEDOCHODUODENOSTOMY

INDICATIONS This is a procedure favored by many in place of the transduodenal approach for stones impacted in the ampulla, and is indicated for the treatment of primary common bile duct stones with a dilated common bile duct, or benign strictures of the distal bile duct. The procedure should not be considered for a nondilated common duct, recurrent pancreatitis, sclerosing cholangitis, or common bile duct stone amenable to endoscopic removal. The procedure of choledochoduodenostomy in properly selected patients may be far safer, with long-term results more satisfactory, than those that follow more complicated procedures for the excision of diverticuli.

PREOPERATIVE PREPARATION Liver function studies are evaluated, and consultation with an endoscopist should be considered. Antibiotics are given preoperatively.

ANESTHESIA General anesthesia is preferred. The anesthesiologist must consider liver function studies as well as age and general condition of the patient in selecting the type of anesthetic to be administered.

POSITION The patient is placed flat on the table with the feet lower than the head. Slight rotation toward the side of the surgeon may improve exposure.

OPERATIVE PREPARATION The skin is prepared from the lower chest to the lower abdomen.

INCISION AND EXPOSURE A right subcostal incision or an upper midline incision is made. Adhesions to the peritoneum are carefully freed up, including those that tend to prevent mobilization of the liver needed for exposure of the common duct.

DETAILS OF PROCEDURE Following a general abdominal exploration, special attention is given to the size of the common duct as well as any evidence of ulcer deformity or acute inflammatory involvement of the first portion of the duodenum. A biopsy of the liver may be considered and needle aspiration of bile from the common duct is obtained for culture to guide appropriate antibiotic therapy. The diameter of the duct is measured and should be 2 to 2½ cm in diameter. If the gallbladder has not been removed previously, it should be excised, particularly if stones are present. The cystic duct and the common duct are carefully palpated for possible calculi. Any calculus, especially in the lower end of the common duct, should be removed when the common duct is opened for the anastomosis. Any inflammatory involvement of the duodenum should be noted, as this may contraindicate the planned procedure.

The duodenum and head of the pancreas should be mobilized by incising the peritoneum from the region of the foramen of the Winslow around to the third portion of the duodenum (FIGURE 1). The entire duodenum should be freed up by the Kocher maneuver and further mobilized by the hand placed under the head of the pancreas.

The anterior aspect of the common duct is cleaned as far down as possible. The surgeon should not be tempted to perform a convenient side-to-side anastomosis between the dilated common duct and the duodenum as the resultant small stoma dooms the procedure to failure. The secret of success is related to the adequate mobilization of the duodenum, the adequate size of the stoma, and finally the triangularization of the anastomosis in accordance with the technique of Gliedman. This type of anastomosis decreases the potential for the development of the sump syndrome due to the collection of food particles and calculi in the blind segment of the lower end of the common duct.

Before making the incision, the mobilized duodenum is brought up alongside the common duct to be certain the anastomosis will be free of tension (FIGURE 2).

An incision about 2.5 cm long is made carefully in the middle of the common duct below the entrance of the cystic duct. The location for the anastomosis obviously will vary depending upon the anatomy presented. A slightly smaller incision is made in the adjacent duodenum in a longitudinal direction.

It should be remembered that the early success of this procedure may rest upon the accuracy of the right-angle approximation of the vertical incision in the common duct to the transverse incision in the duodenum.

Usually three traction sutures (a, b, and c) are placed to ensure that the vertical incision in the common duct will be similar in length to the transverse incision in the duodenum. Special attention must be given to the placement of the first suture (midpoint a), which involves the midportion of the incision in the duodenum and the lower angle of the incision in the common duct. Similar sutures (angles b, c) are placed through either end of the duodenal incision (FIGURE 3). These angle sutures pass from either end of the duodenal stoma fissure from outside to inside and from inside to outside in the midportion of the incision in the common duct.

Traction on these angle sutures (b, c) verifies the triangularization of the stoma in the common duct. Delayed absorbable or nonabsorbable polypropylene sutures may be used. Silk should be avoided as it can result in a focus for infection or stone formation. The proper placement of these early sutures ensures the subsequent accuracy of the anastomosis. The posterior row is approximated using interrupted sutures placed 2–3 mm apart. The knots for the posterior row will be inside the stoma. It is best for the surgeon to start at one end and sew towards him or herself. The sutures are secured with atraumatic clamps until the row has been completed. When the posterior row has been completed, all sutures are tied and then cut except the original angle sutures (b, c) (FIGURE 4).

Before closing the anterior layer, a guide traction suture (midpoint D) may be passed from outside to inside the midportion of the duodenal opening to inside to outside the apex of the longitudinal suture in the common duct. Traction on this suture ensures more accurate placement of the interrupted sutures for closing the anterior layer (FIGURE 5). Again, the sutures are placed 2 to 3 mm apart and held in place with atraumatic clamps with the surgeon sewing towards him or herself. Once all of the sutures have been placed, the knots are tied and then the suture is cut. The sutures should be placed so that the knots will be on the outside of the anterior row (FIGURE 6).

An additional suture is taken at either angle to affix the duodenum either to the capsule of the liver laterally (x) or to the hepatoduodenal ligament medially (x') (FIGURE 7).

The plateau of the stoma is tested by finger compression against the duodenal wall (FIGURE 8). The anastomosis should be free of tension and the angles secure. A closed-suction-system Silastic drain may be placed adjacent to the anastomosis and down into Morison's pouch.

CLOSURE Closure of the abdominal wall is accomplished in a routine manner.

POSTOPERATIVE CARE Antibiotics are given. If there is an insignificant output from the closed-suction drain, it is removed after a few days. Nasogastric suction may be indicated for a day or so. Diet is advanced as tolerated. Liver function tests should be restudied as needed during the postoperative recovery period. ■

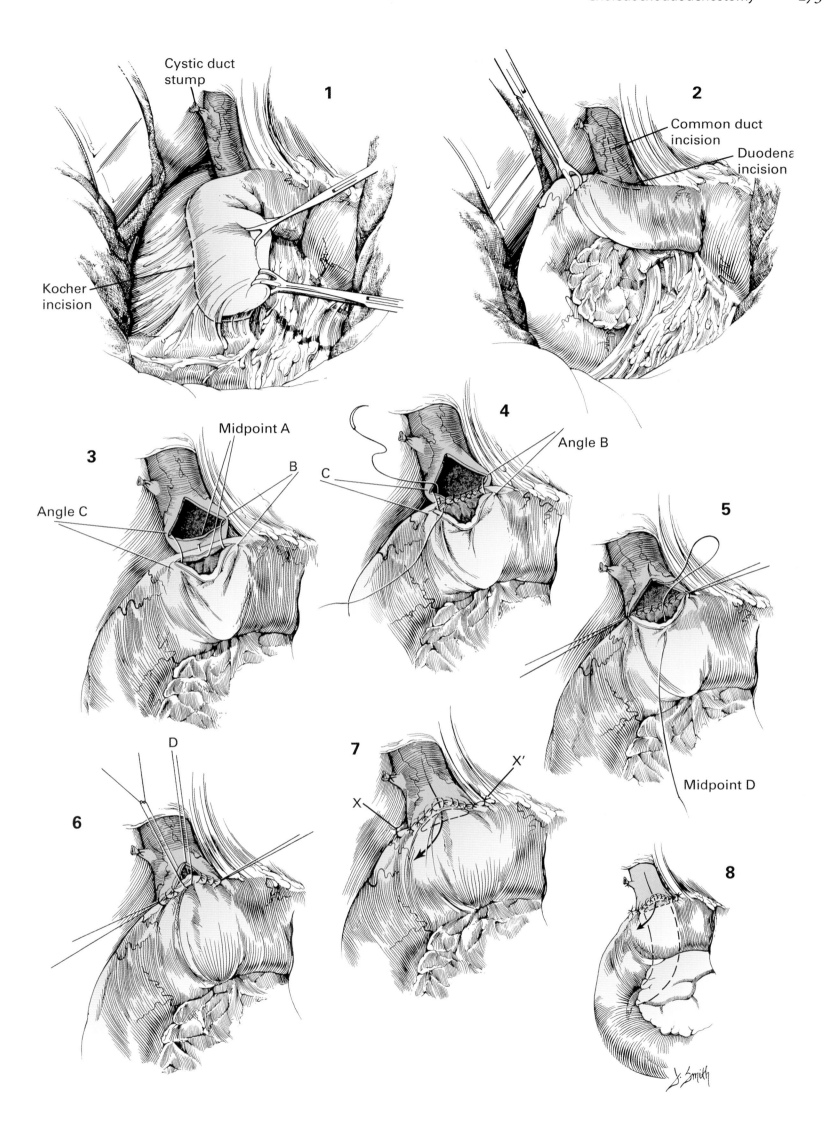

1

Cystic duct stump

Kocher incision

2

Common duct incision

Duodenal incision

3

Midpoint A

B

Angle C

4

Angle B

C

5

Midpoint D

6

D

7

X

X'

8

CHOLECYSTECTOMY, PARTIAL CHOLECYSTECTOMY

A. CHOLECYSTECTOMY FROM FUNDUS DOWNWARD ("Dome-down approach")

INDICATIONS Cholecystectomy from the fundus downward is the desirable method in many cases of acute or gangrenous cholecystitis, where exposure of the cystic duct is difficult and hazardous. Extensive adhesions, a large, thick-walled, acutely inflamed gallbladder, or a large calculus impacted in the neck of the gallbladder makes this the safe and wiser procedure. Better definition of the cystic duct and cystic artery is ensured with far less chance of injury to the common duct. Some prefer this method of cholecystectomy as a routine procedure.

PREOPERATIVE PREPARATION In the presence of acute cholecystitis, the preoperative treatment depends on the severity and duration of the attack. Early operation is indicated in patients seen within 48 hours after the onset, as soon as fluid balance and antibiotic coverage have been established. Frequent clinical and laboratory evaluation over a 24-hour period is necessary. Antibiotic therapy is given. Regardless of the duration of the acute manifestations, surgical intervention is indicated if there is recurrence of pain, a mounting white cell count, or an increase in the signs and symptoms suggesting a perforation. The gallbladder may show advanced acute inflammation despite a normal temperature and white count and negative physical findings. It is generally recommended that patients undergo surgery within 72 hours of the onset of symptoms as delays longer than this are associated with an increased risk of common bile duct injury. Percutaneous cholecystostomy may be considered for patients with a delayed presentation, or for those who are too ill to tolerate surgery. These patients may undergo interval cholecystectomy in 6 weeks.

ANESTHESIA See Chapter 70.

POSITION The patient is placed in the usual position for gallbladder surgery. If local anesthesia is used, the position may be modified slightly to make the patient more comfortable.

OPERATIVE PREPARATION The skin is prepared in the usual manner.

INCISION AND EXPOSURE Incision and exposure are carried out as shown in Chapter 70 The omentum must be separated carefully by either sharp or blunt dissection from the fundus of the gallbladder, care being taken to tie all bleeding points. An oblique incision below the costal margin is preferred, especially if the mass presents rather far laterally.

DETAILS OF PROCEDURE Blunt dissection only is utilized to free the omentum and other structures from the gallbladder wall. It is safer to empty the contents of the gallbladder immediately to decrease the bulk and to give more exposure. A short incision is made through the serosa of the fundus, a trocar introduced, and the liquid contents are removed by suction. Cultures are taken. A fenestrated forceps is introduced deep into the gallbladder to remove any calculi in the ampulla. The opening is closed with a purse-string suture, which prevents further soiling and serves as traction.

Incisions are made into the serosa of the gallbladder along both sides about 1 cm from the liver substance with a scalpel or electrocautery (FIGURE 1); otherwise, excessive traction will result in avulsion of the gallbladder from the liver bed. Separation is accomplished by blunt or scissors dissection, especially since the loose tissue beneath the serosa is edematous in the presence of acute cholecystitis (FIGURE 2). The cuff of gallbladder serosa in the region of the fundus is held with forceps, while the gallbladder is further freed by scissors dissection (FIGURE 3).

As an alternative method, since the contents have been aspirated and are frequently sterile, the opening in the fundus is enlarged, permitting the index finger or a gauze sponge to be inserted to give counter-resistance and to aid in dissecting within the developed cleavage plane.

The serosa is incised on each side down to the ampulla of the gallbladder. Since there may be difficulty from oozing because the cystic artery is intact, all bleeding points should be meticulously clamped or cauterized. As the cuff at the margin of the liver is held by a curved, half-length clamp, a relatively dry field is obtained if the cuff is closed with interrupted sutures as the dissection progresses down to the ampulla (FIGURE 4). Most surgeons, however, leave the cuff edges free. Great care must be taken in mobilizing the infundibulum and neck of the gallbladder. Alternate sharp and gauze dissection is advisable until the majority of adhesions have been separated. The gallbladder is retracted medially and outward to assist in identifying the cystic duct and cystic artery. The cystic duct is isolated with a right-angle clamp cautiously introduced from the lateral side to avoid injury to the common duct and to the right hepatic artery (FIGURE 4). The cystic artery is isolated with any accompanying indurated tissue. The artery may be much larger than normal, and the right hepatic artery may be in an anomalous position. It is safer to isolate the cystic artery as near the gallbladder wall as possible. The cystic artery and adjacent tissues are divided between a half-length and a right-angle clamp (FIGURE 5) and ligated.

The cystic duct is palpated carefully, especially if acute cholecystitis is present, to ensure that a stone has not been overlooked. The common duct is palpated carefully, and exploration is avoided unless cholangiography shows clear-cut evidence of a choledocholithiasis. If common bile duct exploration is not indicated, the cystic duct is divided between right-angle and half-length clamps (FIGURE 6) and tied unless a cholangiogram is planned through the cystic duct. After thorough inspection of the area for oozing, the clamp is removed from the liver margin. Since inflammation and technical difficulties have made this procedure necessary, placement of a drain should be considered, particularly if raw liver parenchyma has been exposed.

B. PARTIAL CHOLECYSTECTOMY

If a classic open cholecystectomy appears hazardous because of advanced inflammation, if the gallbladder is partially buried in the liver, or if structures in the cystic duct region cannot be safely identified, the full thickness of the gallbladder is left within the liver bed. A very specific indication for this procedure occurs in patients with cirrhosis of the liver and portal hypertension. Attempts to remove the back wall of the gallbladder will result in significant hemorrhage that can be extremely difficult to control. The gallbladder is aspirated, and traction is exerted on the fundus. The inferior surface is divided cautiously down to the infundibulum, which may be densely adherent to the adjacent structures (FIGURE 7). Calculi impacted in the neck or cystic duct are removed with fenestrated forceps (FIGURE 8). The gallbladder wall beyond the liver margin is excised, and any bleeding points are controlled with electrocautery or interrupted sutures. The mucosa in the retained portion of the gallbladder head is fulgurated by electrocautery. If the cystic duct can be intubated with a small catheter (FIGURE 9) and a cholangiogram may be performed. Often the gangrenous cystic duct cannot be found and closed suction drains are placed in the general region of the duct. Fortunately, the spiral valves in the retained cystic duct stump usually scar shut. The duct and artery should be ligated if they are identified.

CLOSURE The abdomen is closed in the routine fashion. Drains should be brought out through separate stab wounds.

POSTOPERATIVE CARE NG decompression is rarely used if needed. The patient should be treated with a 5- to 7-day course of broad spectrum antibiotics and intraoperative cultures can be used to guide therapy. Liver function tests should be monitored. The diet is advanced as tolerated, and intravenous fluids are continued until the patient is tolerating adequate oral intake. Drains should be left in until the output is minimal. Cholangiography by MRCP or ERCP should be considered in patients with persistent bilious drainage or elevated liver function tests, although most bile leaks will resolve without the need for intervention. ■

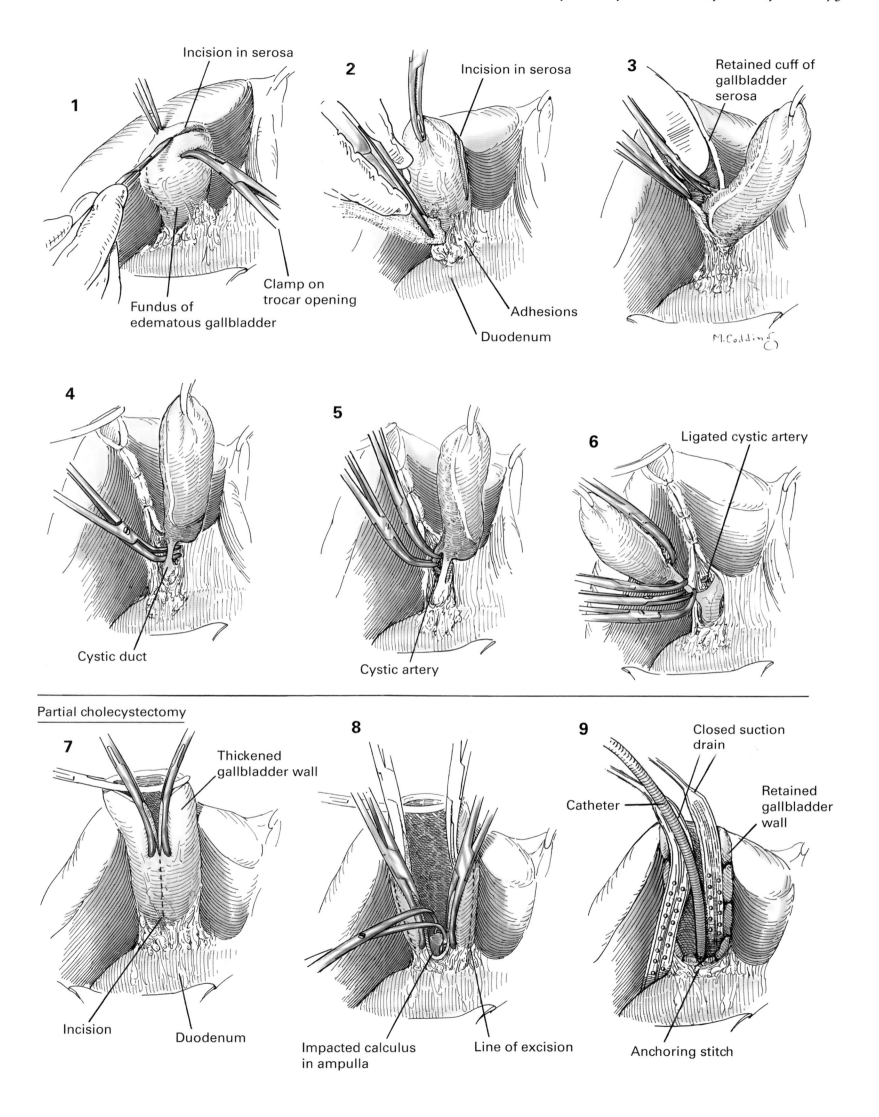

1   Incision in serosa

Fundus of edematous gallbladder

Clamp on trocar opening

2   Incision in serosa

Adhesions

Duodenum

3   Retained cuff of gallbladder serosa

M.Codding

4   Cystic duct

5   Cystic artery

6   Ligated cystic artery

Partial cholecystectomy

7   Thickened gallbladder wall

Incision

Duodenum

8   Impacted calculus in ampulla

Line of excision

9   Closed suction drain

Catheter

Retained gallbladder wall

Anchoring stitch

CHOLECYSTOSTOMY

INDICATIONS Cholecystostomy, while not recognized as routine treatment for cholelithiasis, may be a lifesaving procedure. Today cholecystostomy is usually placed under image guidance by a percutaneous technique. Surgical cholecystostomy may be needed in some situations. It is the operation of choice in some elderly patients with acute cholecystitis, in poor surgical risks who present a well-defined mass, in seriously ill patients in whom minimum surgery is desirable, and when technical difficulties make cholecystectomy hazardous. If there is obstruction of the common duct with long-standing jaundice and a tendency toward hemorrhage that cannot be controlled by vitamin K and transfusions or percutaneous transhepatic biliary tube drainage, preliminary cholecystostomy for decompression may be the procedure of choice.

INCISION AND EXPOSURE A small incision is made with its midportion directly over the maximum point of tenderness in the right upper quadrant. Occasionally, when unsuspected technical difficulties or inflammation more severe than anticipated are encountered, the procedure is carried out through the usual upper right rectus or infracostal incision. The adhesions are not dissected from the undersurface of the gallbladder unless it is thought that cholecystectomy might be feasible (FIGURE 1).

DETAILS OF PROCEDURE The fundus is walled off with gauze before the evacuation of its contents. An incision is made just through the serosa of the bulging fundus (FIGURE 2). A trocar is inserted to remove the liquid contents (FIGURE 3). Suction is maintained adjacent to the incision in the fundus as the trocar is withdrawn. A culture is taken routinely. The edematous wall is then grasped with Babcock forceps, and the opening is extended (FIGURE 4). A purse-string suture of fine absorbable material is placed about the opening in the fundus to control oozing and to close the fundus about the drainage tube. Any liquid or debris remaining in the lumen of the gallbladder is removed by suction. Since there is usually an impacted stone in the neck of the gallbladder, a determined effort is made to remove it to permit drainage of the gallbladder. A small, flexible scoop, such as a Cushing pituitary curette, is directed down to the neck (FIGURE 5). If the scoop cannot dislodge the stones, a fenestrated forceps is used. The lumen of the gallbladder is repeatedly flooded with saline. A small rubber catheter or mushroom catheter is inserted into the lumen of the gallbladder and anchored with an interrupted silk suture (FIGURES 6 and 7) or a Foley catheter may be used. The previously placed purse-string suture is tied snugly about the drainage tube (FIGURE 7). If the inflammation is severe, if an abscess was encountered, or if there has been soiling about the wall, a closed suction drain is inserted along the wall of the gallbladder. The common duct must be decompressed if suppurative cholangitis is suspected.

CLOSURE Stitches are taken to anchor the fundus to the overlying peritoneum to prevent the soiling of the peritoneal cavity before the area is sealed off (FIGURE 8). Routine closure is performed. After a sterile dressing has been applied, the drainage tube is anchored to the skin with a suture or adhesive tape and is connected to a drainage bottle.

POSTOPERATIVE CARE See Chapter 74. Antibiotics should be administered for 5 to 7 days after drainage. While the drainage tube is in place, contrast may be injected and a cholangiogram taken for evidence of overlooked calculi. If the patient is in good condition, and the postoperative recovery is uncomplicated, a subsequent cholecystectomy may be performed through the original wound after 6 weeks. A secondary operation after cholecystostomy is not recommended in the extremely poor-risk patient. For high-risk patients who survive their attack of cholecystitis, the cholecystostomy tube may be removed if cholangiography through the catheter demonstrates a patent cystic duct with good flow of contrast into the duodenum. ■

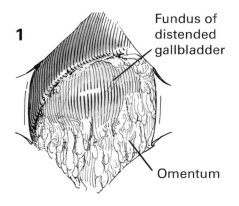

1
Fundus of distended gallbladder

Omentum

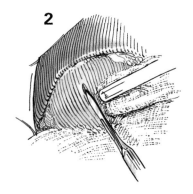

2

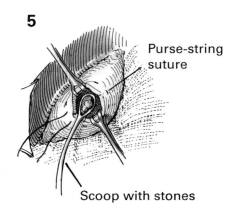

3

Suction

Trocar

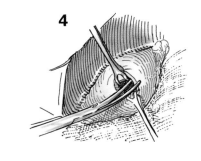

4

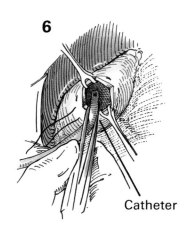

5

Purse-string suture

Scoop with stones

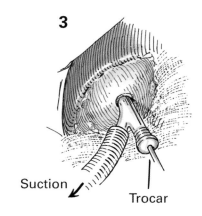

6

Catheter

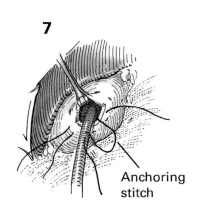

7

Anchoring stitch

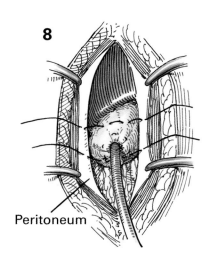

8

Peritoneum

In this chapter two techniques of Roux-en-Y choledochojejunostomy are described. The first is a direct mucosa-to-mucosa anastomosis and is the preferred technique. The alternate procedure of a mucosal graft was described by Sir Rodney Smith in situations where there is a very high structure or injury precluding direct visualization of the proximal biliary tree.

DETAILS OF PROCEDURE The surgeon is occasionally faced with the difficult problem of finding the strictured area or blind end of the hepatic duct. The adhesions between the duodenum and hilus of the liver are divided carefully by sharp and blunt dissection (FIGURE 1). Great care must be exercised to avoid unnecessary bleeding and possible injury to the underlying structures. Usually, it is easier to start the dissection quite far laterally and to free up the superior surface of the right lobe of the liver from the adherent duodenum, hepatic flexure of the colon, and omentum. Sharp dissection is used along the liver margins to avoid tearing the liver capsule, which results in a troublesome ooze. After the edge of the adhesion has been incised, blunt dissection will be more effective and safer in freeing up the undersurface of the liver. The exposure should be directed toward identifying and exposing the foramen of Winslow. The stomach may or may not have to be dissected away from the liver. Usually, the duodenum is drawn up into the old gallbladder bed and fixed by dense adhesions. The second portion of the duodenum is mobilized medially (Kocher maneuver), following division of the peritoneum along its lateral margin (FIGURE 2). As the duodenum is reflected downward the undersurface of the liver is retracted upward. The scar tissue around the porta hepatis may obscure the biliary ductal system. It is best to approach the duct from the lateral side. Identifying the cystic duct stump is helpful in delineating the location of the biliary tree and will facilitate dissection. The upper portion of the dilated duct may be verified by aspiration of bile through a 25-gauge needle (FIGURE 3). A cholangiogram may be performed. Sharp dissection should be used to identify the duct. An effort is made to free up the entire circumference of the ductal system in order to create an end to side anastomosis with the jejunum. A retrocolic Roux-en-Y arm of jejunum is prepared in the usual way using a linear staple to divide the small intestine. If the intestine is divided between clamps then the end of the mobilized jejunal limb is closed with two layers of interrupted silk. On the antimesenteric border of the jejunum about 5 to 10 cm distal to the divided end of the intestine, an incision slightly smaller than the duct opening is made with electrocautery. This should be easily approximated to the hepatic duct with no tension.

DIRECT MUCOSA TO MUCOSA CHOLEDOCHOJEJUNOSTOMY For a direct anastomosis, the duct is identified and the circumference exposed. If the lumen is narrow then an additional opening can be achieved by dissecting the left hepatic duct and opening it longitudinally stopping short of the bifurcation of the left hepatic duct. An enterotomy is made, slightly smaller than the circumference of the bile duct as the opening will tend to enlarge secondary to the elasticity of the intestine. A single layer end duct to side jejunal anastomosis is created. Fine absorbable double-armed sutures are used. These may be 4-0 to 6-0 depending on the caliber of the duct and the tissue thickness. Stay sutures are placed. With gentle traction the posterior wall of the bile duct and the jejunum are visualized. The posterior row of the anastomosis is then completed between the hepatic duct and the jejunum. Sutures are placed full thickness in the bile duct and the jejunum. The knot may be on the inside. (FIGURE 4). These may be held with fine hemostats and tied in sequence as a group (preferred) or tied as you go. Once the posterior anastomosis is completed and if a pigtail catheter was placed to decompress the biliary tree, then it is now repositioned in the intestine by advancing it through the bile duct opening and into the opening made in the jejunum. The anterior row is then completed (FIGURE 5). The Roux-en-Y loop is securely tacked in place beneath the liver by several absorbable sutures placed through the seromuscular coat

In difficult cases in which there is posterior displacement of the duct it may help to place the initial sutures in the anterior wall of the hepatic duct. These are then individually clamped with fine hemostats and placed on the abdominal wall with mild tension so as to lift the anterior duct wall and expose the posterior wall. Once all the anterior sutures are placed, the posterior wall of the duct will be easily exposed by gentle traction of the anterior row. The posterior sutures are then placed. Once these are tied and the posterior row completed then the anterior sutures are tied completing the anastomosis.

MUCOSAL GRAFT CHOLEDOCHOJEJUNOSTOMY, RODNEY SMITH TECHNIQUE In some situations the duct cannot be dissected and in these cases an option would be to use the Rodney Smith mucosal graft technique (FIGURES 6 to 8). In this situation the needle is left in place as a guide and an incision is made alongside the needle until a free flow of bile is obtained. Then a blunt-nosed, curved clamp is inserted upward into the dilated duct and the opening gradually enlarged by dilatation, which may include an additional incision to enlarge the opening. In the mucosal graft technique, the mucosa is intussuscepted well up into the duct without a direct end-to-end anastomosis may be used. (FIGURES 7 and 8). Most patients with a high stricture or injury will have a transhepatic biliary catheter in place that will facilitate the location of the proximal biliary tree and placement of a Silastic stent as described below.

To create a mucosal graft the technique described below is used. Following the opening of the dilated hepatic duct, a long, curved clamp is inserted, usually toward the left side, and extended up through the liver substance. A rubber or preferably a Silastic tube (14 or 16 French) is pulled down through the liver and partially out through the duct opening (FIGURE 6). A transhepatic biliary drain placed preoperatively will facilitate placement of the Silastic stent. Additional holes that will be above and below the anastomosis are made in this tube. Following this, a Roux-en-Y limb of jejunum is prepared as described above. On the antimesenteric border of the jejunum a 5-cm segment of the seromuscular coat is excised approximately 5 cm from the closed end (FIGURE 6). Care should be taken to avoid making any additional openings in the mucosa except in the very apex of the protruding mucosal pocket. The tube that was pulled down through the liver is now directed through the small opening made in the apex of the mucosal pocket and directed down into the arm of the jejunum for 10 cm or more. A purse-string suture of absorbable suture is placed in the mucosa about the tube and tied. After the tube has been passed the desired distance down the Roux-en-Y limb, a 2-0 absorbable suture is passed completely through the jejunal walls and around the tube to fix it in position when tied just distal to the mucosal outpocketing. A centimeter or two distally a similar absorbable suture is taken to ensure further fixation. These are the only sutures utilized to fix the tube to the wall of the jejunum (FIGURE 8). These sutures ensure fixation of the jejunal mucosa to the tube as it is withdrawn. Several holes are cut around the tube just above the mucosal graft to ensure drainage of the right as well as the left hepatic duct. Traction then is placed on the end of the tube coming out of the dome of the liver in order to pull the mucosal graft carefully and firmly up into place inside the common hepatic duct. This provides an intussusception of the jejunal mucosa up into the dilated common hepatic duct and ensures direct mucosa-to-mucosa approximation (FIGURE 8). In very high strictures it may be necessary to use a tube into the left as well as the right hepatic radical. The Roux-en-Y loop is securely anchored in place beneath the liver by several absorbable sutures placed through the seromuscular coat and the scar tissue around the opening into the duct system (FIGURE 7). The tube is brought out through a separate stab wound to one side or the other of the incision and anchored securely in place with nonabsorbable suture material. A closed suction drain is placed.

Rarely the situation may warrant an end-to-end anastomosis or primary repair of the common duct. This is associated with a greater stricture rate than Roux-en-Y reconstruction and hence not used very often. Please refer to the electronic supplement for a description of this procedure.

CLOSURE The wound is closed in layers after suction drainage is instituted to the undersurface of the liver by a plastic tube with many perforations.

POSTOPERATIVE CARE The tube going through the anastomosis is placed on gravity drainage to divert bile until the newly made junction is healed. The drain is removed when there is no evidence of bile leakage. The appropriate antibiotic therapy should be adjusted following culture and sensitivity studies of the bile. The tube may be irrigated with saline intermittently to wash out all debris or small calculi. In addition, the tube provides a means of taking postoperative transhepatic cholangiograms from time to time to evaluate the security of the anastomosis and the evidence of regression in the size of the formerly obstructed ducts. Ordinarily, the tube is left in place for a minimum of 4 months. A complete evaluation with liver function studies and several cultures of the bile should be made, as well as a cholangiogram, before it is advisable to remove the tube. ■

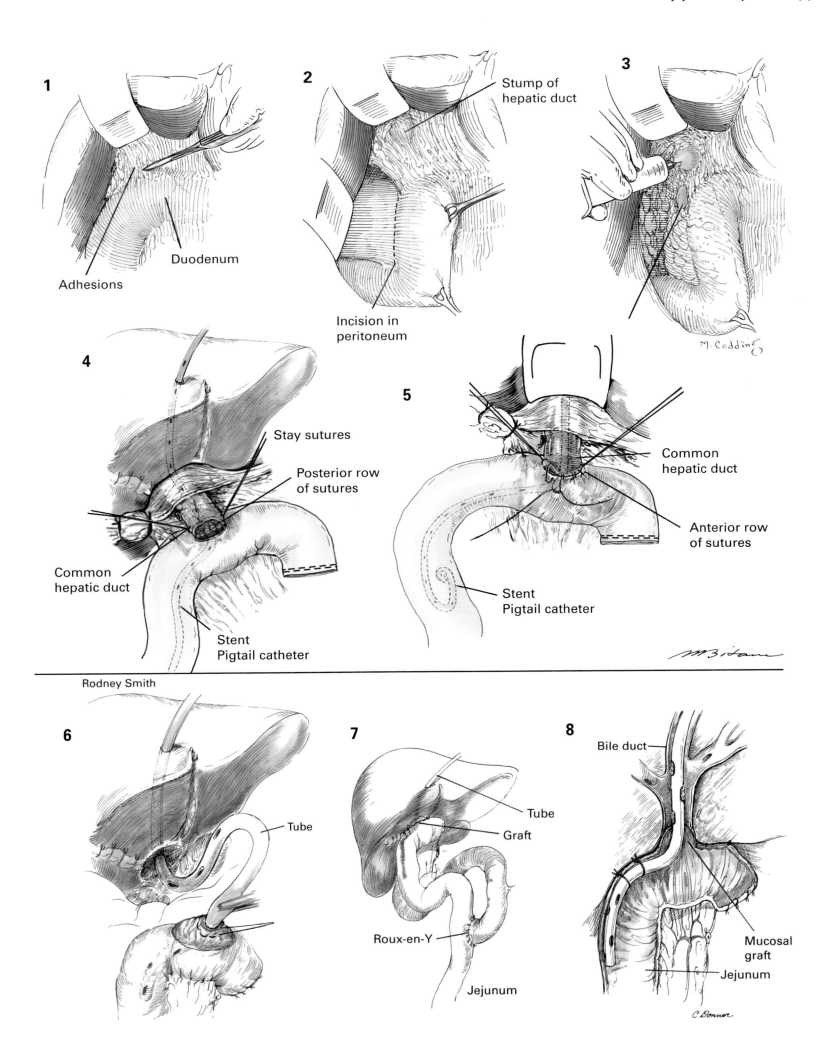

1

Adhesions
Duodenum

2

Stump of hepatic duct
Incision in peritoneum

3

M. Codding

4

Stay sutures
Posterior row of sutures
Common hepatic duct
Stent Pigtail catheter

5

Common hepatic duct
Anterior row of sutures
Stent Pigtail catheter

Rodney Smith

6

Tube

7

Tube
Graft
Roux-en-Y
Jejunum

8

Bile duct
Mucosal graft
Jejunum

C Bonner

INDICATIONS Cholangiocarcinomas arising at or near the confluence of the right and left hepatic ducts, commonly referred to as *Klatskin tumors*, are being diagnosed earlier and treated more promptly by palliative or curative surgical procedures. These may be termed hepatic duct bifurcation tumors or hilar tumors. The majority of patients exhibit jaundice of increasing intensity and many have had recent biliary exploration, where the diagnosis was suggested by operative cholangiography. There is a wide patient age range and occasionally a preceding history of ulcerative colitis or sclerosing cholangitis. Although the number who can be cured is limited, many patients are benefited by palliative procedures.

PREOPERATIVE PREPARATION The seriousness of the lesion, the difficulty in determining the extent of involvement, and the necessity for avoiding infection from preoperative studies in an obstructed jaundiced patient requires meticulous preoperative evaluation. Early endoscopy of the common duct and consultation with an expert in interventional radiology are essential in planning when and if access to the biliary tree is necessary. The decision to instrument the obstructed biliary tree should be made only after treatment goals are defined. The jaundiced patient selected for biliary decompression should undergo percutaneous transhepatic cholangiography with appropriate prophylactic antibiotics given. These procedures should be undertaken by an experienced interventional radiologist. Following cholangiography, pigtail catheters may be placed bilaterally (although unilateral is usually sufficient), directed if possible through the obstructing lesion into the duodenum for palliation of the jaundice (FIGURE 1). If there is cholangiographic evidence of tumor extending into the right or left hepatic ducts, the patient may eventually be explored to relieve the obstruction on the side of the involved duct. Palliation, however, is usually possible with internal drainage into the duodenum through the pigtail catheters. The catheters also serve as invaluable technical aids to the surgeon at the time of laparotomy.

High-resolution cross-sectional imaging is mandatory for evaluating hilar vasculature prior to any attempt at resection. MRI/MRCP with contrast enhancement and delayed imaging (i.e., cholangiocarcinoma protocol) is ideal at identifying occlusion of the hepatic artery or encasement of the main portal vein, either of which complicates and may contraindicate attempt at resection of the tumor. The vast majority of patients will show a stage of tumor involvement that makes attempts at surgical excision impossible.

Appropriate antibiotic therapy, intravenous alimentation, and vitamin K are given, and blood volume deficits are corrected.

ANESTHESIA The deeply jaundiced patient should be considered a poor surgical risk meriting special consideration by the anesthesiologist in planning the anesthesia.

POSITION The patient is placed on the table in a slightly reversed Trendelenburg position. Intravenous catheters should be placed in both arms. Catheter drainage of the bladder may be advisable as well as nasogastric suction.

OPERATIVE PREPARATION The skin of the lower chest and upper abdomen as well as the right flank should be prepared.

INCISION AND EXPOSURE Either a liberal bilateral subcostal incision or a midline incision from over the xiphoid to below the umbilicus is made.

DETAILS OF PROCEDURE Bimanual palpation of the liver and peritoneal surfaces is carried out in a search for possible metastases. Metastatic adenopathy at the root of the mesentery can impede reconstruction so should be evaluated early. Despite the history of deep jaundice, the gallbladder and common duct appear normal. Any enlarged lymph nodes are excised for immediate frozen section examination if outside of the porta hepatis. The tumor tends to be well hidden and careful palpation of the previously placed pigtail catheters is performed up into the hilus of the liver until the tumor is localized. The distortion of the pigtail catheters is helpful in localizing the area of tumor involvement.

Before proceeding with the tumor excision, some prefer to divide the falciform ligament and ligate both ends with a transfixing suture. This procedure may enhance the exposure (FIGURE 2). If a hepatic bridge or plate is present, it is divided. The exposure of the tumor area is further improved by dividing and ligating the cystic duct followed by enucleation of the gallbladder from the liver bed.

A Kelly hemostat is applied to the fundus of the attached gallbladder to be used for improved traction of the common duct. The duodenum is thoroughly mobilized by the Kocher maneuver and the common duct dissected free as far downward as possible.

The anterior wall of the lower most portion of the common duct is opened and the ends of the pigtail catheters brought out (FIGURE 3). The common duct is divided and the distal end is oversewn at the level of the head of the pancreas.

The gallbladder and end of the common duct are reflected upward to expose the posterior aspects of the region of the tumor (FIGURE 4). This is the most delicate portion of the procedure. Very gently the adhesions above the posterior aspects of the tumor and adjacent structures, such as branches of the hepatic artery, must be gently determined and divided. Likewise the portal vein is very close as well as the caudate lobe of the liver. Involvement of the caudate lobe of the liver with tumor is commonplace with prompt recurrences of the tumor if overlooked. The possibility of removing the caudate lobe should be considered standard.

All bleeding is controlled by metal clips or ligature. The lower small hepatic vein going to the caudate lobe may be ligated.

The tissue about the left hepatic duct is carefully divided to provide sufficient exposure of the left duct for a right-angle clamp to be carefully inserted under the duct to permit the placement of a blood vessel loop for possible traction (FIGURE 5). The duct should be palpated for possible tumor involvement. This maneuver should be considered carefully as aberrant biliary anatomy is common. **CONTINUES▶**

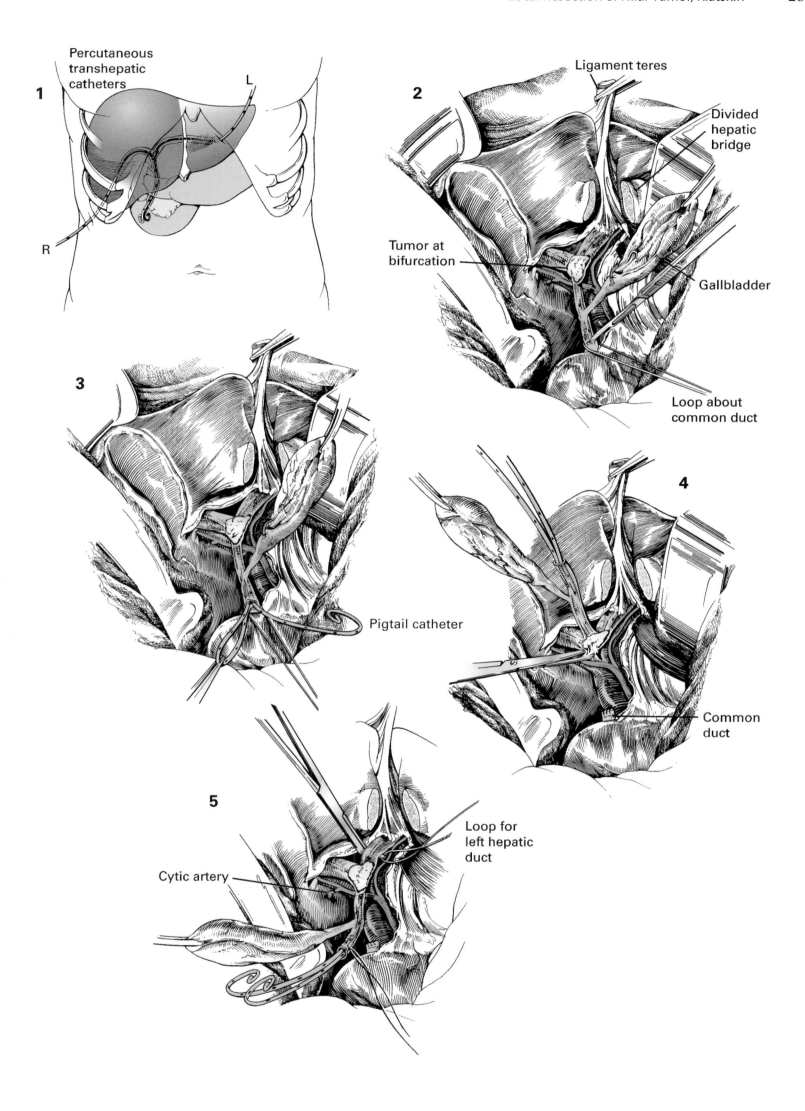

1 Percutaneous transhepatic catheters
L
R

2 Ligament teres
Divided hepatic bridge
Tumor at bifurcation
Gallbladder
Loop about common duct

3 Pigtail catheter

4 Common duct

5 Cytic artery
Loop for left hepatic duct

DETAILS OF PROCEDURE `CONTINUED` The right duct is freed up a short distance and a blood vessel loop passed around it for traction (FIGURE 6). If the tumor has involved the wall of either major duct with probable extension into the liver, the need for added lobectomy must be seriously considered. Occasionally, a third large duct, or even more, may be found on the right side, which must be conserved for implantation. Traction sutures are placed in the major ducts at the point of division for each duct (FIGURE 7).

The two ducts of the specimen should be marked with different colored sutures for specific identification by the pathologist of possible infiltration of tumor at the point of division. Should this be found on frozen section study, more duct must be resected.

The Silastic transhepatic biliary stents are positioned using a Coudé catheter as a preceding dilator that is drawn up the ducts and through the liver by the pigtail catheters. First, the pigtail catheters with the guide wires inside are brought out the open left and right hepatic ducts. Each curled (pigtail) end is cut off and the remaining straight pigtail catheter is placed into the cut leading end of a No. 16 French Coudé catheter. Each pigtail catheter is then secured with a mattress suture through itself and the Coudé. Both catheters are pulled up into the ducts (FIGURE 8) using traction on the pigtail catheter at the surface of the liver. The Coudé catheters may need to be manipulated back and forth so as to dilate the ductal systems.

A No. 14 French Silastic transhepatic biliary stent is positioned in the open end of the No. 16 Coudé French catheter and anchored with mattress sutures of silk which are passed through the wall of the Coudé catheter. With traction on the Coudé catheters the Silastic stents with multiple holes are drawn into the liver in a position with no holes beyond the exit of the plastic tubes (FIGURE 9). Thus, there are holes present within the liver and the portion that projects into the Roux-en-Y of the jejunum. Short horizontal mattress sutures of absorbable material are placed around the stents on the surface of the liver at their point of exit. The liver is compressed without disruption about each catheter. `CONTINUES`

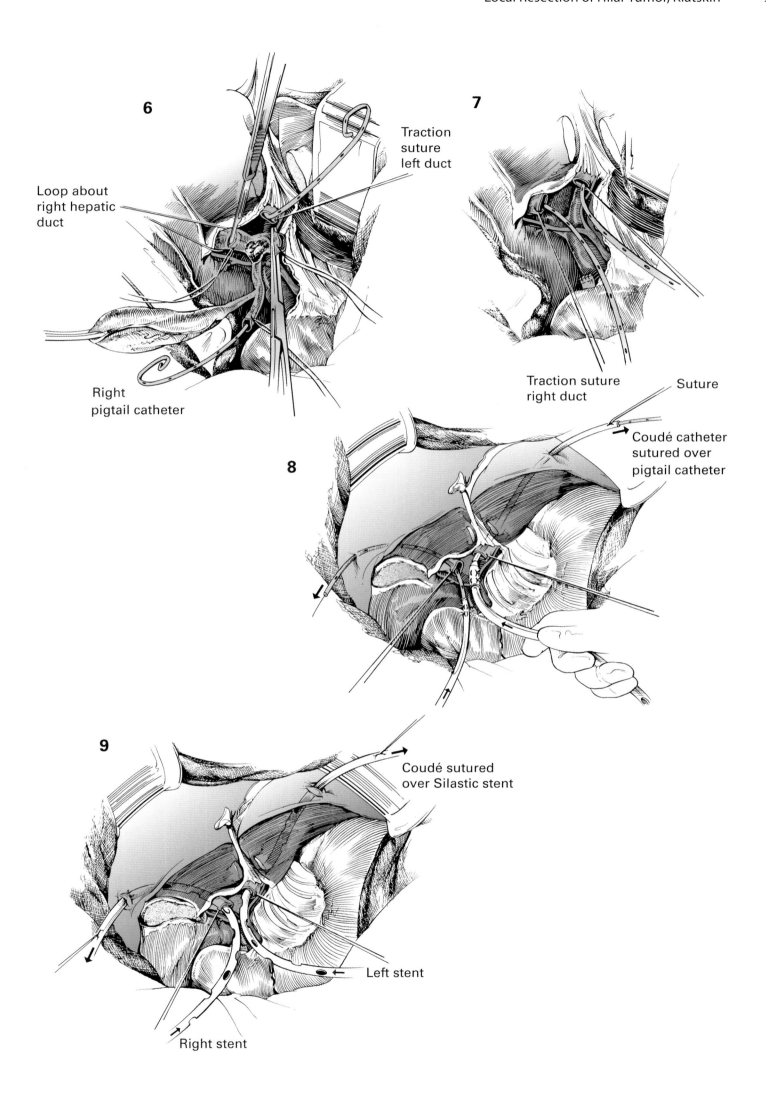

6

Loop about
right hepatic
duct

Traction
suture
left duct

Right
pigtail catheter

7

Traction suture
right duct

Suture

Coudé catheter
sutured over
pigtail catheter

8

9

Coudé sutured
over Silastic stent

Left stent

Right stent

DETAILS OF PROCEDURE ◄CONTINUED► A Roux-en-Y loop of upper jejunum is brought into the right upper quadrant through an avascular area of the mesocolon and anterior to the second and third portions of the duodenum. The opening in the mesocolon is closed about the jejunum and its mesentery after making certain the end of the Roux-en-Y extends up to and slightly beyond the hepatic duct openings. The end of the jejunum is closed with staples or in layers of running or interrupted sutures. The posterior wall of the jejunum in the region of the anastomosis should be anchored to the capsule of the liver or adjacent tissue.

It is helpful to insert interrupted sutures through the lateral angles of each open duct for positioning and sizing an accurate anastomosis on the jejunum (FIGURE 10). A posterior row of absorbable sutures is placed using the full thickness of each duct. None of these sutures is tied until all posterior sutures are in place for each duct. The middle suture in the posterior row may also be used to tie about the stent, so as to help prevent migration of this tube.

The knot of the back suture line will be on the inside. The sutures are cut at the knot, except for the suture at each angle. A small incision parallel to the posterior suture line is made in the jejunum (FIGURE 11).

The ends of the Silastic biliary stents are gently introduced into the lumen of the jejunum (FIGURE 12). Anterior, full-thickness suture lines are closed on both ducts (FIGURES 13 and 14). Finally, the jejunum is anchored to the adjacent liver. Regional closed-system Silastic suction catheters are placed and the Silastic transhepatic stents are doubly sutured to the skin with 5-0 nylon (FIGURE 15). The abdomen is closed in a routine manner and the stents are connected to a sterile plastic bag to allow drainage by gravity.

POSTOPERATIVE CARE The closed system Silastic suction drains are removed early in the postoperative course unless there is a significant bile output or a leak is shown on cholangiography. If no leaks are found from the superior surface of the liver or the anastomosis, three-way stopcocks are attached to the end of the catheters. The patients are trained to self-administer injections of sterile saline into the stents three times per day. The stents can be removed as an outpatient 4 to 6 weeks after surgery. Consultation with radiation medicine and medical oncology is recommended to guide the next steps in therapy. ■

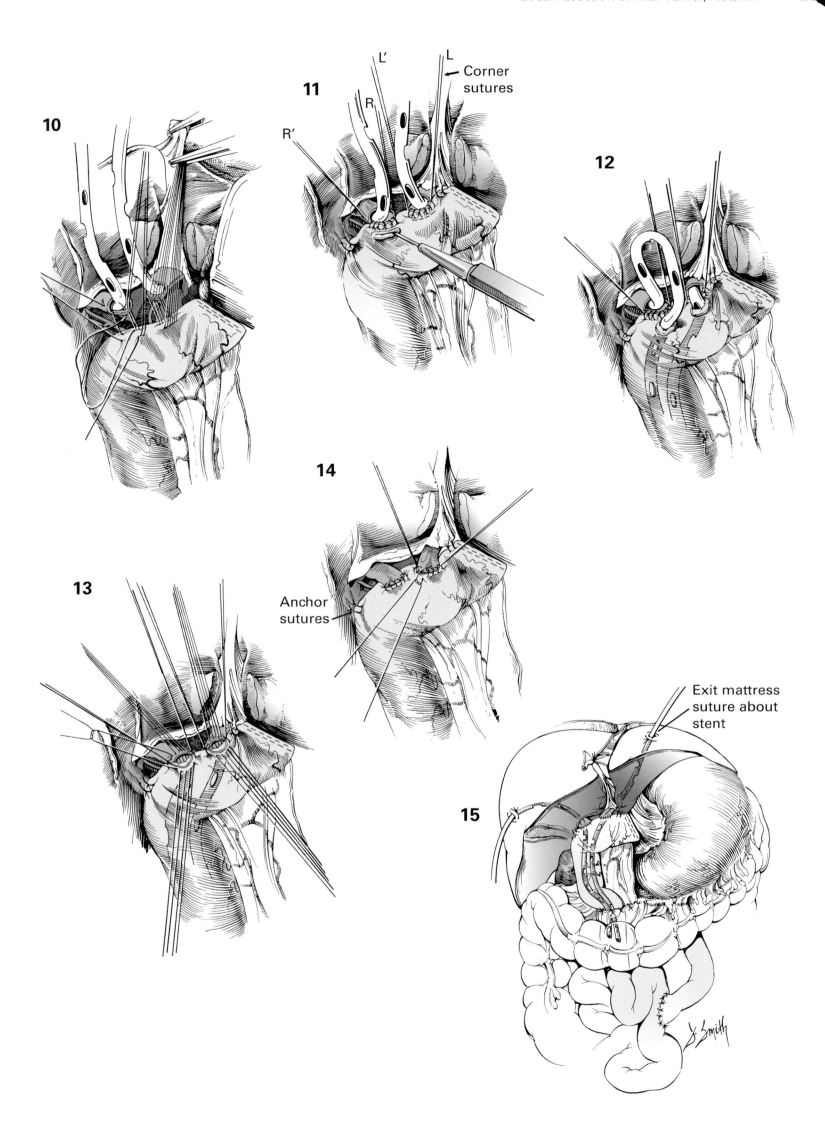

10

11 L′ L Corner sutures

R R′

12

14 Anchor sutures

13

15 Exit mattress suture about stent

J. Smith

S It is not uncommon during an exploratory laparotomy to
re... .all fragment of the liver for histologic study. Biopsy of the liver
is indicated in most patients who have a history of splenic or liver disease,
or in the presence of a metastatic nodule. The specimen should not be taken
from an area near the gallbladder, since the vascular and lymphatic connec-
tions between the liver and gallbladder are such that a pathologic process
involving the gallbladder may have spread to the neighboring liver, and as a
result the biopsy would not give a true picture of the liver as a whole.

DETAILS OF PROCEDURE Two deep 2-0 absorbable sutures, a and b, are
placed about 2 cm apart at the liver border (FIGURE 1A) using an atraumatic
type of needle. The suture is passed through the edge of the liver and back
through again to include about one-half the original distance (FIGURE 1B).
This prevents the suture from slipping off the biopsy margin with resultant

bleeding. These sutures are tied with a surgeon's knot, which will not slip
between the tying of the first and second parts (FIGURE 1B). The suture
should be tied as snugly as possible without cutting into the liver, for the
tension under which these knots are tied is the important factor in the procedure. Such sutures control the blood supply to the intervening liver substance. The two sutures are placed not more than 2 cm apart, deep in the liver
substance; yet as they are tied, at least 2 cm of liver are included at the free
margin to increase the size of the biopsy by making it triangular in shape. An
additional mattress suture, c, may be taken at the tip of the triangular wound
(FIGURE 2). After the biopsy is removed with a scalpel (FIGURE 3), the wound
is closed by tying together the sutures, a and b, or by placing an additional
mattress suture (2-0 absorbable), d, beyond the limits of the original sutures
(FIGURES 4 and 5). The area of biopsy is covered with some type of anticoagulant matrix and omentum. ∎

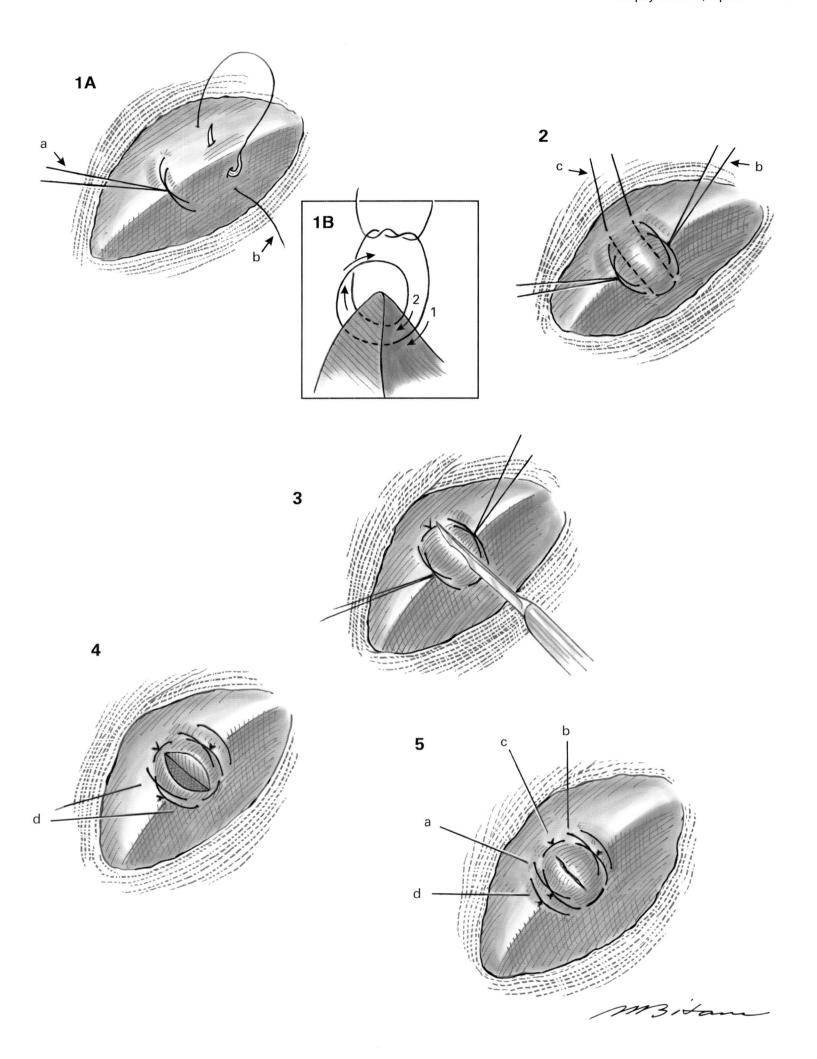

1A

a

b

1B

2

1

2

c

b

3

4

d

5

c

b

a

d

ANATOMY OF LIVER The liver is divided into eight major areas or sectors (including the caudate lobe), with the principal line (Cantlie's line) of division between the right and left sides extending cephalad and obliquely from the middle of the gallbladder fossa to the center of the inferior vena cava between the right and left main hepatic veins (FIGURE 1, A–A'). The true anatomic left lobe thus defined is divided into medial (segment IV) and lateral segments (segments II and III) approximately along the line of the falciform or round ligament, and each of these segments is then subdivided into a superior (cephalad, II) area and an inferior (caudad, III) sector (FIGURE 2). In contrast, the right lobe (segments V–VIII) is divided into anterior and posterior segments by a plane from the anteroinferior edge of the liver that extends both superiorly and posteriorly. This cleavage is similar to the oblique fissure above the right lower lobe of the lung, and it is roughly parallel to it. These segments of the right hepatic lobe are then split into superior (segments VII and VIII) and inferior (segments V and VI) areas similar to those on the left (FIGURE 2).

Although the segmentation of the liver appears straightforward, successful segmentectomy or lobectomy depends upon a thorough understanding of the difference between the portal vein, biliary duct, and hepatic artery distribution as opposed to the hepatic vein drainage. In general, the portal triad structures bifurcate in a serial manner and ultimately lead directly into each of the eight sectors. The specific exception to this rule is the paraumbilicalis of the left hepatic branch of the portal vein, as this structure straddles the division between the left inferior medial (IV) and lateral (III) segments. Thus, it lies roughly under the round ligament (FIGURE 1, #7). The superior and inferior areas of the left lateral lobe have a portal venous supply from either end of the paraumbilicalis (FIGURE 1, #9 and #10); however, special note should be made of the paired medial supply to the superior and inferior areas of the medial segment (FIGURE 1, #8 and #12). It is equally important at this point to examine the biliary and arterial supply of this area (FIGURE 6). The main left hepatic duct and artery proceed with the expected bifurcations out through the superior and inferior divisions of the left lateral segment; however, the left medial segment duct and artery (FIGURE 6, #13) do not divide and send a large branch to the superior and inferior areas, but rather send long, paired structures out in each direction from the junction of the two areas (FIGURE 6, #12 and #13).

In contrast, the portal triad distribution to the right hepatic lobe is by a straightforward arborization with major divisions first into anterior and posterior segments, followed by secondary divisions into superior and inferior subsegmental vessels (FIGURE 1, #2 through #5). Interestingly, the caudate lobe straddles the major right and left cleavage plane and simply receives its portal supply directly from the right and left main branches of the portal vein, hepatic arteries, and biliary ducts. Its venous return, however, is usually a single caudate lobe hepatic vein that enters the inferior vena cava on its left side just caudal to the main hepatic veins (FIGURE 1, #11).

The hepatic veins, in general, run between the hepatic segments in a manner analogous to the pulmonary veins. The right hepatic vein lies in the major cleft between the anterior and posterior segments on that side (FIGURE 1, #14). The left hepatic vein (FIGURE 1, #15) drains predominantly the lateral segment, while the middle hepatic vein (FIGURE 1, #16) crosses between the left medial segment and the right lobe. It is imperative to know that this middle vein is variable where it joins the main left hepatic vein within a few centimeters of the junction with the vena cava and that this vein has two major tributaries that cross over into the right anterior inferior and the left medial inferior areas (FIGURE 1, #17). Appropriate preservation of these channels is, of course, important in specific segmental resections, as hepatic venous occlusion may result in congestion of the entire area(s) involved. Two common variations in the termination of the middle hepatic vein may be found. The first is shown in this chapter where it joins the left hepatic vein (FIGURE 1). The other variation is shown in Chapter 83 (FIGURE 8, page 303) where it has an entrance into the inferior vena cava that is separate from the left hepatic vein.

The remaining figures demonstrate the four most common hepatic resections, whose specific details are covered in the operative text (Chapters 80 to 83). Of specific note are the "danger points" along the paraumbilicalis of the left branch of the portal vein (FIGURES 3, 4, and 5). It is in these areas that the surgeon must be certain of the integrity of the hepatic venous drainage before dividing any major venous branches. Also shown is the use of interlocking full-thickness mattress sutures for hemostasis in the partial and total left lateral segmentectomies, a common technique (FIGURE 3), as is the finger-fracture technique. ■

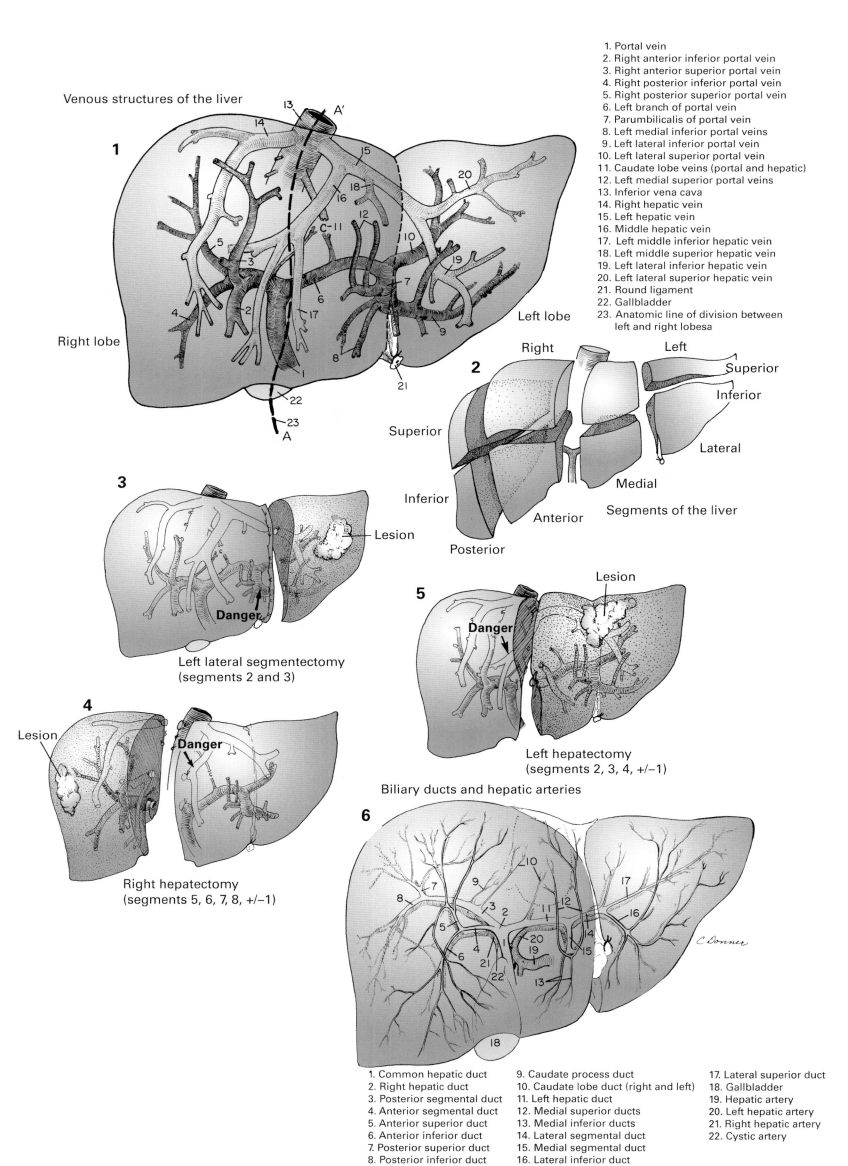

Venous structures of the liver

1

Right lobe

Left lobe

1. Portal vein
2. Right anterior inferior portal vein
3. Right anterior superior portal vein
4. Right posterior inferior portal vein
5. Right posterior superior portal vein
6. Left branch of portal vein
7. Parumbilicalis of portal vein
8. Left medial inferior portal veins
9. Left lateral inferior portal vein
10. Left lateral superior portal vein
11. Caudate lobe veins (portal and hepatic)
12. Left medial superior portal veins
13. Inferior vena cava
14. Right hepatic vein
15. Left hepatic vein
16. Middle hepatic vein
17. Left middle inferior hepatic vein
18. Left middle superior hepatic vein
19. Left lateral inferior hepatic vein
20. Left lateral superior hepatic vein
21. Round ligament
22. Gallbladder
23. Anatomic line of division between left and right lobesa

2

Right   Left

Superior

Inferior

Lateral

Superior

Inferior

Medial

Anterior

Posterior

Segments of the liver

3

Lesion

Danger

Left lateral segmentectomy
(segments 2 and 3)

5

Lesion

Danger

Left hepatectomy
(segments 2, 3, 4, +/−1)

4

Lesion

Danger

Right hepatectomy
(segments 5, 6, 7, 8, +/−1)

Biliary ducts and hepatic arteries

6

C Donner

1. Common hepatic duct
2. Right hepatic duct
3. Posterior segmental duct
4. Anterior segmental duct
5. Anterior superior duct
6. Anterior inferior duct
7. Posterior superior duct
8. Posterior inferior duct

9. Caudate process duct
10. Caudate lobe duct (right and left)
11. Left hepatic duct
12. Medial superior ducts
13. Medial inferior ducts
14. Lateral segmental duct
15. Medial segmental duct
16. Lateral inferior duct

17. Lateral superior duct
18. Gallbladder
19. Hepatic artery
20. Left hepatic artery
21. Right hepatic artery
22. Cystic artery

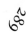
persistent rise in the carcinoembryonic antigen (CEA) very 2 to 3 months during the postoperative years follow- of a colorectal malignancy is an indication for a thorough search possible recurrence. The original operation and pathologic reports are reviewed because they may provide a clue as to where the recurrence is located. A complete survey of the colon and rectum is done and the liver is fully studied with liver function tests and imaging scans (CT, MRI, PET-CT) as it is the principal site for metastatic disease. Evidence of metastases to the lungs or diffuse involvement of the abdomen or bone generally contraindicates surgical intervention, but local excision is usually considered in a good risk patient with a definite steady increase in the CEA level. Further, a hepatic lobectomy may be considered for a metastasis too large for local excision. The 5-year survival rates following the removal of hepatic metastases tend to be encouraging. The patient should be fully informed of the uncertainty of being cured of recurrence of malignancy.

PREOPERATIVE PREPARATION Multivitamins and adequate caloric intake are urged during the days of preoperative investigation. Antibiotics are given.

ANESTHESIA A general endotracheal anesthetic is given. Catheters are placed in both arms for replacement of fluid and blood products if required.

POSITION The patient is placed supine on the operating table in a slightly reverse Trendelenburg position.

OPERATIVE PREPARATION The skin is prepared over the chest and abdomen down to the pubis.

INCISION AND EXPOSURE An extended or bilateral subcostal incision can provide excellent exposure. Alternatively a liberal midline incision beginning over the xiphoid may be used.

DETAILS OF PROCEDURE The peritoneum, the small and large intestines, the cul de sac, mesentery, and omentum are all inspected for evidence of metastases. The major concern will be the liver, especially if preoperative studies indicate probable liver involvement. If only one or two very small metastases are found in readily accessible locations, they can be excised or destroyed by cauterization. Diffuse multiple metastases should be considered to contraindicate extensive attempts at surgical excision of many sites of recurrence. Formal lobectomy may be considered in such circumstances.

The liver is carefully inspected and palpated bimanually. In addition, the use of hand-held intraoperative ultrasound is very useful in the search for deep metastases and to map out the internal anatomy of the liver. Sufficient mobilization of the liver is advisable to visualize the dome and posterior aspects of the liver. The falciform and triangular ligaments are divided to ensure direct vision of all aspects of the liver. Fixation of the liver with tumor invading into the diaphragm posteriorly complicates the resection and should only be undertaken in experienced hands with great trepidation.

The size and location of the metastases as well as the age and general condition of the patient are factors to be considered in determining whether local excision or lobectomy are to be performed. A metastasis tends to be spherical but usually is not as deep as it is wide. The technique for liver biopsy is shown in Chapter 78.

Local excision is usually performed when the lesion can be completely excised with expectation of negative margins without injury to major central vascular or biliary structures.

When the metastatic nodule is near the margin of the left lobe of the liver, a wedge resection is easily performed (FIGURE 1). A safety zone of at least 1 or preferably 2 cm is outlined with an electrocautery around the metastatic nodule, since at least 1 cm of normal liver should be excised with the lesion.

Distal to the cautery line and parallel to it, a series of deeply placed chromic mattress sutures on slightly curved large thin needles are placed in the liver tissue to provide hemostasis (FIGURE 2). These chromic sutures are carefully tied to compress the liver tissue without lacerating the surface of the liver.

One or more traction sutures (A) may be placed in the safety zone between the tumor and the line of compression sutures. The traction sutures should never be placed through the tumor, since seeding may take place. Such sutures are valuable in lifting up the tumor as the dissection progresses (FIGURE 3). Traction on these sutures helps in keeping a safe distance from the metastasis as the tumor nodule is retracted upward. Every precaution is taken to ensure a safe zone of normal liver tissue beyond the neoplasm, especially in the deepest portion of the resection. Electrocautery may be used for the division of the liver tissue as well as to control bleeding. Some surgeons use the Cavitron Ultrasonic Surgical Aspirator (CUSA) ultrasonic instrument for dissection, while others find the Argon beam electrocoagulator very useful for obtaining hemostasis. Several other modern energy devices are available and should be used at the discretion of the surgeon.

Any visible vessels or bile ducts may be clipped (FIGURE 4). However, most liver surgeons prefer individual ligation of vessels and ducts. Evaluation of the completeness of the resection by the pathologist prior to closure is often beneficial.

Sometimes several metastases of various sizes may be excised in a similar fashion. Some prefer to pack the cavity left by the excision for a few minutes with a hemostatic agent. Blood loss is rarely a troublesome factor in the excision of liver metastases, unless the lesion is located rather deep and near a sizable blood vessel in an unusual location. The risk of excising such lesions must be carefully weighed against the potential gain of their removal. In such instances, anatomic resection with pedicle control may be a safer option.

CLOSURE If the field is dry, drainage is not necessary (FIGURE 5), otherwise, Silastic closed-system suction drains are inserted in the area. If bile is noted to escape into the liver tissue, an effort should be made to ligate the area of drainage and consider closed suction drainage.

When the margins of the metastasis are questionable, additional liver tissue is excised for study by the pathologist.

POSTOPERATIVE CARE Patients with proven metastases might be considered candidates for chemotherapy. The CEA levels are measured every 2 or 3 months, and the patient is surveyed for evidence of other recurrences. Measurements should be continued indefinitely, although the interval between tests can be lengthened after several years if the CEA level and CT scans as well as other evaluation procedures remain within a normal range. ■

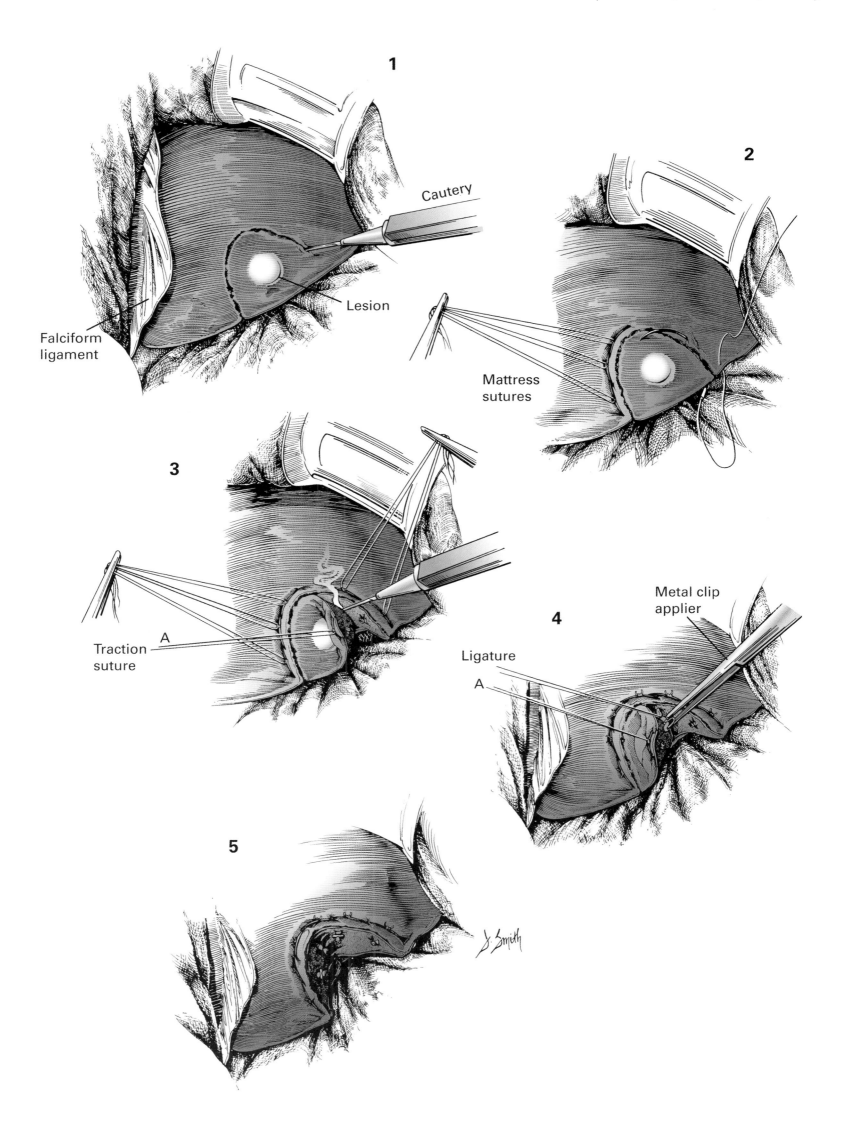

1

Cautery

Lesion

Falciform
ligament

2

Mattress
sutures

3

Traction
suture

A

4

Metal clip
applier

Ligature

A

5

D. Smith

CHAPTER 81

RIGHT HEPATECTOMY
(SEGMENTS 5, 6, 7, 8 ± SEGMENT 1)

INDICATIONS The successful local excision of benign liver tumors has fostered a more aggressive surgical approach to the excision of hepatic metastases of colorectal malignancies. During the first 2 or more years after the removal of a colorectal tumor, carcinoembryonic antigen (CEA) levels are measured every 3 months. When the CEA level begins to rise, recurrence must be considered. In the absence of proof of metastasis or recurrence in the rectum, colon, lung, or peritoneal cavity, a search is made for hepatic metastases. Imaging by CT, MRI, or PET scans is performed. Hepatic angiography is usually not necessary and has been replaced by CT or MRI with coronal reconstruction to define regional anatomy. Any evidence of liver metastases requires an evaluation of the number, size, and location of the metastases. It is hoped that none or only one or two solitary metastases will be verified in locations easily accessible to the surgeon. The age and general condition of the patient, as well as the size, number, and locations of metastases, are considered in making a decision to attempt curative resection. Given the sensitivity of modern imaging, "blind" abdominal exploration for rising CEA in the absence of radiographic abnormalities is discouraged. The patient should be fully informed and should participate in making a decision to re-operate. The patient should be made aware that a major portion of the liver may need to be excised. A residual of 20% or more of normal liver tissue remaining in the left lobe is essential for survival but this number may exceed 30% if heavily pretreated with chemotherapy.

PREOPERATIVE PREPARATION Perioperative antibiotics are given, and any blood deficiency is corrected. Studies should have ruled out metastases to the lungs and general peritoneal cavity insofar as possible.

ANESTHESIA A general anesthetic that has minimal potential to harm the liver is required.

POSITION The patient is placed flat on the table with arms extended and accessible to the anesthesiologist.

OPERATIVE PREPARATION The skin of the thorax and abdomen is prepared, since the incision may extend from over the lower sternum to below the umbilicus. Bilateral large bore IVs are mandatory in anticipation of substantial blood loss. Central venous catheters should be considered standard for major liver surgery and intraoperative monitoring of central venous pressure is helpful. Resistance to large volume resuscitation so as to maintain a CVP <6 greatly reduces blood loss. Once parenchymal transection is complete and large bleeding points addressed, aggressive fluid resuscitation should be undertaken. Continuous arterial pressure monitoring is mandatory.

INCISION AND EXPOSURE A long right subcostal incision that extends across the midline as a bilateral subcostal incision provides excellent exposure. Alternatively, a liberal midline incision extending from well above the xiphoid to or below the umbilicus may be used but makes mobilization of a large liver lobe much more difficult, particularly in a larger patient.

DETAILS OF PROCEDURE The extent of tumor involvement in the right lobe is verified by inspection and bimanual palpation (FIGURE 1). The imaging scans available in the operative room are reviewed to reconfirm the location of the lesion. In patients with colorectal metastases, it is essential to palpate and visualize the pouch of Douglas for metastases as well as the entire colon, small bowel, mesentery, omentum, and peritoneum. If there is suspicion of intraperitoneal spread, many surgeons will first view the peritoneal space with a diagnostic laparoscopy. Multiple seeding would cancel the procedure, although some prefer to excise an occasional small metastasis and proceed with the liver section. The extent and location of all hepatic metastases is noted using ultrasound directly on the liver surface. Understanding the relationship of lesions in question with major vascular structures is essential to minimizing blood loss.

The liver is mobilized by dividing the falciform and right triangular ligaments as well as freeing the liver posteriorly from the diaphragm (FIGURE 2). Some surgeons prefer not to cut the triangular ligament, as it provides stabilization and support for the left lobe. The cystic artery and cystic duct are ligated and the gallbladder removed, since the gallbladder bed is the dividing line between the left and right lobes of the liver. The right hepatic duct is easier to visualize after removal of the gallbladder. A clear exposure of the right hepatic duct is the safest way to avoid interference with the area of confluence with the left hepatic duct.

The right hepatic duct is divided under clear vision and double-sutured with one or more transfixing sutures (FIGURE 3). Great care must be taken when passing a clamp behind the right hepatic duct as aberrant insertion of the left hepatic duct can be inadvertently injured. After the right duct is divided, the variable arterial supply is exposed. The surgeon should at this time review imaging, alert to the possibility that the right hepatic artery may arise from the superior mesenteric artery. The right hepatic artery is ligated and divided (FIGURE 4). The left hepatic artery must be visualized to be certain it has not been obstructed or compromised in any way. Variations in the arterial blood supply between the right and left lobes of the liver should be remembered by the surgeon during the dissection in this area.

The right and left branches of the portal vein are clearly exposed before the right branch of the portal vein is doubly clamped with straight Cooley vascular clamps. Both ends of the portal vein are oversewn with a continuous 4-0 nonabsorbable suture. For additional security, the end of the proximal vein may be doubly closed with horizontal mattress sutures (FIGURE 5A). Alternatively, the right portal vein may be divided using a vascular stapler (FIGURE 5B).

Special attention must be given to taking down the hilar plate, followed by freeing up the left hepatic duct, the left hepatic artery, and the left branch of the portal vein from the undersurface of the overlying liver. These vessels enter the liver near the falciform ligament. After the vessels and other structures are gently dissected away from the liver, a logical area is exposed for the division between the right lobe and the medial segment of the left lobe of the liver. **CONTINUES**

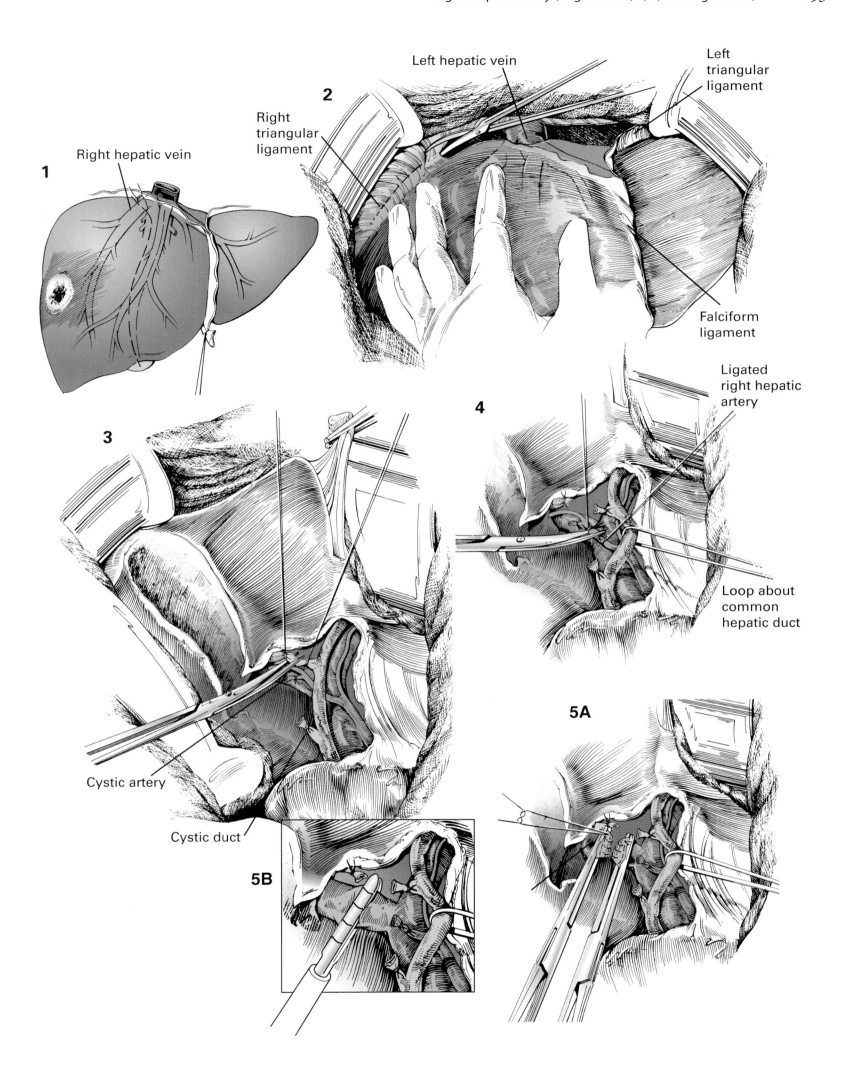

1

Right hepatic vein

2

Left hepatic vein

Left triangular ligament

Right triangular ligament

Falciform ligament

3

4

Ligated right hepatic artery

Loop about common hepatic duct

Cystic artery

Cystic duct

5A

5B

DETAILS OF PROCEDURE CONTINUED The right hepatic lobe is freed up from the diaphragm and rotated medially away from the diaphragm, exposing the small hepatic veins communicating with the inferior vena cava (IVC). These small vessels are carefully and securely ligated (FIGURE 6A). The caval ligament must be divided to expose the inferior border of the right hepatic vein. Caution must be executed as an accessory right hepatic vein may traverse this ligament and drain into the IVC (FIGURE 6B). The main right hepatic vein is exposed.

A loop is passed around the large right hepatic vein, and the liver tissue gently pushed away to permit the application of two curved Cooley vascular clamps to the vein. Sufficient vein must extend beyond the vascular clamps in order to secure the open ends. After the vein has been divided, two rows of nonabsorbable vascular sutures are used to secure the ends of the right hepatic vein (FIGURE 7A). Alternatively a vascular stapler may be used (FIGURE 7B).

The concave line of demarcation following the color change subsequent to ligation of the blood supply may be superficially outlined with a cautery. Starting at the inferior border of the line of demarcation, deeply placed mattress sutures may be inserted to control bleeding. The mattress sutures are tied to compress the liver substance but not to crush it, thus leading to more bleeding. After three or four mattress sutures are placed on either side of the lower end of the zone of demarcation, the liver tissue is divided with an ultrasound dissector, electrocautery unit, or other energy device (FIGURE 8). Larger vessels and branches from the middle hepatic vein may require double ligation. Surface coagulation may be obtained with an argon beam electrocautery device. Alternatively, the hepatic parenchyma can be transected using multiple applications of an endoscopic cutting linear stapler with vascular loads. This approach should only be used after clear mapping of the internal vascular anatomy using the ultrasound probe. After all bleeding and bile leakage has been controlled (FIGURE 9), the omentum may be brought up to cover the raw surface of the left lobe. Sufficient sutures are taken to secure the omentum in place.

If low CVP was utilized throughout the dissection and parenchymal transection, time should be given to allow volume resuscitation (often ~2 L) and restoration of the natural liver turgor prior to closure as new points of bleeding may become evident.

The pathologist examines the specimen to determine adequate clear margin. The structures going into the left lobe are inspected to ensure that no structures are obstructed by angulation.

The falciform ligament is reapproximated to ensure stability of the left liver lobe. Closed system Silastic suction drainage is used selectively when there is concern about bile leakage.

CLOSURE Routine surgical closure procedures are followed.

POSTOPERATIVE CARE Daily blood and liver function studies should be carried out. Significant blood loss may require replacement. Meticulous attention must be paid to minimizing infectious risks. Leakage of fluid from the wound should not be tolerated and aggressively corrected. If there is a bile leak of greater than 100 mL/day, then an endoscopic biliary stent should be considered. If there is an ascites leak, the wound should be revised. Long-term follow-up should include frequent examinations with periodic liver function tests and CEA assays for patients with colon cancer. Rising abnormal values will signal the need for complete reevaluation, as described under Indications. ■

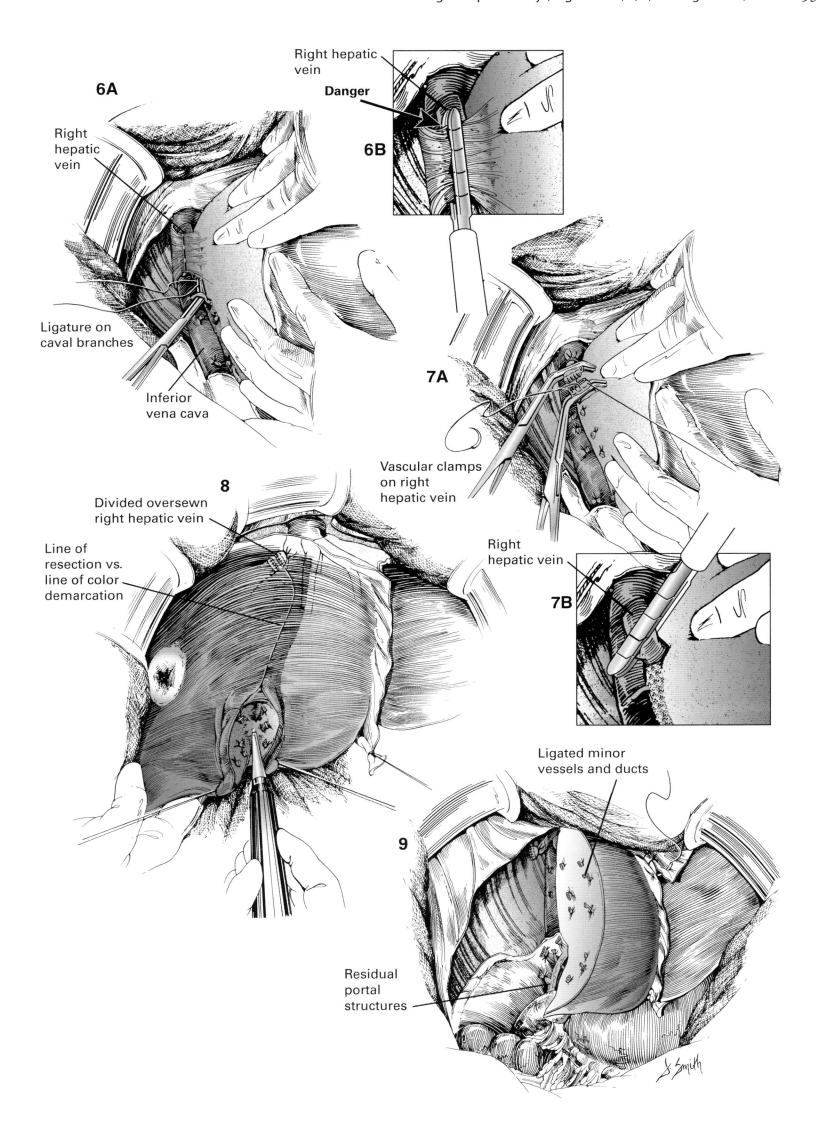

6A

Right
hepatic
vein

Ligature on
caval branches

Inferior
vena cava

Right hepatic
vein

Danger

6B

7A

Vascular clamps
on right
hepatic vein

Right
hepatic vein

7B

8

Divided oversewn
right hepatic vein

Line of
resection vs.
line of color
demarcation

Ligated minor
vessels and ducts

9

Residual
portal
structures

S. Smith

LEFT HEPATECTOMY (SEGMENTS 2, 3, 4 ± SEGMENT 1)

INDICATIONS There are a number of indications for removal of all or part of the left lobe of the liver. The most common indication is evidence of one or more metastases from a previously resected colorectal cancer. The diagnosis is supported by a rising carcinoembryonic antigen (CEA) level during repeated postoperative evaluations. Liver function studies are performed and evaluated. Imaging scans verify the location, size, and probable number of metastases. The initial operative notes and the pathologist's report should be carefully studied for evidence of metastasis at the time of the initial operation. Studies to identify abdominal and lung metastases, including colonoscopy, must be negative. A period of delay may be chosen to reassess the trend of the CEA levels and CT scans, as well as to evaluate the risk of a second-look procedure in an elderly patient. PET/CT to identify occult intra- and extrahepatic disease should be undertaken.

PREOPERATIVE PREPARATION An informative discussion with the patient and the family is part of the preoperative preparation. Antibiotics are given and cross-matched blood is made available.

ANESTHESIA A general anesthetic agent with the minimum of potential for injuring the liver is administered.

OPERATIVE PREPARATION The skin is prepared over the entire abdomen and the chest. Bilateral large bore IVs are mandatory in anticipation of substantial blood loss. Central venous catheters should be considered standard for major liver surgery and intraoperative monitoring of central venous pressure is helpful. Resistance to large volume resuscitation so as to maintain a CVP <6 greatly reduces blood loss. Once parenchymal transection is complete and large bleeding points addressed, aggressive fluid resuscitation should be undertaken. Continuous arterial pressure monitoring is mandatory.

INCISION AND EXPOSURE Various incisions have been used, but the bilateral subcostal incision provides excellent exposure. Extra assistants may be needed, unless special self-retaining retractors are available to retract the left costal margin. Alternatively, a long midline incision that can be extended can be used.

DETAILS OF PROCEDURE The abdominal cavity is carefully inspected for evidence of pinpoint or large metastases in the pouch of Douglas, colon, mesentery, small bowel, omentum, or peritoneum. Any suspicious areas are excised for frozen section examination. The liver surface is inspected for evidence of metastases, followed by bimanual palpation to verify the diagnostic procedures suggesting metastasis in the left lobe of the liver. Metastases deep within the left lobe rather than superficially are best evaluated with a hand-held ultrasound probe. Metastases readily seen on the surface of the left lobe can be locally excised with a 1-cm margin. Metastases near the inferior liver margin can be removed by wedge incision.

The line of transection is outlined extending into the bed of the gallbladder. The left hepatic vein is the major vessel in the dome of the left lobe (FIGURE 1). When the tumor is located deep in the left lobe, the left lobe is mobilized by division of the falciform and coronary ligaments (FIGURE 2).

Since the median margin of the left lobe extends into the gallbladder bed, a cholecystectomy is performed after ligation and division of the cystic artery and cystic duct. Removal of the gallbladder improves the exposure for the identification of the major hepatic ducts and vessels to be divided and ligated (FIGURE 3).

The hilar plate is incised and the bridge of liver parenchyma overlying the umbilical fissure, if present, is divided to enhance the exposure of the structures entering the left lobe. The left hepatic duct is freed up for the sufficient distance to allow passage of a right-angle clamp. This is done carefully so as to not injure any aberrant ducts which may be inserting from the right lobe of the liver. The duct is doubly ligated and then divided (FIGURE 4). The division of the left hepatic duct exposes the underlying left hepatic artery, which usually arises from the proper hepatic artery. The surgeon should seek out the presence of aberrant arterial anatomy. The most common variation is the abnormal origin of the left hepatic artery from the left gastric artery. In this case, the left hepatic artery will run through the cranial portion of the hepatogastric ligament (pars densa) in the lesser omentum.

The left hepatic artery is gently freed up a short distance from its point of origin and doubly tied with 2-0 nonabsorbable sutures proximally (FIGURE 5). The area of the arterial bifurcation is inspected to be certain the blood supply to the right lobe is intact and then the artery is divided between the ligatures. CONTINUES ▶

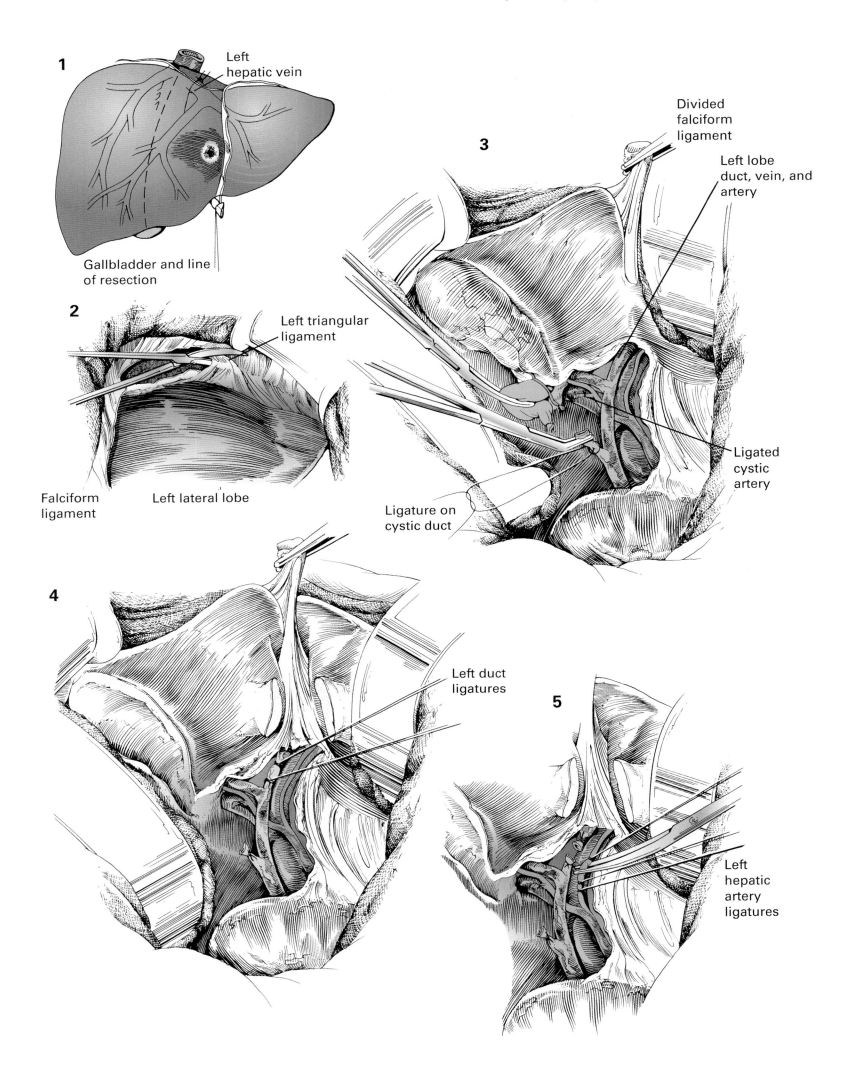

1

Left hepatic vein

Gallbladder and line of resection

2

Left triangular ligament

Falciform ligament   Left lateral lobe

3

Divided falciform ligament

Left lobe duct, vein, and artery

Ligated cystic artery

Ligature on cystic duct

4

Left duct ligatures

5

Left hepatic artery ligatures

DETAILS OF PROCEDURE CONTINUED The left branch of the portal vein is now exposed. The area of the bifurcation of the portal vein is carefully freed up and the left branch mobilized for a sufficient distance to permit the application of a pair of curved Cooley vascular clamps without compromising the bifurcation of the portal vein. The left branch of the portal vein is divided a short distance beyond the clamps to permit closure of the proximal end of the branch of the portal vein with a continuous horizontal mattress suture of 4-0 synthetic nonabsorbable suture that is then run back as an over-and-over suture after the method of Cameron (FIGURE 6). If the caudate (Segment 1) is to be preserved, the surgeon must take care to divide the left portal vein distal to the caudate branch at the base of the umbilical fissure. Alternatively, the portal vein can be divided using a vascular stapler. A final inspection determines that the blood supply to the right lobe is functioning normally.

The blood loss should be lessened if the left hepatic vein is ligated before the liver tissue is divided. The left hepatic vein is freed of liver substance until a sufficient distance is gained to permit the application of a pair of long curved Cooley vascular clamps. The left lateral segment (Segments 2 and 3) can be lifted to expose the ligamentum venosum. When this is divided at its most cranial extent, a window is opened along the inferior border of the left hepatic vein as well as the middle hepatic vein depending upon their point of convergence. The path of the middle hepatic vein must be visualized as separate from the left hepatic vein. The end of the vein projecting beyond the clamps is closed first with a continuous mattress suture and then back with an over-and-over suture (FIGURE 7). The clamps are removed and a final check is made that the proximal caval end of the divided left hepatic vein is secure. A vascular stapler may be utilized to control the left hepatic vein.

A line of demarcation between the right and left lobes develops after the portal structures have been divided. This line tends to curve in a concave manner to the left until the dome of the liver is reached. Ultrasonic dissecting instruments are available for dividing (FIGURE 8) and aspirating the liver tissue with easier exposure for ligation of the larger ducts and vessels, especially the venous branches of the median hepatic vein. Alternatively, an electrocautery or other energy device may be used to divide the liver parenchyma or an endoscopic GIA stapler can be used once the internal vascular anatomy is clearly definedsonographically.

Some have used deeply placed absorbable mattress sutures, starting at the anterior lower liver edge and progressing upward along the line of demarcation. The liver tissue should be compressed with the capsule intact and not crushed. The liver may be divided in a variety of ways but ligatures or clips must be applied to the larger vessels or bile ducts on the cut surface of the right lobe. Clips are usually adequate on the left lobe side, which is to be resected. The deeply placed interrupted sutures near the dome of the liver do not go completely through all the liver tissue in the region of the dome.

The raw surface of the right lobe is carefully inspected for bleeding points as well as for bile leakage, which may require a suture ligature (FIGURE 9). Surface coagulation may be obtained with an argon beam electrocautery system. This may lessen the need for application of various hemostatic materials to the cut surface of the residual liver. The omentum can be mobilized and anchored over the divided surface of the right lobe. Closed-system Silastic suction drains can be considered if there is concern for bile leakage.

Resuscitation should be initiated by the anesthesiologist until normal liver turgor has returned while the abdomen is still open as small bleeding points may develop.

CLOSURE A routine closure of the abdominal wall is performed.

POSTOPERATIVE CARE Antibiotics are given and the amount of blood or bile drainage is recorded daily. ■

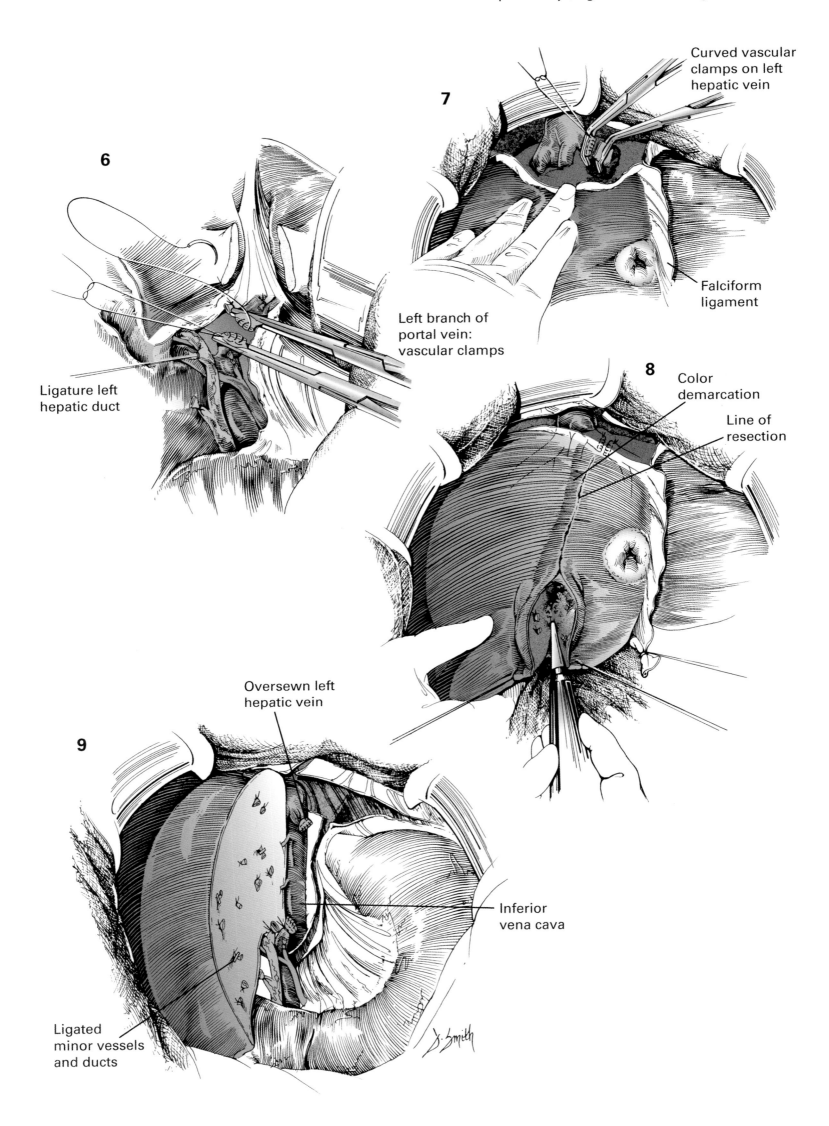

6

Ligature left hepatic duct

7

Curved vascular clamps on left hepatic vein

Left branch of portal vein: vascular clamps

Falciform ligament

8

Color demarcation

Line of resection

9

Oversewn left hepatic vein

Inferior vena cava

Ligated minor vessels and ducts

EXTENDED RIGHT HEPATECTOMY
(SEGMENTS 4, 5, 6, 7, 8 ± SEGMENT 1)

INDICATIONS Malignant tumors involving a large part of the right lobe with extension into the medial segment of the left lobe are a possible indication for extended right hepatectomy (or trisegmentectomy). Lesions straddling midway between the right and left lobes will require trisegmentectomy. This is a major surgical procedure that requires a highly skilled team trained in this field.

PREOPERATIVE PREPARATION Antibiotics are given and any blood deficiency is corrected. Imaging scans (CT, MRI, or PET-CT) localize the metastases in the liver. Hepatic angiography is not routinely necessary. The lungs must be free of metastases, and studies should not have demonstrated any gross abdominal or colorectal recurrence. The patient must be made aware that a major portion of the liver may need to be excised. Survival of the patient can be anticipated if 20% or more of normal liver tissue remains in the left lobe. If the volume of the remaining live is estimated by three-dimensional reconstruction to be less than 20%, then right portal vein embolization may be performed in order to enhance the residual liver volume through post-embolization hypertrophy of the left lateral segment. If pretreated with greater six cycles of chemotherapy at least 30% of the liver should be retained as the remnant.

ANESTHESIA A general anesthetic is required. Bilateral large bore IVs are mandatory in anticipation of substantial blood loss. Central venous catheters should be considered standard for major liver surgery and intraoperative monitoring of central venous pressure is helpful. Resistance to large volume resuscitation so as to maintain a CVP <6 greatly reduces blood loss. Once parenchymal transection is complete and large bleeding points addressed, aggressive fluid resuscitation should be undertaken. Continuous arterial pressure monitoring is mandatory.

POSITION The patient is placed supine on the operating table with arms extended for access as needed by the anesthesiologist.

OPERATIVE PREPARATION The skin of the thorax and abdomen is prepared, since the incision may extend from over the lower sternum to below the umbilicus.

INCISION AND EXPOSURE A long right subcostal incision that extends across the left subcostal region provides excellent exposure. Alternatively, a long midline incision starting above the xiphoid and extending below the umbilicus may be used. This procedure requires liberal exposure.

DETAILS OF PROCEDURE The extent of tumor involvement of both the right lobe and the medial portion of the left lobe is verified by inspection, bimanual palpation, and ultrasonic imaging (FIGURE 1).

The scans are reviewed to reconfirm the location of the lesion and review the vascular supply to the liver. In patients with colorectal metastases, it is essential to palpate and visualize the pouch of Douglas for metastases as well as the entire colon, small bowel, mesentery, omentum, and peritoneum. Multiple seeding would cancel the procedure, although some prefer to excise an occasional very small metastasis and proceed with the liver resection.

The liver is mobilized by dividing the falciform and both triangular ligaments as well as freeing up the liver posteriorly from the diaphragm (FIGURE 2).

When mobilization of the liver has been completed by dividing the right coronary ligament, the procedure outlined for a right hepatectomy is followed. Ligation of the cystic artery and cystic duct is performed, and the gallbladder is removed, resulting in a better exposure of the deeper structures that are to be divided. A clear exposure of the right hepatic duct is essential to confirm the absence of interference with the area of confluence with the left hepatic duct (FIGURE 3).

After the right duct is divided, the variable arterial supply is exposed. The surgeon should be alerted to the possibility that the right hepatic artery may arise directly from the superior mesenteric artery. The left hepatic artery must be visualized to be certain it has not been obstructed or interfered with in any way. The variability of the arterial blood supply between the right and left lobes should be kept in mind by the surgeon during the dissection in this area. Under clear vision, the right hepatic artery is divided and double-tied with a transfixing suture (FIGURE 4).

The right and left branches of the portal vein are clearly exposed before the right branch of the portal vein is doubly clamped with straight Cooley vascular clamps. Both open ends of the portal vein are oversewn with a continuous 4-0 nonabsorbable vascular suture. The ends of the proximal vein are also approximated with horizontal mattress sutures. The end going to the right lobe is doubly ligated or oversewn (FIGURE 5). Alternatively, the right portal vein may be divided using a vascular stapler. **CONTINUES ▸**

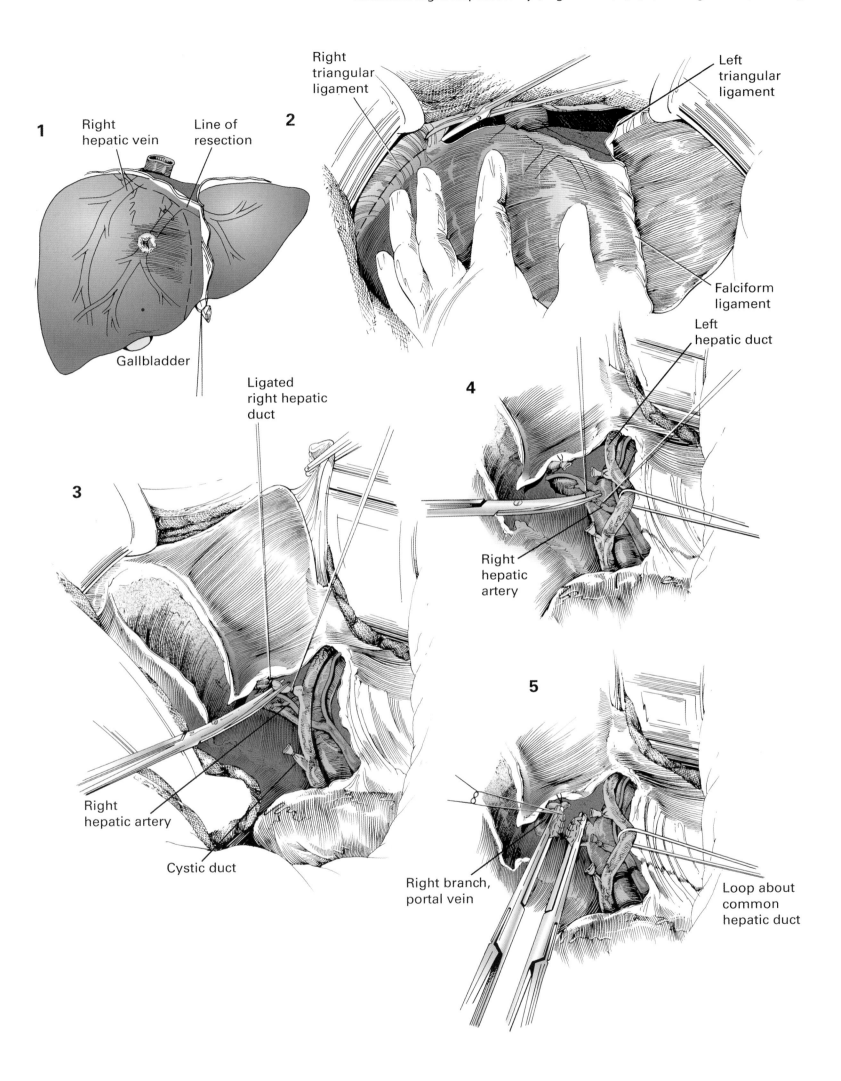

1 Right hepatic vein   Line of resection

Gallbladder

2 Right triangular ligament   Left triangular ligament

Falciform ligament

Ligated right hepatic duct

Left hepatic duct

4 Right hepatic artery

3 Right hepatic artery

Cystic duct

5 Right branch, portal vein

Loop about common hepatic duct

DETAILS OF PROCEDURE **CONTINUED** Special attention must be given to taking down the hilar plate, followed by carefully mobilizing the left hepatic duct, the left hepatic artery, and the left branch of the portal vein from the undersurface of the overlying liver. These vessels enter the liver at the base of the umbilical fissure. After the vessels and other structures are gently dissected away from the liver, an area is exposed for the incision between the medial and lateral segments of the left lobe of the liver (FIGURE 6). The bridge of hepatic parenchyma across the umbilical fissure does not contain a major vascular structure and can be divided with electrocautery. Branches to Segment 4 from the left portal vein can be individually controlled along the right border of the round ligament as it traverses the umbilical fissure.

The right lobe is rotated medially away from the diaphragm, exposing the small hepatic veins communicating with the inferior vena cava. These small vessels are carefully and securely ligated, followed by exposure of the main right hepatic vein (FIGURE 7). As in right hepatectomy, the caval ligament is carefully divided to expose the right hepatic vein.

A vessel loop is passed around the large right hepatic vein, and the liver tissue gently pushed away from this large vein to permit the application of two curved Cooley vascular clamps to the vein. Sufficient vein must extend beyond the vascular clamp to enable oversewing of the open ends after the vein has been divided. Two rows of nonabsorbable vascular sutures are used to secure the end of the right hepatic vein. The middle hepatic vein can be treated in a similar manner or its branches ligated individually as the medial and lateral segments are divided (FIGURE 8). The hepatic veins can similarly be controlled using a vascular stapler.

The division of the liver lobes is made nearer the falciform ligament, rather than in the line of the vascular demarcation between the right and left lobes. Deeply placed stay sutures are placed parallel a few centimeters away from the falciform ligament. These sutures are placed on either side of the incision and tied to control the bleeding, but care is taken not to crush the liver substance. The liver is divided with an ultrasound dissector or electrocautery unit between the area supplied by the middle hepatic vein and medial to the left hepatic vein. Any structures losing blood or leaking bile are ligated with a transfixing suture or clips (FIGURE 9). Alternatively, the hepatic parenchyma can be transacted using multiple applications of endoscopic cutting linear stapler (GIA) with vascular loads. Great care must be taken along the inferior border of Segment 4B so as not to compromise the integrity or vascular supply of the left hepatic duct.

After removal of the right lobe and involved portion of the left medial lobe, the falciform ligament is reapproximated to ensure stability of the remaining portion of the left lobe (FIGURE 10). Special care is taken to avoid injuring the ducts and blood vessels that may be exposed as they enter the smaller residual left lobe.

The pathologist examines the specimen to determine that adequate margins are present and free of tumor.

A variety of materials ranging from tissue glue to prepared hemostatic sterile dressings, as well as omentum are used to cover the raw surfaces of the remaining left lobe of the liver. Closed-system Silastic suction drains should be considered.

Volume resuscitation should be initiated until the liver has returned to normal turgor prior to closure as new bleeding points may become evident.

CLOSURE A routine surgical closure is used. Closed-system Silastic suction drains are inserted.

POSTOPERATIVE CARE Antibiotics are discontinued within 24 hours. Blood and liver function studies should be done on a daily basis postoperatively. Blood losses from drains should be replaced. Patients can do well despite extensive hepatic resection. Meticulous attention should be paid to minimizing infectious risks. (Leakage of fluid from the wound should not be tolerated and should be aggressively corrected.) ∎

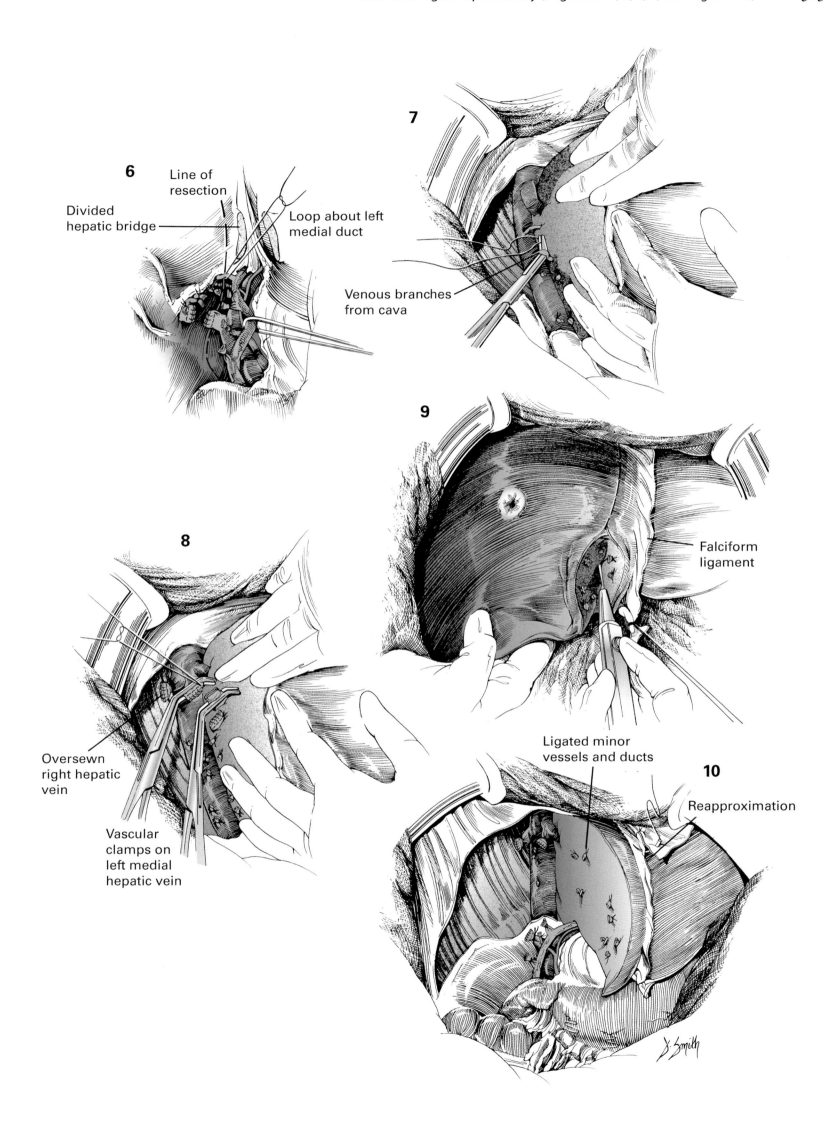

6

Line of resection

Divided hepatic bridge

Loop about left medial duct

7

Venous branches from cava

8

Oversewn right hepatic vein

Vascular clamps on left medial hepatic vein

9

Falciform ligament

Ligated minor vessels and ducts

10

Reapproximation

SECTION VII
PANCREAS AND SPLEEN

CHAPTER 84

DRAINAGE OF CYST OR PSEUDOCYST OF THE PANCREAS

INDICATIONS Pseudocysts of the pancreas are not an uncommon sequela of acute pancreatitis, chronic pancreatitis, and blunt abdominal trauma with resultant traumatic pancreatitis. Pancreatic pseudocysts should be suspected when the serum amylase remains elevated after apparently satisfactory response to treatment of the acute episode. However, the serum amylase may be normal, and quantitative urinary amylases may establish the diagnosis. Blood calcium levels should be followed during severe episodes. A palpable mass can usually be detected in the upper abdomen, most frequently in the mid-epigastrium or the left upper quadrant. These cysts do not have an epithelial lining as do the true pancreatic cysts. They are most commonly found in the body and tail of the pancreas but also may be found in the neck and head of the pancreas. Ultrasonography, computerized tomographic scans, and retrograde cannulation of the pancreatic duct with injection of dye and x-ray opacification (endoscopic retrograde cholangiopancreatography or ERCP) may demonstrate a pseudocyst. Films of the chest and abdomen may demonstrate elevation of the left hemidiaphragm with or without basilar atelectasis or pleural effusion. Treatment of cysts that do not regress spontaneously consists most commonly of internal drainage via the stomach, duodenum, or jejunum. External tube drainage with subsequent fistula may be rarely indicated. Alternatively, some radiologists may drain mature pseudocysts attached to the posterior wall of the stomach using computerized axial tomography. A transgastric needle and then catheter is introduced via a gastrostomy usually created by the percutaneous endoscopic gastrostomy technique (Chapter 18).

The ideal time to drain these pseudocysts internally is 6 to 8 weeks after their appearance, when the cyst is intimately attached to the surrounding structures and the surrounding inflammatory reaction is quiescent. At this time the cyst wall is strong enough for the technical anastomosis. External tube drainage of the cyst may be necessary if the cyst wall is friable or if the patient is septic or has a rapidly expanding pseudocyst. In all cases the interior of the cyst should be thoroughly examined and the cyst wall biopsied. Externally drained cysts usually close spontaneously, but pancreatic fistulas can occur. Cysts may resolve gradually, particularly those associated with stones in the common duct and acute pancreatitis. In general, patency of the ampulla and the proximal pancreatic duct should be established by ERCP prior to any operative procedure.

PREOPERATIVE PREPARATION It is most important that these patients be in satisfactory metabolic condition before surgery. Accordingly, deficiencies in electrolytes, red cell mass, serum protein, or prothrombin levels are corrected preoperatively, and total parenteral nutrition should be considered. A clear liquid diet is given on the day before surgery, and the colon is emptied by the use of oral cathartics.

ANESTHESIA General anesthesia with intratracheal intubation is satisfactory.

POSITION The patient is placed in a comfortable supine position as near the operator's side as possible. The knees are flexed on a pillow. Moderate elevation of the head of the table facilitates exposure. Facilities for operative pancreatic cystogram as well as cholangiogram should be available.

OPERATIVE PREPARATION The lower thorax and abdomen are prepared in the usual manner.

INCISION AND EXPOSURE An epigastric midline incision can be used for this procedure. Resection of the xiphoid process will give an additional 5 to 7.5 cm of exposure if necessary.

DETAILS OF PROCEDURE After the peritoneal cavity is entered, thorough exploration is carried out with particular emphasis on the gallbladder and common duct. Fat necrosis in the omentum or transverse mesocolon is commonly found. The cysts of the pancreas are best drained into that portion of the upper gastrointestinal tract most intimately adherent to the cyst, as shown in FIGURE 1A. Cystogastrostomy or cystoduodenostomy is quite satisfactory when it can be performed easily. Loop cystojejunostomy or Roux-en-Y cystojejunostomy may be performed also (FIGURE 1B). The Roux-en-Y is the preferred method for drainage unless the cyst is intimately attached to the posterior gastric wall. It has the added advantage of preventing reflux of intestinal contents into the cyst, with less chance of leakage about the suture line.

After the field is walled off by gauze pads, the omentum overlying the cyst is opened and all bleeding points ligated (FIGURE 2). The diagnosis of a cyst is confirmed by needle aspiration of the suspected area. The cyst is then partly aspirated, permitting the operator to determine the thickness of the cyst wall and confirm the diagnosis (FIGURE 3). Specimens of the cyst contents are sent for culture and sensitivity, amylase and electrolyte determination. At this time operative cystography can be performed. Since the cyst fluid will dilute the contrast medium, it is better to inject 5 to 10 mL of an undiluted contrast medium into the cyst.

Guide sutures A and B are placed into the wall of the cyst, and a 2- to 3-cm opening is made at the desired level for drainage (FIGURE 4). Suction should be available for aspirating the cyst contents. A full thickness biopsy of the cyst wall must be taken to rule out any malignancy (FIGURE 4).

The surgeon should explore the interior of the cyst with the index finger, carefully checking for coexistent neoplasm and pocketing within the cystic cavity (FIGURE 5). To prevent tension on the cystoduodenostomy, it is advisable to perform a Kocher maneuver to mobilize the duodenum. **CONTINUES**

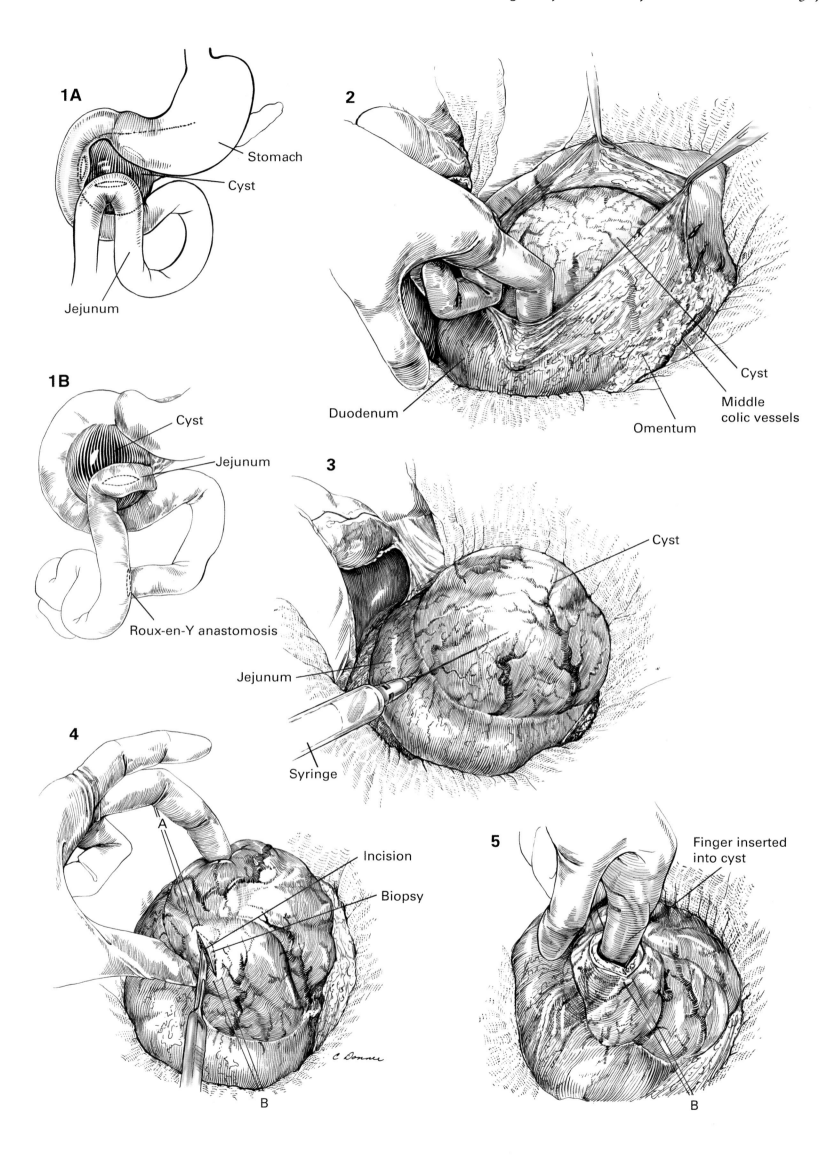

1A

Stomach

Cyst

Jejunum

1B

Cyst

Jejunum

Roux-en-Y anastomosis

2

Duodenum

Cyst

Middle
colic vessels

Omentum

3

Cyst

Jejunum

Syringe

4

A

Incision

Biopsy

B

5

Finger inserted
into cyst

B

C Donner

DETAILS OF PROCEDURE ◄**CONTINUED** Gentle tension is put on the duodenum with non-crushing clamps, and a posterior row of oo interrupted silk horizontal mattress sutures is placed (FIGURE 6).

Traction angle sutures are placed at the angles of the proposed opening in the duodenum. The incision into the duodenum is made slightly smaller than that in the cyst. All bleeding points are meticulously ligated with oooo silk (FIGURE 6). The full thickness of the cyst wall is approximated to the full thickness of the duodenal incision, using interrupted oooo silk sutures (FIGURE 7). Through the duodenal incision, adequate exposure of the ampulla of Vater can be obtained. If a sphincterotomy is considered, a small probe or French woven whistle-tip catheter, No. 10 or No. 12 French, is passed through the papilla of Vater into the duct (FIGURE 8). The patency of the common bile duct as well as the pancreatic duct is determined. Contrast medium is injected in a search for calculi or area of stenosis, as well as documentation of the size of the ducts. The superior margins of the ampulla are grasped by straight mosquito forceps. These clamps are placed in an anterolateral position to avoid injuring the pancreatic duct which enters on the medial side (FIGURE 9). A full thickness of tissue between the clamps can be excised for a biopsy. The contents of the clamps are oversewn with fine atraumatic sutures.

The mosquito clamps are applied again and include only several millimeters of common duct and duodenal wall at a time. The procedure is repeated until the opening is the approximate size of the common duct. Because of the wide range in the length of the intramural course of the ducts, the length of the incision will vary from 6 to 10 mm. The opening must be free of constriction when tested with a catheter or Bakes dilator. It is absolutely essential that one or more figure-of-eight stitches be taken in the apex of the incision to avoid duodenal leakage at this point.

The avascular septum between the lower end of the pancreatic duct and the common duct is divided after the introduction of a small catheter into the pancreatic duct. The septum should be divided in patients who have had recurrent pancreatitis (FIGURE 10). After hemostasis has been obtained and an adequate flow of bile observed upon compressing the gallbladder, the pancreatic duct likewise is probed. The septum between the common bile duct and the pancreatic duct may be divided if stenosis is present. A biopsy of tissue is taken from the ampulla and ductal walls at the time of the sphincteroplasty. After the patency of the ducts has been determined, the full thickness of the cyst wall and the full thickness of the duodenum are approximated with interrupted oooo delayed absorbable suture as inverting sutures (FIGURE 11). The seromuscular layer of the duodenum is approximated to the cyst wall in order to provide the outer layer of the two-layer anastomosis (FIGURE 12). This layer is carried well beyond the margins of the interior anastomosis in order to prevent tension on the anastomosis. **CONTINUES**►

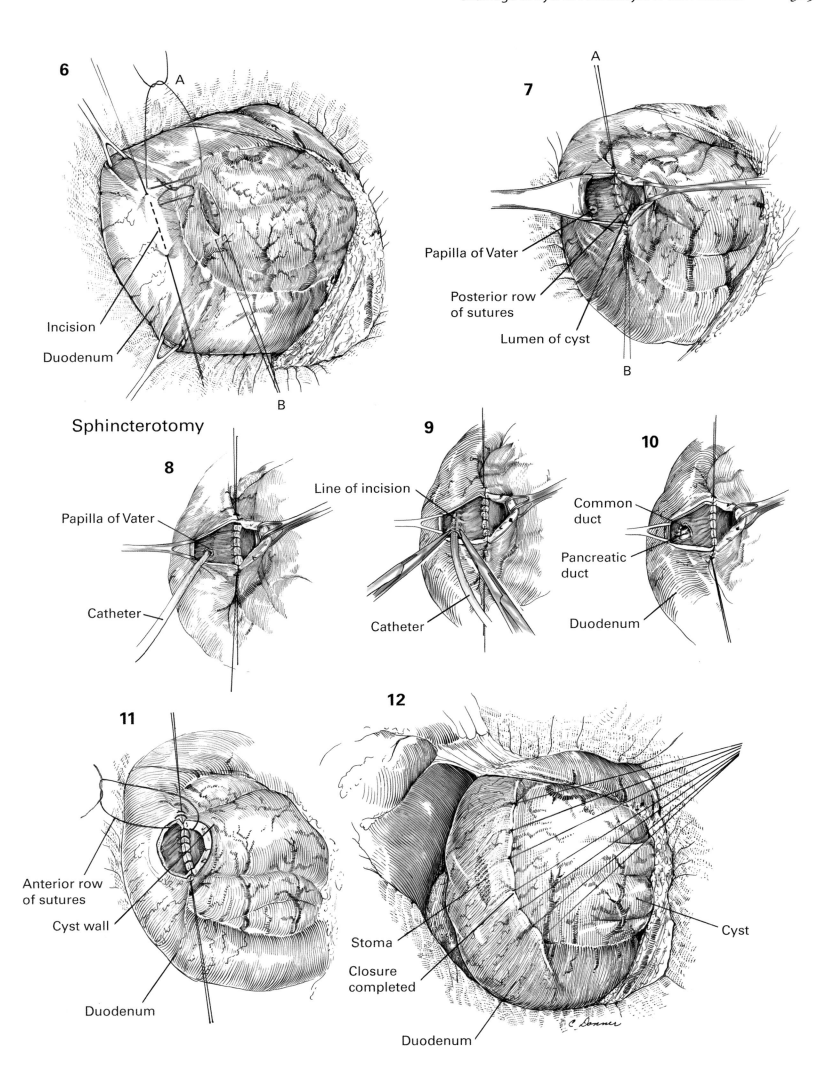

6

Incision

Duodenum

A

B

7

Papilla of Vater

Posterior row
of sutures

Lumen of cyst

A

B

Sphincterotomy

8

Papilla of Vater

Catheter

9

Line of incision

Catheter

10

Common
duct

Pancreatic
duct

Duodenum

11

Anterior row
of sutures

Cyst wall

Duodenum

12

Stoma

Closure
completed

Duodenum

Cyst

DETAILS OF PROCEDURE CONTINUED Pseudocysts of the body and tail of the pancreas usually are drained most easily by transgastric cystogastrostomy (FIGURE 13). The lesser sac is explored carefully to determine where the posterior stomach wall is adherent to the pancreas. This can be done either above the lesser curvature or by separating the greater omentum from the mid-transverse colon for a short distance. As shown in FIGURE 14, the field is walled off with gauze pads, and guide sutures are placed in the anterior wall of the stomach over the most prominent portion of the palpated cyst and where the cyst is most adherent to the stomach. An incision is made in the anterior gastric wall parallel to the blood supply. The margins of the gastrotomy are grasped with noncrushing clamps for exposure as well as hemostasis.

The cyst is localized by partial aspiration through the posterior wall of the stomach at the point where the cyst and stomach are intimately attached. Aspiration confirms the diagnosis and provides a specimen of the cyst fluid for culture as well as amylase and electrolyte determination (FIGURE 15). At this point, operative cystography can be performed to determine the size and extent of the cyst. The mucosa of the posterior wall of the stomach is grasped gently with fine-toothed forceps by the surgeon and the assistant, and the full thickness of the posterior wall of the stomach and the full thickness of the cyst wall are then incised (FIGURE 16) as a wedge biopsy. The contents of the cyst cavity are then aspirated with suction. The interior of the cyst is explored with the index finger, and biopsy of the cyst wall performed. All bleeding points are ligated with 0000 silk or absorbable sutures and a full thickness biopsy of the cyst wall must be taken to rule out any malignancy. Firm attachment between the cyst wall and stomach is essential rather than dependence upon suture approximation. All bleeding points should be suture ligated. A one-layer anastomosis using interrupted 00 or running 00 nonabsorbable sutures is performed (FIGURE 17A). It is imperative that the full thickness of the stomach as well as the full thickness of the cyst wall be included in each suture (FIGURE 17B).

Upon completion of the cystogastrostomy anastomosis, the gastrotomy is closed in two layers, using an inner layer of absorbable sutures and an outer layer of interrupted 00 horizontal mattress sutures (FIGURE 18). Cholecystectomy may be performed in good-risk patients with calculi, as may operative cholangiography.

CLOSURE The abdomen is then closed in the usual manner.

POSTOPERATIVE CARE Nasogastric suction is maintained until gastrointestinal function resumes. Frequent blood amylase determinations are made. The initial liquid diet is advanced as tolerated; however, frequent small bland feedings without stimulants are recommended to place the pancreas as rest. ■

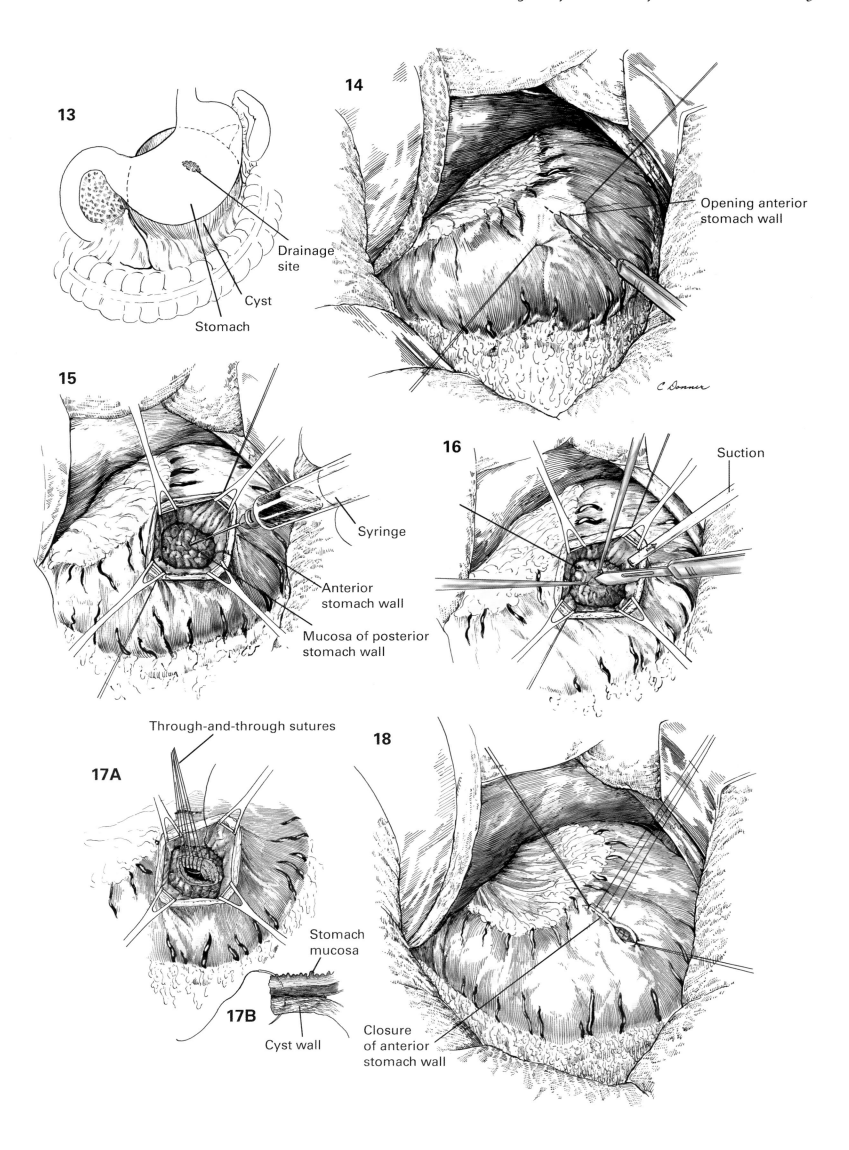

13

Drainage site

Cyst

Stomach

14

Opening anterior stomach wall

C Donner

15

Syringe

Anterior stomach wall

Mucosa of posterior stomach wall

16

Suction

Through-and-through sutures

17A

Stomach mucosa

17B

Cyst wall

18

Closure of anterior stomach wall

CHAPTER 85

PANCREATICOJEJUNOSTOMY (PUESTOW–GILLESBY PROCEDURE)

INDICATIONS Drainage of the pancreatic duct by anastomosis to the jejunum may be indicated in the treatment of symptomatic chronic recurrent calcific pancreatitis. Before this procedure is carried out, all stones from the biliary tract should be removed by cholecystectomy and choledochostomy. There should be evidence of free drainage of bile through the papilla of Vater into the duodenum. Decompression of the obstructed pancreatic duct should be considered because of recurrent or persistent pain and evidence of progressive destruction of the pancreas.

PREOPERATIVE PREPARATION All too often, these patients are addicted to alcohol and/or narcotics because of persistent pain. Evidence of advanced pancreatic disease may be diabetes, steatorrhea, and poor nutrition. The entire gastrointestinal tract should be surveyed with barium studies or endoscopy. The pancreatic and biliary systems are evaluated with endoscopic retrograde cholangiopancreatography (ERCP) and with dye study of both duct systems. Stones in the gallbladder or the common duct should be suspected, and ulceration of the duodenum is not uncommon. Evidence for or against gastric hypersecretion should be determined by secretion studies. The stools should be examined to determine the degree of pancreatic insufficiency, insofar as fats are concerned. Particular attention should be given to restoring the blood volume and controlling existing diabetes. Blood calcium and phosphorus levels should be determined to rule out a parathyroid adenoma.

ANESTHESIA General anesthesia is used.

POSITION The patient is placed supine on the table that is positioned for a cholangiogram or pancreatogram.

OPERATIVE PREPARATION The upper abdomen is prepared in the usual manner.

INCISION AND EXPOSURE A curved incision following the costal margin on the left and extending across the midline around to the right or a long midline incision, which may extend below the umbilicus on the left side, may be used. An upper midline incision may be used.

DETAILS OF PROCEDURE The stomach and duodenum should be evaluated thoroughly for evidence of an ulcer. Likewise, the gallbladder should be palpated carefully for evidence of stones, and the size of the common duct determined. In the presence of stones the gallbladder is removed and a cholangiogram is taken through the cystic duct. A small amount of contrast medium (5 mL) is first injected to avoid a dense shadow, which may hide small calculi in the common duct. Sufficient contrast medium should be injected subsequently to determine the patency of the papilla of Vater by visualization of the duodenum. It is advisable to carry out a Kocher maneuver to palpate the head of the pancreas, especially if there is radiographic evidence of an enlarged C-loop. Under such circumstances, needle aspiration may be carried out to search for evidence of a pancreatic cyst. The omentum, which is often quite vascular, is freed in the usual fashion from the transverse colon across to the region of the splenic flexure. The lesser sac may be obliterated, and sharp dissection may be required to separate the adhesions between the stomach and the pancreas that may be due to chronic pancreatitis. The stomach should be freed until the entire length of the fibrotic and lobulated pancreas can be explored easily (FIGURE 1). The transverse colon is returned to the peritoneal cavity, while the stomach is retracted upward with a large S retractor. The posterior wall of the antrum should be freed from the pancreas so that the pancreatic duct can be palpated and opened as far to the right as possible to remove any calculi that might be impacted in the duodenal end (FIGURE 2). After the lobulated fibrotic pancreas has been exposed clearly, an effort is made to identify the location of the pancreatic duct by needle aspiration (FIGURE 1). Occasionally, it is desirable to aspirate pancreatic juice from the dilated pancreatic duct and then to inject a limited amount of contrast medium to ensure x-ray visualization of the pancreatic duct. Evidence of calculi in the duct is obtained as well as evidence to indicate whether the papilla of Vater is blocked or patent.

If there is evidence of a large and obstructed pancreatic duct, decompression is performed by anastomosing it to the jejunum. The capsule of the pancreas is incised directly over the needle (FIGURE 3). This is done with a small scalpel or with an electrocautery unit. Some prefer the electrocautery unit to control the bleeding; otherwise, the bleeding points need to be grasped with fine forceps and ligated as the fibrotic pancreas overlying the duct is divided. **CONTINUES ▶**

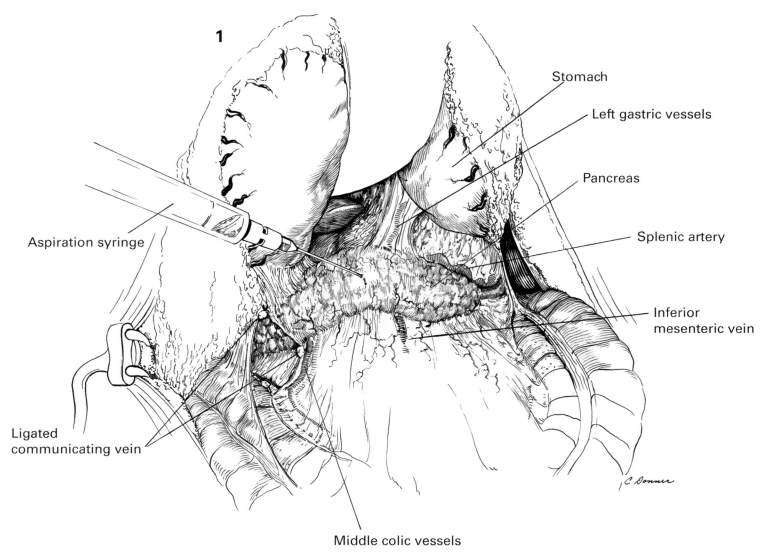

1

Stomach

Left gastric vessels

Pancreas

Splenic artery

Inferior
mesenteric vein

Aspiration syringe

Ligated
communicating vein

Middle colic vessels

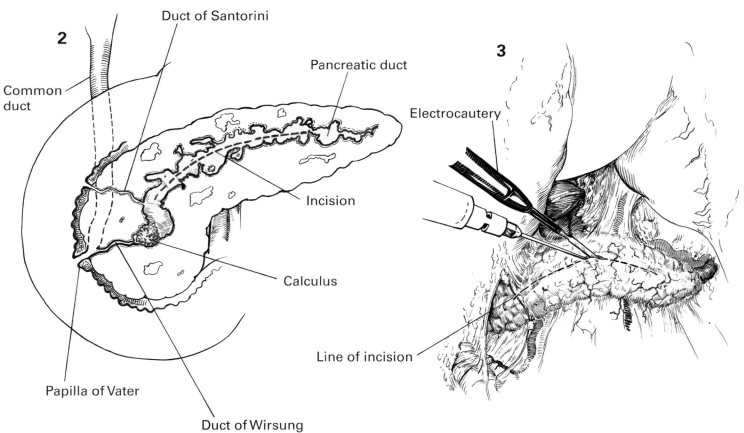

2

Duct of Santorini

Pancreatic duct

Common
duct

Incision

Calculus

Papilla of Vater

Duct of Wirsung

3

Electrocautery

Line of incision

DETAILS OF PROCEDURE ◂**CONTINUED** A rather liberal incision is made in the pancreatic duct and carried over toward the right side but not up against the posterior wall of the duodenum, lest the pancreaticoduodenal vessels be divided and massive hemorrhage occur. A dilated pancreatic duct is usually encountered, and intermittent lakes or segmental dilatations may be found (FIGURE 4). As the pancreatic duct is divided, the fibrotic margins are grasped by Allis forceps, and all bleeding points are controlled (FIGURE 4). An effort can be made to establish the patency between the remaining segment of the pancreatic duct in the head of the pancreas and the lumen of the duodenum through the papilla of Vater. Frequently one or more calculi may need to be dislodged with a gallbladder type of scoop or small, fenestrated type of forceps commonly used to remove ureteral calculi (FIGURE 4). Considerable time may be consumed in clearing the major pancreatic duct of calculi. A French woven catheter can be directed into the pancreatic duct to determine the patency of the papilla of Vater (FIGURE 5). Patency can be proved by distention of the duodenum after an injection of saline. In case of doubt, it may be advisable to inject contrast medium followed by a roentgenogram to visualize the remaining short segment of the pancreatic duct.

Ordinarily, the pancreatic duct is opened for 6 to 8 cm, and a decision then must be made as to the type of anastomosis that will be carried out: the Roux-en-Y arm as in a jejunal "fishmouth" lateral anastomosis, full-width side-to-side anastomosis, or implantation of the mobilized pancreas into the lumen of the jejunal segment. The jejunum is prepared for the Roux-en-Y anastomosis by dividing it 10 to 15 cm below the ligament of Treitz (Chapter 31, FIGURES 16–21). The vessels in the mesentery of the upper jejunum are visualized, and several vascular arcades are divided some distance from the mesenteric border. This permits mobilization of a sufficient length of jejunum to allow it to reach up into the region of the pancreas. An opening is made in the mesocolon to the left of the middle colic vessels in an avascular portion near the base of the mesentery. The arm of the jejunum is then tested for length and is turned with the open end to the right as well as to the left to determine which position of the mobilized jejunum produces the least interference with the blood supply. Many procedures can be followed in accomplishing the pancreaticojejunostomy.

FIRST TECHNIQUE: LATERAL FISHMOUTH ANASTOMOSIS The antimesenteric border of the Roux limb may be opened with a cutting linear stapler stapling instrument. The distance required is longer than that for the opening in the pancreatic duct (FIGURE 6). This usually requires two firings of the cutting linear stapler. Any active bleeding sites along the stapled cut edge are secured with fine silk sutures (FIGURE 7).

The pancreas is anchored to the opened jejunum with one layer of interrupted oo silk or nonabsorbable sutures (FIGURE 8). These sutures go through the entire wall of the jejunum but through only the capsule of the pancreas. The full thickness of the fibrotic pancreatic wall down to the opened pancreatic duct should not be sutured because there are numerous intramural smaller ducts that would be blocked and then would deliver pancreatic secretions into the peripancreatic tissue instead of to the intestinal lumen. **CONTINUES**▸

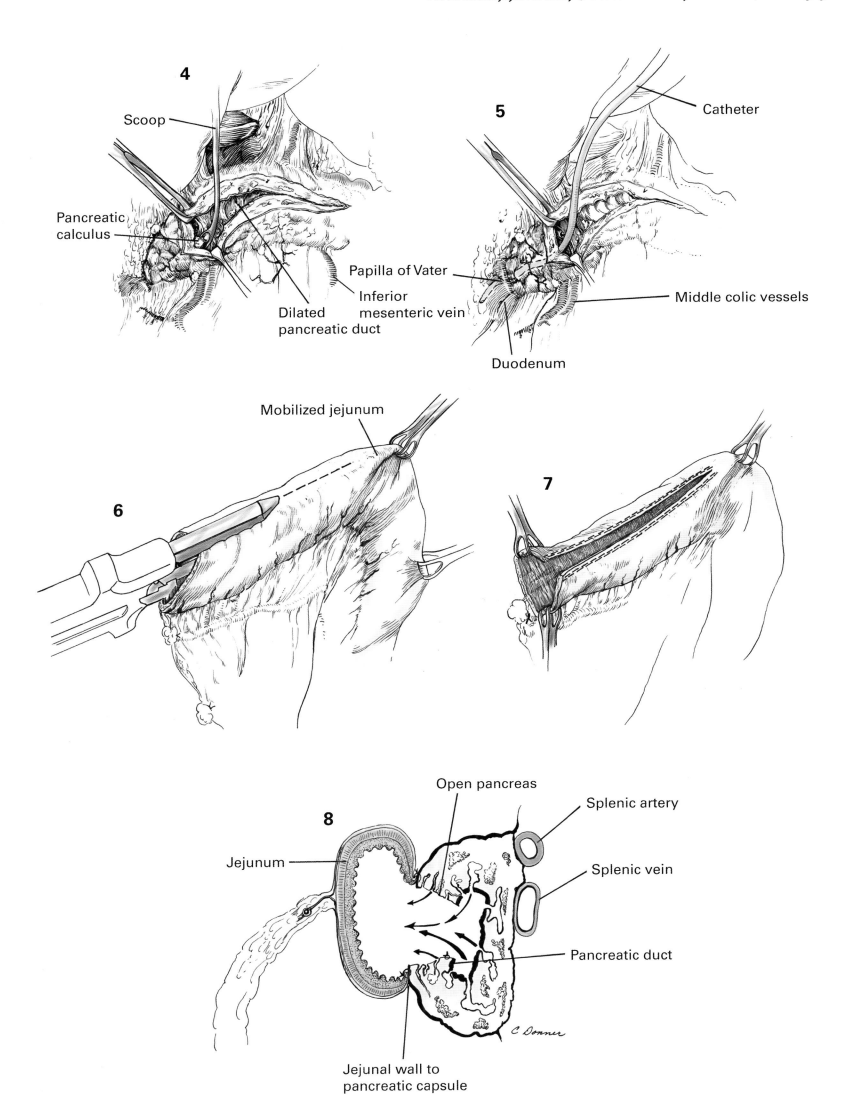

4

Scoop

Pancreatic calculus

Dilated pancreatic duct

Papilla of Vater

Inferior mesenteric vein

5

Catheter

Middle colic vessels

Duodenum

Mobilized jejunum

6

7

8

Open pancreas

Splenic artery

Jejunum

Splenic vein

Pancreatic duct

Jejunal wall to pancreatic capsule

C Donner

FIRST TECHNIQUE: LATERAL FISHMOUTH ANASTOMOSIS ◀CONTINUED
The open end of the jejunal arm is anastomosed over the opened pancreatic duct (FIGURE 9). The jejunum is anchored to the capsule of the tail of the fibrotic pancreas just beyond the end of the incision into the duct, and the full thickness of the jejunal wall is anchored to the cut margins of the capsule of the pancreas throughout the full length of the opened pancreatic duct. The open (fishmouth) end of the jejunum may need to be tailored from time to time, as outlined by the dotted lines (FIGURE 9), to ensure a sealed anastomosis around the duct. Again, only the capsule is included in these sutures, and the fibrotic wall of the pancreas is left free to promote drainage of the fine ducts, many of which are filled with small calculi. The anterior layer is also made with interrupted sutures, and the free end of the jejunum is anchored to the capsule with three or four additional sutures toward the tail of the pancreas (FIGURE 10). When the pancreas is shortened and thickened, a splenectomy may be necessary to adequately mobilize the pancreas and facilitate this anastomosis.

SECOND TECHNIQUE: FULL-WIDTH SIDE-TO-SIDE ANASTOMOSIS Some prefer to close the end of the Roux-en-Y arm of jejunum with two layers of interrupted silk sutures (Chapter 31, FIGURES 18 and 19) and anastomose the jejunum to the pancreas in a manner similar to a lateral anastomosis of small intestine (FIGURES 11 and 12). Only one layer of sutures is used, but they must be placed accurately and close enough together to prevent subsequent leakage.

When the Roux-en-Y principle is used, the jejunum near the ligament of Treitz is anastomosed to the arm of the jejunum going to the pancreas by an end-to-side anastomosis (FIGURE 13). The free margin of the mesentery should be secured by interrupted sutures (A) to the ascending jejunum to obliterate any opening for the subsequent development of an internal hernia (FIGURE 13). The opening in the mesocolon is closed about the jejunal arm. CONTINUES▶

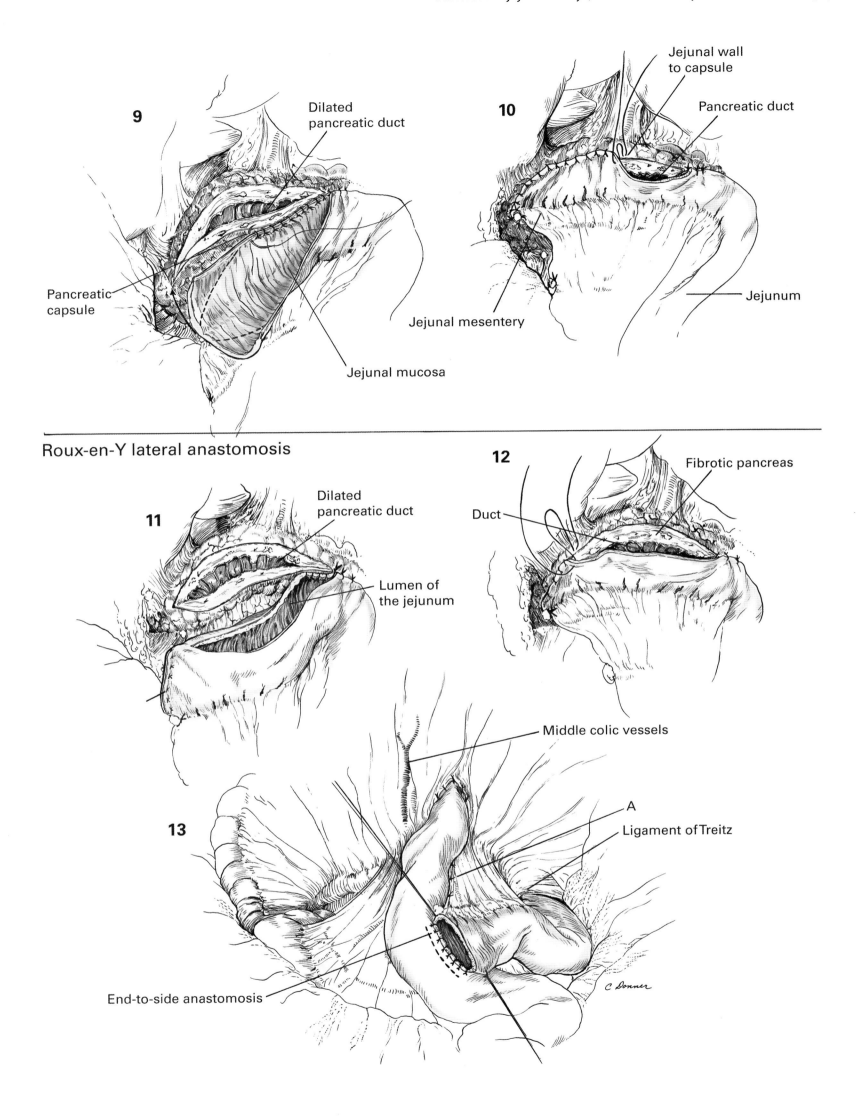

9 Dilated pancreatic duct

Pancreatic capsule

Jejunal mucosa

10 Jejunal wall to capsule

Pancreatic duct

Jejunum

Jejunal mesentery

Roux-en-Y lateral anastomosis

11 Dilated pancreatic duct

Lumen of the jejunum

12 Fibrotic pancreas

Duct

Middle colic vessels

13 A

Ligament of Treitz

End-to-side anastomosis

C. Donner

THIRD TECHNIQUE: PANCREATIC IMPLANTATION WITHIN JEJUNUM
CONTINUED In addition to the previous procedures described, drainage of the body and tail of the pancreas may be accomplished by implanting the left end of the pancreas into the open end of the arm of jejunum that has been brought up for a Roux-en-Y type of anastomosis.

When the pancreas is severely inflamed, small, and contracted, it may be advisable to mobilize as much of the tail and body as possible and to remove the spleen in anticipation of implantation into the jejunum. Once the presence or absence of a dilated duct is confirmed by needle aspiration and palpation (FIGURE 14), the peritoneum is incised superior and inferior to the body and tail of the pancreas, care being taken not to injure the inferior mesenteric vein (FIGURE 14). After the peritoneum has been incised, the surgeon inserts his index finger behind the pancreas and can very easily, by a backward and forward motion, free the posterior wall of the body and tail of the pancreas from adjacent tissues. The finger is inserted completely around the pancreas, including the splenic artery and vein, which run along the superior surface of the pancreas (FIGURE 15). A rubber drain is passed through this opening in order to provide gentle traction on the pancreas for the dissection of the tail and exposure during the freeing of the remainder of the pancreas and the splenectomy (FIGURE 16). The gastrosplenic ligament is divided, and the blood supply along the greater curvature of the stomach is transfixed to the gastric wall with interrupted oo sutures. Alternatively, an ultrasonic dissector can be used to coagulate and divide the short gastric vessels. Any attachments between the superior pole of the spleen and the diaphragm are divided, and the spleen is mobilized well into the wound. The pedicle of the attachments between the inferior surface of the spleen and the colon is likewise divided, as is the posterior splenorenal ligament (see Chapter 90). The blood supply to the spleen is divided and ligated. The vessels then are doubly ligated with oo nonabsorbable ligatures (FIGURE 17). In the younger age-groups, it is desirable to make every effort to save the spleen because of the risk of subsequent sepsis. The mobilization of a chronically inflamed tail and body of the pancreas requires ligation of numerous small blood vessels entering the major splenic blood supply. CONTINUES

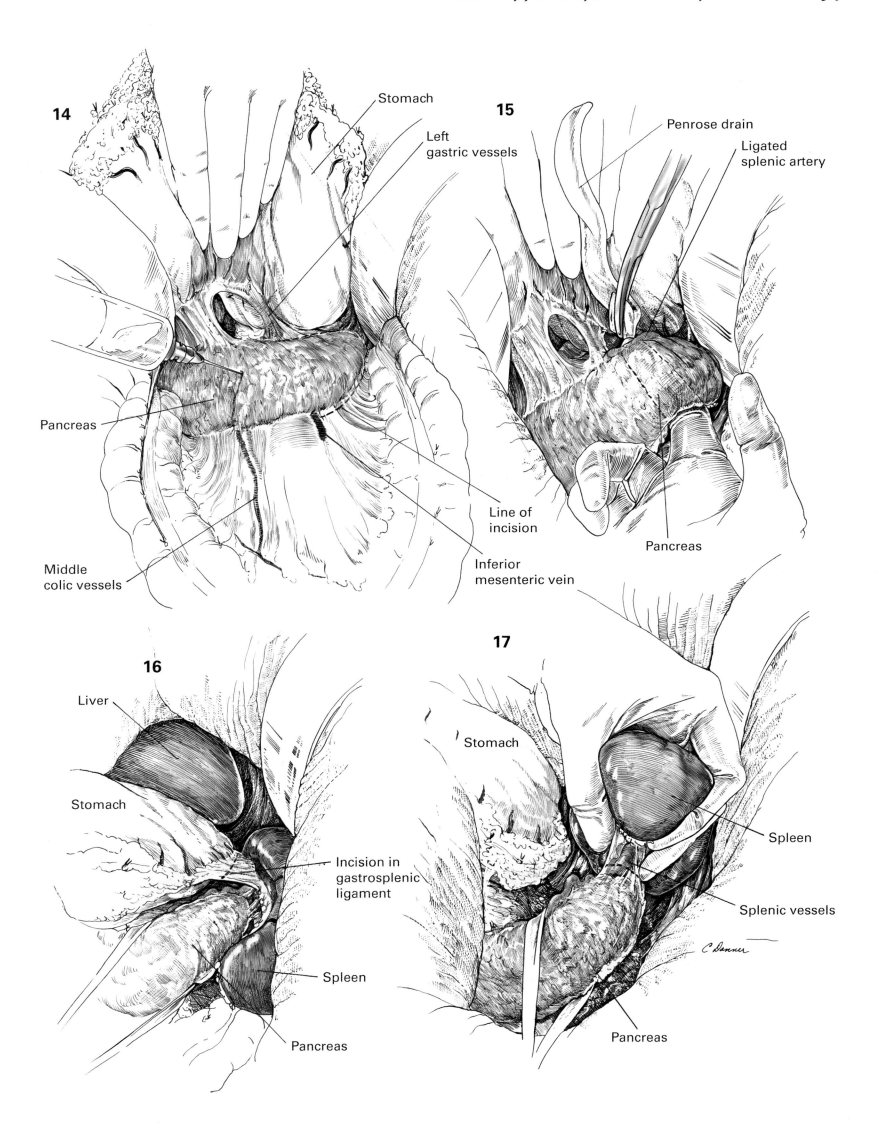

14

Stomach

Left gastric vessels

Pancreas

Middle colic vessels

Line of incision

Inferior mesenteric vein

15

Penrose drain

Ligated splenic artery

Pancreas

16

Liver

Stomach

Incision in gastrosplenic ligament

Spleen

Pancreas

17

Stomach

Spleen

Splenic vessels

Pancreas

C. Danner

THIRD TECHNIQUE: PANCREATIC IMPLANTATION WITHIN JEJUNUM
CONTINUED The tail and body of the pancreas, now freely mobilized, are rotated toward the midline so that the courses of the splenic artery and vein are clearly visualized (FIGURE 18). The splenic artery should be doubly ligated and divided near its point of origin. It is advisable to remove the artery from this point of ligature out to the tip of the pancreas. Likewise, the splenic vein should be carefully dissected free of the adjacent pancreas and doubly ligated very near its junction with the inferior mesenteric vein (FIGURE 18). After the artery and vein have been removed from the distal half of the pancreas, the tail of the pancreas is stabilized with a suture or Allis forceps, and the end of the pancreas is transected carefully until the pancreatic duct is identified (FIGURE 19). The small amount of bleeding that occurs can be controlled easily by compressing the pancreas between the thumb and index finger, clamping the individual bleeding points, and then ligating them with 0000 silk (FIGURE 19). As soon as the pancreatic duct is located, a probe is inserted into the duct (FIGURE 20). The duct is usually a little nearer to the superior than to the inferior margin of the pancreas. The surgeon then grasps the pancreas with the thumb and index finger and makes an incision directly down onto the probe, completely exteriorizing the major pancreatic duct (FIGURE 21). The incision should be carried medially, and soon the pancreatic duct will greatly enlarge. With intermittent strictures and dilatations, there is a tendency of the duct to form a chain of individual lakes. Multiple calculi may be encountered and small calcifications noted in many small ducts within the wall of the fibrosed pancreas. The incision is carried from the tail of the pancreas downward as near as possible to the medial border of the duodenum (FIGURE 22). This is accomplished by stabilizing the pancreas with the left hand and inserting scissors into the lumen of the duct and carrying the dissection medially (FIGURE 22). The finger is inserted into the enlarged proximal portion of the dilated duct, and any calculi are removed. A small probe may be introduced into this area to determine whether or not there is free communication between the pancreatic duct and the duodenum through the ampulla, but this is not absolutely necessary (FIGURE 23). During the dissection the fibrotic wall of the pancreas is grasped with multiple Allis forceps, usually at the points of active bleeding. When these clamps are removed, the individual points are carefully ligated with interrupted absorbable sutures. No effort is made to approximate the wall of the duct and the fibrous capsule so that free drainage from the smaller ducts will be possible. **CONTINUES**

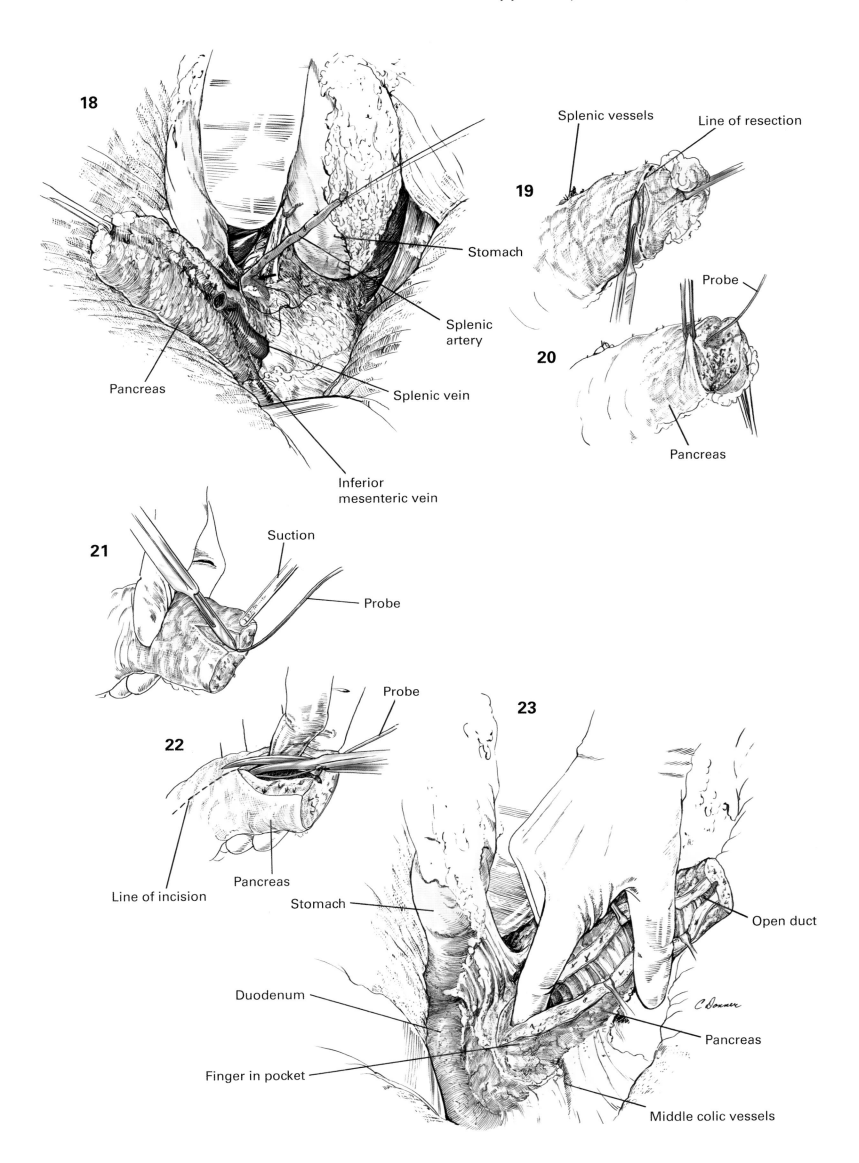

18

Pancreas

19 Splenic vessels   Line of resection

Stomach

Splenic artery

Splenic vein

20 Probe

Pancreas

Inferior mesenteric vein

21 Suction

Probe

22 Probe

23

Line of incision

Pancreas

Stomach   Open duct

Duodenum

Pancreas

Finger in pocket

Middle colic vessels

THIRD TECHNIQUE: PANCREATIC IMPLANTATION WITHIN JEJUNUM

CONTINUED The jejunum is held up out of the wound. By transillumination, the surgeon can study the vascular arcades and select more accurately the blood vessels to be divided for mobilizing the arm of the jejunum to be brought up to the pancreas (Chapter 31). The jejunum is divided at a point 10 to 15 cm beyond the ligament of Treitz. A small opening is made in the mesocolon to the left of the middle colic vessels, just over the ligament of Treitz. The jejunum is pulled through this opening and measured along the full length of the pancreas (FIGURE 24). The length of the pancreas from just beyond the end of the opened duct to the end of its tail is marked, point X, on the jejunum, by Babcock forceps placed on its antimesenteric border (FIGURE 24). The tail of the pancreas will be drawn into the bowel lumen and approximated to point X. Here the surgeon must be certain that there is adequate jejunal length and that the mesenteric vascular pedicle will reach easily without angulation. Traction sutures (A and B) of oo silk are placed on the superior and inferior borders of the capsule of the pancreas (FIGURE 25) to aid in pulling the tail to point X. The Potts forceps are removed from the open end of the jejunum and replaced by Babcock forceps at the antimesenteric border. The jejunum is gently stretched between the two Babcock forceps as the needles, with attached traction sutures A and B, are introduced into the lumen of the bowel. During insertion the needles are held parallel to the long axis of the holder with points backward to ensure that the bowel wall is not punctured (FIGURE 26A). At point X, the needle is sharply retracted to puncture the wall and carry the suture externally (FIGURE 26B). Gentle traction is maintained upon these sutures to aid in pulling the pancreas up into the jejunum. When the pancreas is completely encased inside the bowel, sutures A and B are tied together, bringing the tail to point X (FIGURE 27). The opened end of the jejunum is then circumferentially tracked down to the capsule with interrupted nonabsorbable oo sutures. The posterior row is placed first, beginning at the mesenteric border and proceeding superiorly to the antimesenteric surface.

The anterior row is also begun at the mesenteric border of the jejunum. If the jejunal circumference is too small, the bowel may be longitudinally incised to accommodate the girth of the pancreas (FIGURE 27).

The adequacy of the blood supply of the jejunum is repeatedly checked. Intestinal continuity is established through a Roux-en-Y jejunojejunostomy, beyond the ligament of Treitz, using two layers of fine nonabsorbable sutures (FIGURE 28). All free edges of the mesentery should be closed with interrupted oooo silk sutures, care being taken that the marginal blood supply within the mesentery is not compromised. Before closure the blood supply of the jejunum should be rechecked carefully. A few sutures are taken to anchor the vascular margin of the mesentery to adjacent structures to prevent its rotation and the formation of an internal hernia. The window in the mesocolon is also secured to the pancreatic arm of the Roux-en-Y.

CLOSURE If biliary tract surgery has been performed simultaneously, a closed-system suction catheter made of Silastic is inserted in the foramen of Winslow. If T-tube drainage of the common duct has been instituted, the tube is brought out through a separate stab wound on the right side. Drainage is unnecessary for the pancreaticojejunostomy itself. The incision is closed in a routine manner. In the presence of impaired nutrition, it may be advisable to supplement the closure with retention sutures.

POSTOPERATIVE CARE Although varying degrees of pancreatitis can be anticipated following this procedure, the postoperative course is surprisingly mild. Blood amylase and sugar levels are determined and attention given to the narcotic requirements. These patients tend to be addicted to narcotics and may be difficult to sedate because of chronic alcoholism. Pancreatic enzyme therapy should be instituted, the diabetic tendency should be regulated, and any previous addiction should be corrected, if possible, before the patient is discharged from the hospital. An ulcer type of dietary program should be followed, with a gradual return to a more liberal diet. ■

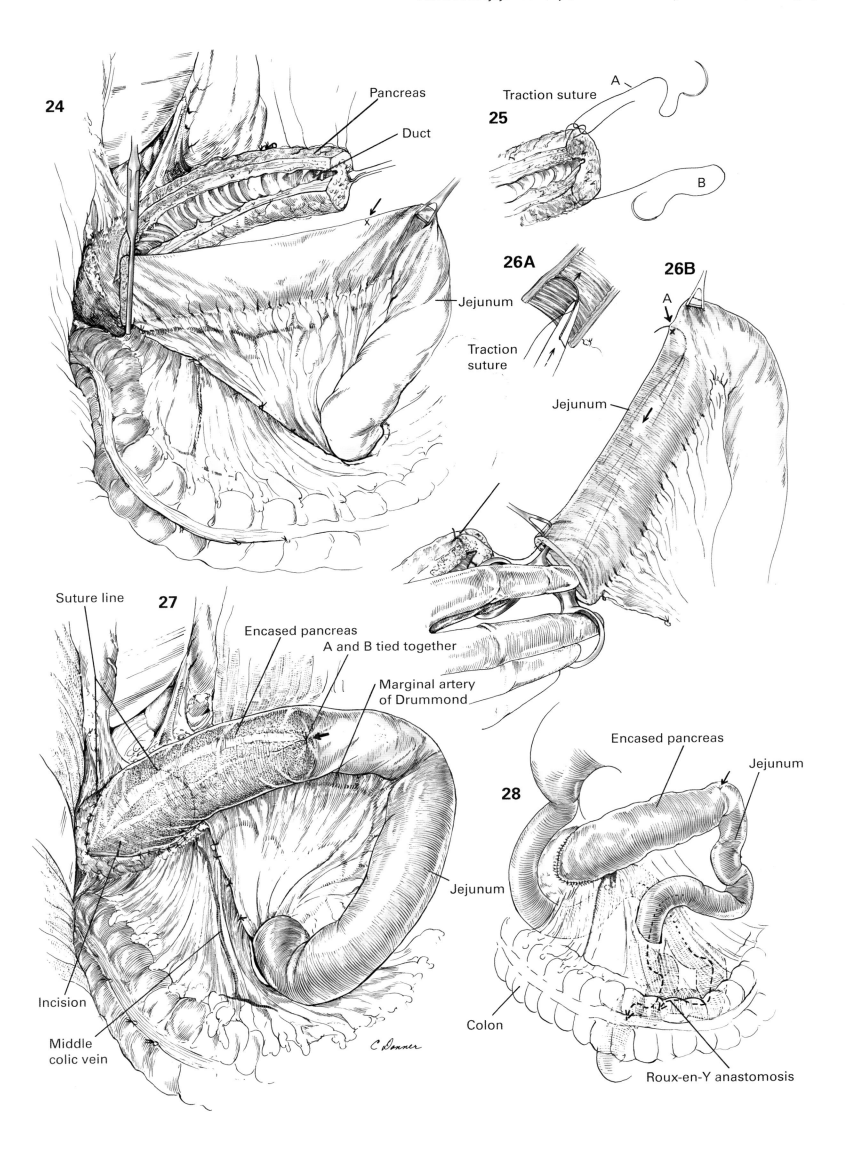

24
Pancreas
Duct
Jejunum

25
Traction suture
A
B

26A
Traction suture

26B
A
Jejunum

27
Suture line
Encased pancreas
A and B tied together
Marginal artery of Drummond
Jejunum
Incision
Middle colic vein

C Donner

28
Encased pancreas
Jejunum
Colon
Roux-en-Y anastomosis

INDICATIONS The more common indications for resecting the body and tail of the pancreas include localized adenocarcinoma in this area, islet cell adenomas, cysts, and chronic calcific pancreatitis. This procedure may be the initial approach for total pancreatectomy for carcinoma of the pancreas.

PREOPERATIVE PREPARATION The preparation is related to the preoperative diagnosis. If splenectomy is contemplated then vaccines for pneumococcus, haemophilus influenza, and meningococcus should be administered prior to the surgery.

The patient with an insulinoma, suggested by repeated fasting blood sugars of below 50 mg/dL, requires supplementary glucose by mouth or intravenously at regular intervals for 24 hours preceding surgery and intravenously during surgery.

When an ulcerogenic tumor is suspected, the fluid and electrolyte balance should be corrected, particularly if there have been large losses of gastric secretion or losses from enteritis. Serum gastrin levels may establish the diagnosis, and the patient may require a total gastrectomy in the future. Every effort should be made to localize one or more endocrine tumors by CT, MRI, somatostatin scintigraphy, or selective arteriography and selective arterial stimulation with either secretin (for gastrinoma) or calcium (for insulinoma).

ANESTHESIA General anesthesia with endotracheal intubation is used.

POSITION Supine position with the feet lower than the head.

OPERATIVE PREPARATION The skin is shaved from the level of the nipples well out over the chest wall and down over the abdomen, including the flanks. The skin is prepared in the routine manner.

INCISION AND EXPOSURE Either a long vertical midline or an extensive curved incision parallel to the costal margins, as described for pancreaticoduodenectomy (Chapter 88).

DETAILS OF PROCEDURE When the procedure is carried out for an inflammatory lesion of the body and tail of the pancreas, a direct exploration of this region is performed. When the procedure is carried out for tumor, a thorough exploration of the abdomen, with particular reference to the liver and the gastrohepatic ligament in the region of the celiac plexus, should be made for evidence of metastasis. A possible microscopic diagnosis of adenocarcinoma is sought by biopsy before proceeding with a total pancreatectomy from the left-side approach. Since the adenomas can be distributed throughout the pancreas, the head of the pancreas must be thoroughly explored by visualization and palpation preliminary to a definitive type of procedure on the left half of the pancreas. Evidence of gastric hypersecretion, as indicated by increased vascularity and thickening of the gastric wall, along with a hyperemic and hypertrophic duodenum and an ulcer in the duodenum or beyond the ligament of Treitz, adds support to the potential diagnosis of gastrinoma tumor of the pancreas. Likewise, the inner wall of the duodenum should be carefully palpated in the search for small adenomas extending into the lumen of the duodenum from the pancreatic side. Finally, a sterile ultrasound probe for intraoperative scanning of nonpalpable lesions is advocated by most surgeons.

After the abdomen has been explored and the region of the head of the pancreas evaluated, the greater omentum is reflected upward, and downward traction is maintained on the transverse colon as the omentum is separated by sharp dissection and the lesser sac entered (FIGURE 1). Usually, the stomach is easily separated from the pancreas, but sharp dissection may be required to separate it from the capsule of the pancreas, especially if there have been repeated bouts of acute inflammation. Sharp as well as blunt dissection is used to sweep the posterior gastric wall away from the pancreas, particularly in the region of the antrum, to make certain the middle colic vessels have not been angulated upward and attached to the posterior gastric wall. A clear view must be ensured of the entire pancreas and the first part of the duodenum all the way over to the hilus of the spleen (FIGURE 1). To avoid troublesome bleeding, it is usually desirable to divide the communicating vein between the right gastroepiploic vessels and the middle colic vein inferior to the pylorus. This permits better mobilization in the region of the antrum. Large S retractors can be used to retract the stomach upward as the transverse colon is either pulled downward outside the wound or returned to the abdomen and packed away. The pancreas should be inspected thoroughly and palpated to verify the pathology. It is safer and far easier to mobilize and remove the spleen rather than attempt to separate the pancreas from the splenic artery and vein running along the superior surface of the body and tail of this organ.

In carcinoma the tumor's mobility and the presence or absence of regional metastasis must be determined before a radical resection is planned. It is less uncommon to find a resectable carcinoma involving the tail or body of the pancreas. In insulinomas it is more common to find only one tumor; this may be enucleated without removing a large segment of the pancreas, depending on the adenoma's location and relationship to the major pancreatic duct and vessels. Finding a solitary gastrinoma of considerable size may tempt the surgeon to do a local excision only, followed by vagotomy, pyloroplasty, and proton pump inhibitor therapy postoperatively. Any enlarged lymph nodes around the pancreas are excised for frozen section examination searching for evidence of metastases. For gastrinoma, the duodenum must be opened and explored to search and remove a possible duodenal primary lesion.

When the lesion cannot be seen or palpated by digital examination of the anterior surface of the gland, the body and tail must be mobilized for direct palpation with the thumb and index finger and for visualization of the under-side of the pancreas. This is accomplished by incising the peritoneum along the inferior surface of the pancreas (FIGURE 2). Only a few small blood vessels are encountered. The inferior mesenteric vein should be identified, and the incision should avoid it as well as the middle colic vessels. After the inferior surface of the peritoneum has been incised, a finger can be introduced rather easily underneath the pancreas, and the substance of the gland can be palpated quite easily between the thumb and index finger (FIGURE 3). As a matter of fact, the finger can be inserted completely around the pancreas following the incision in the peritoneum just above the splenic artery and vein. Finally, a hand-held ultrasound unit is very useful in finding nonpalpable lesions within the pancreas. CONTINUES ▶

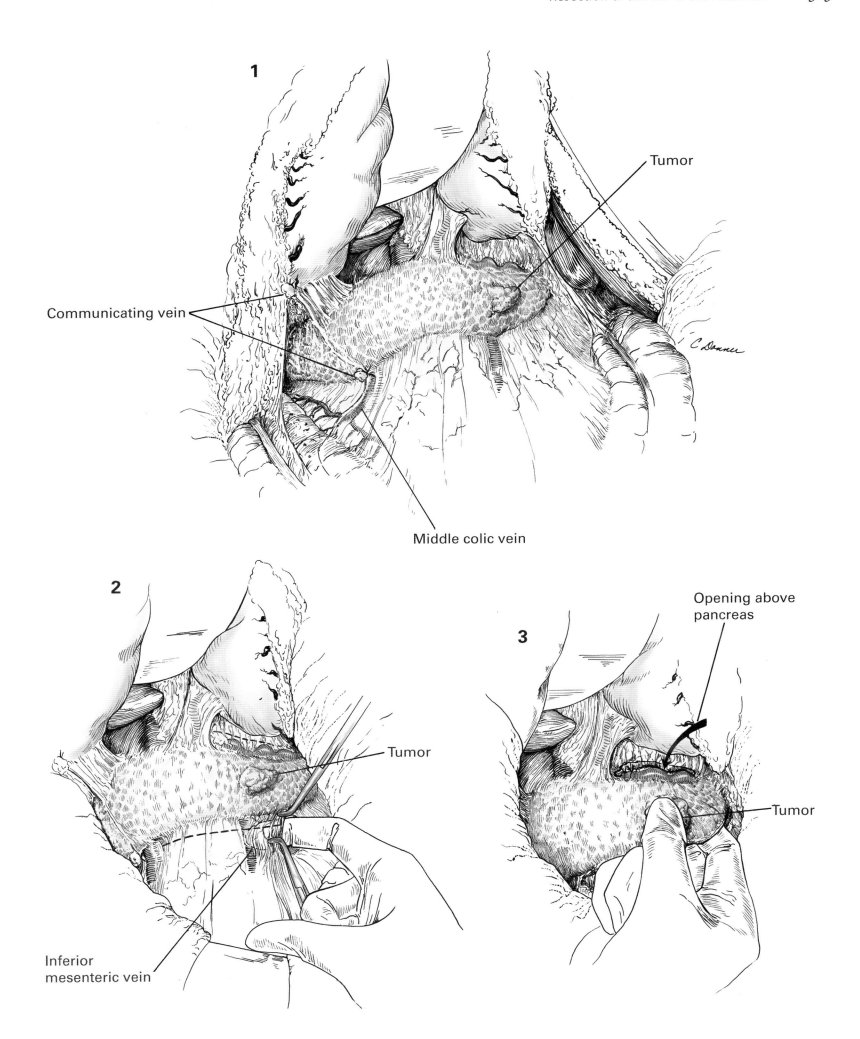

1

Tumor

Communicating vein

Middle colic vein

C Danner

2

Tumor

Inferior
mesenteric vein

3

Opening above
pancreas

Tumor

DETAILS OF PROCEDURE ◄CONTINUED In the presence of a tumor that necessitates removal of the left half or all of the pancreas, steps should be taken to mobilize and remove the spleen. The splenic artery is doubly ligated with oo silk near its point of origin. This tends to decrease the blood loss following manipulation of the spleen and permits blood to drain from this organ into the systemic circulation during the subsequent steps of its removal. The left gastroepiploic vessel is doubly clamped and ligated, and the short gastric vessels are then divided all the way up to the diaphragm. The blood supply on the greater curvature should be ligated by transfixing sutures that incorporate a bite of the gastric wall to prevent hemorrhage if gastric distention should occur and the ligature slip off the gastric side (FIGURE 4). Alternatively, the ultrasonic dissector can be used to coagulate and divide the short gastric vessels. The splenorenal ligament is divided as the surgeon pulls the spleen medially with his left hand (FIGURE 5). Blunt and sharp dissection may be carried out to free the tail of the pancreas, but this is rather easily done by finger dissection as the organ is reflected medially (FIGURE 6). The left adrenal and kidney are clearly visualized as well as a segment of the left renal vein. The inferior mesenteric vein is ligated and divided (FIGURE 6) at the inferior border of the pancreas. The splenic artery is divided near its point of origin and ligated and then transfixed distally with double ties of oo silk. The splenic vein is cleared and separated from the posterior surface of the pancreas and is followed over to the point where it joins the superior mesenteric vein to form the portal vein (FIGURE 7). The splenic vein is gently freed from the pancreas, using blunt-nosed right-angle clamps (FIGURE 7). The vessel is ligated and is transfixed proximally to this tie to avoid any possible late hemorrhage. The spleen and body of the pancreas can then be mobilized sufficiently to be brought outside the peritoneal cavity.

This approach is useful in performing a total pancreatectomy since it ensures a good exposure for the identification of veins coming off the medial aspect of the portal vein. The superior surface of the portal vein is free of venous tributaries. However, the resection may be restricted due to involvement of the portal vein by adenocarcinoma. CONTINUES►

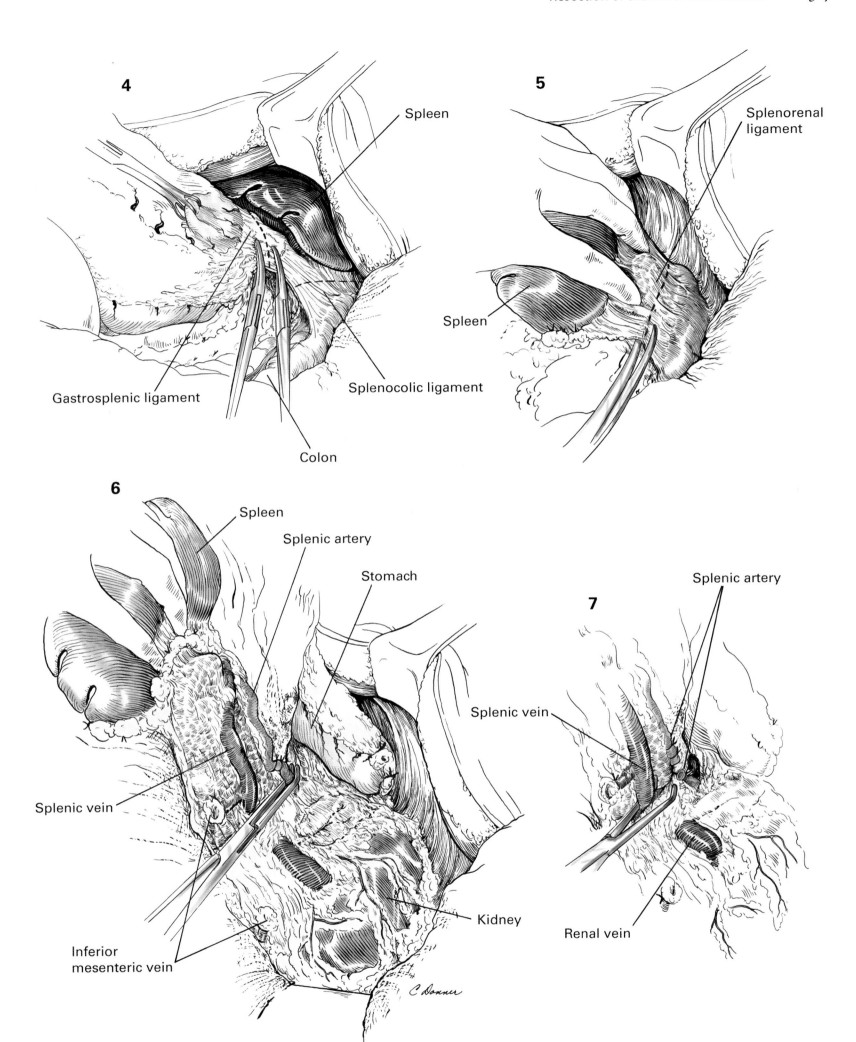

4

Spleen

Gastrosplenic ligament

Splenocolic ligament

Colon

5

Splenorenal ligament

Spleen

6

Spleen

Splenic artery

Stomach

Splenic vein

Inferior mesenteric vein

Kidney

7

Splenic artery

Splenic vein

Renal vein

C. Donner

DETAILS OF PROCEDURE ◄CONTINUED After the spleen and the tail of the pancreas have been mobilized outside the peritoneal cavity, the entire pancreas is palpated once again for evidence of tumor involvement. The pancreas can be divided with electrocautery to the left of the portal vein or, if need be, even to the right side of the portal vein, provided that a finger has been introduced between the vein and the pancreas to free its anterior margin (FIGURE 8).

The surgeon usually finds it advisable to make multiple serial sections of the pancreas in searching for additional adenomas and in determining whether his line of incision is free of tumor. Frozen section consultations may be obtained, although pancreatic tissue is difficult to evaluate under these circumstances, and the final diagnosis may have to be delayed until the permanent sections have been made.

The cut end of the pancreas is examined and the pancreatic duct is identified. The pancreatic duct is closed with a 0000 nonabsorbable monofilament suture (FIGURE 9A). The end of the pancreas is closed with interrupted overlapping 000 silk sutures of the mattress type (FIGURE 9B). Additional sutures are taken, particularly where there is persistent bleeding (FIGURE 10). Alternatively, the pancreas may be divided and secured with staples using a linear stapler.

CLOSURE A closed-system suction catheter made of Silastic is used to drain the stump of the pancreas. The drain is brought out either directly through a stab wound in the midportion of the abdomen or to either side through a separate stab wound incision. The incision is closed in the routine manner.

POSTOPERATIVE CARE The postoperative care is routine except for repeated laboratory checks on the blood sugar and amylase levels. A mild degree of pancreatitis may occur, and colloids and other solutions should be given in adequate amount. A transient diabetic tendency may occur; on the other hand, it is difficult to determine in the immediate postoperative period what effect the surgical procedure will have on total pancreatic function. Oral replacement of pancreatic enzymes may be indicated. Determination of amylase in the drain output is necessary prior to drain removal. An amylase concentration less than serum is generally required for the closed-suction drain to be removed.

When total pancreatectomy is planned, the pancreas is not divided but used for traction as the head of the pancreas and the duodenum are excised in the Whipple operation. Systemic symptoms associated with the gastrinoma, a hormone-producing islet cell tumor, may be controlled partially, but rarely completely, for years by resection of a solitary tumor. Those associated with other apudomas (vipoma, glucagonoma, insulinoma, and so forth) may respond to local excision in the absence of malignancy and metastases. ■

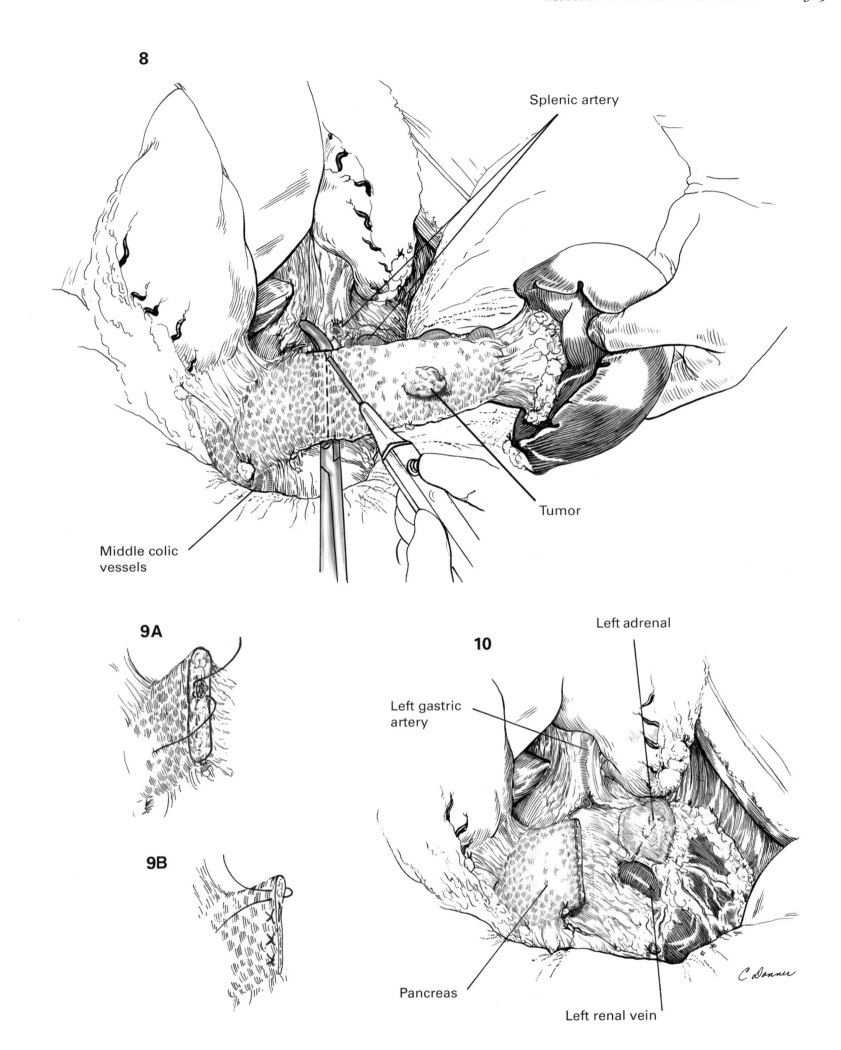

8

Splenic artery

Tumor

Middle colic
vessels

9A

9B

10

Left adrenal

Left gastric
artery

Pancreas

Left renal vein

C. Donner

RESECTION OF THE TAIL OF THE PANCREAS WITH SPLENIC PRESERVATION, LAPAROSCOPIC

INDICATIONS Laparoscopic resection of the body and tail of the pancreas is limited to certain pancreatic neoplastic diseases including pancreatic neuroendocrine tumors such as insulinomas, pancreatic cystic neoplasms, and pseudopapillary tumors. The approach is not recommended for chronic calcific pancreatitis. For adenocarcinoma of the body and tail of the pancreas, splenectomy should be performed. Splenic preservation is recommended and should be attempted in the absence of a malignant neoplasm.

PREOPERATIVE PREPARATION The preparation is related to the preoperative diagnosis. As splenic preservation is not always possible, it is recommended to vaccinate the patient 2 weeks prior to the surgery against encapsulated organisms including pneumococcus, haemophilus influenza, and meningococcus.

ANESTHESIA General anesthesia with endotracheal intubation is required.

POSITION A cushioned beanbag should be placed on the operating table prior to bringing the patient into the room. After insertion of a bladder catheter, the patient should be positioned in a partial lateral position at about 45 degrees with the left arm crossing the chest and supported on an arm board or pillows (FIGURE 1A). The right arm is placed on an arm board and an axillary roll is used. Liberal padding is used between and around both arms. The abdomen and flank area should be exposed. The left knee is flexed, with a padding of blankets or pillows between the legs. Alternatively, the patient may be positioned in a modified lithotomy position, also using a cushioned beanbag and taking care not to flex the thighs excessively so as to avoid interference with the range of motion of the instruments.

OPERATIVE PREPARATION Hair removal is accomplished with skin clippers from the level of the nipples well out over the chest wall and down over the abdomen, including the flanks. The skin is prepared in the routine manner.

INCISION AND EXPOSURE The surgeon stands on the patient's right side similar to a laparoscopic left adrenalectomy (FIGURE 1A). The camera operator stands to the right of the surgeon and the assistant on the left side of the patient. If the modified lithotomy position is employed, the surgeon is positioned between the legs and the camera operator to the patient's right and the assistant to the patient's left. Port placement is shown in FIGURE 1B. A 10-mm 30-degree laparoscope is placed above the umbilicus using the open technique of Hasson as described in Chapter 11. The abdomen is insufflated to 15 mm Hg pressure. The laparoscope is introduced and all four quadrants of the abdomen are examined for metastatic disease. Two 5-mm ports are placed: one in the midline and one to the left side midway between the umbilicus and the xiphoid process at the midclavicular line. The ports are place about 5 to 8 cm apart in the craniocaudal orientation to permit bimanual operation without physical restriction. A 10–12 or 15-mm port is placed on the left side at the level of the umbilicus in the anterior axillary line. An additional 5-mm port is placed just below the right subcostal margin in the midclavicular line. A 15-mm port is required for an endoscopic stapler with 4.8-mm staples that may be used to divide a thicker pancreas, whereas a stapler with 3.8-mm staples or less will be able to be introduced through a 12-mm port.

DETAILS OF PROCEDURE The stomach is grasped with an atraumatic laparoscopic clamp and retracted superiorly. The lesser sac is then entered using a harmonic scalpel to divide the omentum along the greater curvature of the stomach (FIGURE 2). The opening in the lesser sac should be generous and allow exposure of the body and tail of the pancreas. The lateral extent of the incision is carried to the level of the short gastrics. The short gastric vessels are not divided when planning splenic preservation. Medial exposure is essential; therefore, the opening in the omentum is carried to the right gastroepiploic vessels. Sharp as well as blunt dissection is used to sweep the posterior gastric wall away from the pancreas, particularly in the region of the antrum, to make certain the middle colic vessels have not been angulated upward and attached to the posterior gastric wall. The surgeon must ensure a clear view of the entire pancreas and the first part of the duodenum all the way over to the hilus of the spleen (FIGURE 2). To avoid troublesome bleeding, it is usually desirable to divide the communicating vein between the right gastroepiploic vessels and the middle colic vein inferior to the pylorus. This permits better mobilization in the region of the antrum. The pancreas should be visually inspected to identify the pathology. Intraoperative ultrasound may be helpful.

The operation will be carried out in a medial to lateral direction, as opposed to the lateral to medial direction for an open distal pancreatectomy as shown in the preceding Chapter 86. An incision is made in the peritoneum along the inferior border of the body and tail of the pancreas (FIGURE 2). Gentle dissection along the neck of the pancreas will expose the superior mesenteric vein and the portal vein (FIGURE 3). The splenic vein is identified. An incision is then made along the superior edge of the pancreas to the left of the gastroduodenal artery

and inferior to the hepatic artery. A plane between the portal vein and the neck of the pancreas is created by gentle blunt dissection in the inferior to superior direction with a blunt nose laparoscopic dissector (FIGURE 4). Once the opening is complete and the blunt-tipped dissector can be seen protruding from the superior edge of the pancreas, a half-inch Penrose drain shortened to 12 cm is placed into the abdominal cavity through the 12- or 15-mm port. It is then passed underneath the neck of the pancreas and the ends are secured with an endoloop (FIGURE 5). This will allow anterior traction of the pancreas, which is essential to dissecting the plane along the superior mesenteric vein and the neck of the pancreas, and will also facilitate mobilization of the splenic vein away from the proximal body of the pancreas. The assistant grasps the Penrose drain and pulls it superiorly and anteriorly. The surgeon then begins to gently dissect the mesenteric vessels and portal vein away from the neck. The splenic vein will come into view, and prior to division of the pancreas, small branches of the vein are divided with the ultrasonic dissector and larger branches are clipped. This dissection is carried out in the medial to lateral direction for 2 to 3 cm. It may be necessary to place a shortened vessel loop around the splenic vein to provide countertraction and proximal vascular control. Once 2 to 3 cm of the vein has been dissected free, the neck of the pancreas is divided. This is accomplished with a reticulated endoscopic stapling device with 3.8- or 4.8-mm staples. The staple line may be reinforced with a commercial material (FIGURE 6). Both the proximal and the distal staple lines are inspected for bleeding, and if bleeding is found, it is controlled with electrocautery or the ultrasonic dissector. The Penrose drain may be removed at this point, as retraction of the pancreas may be obtained by grasping the distal staple line. Once the pancreas is divided, the body of the pancreas is retracted superiorly (FIGURE 7). This will permit the branches of the splenic artery to be divided. The splenic artery will come into view superior to the splenic vein. Small braches of the splenic artery are then divided with the ultrasonic dissector and larger branches are clipped. (FIGURE 7). A second shortened vessel loop may be passed around the splenic artery in order to provide counter traction as well as proximal vascular control. Once the branches of the proximal splenic artery are divided, the remaining branches of the splenic vein are ligated. The distal pancreas is pulled downward to further expose the splenic artery (FIGURE 8). The branches of both the artery and the vein are very fragile and unavoidable avulsion will occasionally occur. For small branches, bleeding may be controlled with pressure. Larger branches should be grasped with a Maryland dissector to control the bleeding and then clipped if there is sufficient length or ligated with a 4-0 or 5-0 monofilament suture if their length is insufficient. The peritoneum is further divided along the inferior edge of the pancreas. The posterior margin of the dissection will be the splenic vein and artery. The proximal jejunum may be seen and should be retracted inferiorly. Defects in the mesocolon should be closed with sutures to prevent internal hernias. The peritoneum is also divided along the superior edge of the pancreas with the ultrasonic dissector. As dissection proceeds, the vein will next be seen as it exits the splenic hilum. Shortly thereafter, the artery will be seen entering the spleen. The distance between the end of the tail of the pancreas and the spleen is variable. The final attachments are divided with the harmonic ultrasonic dissector. The specimen is extracted from the abdominal cavity using a specimen retrieval bag or similar device (FIGURE 9). It is removed from the abdominal cavity from the umbilical port. Once it is removed, the abdomen is reinsufflated and the lesser sac exposed to permit inspection of the splenic artery and vein for bleeding. If vessel loops have been used, they are removed at this point.

CLOSURE The specimen should be examined to determine that the pathology has been removed. A frozen section at the margin should be obtained for pancreatic cystic tumors and intraductal mucinous neoplasms. A closed-suction Silastic drain may be placed by passing the external portion of the drain through the 12- or 15-mm port and withdrawing from one of the 5-mm port sites. The 12- or 15-mm port site is closed with #1 absorbable suture. The umbilical port site is closed with #1 absorbable suture.

POSTOPERATIVE CARE A nasogastric tube is not necessary. Crystalloids should be given in an adequate amount. Pain management will require intravenous narcotic analgesics for 1 to 2 days. Antibiotics are discontinued within 24 hours. Glucose monitoring should be performed as a transient diabetic state may occur. The hemoglobin and electrolytes should be checked on the first postoperative day and repeated as deemed necessary by the clinical course. An initial postoperative diet may be started on the first postoperative day. The drain amylase should be measured prior to removing the closed-suction drain. The drain should not be removed if the amylase is greater than two times the upper limit of normal. Supplemental pancreatic enzymes are usually not necessary. The patient is discharged when tolerating a diet. ■

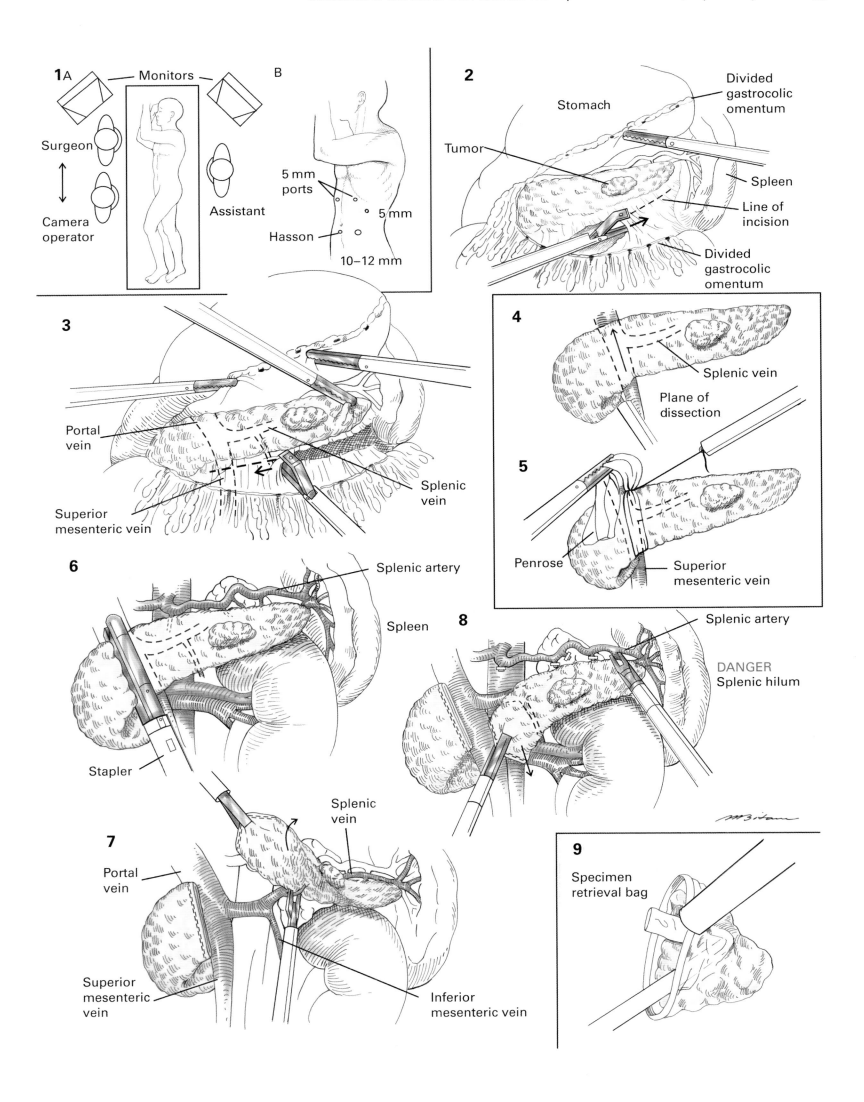

CHAPTER 88

PANCREATICODUODENECTOMY (WHIPPLE PROCEDURE)

INDICATIONS The head of the pancreas is usually removed for malignancy involving the ampulla of Vater, the lower end of the common duct, the head of the pancreas, or the duodenum. With increasing frequency, Whipple is indicated for the risk of malignancy associated with the presence of a cystic neoplasm with worrisome features. Far less frequently, the procedure is carried out to manage intractable pain associated with a chronic calcific pancreatitis or for massive trauma when there has been irreparable "burst" damage to the head of the pancreas, the ductal structures, and the duodenum. In the presence of malignancy, the resection is indicated in the absence of proven metastases and if the tumor is of such a limited size that the portal vein is not involved beyond the ability of the surgeon to accomplish a safe vascular resection and repair. Total pancreatectomy may be considered in some cases due to central location of a malignant tumor or extensive main duct involvement by papillary mucinous epithelium (IPMN). While, total pancreatectomy decreases the incidence of postoperative complications related to the leakage of pancreatic juice from an anastomosis, the subsequent endocrinopathy can be profound. The patient should be made aware of the problem of diabetes mellitus after operation as well as the need for daily pancreatic enzyme replacement.

PREOPERATIVE PREPARATION Patients will have had imaging including CT, MRI, and possibly endoscopic ultrasound prior to the procedure. Some patients may have had biliary stents placed by an endoscopic or transhepatic route. The electrolyte levels should be returned to normal and particular care should be taken that the INR is normal and that renal function is not impaired, as shown by creatinine and blood urea nitrogen levels. Patients with jaundice may have occult vitamin K deficiency that may not become apparent until blood loss occurs. Unexpected blood loss can be substantial so blood should be available for transfusion as needed, preferably via a central venous catheter. It is advisable to have a catheter in the bladder in order to follow the postoperative hourly output of urine. Antibiotic therapy should be started prior to operation. This is particularly important for patients with stents, as they are prone to wound infections.

ANESTHESIA A nasogastric tube is inserted. General anesthesia with endotracheal intubation is recommended.

POSITION The patient is placed supine on the table with the feet slightly lower than the head. Facilities should be available for performing a cholangiogram or pancreaticogram.

OPERATIVE PREPARATION The skin should be shaved from the level of the nipples well out over the chest wall and down over the abdomen, including the flanks.

INCISION AND EXPOSURE Diagnostic laparoscopy is indicated in some patients to identify metastatic disease that may have been missed by preoperative imaging. Pancreaticoduodenectomy for pancreatic or periampullary adenocarcinoma should not be performed if there are liver or peritoneal metastasis. A type of incision should be selected that will ensure the extensive

and free visualization of the upper abdomen, especially on the right side. While an upper midline (FIGURE 1A) incision that may extend below the umbilicus is useful, many prefer an oblique or curved incision that parallels the costal margins (FIGURE 1B). When the xiphoid is long and the xiphocostal angle narrow, further exposure may be obtained by excision of the xiphoid process. On the other hand, very good exposures can usually be obtained by the oblique or curved incision, first carried out over the right upper quadrant and then extended across the midline and as far to the left as the surgeon believes necessary to ensure a liberal exposure. All bleeding points must be carefully controlled to keep blood loss at a minimum, especially in jaundiced patients. Regardless of the type of incision used, the round ligament is divided (FIGURE 2). The contents of the curved clamps must be securely ligated or divided with an energy device to avoid bleeding from a vessel in the round ligament. Further mobility of the liver can be obtained if the falciform ligament is divided well up over the dome of the liver but is often not necessary (FIGURE 2). After the falciform ligament has been divided, a self-retaining retractor can be inserted.

DETAILS OF PROCEDURE The type, location, and extent of the pathologic process now must be determined by thorough exploration. Evidence of metastatic spread to the peritoneum, liver, the lymph nodes around the celiac axis, and the region above the pancreas, as well as in the hepatoduodenal ligament, should be sought by careful exploration.

Initial determination of resection begins with mobilization of the duodenum and head of the pancreas by the Kocher maneuver (FIGURE 3). The duodenum is grasped with one or more Babcock forceps and retracted medially as the peritoneum along the lateral wall of the duodenum is incised. Usually, it is not necessary to ligate vessels in this area; in the presence of jaundice; however, it is advisable to carry out a meticulous hemostasis. Finger or gauze dissection is used to push the posterior wall of the pancreas from the underlying vena cava and right kidney. An avascular cleavage plane can easily be developed (FIGURE 4). A column of peritoneum that remains forms the lower boundary of the foramen of Winslow (FIGURE 5). The surgeon can place this column of peritoneum under tension by inserting the index and middle fingers on either side of the peritoneum and should incise it very carefully, avoiding injury to the underlying vena cava. In the presence of recurrent ulceration in the region of the second part of the duodenum, considerable scarring and fixation in this area may be encountered. Attention should be paid to avoid injury to an aberrant right hepatic artery, if present, traversing the posterior hepatoduodenal ligament from the superior mesenteric artery.

After the posterior wall of the duodenum and head of the pancreas have been inspected carefully for evidence of tumor or metastatic involvement, further freeing of the second or third part of the duodenum is indicated to determine whether the lesion is operable. Care should be exercised in sweeping away the middle colic vessels that, surprisingly enough, frequently cross to the hepatic flexure of the colon high up over the second part of the duodenum (FIGURE 6). **CONTINUES**

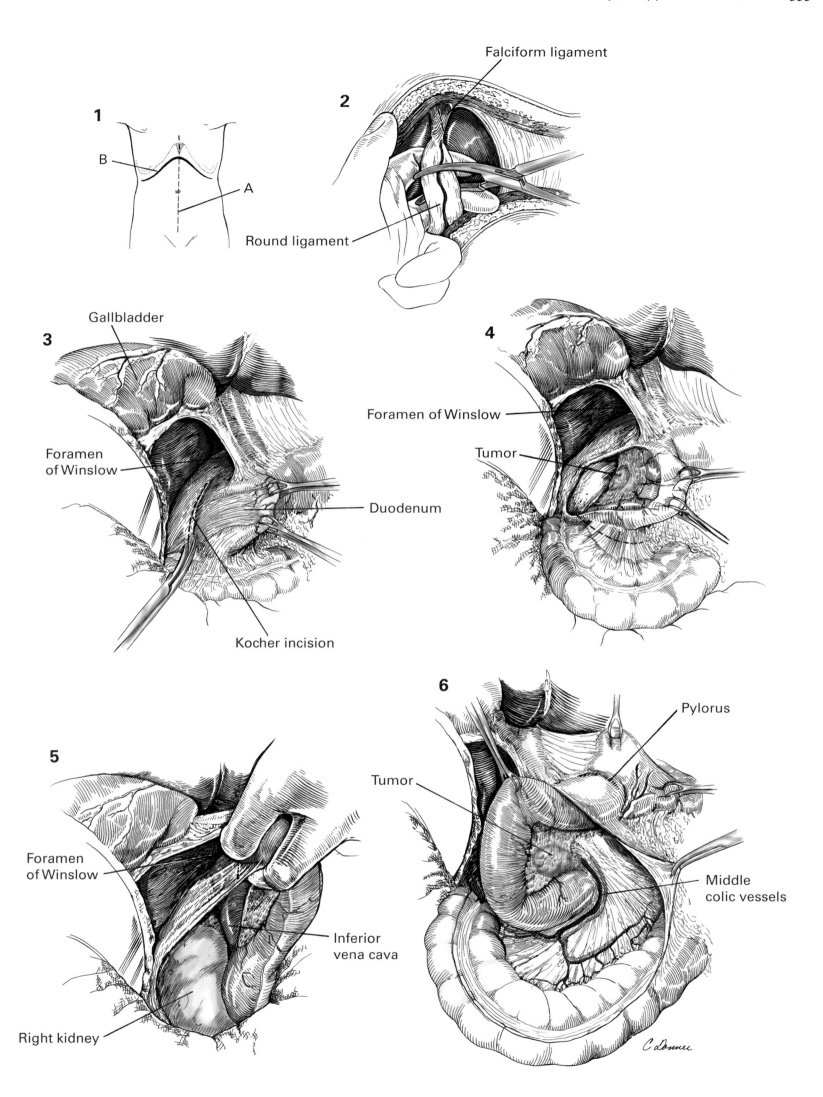

1

B
A

2

Falciform ligament

Round ligament

3

Gallbladder

Foramen
of Winslow

Duodenum

Kocher incision

4

Foramen of Winslow

Tumor

5

Foramen
of Winslow

Right kidney

Inferior
vena cava

6

Pylorus

Tumor

Middle
colic vessels

DETAILS OF PROCEDURE ◀CONTINUED The gallbladder, antrum of the stomach, head of the pancreas, and duodenum have been separated to call attention to the various relationships, including the blood vessels that must be ligated in this procedure. These structures are numbered for convenient identification. The gallbladder is rendered nonfunctional so is routinely removed. To ensure adequate lymphadenectomy of the hepatoduodenal ligament, the common hepatic duct should be divided just below the confluence, well above the cystic duct junction. The common hepatic artery and its branches must be identified carefully. The right gastric artery may be divided, even when pylorus preservation is planned. The gastroduodenal artery (GDA) is controlled with suture ligatures after test occlusion assures that distal hepatic artery flow is not dependent upon collateral flow arising from the SMA. Once the GDA is divided this gives access to the region of the portal vein just above the neck of the pancreas. Since no vessels enter at the anterior surface of the portal vein, this is the logical point for dividing the head of the pancreas from the body and tail. A number of pancreatic veins enter at the lateral border of the portal vein opposite the point where the splenic vein joins the superior mesenteric to form the portal vein. The middle colic artery and vein should be preserved but the vein may be safely divided in most cases, if necessary, for exposure of the superior mesenteric vein.

Before the blood supply of the head of the pancreas is compromised, the antrum of the stomach is transected, using the landmarks for hemigastrectomy (see Chapter 24). If a pyloric-sparing anastomosis is planned, the first portion of the duodenum is divided. Otherwise, the antrum is transected. Either of these divisions provides a direct approach to the pancreas in the region of the portal vein.

The pancreatic duct varies in size, depending on the amount of obstruction that may have occurred as a result of a prolonged block by calculi or tumor formation. If it is quite small, direct implantation of the duct may not be possible, and direct implantation of the tail of the pancreas into the lumen of the jejunum or back of the stomach can be carried out. Usually, there is one blood vessel that needs to be ligated above the pancreatic duct in the substance of the gland and two below.

Since marginal peptic ulceration may occur in a prolonged survival, the ability of the stomach to produce acid may be controlled with truncal vagotomy and by removing the entire antrum of the stomach. The latter can be accomplished by hemigastrectomy, selecting as the point of division the stomach at the level of the third vein on the lesser curvature and the point on the greater curvature where the epiploic vessels are nearest the gastric wall (see Chapter 24). Patients should routinely be treated with lifelong acid-reducing medication.

One of the most difficult parts of the procedure is the freeing of the third part of the duodenum, because of the short mesentery in this area. A portion of the upper jejunum should be resected along with the duodenum to ensure free mobilization of the upper jejunum, which is to be brought through the opening in the mesentery to the right of the middle colic vessel. CONTINUES▶

1. Tumor
2. Duodenum
3. Pancreaticoduodenal artery and vein: (a) Superior (b) Inferior
4. Right gastroepiploic artery and vein
5. Right gastric artery
6. Right gastric vein
7. Gastroduodenal artery

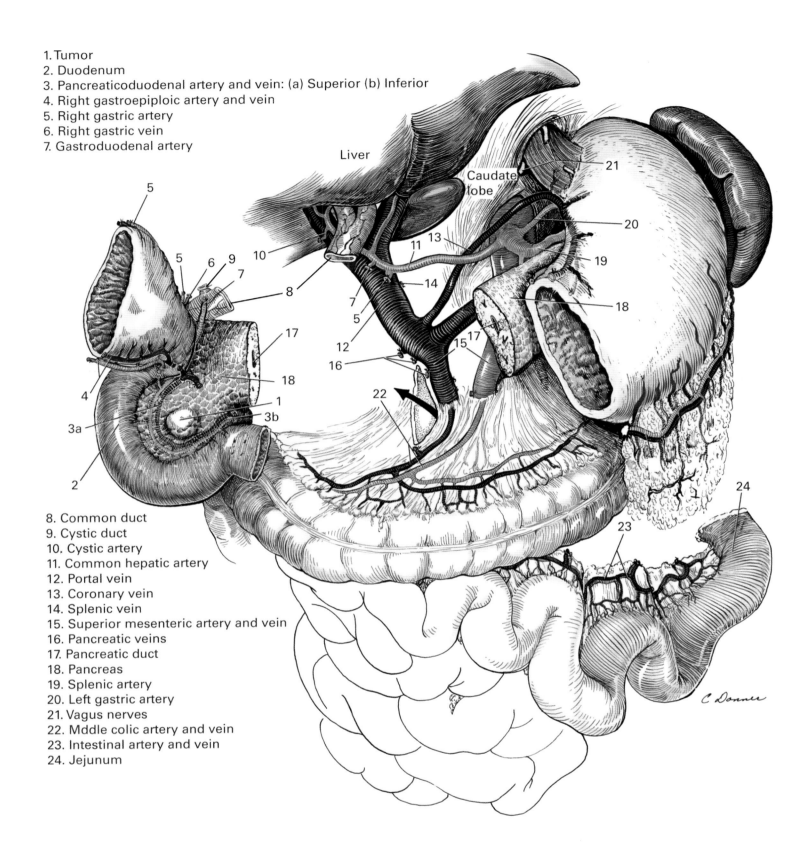

Liver

Caudate lobe

8. Common duct
9. Cystic duct
10. Cystic artery
11. Common hepatic artery
12. Portal vein
13. Coronary vein
14. Splenic vein
15. Superior mesenteric artery and vein
16. Pancreatic veins
17. Pancreatic duct
18. Pancreas
19. Splenic artery
20. Left gastric artery
21. Vagus nerves
22. Mddle colic artery and vein
23. Intestinal artery and vein
24. Jejunum

C. Donner

DETAILS OF PROCEDURE ◄CONTINUED When the second and third parts of the duodenum are well mobilized, the surgeon may or may not have proved the presence and the extent of a tumor. Additional information can be obtained by palpating the head of the pancreas between the thumb and index finger (FIGURE 7). It should be remembered that pancreatic lesions are occasionally found extending into the wall of the duodenum on the inner curvature side. The presence of a tumor involving the lower end of the common duct, and particularly ulceration with tumor involvement in the region of the ampulla of Vater, may be verified by palpation. A major concern when a tumor is felt or visualized is to determine whether it is a benign or malignant lesion and whether the portal vein is involved. Unless the surgeon is skilled in potential resection and repair of the portal vein, there should be good evidence that the tumor does not extend into or about the portal vein before deciding to proceed with the radical extirpation of the head of the pancreas.

It is not unusual to have considerable difficulty in proving the presence or absence of a malignant tumor deep in the head of the pancreas that is producing an obstructive jaundice. A surgeon is often reluctant to mobilize the head of the pancreas adequately and to carry out a biopsy to prove the presence of tumor because of potential complications, such as hemorrhage or a pancreatic fistula and because of the poor accuracy of frozen section in differentiating between adenocarcinoma and chronic pancreatitis. A transduodenal needle biopsy is utilized by some to obtain sufficient material for frozen-section diagnosis. Proof of the diagnosis may not be possible before proceeding with pancreaticoduodenectomy. The surgeon must use his judgment to establish a reasonable diagnosis based on the gross findings. If the lesion is not resectable and definitive diagnosis was not obtained preoperatively, then microscopic proof of cancer diagnosis is required. Biopsy of a mass in the head of the pancreas should be undertaken using a Tru-Cut needle via a transduodenal approach (FIGURE 8). Careful guidance with the tumor in hand should prevent inadvertent puncture of retropancreatic structures. The puncture site in the duodenum can be oversewn with a figure-of-eight or purse-string suture.

Next, the surgeon should proceed with further mobilization of the pancreas by entering the lesser sac (FIGURE 9). The omentum is retracted upward and the incision made into the lesser sac for more thorough evaluation of potential metastases above the pancreas and about the region of the celiac axis. Since some tumors of the pancreas are multiple, it is important that the entire pancreas be visualized and palpated, especially if a diagnosis of gastrinoma has been considered. It is usually advisable to open the lesser sac completely by freeing the omentum from the underlying transverse colon all the way over to and including the region of the splenic flexure of the colon (FIGURE 10). It should be kept in mind that the blood vessels to the colon may be angulated upward and attached for several centimeters to the undersurface of the omentum. The incision, therefore, should be made several centimeters away from the visualized bowel wall, as shown in FIGURE 10. It may be necessary to free the spleen, especially during the exploration of the pancreas for islet cell adenomas. Next, the surgeon explores the structures above the first part of the duodenum (FIGURE 11). The contents of the enlarged gallbladder can be aspirated if exposure is limited. The peritoneum is incised over the superior border of the duodenum, which is an initial step in isolating the common duct from the adjacent vascular structures. CONTINUES▶

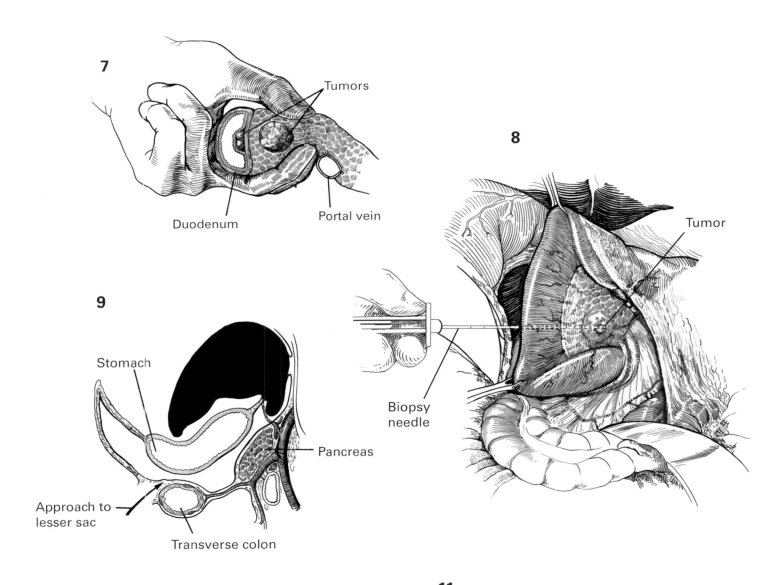

7

Tumors

Duodenum

Portal vein

8

Tumor

Biopsy
needle

9

Stomach

Pancreas

Approach to
lesser sac

Transverse colon

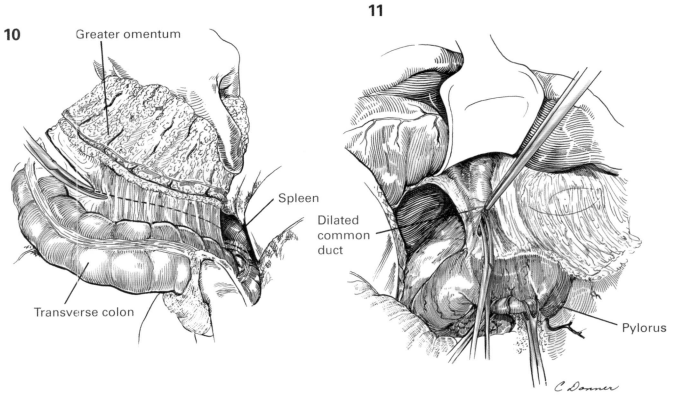

10   Greater omentum

Spleen

Transverse colon

11

Dilated
common
duct

Pylorus

C. Donner

DETAILS OF PROCEDURE ◄**CONTINUED** Mobilization of the superior part of the duodenum is continued in an effort to isolate as long a segment of the common duct as possible. This can be accomplished by gently spreading a right-angle clamp about the dilated common duct and meticulously controlling all bleeding (FIGURE 12).

An effort should be made to free this portion of the common duct completely and it is encircled with a vessel loop. The surgeon can then palpate behind the duodenum with the index finger in an effort to develop a cleavage plane between the duodenum and portal vein, and at the same time to determine more accurately whether there is fixation by the tumor to this vein. Once the surgeon is sure that resection is safe without injury to the portal vein, he or she proceeds to ligate the blood supply necessary for antrectomy. The right gastroepiploic vessels should be ligated and tied (FIGURE 13). Following this, the antrum can be encircled with tape, gentle medial and downward traction is applied to the stomach, and the right gastric vessels are identified (FIGURE 14). An alternate procedure that saves the antrum and pylorus may be chosen at this point. The duodenum is transected a few centimeters beyond the pylorus and later anastomosed, as shown in FIGURE 15 and 16A.

It is helpful to insert a straight clamp above the duodenum and spread the clamp parallel to the small right gastric vessels in order to better define the vascular pedicle to be divided (FIGURE 14). In the standard whipple procedure the antrum is resected. The stomach is therefore divided as shown in FIGURE 15. In the illustration the antrum is resected prior to the duodenum and head of the pancreas (FIGURE 16). It may be resected en bloc with the duodenum and head of the pancreas (FIGURE 15). If there is a question about resectability, the division of the stomach should be deferred until the plan is established between the rest of the pancreas and the portal vein. Since peptic ulceration is one of the late complications following radical amputation of the head of the pancreas and duodenum, it is essential to control the acid-producing ability of the remaining stomach. This can be accomplished by use of proton pump inhibitors or other medications to suppress acid production after surgery or by truncal vagotomy and hemigastrectomy, which ensures complete removal of the antrum. This is accomplished if the resection includes all of the stomach distal to the third vein on the lesser curvature and the area on the greater curvature where the gastroepiploic vessels are nearest the gastric wall. Some prefer to add vagotomy to the hemigastrectomy. Others prefer to conserve the entire stomach, including the pylorus and a short segment of the duodenum without vagotomy. The usual reconstruction after a pylorus-sparing Whipple procedure is shown in FIGURE 16A. An area the width of the index finger should be cleared on either curvature to prepare for the anastomosis after the blood supply has been controlled (FIGURE 16). The linear cutting stapler is applied adjacent to the traction sutures, which are left in place to define the areas prepared for anastomosis (FIGURE 16). The removal of the antrum greatly assists in the subsequent exposure of the more difficult portion of the resection. Most surgeons now use a linear stapling instrument or a cutting linear stapler with deeper gastric staples. A truncal vagotomy is sometimes performed (Chapter 23). **CONTINUES►**

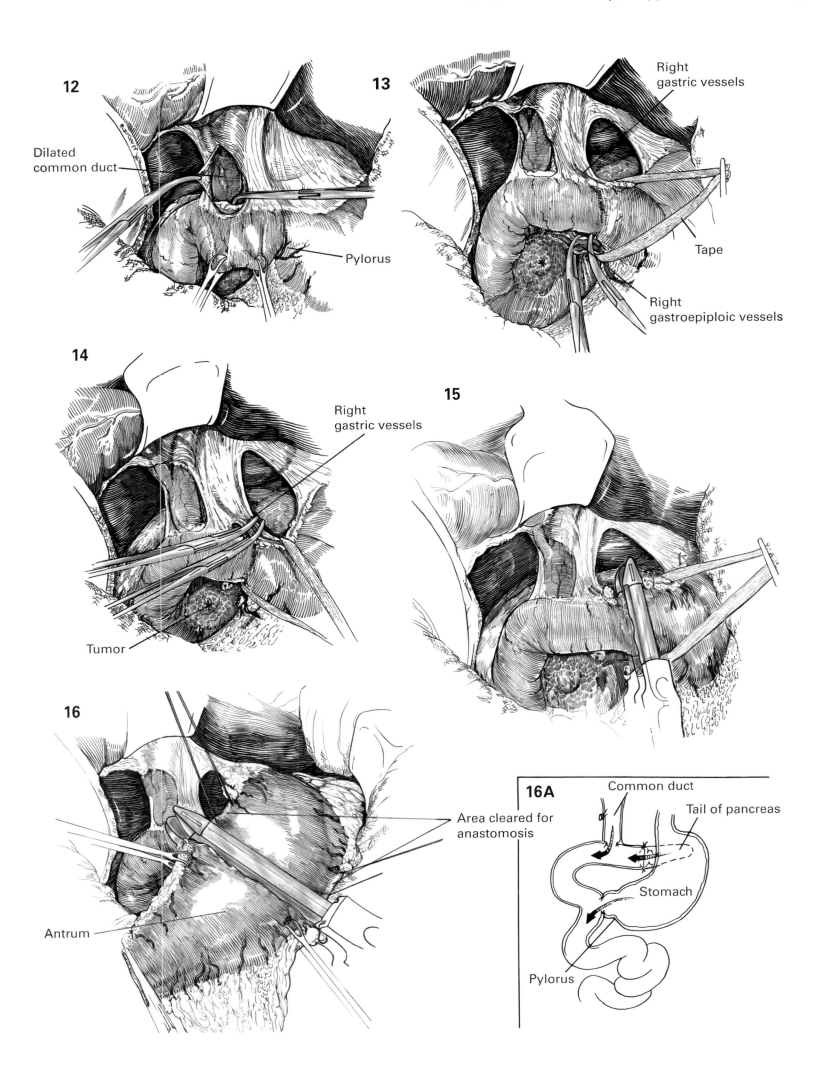

12

Dilated common duct

Pylorus

13

Right gastric vessels

Tape

Right gastroepiploic vessels

14

Right gastric vessels

Tumor

15

16

Area cleared for anastomosis

Antrum

16A

Common duct

Tail of pancreas

Stomach

Pylorus

DETACHS OF PROCEDURE **CONTINUED** If there is oozing between the staples, it is controlled by interrupted sutures of 0000 silk. The upper half of the approximated gastric outlet is inverted by a layer of interrupted 00 silk mattress sutures (FIGURE 17). A sufficient length of the gastric outlet near the greater curvature is retained to provide a stoma approximately two to three fingers wide. This portion of the gastric wall should not be excised until the final steps of the anastomosis, although it may be necessary to apply several sutures along the line of the clips to control oozing.

A very critical point now involves the identification of the common hepatic artery and the gastroduodenal artery, which runs downward over the pancreas behind the duodenum (FIGURE 18A). The common hepatic artery may be located by palpation just above the pancreas. The peritoneum over it is carefully incised and this major artery clearly visualized in order to avoid its injury. By careful dissection, the surrounding tissue is separated until the origin of the gastroduodenal artery is visualized. This vessel must be identified clearly and doubly ligated (FIGURE 18B). The lumen of the common hepatic artery must not be encroached upon. The tissues about the right gastric artery also must be freed gently and separated upward, as shown by the dotted line (FIGURE 18B). Following the ligation of these two vessels, blunt dissection with a long right-angle clamp may be undertaken to further free the region of the common duct and portal vein (FIGURE 19). Since these patients are often rather emaciated, there is relatively little tissue to be separated away from the portal vein. Great care should be taken gently to develop a cleavage plane over the portal vein, which will permit the surgeon to introduce carefully a blunt-nosed clamp, such as a right-angle clamp, behind the pancreas and to open and close the clamp as the tissues are separated from the underlying portal vein. It may be safer and easier for the surgeon to introduce the index finger directly behind the pancreas and over the portal vein. Considerable time should be spent in manipulating the pancreas off the portal vein. This can be done since no vessels enter from the anterior surface of the portal vein. The tissues about the inferior surface of the pancreas may need to be incised so that the finger can be introduced completely underneath the pancreas and come out inferiorly near the region of the middle colic vein (FIGURE 20).

Better exposure is gained if the body and tail of the pancreas have been mobilized to serve as traction for the delicate dissection around the portal vein. Otherwise, the subsequent technical details of the procedure can be enhanced if the pancreas is divided at this point. A blunt-nosed right-angle clamp is passed between the anterior surface of the portal vein and the neck of the pancreas. The pancreas is divided with electrocautery (FIGURE 21). There is usually one sizable bleeding point above the pancreatic duct (FIGURE 22) and at least two other vessels below the pancreatic duct. These are controlled with suture ligatures of fine silk or electrocautery, making certain not to occlude the pancreatic duct. Although there is debate about the value of obtaining a negative microscopic margin at the neck, some surgeons continue to obtain a tissue sample for frozen section. In this case a knife is used to take a 2-mm cross section of the divided pancreas for frozen section to ensure negative margins. If the margin is positive, additional pancreas may be removed. The duodenum and head of the pancreas to be excised are grasped primarily with the surgeon's left hand as the friable vessels entering the head of the pancreas from the right side of the portal vein are identified. **CONTINUES**

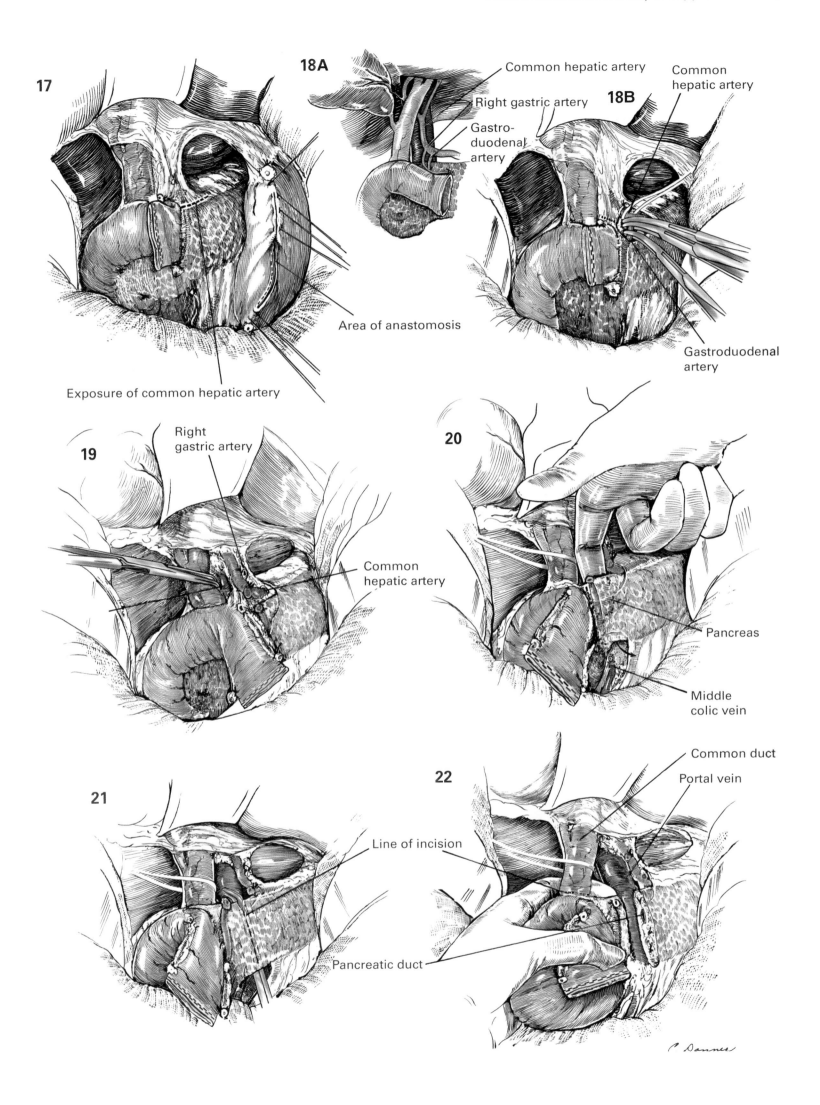

17

Exposure of common hepatic artery

Area of anastomosis

18A

Common hepatic artery

Right gastric artery

Gastro-duodenal artery

18B

Common hepatic artery

Gastroduodenal artery

19

Right gastric artery

Common hepatic artery

20

Pancreas

Middle colic vein

21

Line of incision

Pancreatic duct

22

Common duct

Portal vein

DETAILS OF PROCEDURE ◀ CONTINUED With the index finger of the left hand above and the thumb below compressing the specimen to be excised, the surgeon applies right-angle clamps in pairs to the strand of tissue that extends from the portal vein into the pancreas (FIGURE 23). Within this strand of tissue, there are a number of small veins that must be ligated very carefully lest troublesome bleeding occur. All areas should be ligated to keep the specimen as free of clamps as possible while the third portion of the duodenum is freed from the region of the ligament of Treitz and the superior mesenteric vein and artery (FIGURE 24). This can be one of the most difficult steps in the procedure. An incision into the peritoneum about the third portion of the duodenum produces an opening directly into the general peritoneal cavity, through which the upper jejunum eventually will be pulled for the anastomosis (FIGURE 24). The blood supply in the mesentery to the third part of the duodenum and adjacent jejunum is very short, and it is often difficult to mobilize the area about the ligament of Treitz with a minimal loss of blood. Small bits of the mesentery near the duodenal wall are incorporated between pairs of small curved clamps, and the contents are ligated as this area of the duodenum is further freed (FIGURE 25). The attachment of the duodenum that tends to fix the duodenum beneath the inferior mesenteric vein may be identified more easily and clamped if a portion of the upper jejunum is pulled through the opening made in the transverse mesocolon in the region of the ligament of Treitz (FIGURE 26). The remaining short mesenteric attachments, including arterial branches going into the inferior mesenteric artery, can then be clamped carefully with curved clamps if a portion of the upper jejunum is pulled through the opening made in the mesocolon (FIGURE 27). Alternatively, the surgeon may choose to dissect the ligament of Treitz and proximal jejunum from the left side of the mesentery. This approach is preferred in obese patients in whom exposure in this area is difficult. CONTINUES ▶

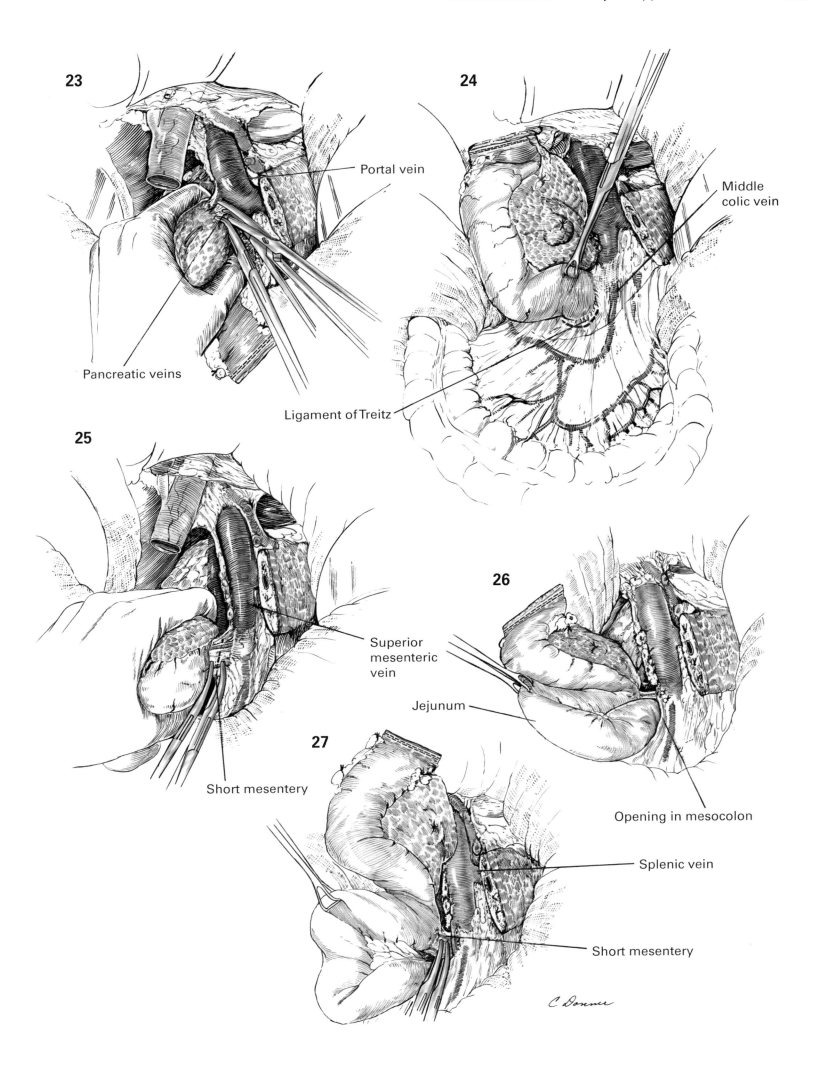

23

Portal vein

Pancreatic veins

24

Middle colic vein

Ligament of Treitz

25

Superior mesenteric vein

Short mesentery

26

Jejunum

Opening in mesocolon

27

Splenic vein

Short mesentery

C Donner

DETAILS OF PROCEDURE ◄ CONTINUED Since the gallbladder is often quite large and distended, it should be removed to provide additional room and prevent late complication from gallstone formation (FIGURE 28). Many surgeons prefer to remove the gallbladder prior to dissection of the porta hepatis and identification of the common bile duct. Attention is now directed toward further mobilization of the upper jejunum in the region of the ligament of Treitz (FIGURE 29). Usually, the peritoneum has been opened from above the colon, just about where the dotted line is shown. The upper jejunum is grasped with Babcock forceps and the bowel held up in order to enhance the visualization of the arcades providing the rich blood supply to the jejunum. Incisions are made through the avascular portion of these arcades, so that two or three of the basic arcades can be divided and double ligated to enhance the mobilization of the upper jejunum (FIGURE 30). The final result is shown in FIGURE 30; whereas FIGURE 12, Chapter 89 provides additional guidance as to the area of mesenteric division below the proximal jejunal vascular arcade. The arcade to be divided must be identified very carefully, and no vessels should be ligated in the mesentery near the mesenteric border of the bowel, since the blood supply to that segment may be compromised. When a segment of the mesentery of the upper jejunum has been divided, the jejunum is brought up through the opening in the mesocolon (FIGURE 30). A point to divide the bowel is selected where the mesenteric blood supply is obviously good (FIGURE 30). About 1 cm of the mesenteric border is freed of blood supply and the jejunum divided with a cutting linear stapler (GIA). The specimen is removed and the jejunal arm is brought up through the opening in the mesocolon. It must be long enough to reach well up into the gallbladder fossa without undue tension or compromise of the blood supply. If there appears to be considerable tension, the bowel should be returned below the colon and additional mesentery divided. CONTINUES►

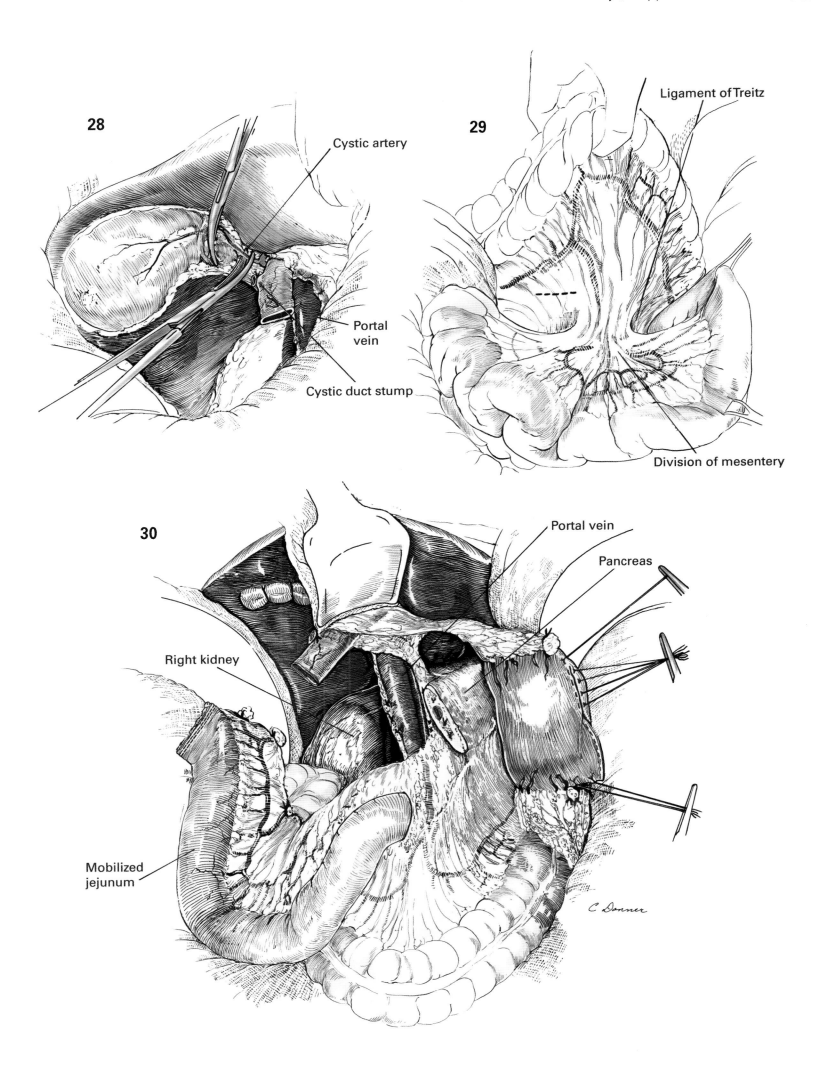

28
Cystic artery
Portal vein
Cystic duct stump

29
Ligament of Treitz
Division of mesentery

30
Portal vein
Pancreas
Right kidney
Mobilized jejunum

C Donner

DETAILS OF PROCEDURE CONTINUED The diagrams in FIGURES 31 and 32 outline two of the many variations of reconstruction after removal of the duodenum and head of the pancreas that have been developed. When total pancreatectomy is performed, only the common duct and end of the stomach, or the first portion of the duodenum if the entire stomach is preserved, are anastomosed to the jejunum. The bile and pancreatic ducts are arranged to empty their alkaline juices into the jejunum before the acid gastric juice as a measure of protection against peptic ulceration. The mobilized jejunum can be used safely in a variety of ways for the several anastomoses required. The end of the jejunum should come to rest without tension in the right upper quadrant after being passed through a rent in the transverse mesocolon to the right of the middle colic vessels. Alternatively, this limb can be passed through the retroperitoneal space vacated by the duodenum behind the mesenteric vessels. The jejunal limb is oriented such that the cut end lies near the cut edge of the pancreas. The limb then makes a gentle counterclockwise bend to abut the bile duct downstream from the pancreas anastomosis. The jejunum is then anastomosed to the partly closed end of the gastric pouch (FIGURE 31). Some prefer to implant the open end of the pancreas directly into the open end of the jejunum (FIGURE 32). Alternatively, a pancreaticogastrostomy may be performed in the case of a small pancreatic duct. With this configuration, the common hepatic duct then is anastomosed to the jejunum and, at an easy point of approximation, to the stomach. FIGURES 33 and 34 demonstrate details of the technique shown in FIGURE 31. The jejunal loop is positioned without tension near the cut end of the pancreas and the bile duct. The posterior capsule of the pancreas is anchored with interrupted 000 sutures to the serosa of the jejunum

(FIGURE 34). There should be no tension and preferably some redundancy of the jejunum between the several sites of anastomosis. The patency and size of the pancreatic duct are determined by inserting a soft rubber catheter. With the catheter in place to serve as a stent, the margins of the duct are freed for a short distance to facilitate an accurate anastomosis to the jejunal mucosa (FIGURE 35).

Some prefer to insert the open end of the pancreas into the open end of the jejunum, especially when the pancreatic duct is quite small (FIGURE 36A). This alternative technique is schematically shown in FIGURE 32. The open end of the pancreas is placed into open end of the jejunum as shown in FIGURE 36A and B. The margins near the cut end of the pancreas should be freed for several centimeters in preparation for telescoping the end of the jejunum over it, and all bleeding points should be ligated carefully. The end of the jejunum is usually large enough to admit the end of the pancreas. If not, it may be necessary to incise the full thickness of the jejunum along the antimesenteric border to make the opening large enough to match easily the size of the end of the pancreas. After all bleeding is controlled, the mucosa of the jejunum is sewed to the capsule of the pancreas in a manner similar to an end-to-end anastomosis. A small, soft rubber catheter can be inserted into the lumen of the pancreatic duct to ensure its patency during the completion of the anastomosis. It is subsequently removed before closure of the gastrojejunostomy. An additional one or two layers of interrupted nonabsorbable sutures are placed to pull the jejunal wall up over the capsule of the pancreas for approximately 1 cm (FIGURE 36B). Next the choledochojejunostomy is created as shown in FIGURE 37 and described in further detail on the next page. CONTINUES

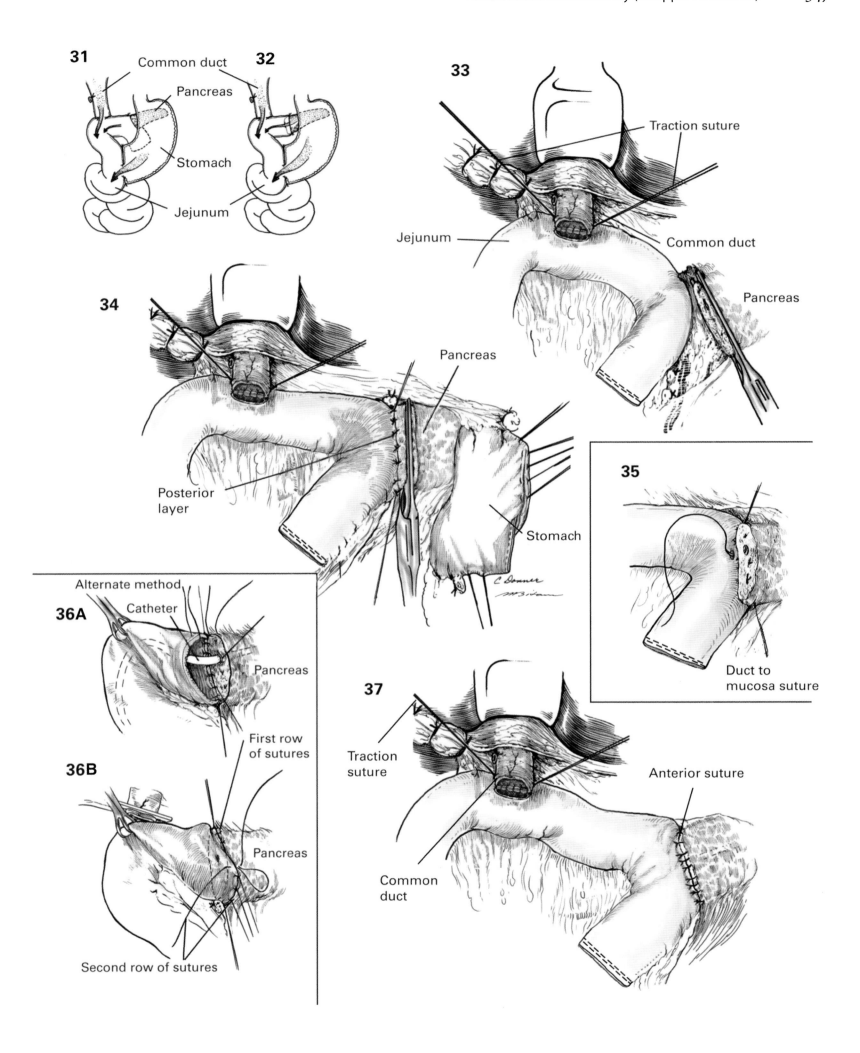

31 Common duct
Pancreas
32
Stomach
Jejunum

33 Traction suture
Jejunum
Common duct
Pancreas

34 Pancreas
Posterior layer
Pancreas
Stomach

35 Duct to mucosa suture

36A Alternate method
Catheter
Pancreas
First row of sutures

36B Pancreas
Second row of sutures

37 Traction suture
Common duct
Anterior suture

DETAILS OF PROCEDURE ◄CONTINUED The cholechojejunostomy is a single-layer anastomosis. The end of the jejunum then should be anchored to the tissues medial to the common duct or even up into the lower portion of the closed liver bed. Great care should be taken, however, that sutures do not include the right hepatic artery, which may curve upward into this area. An incision is made into the adjacent jejunal wall a little shorter than the diameter of the lumen of the common duct. Sutures of 0000 size are used to fix either side of the end of the common duct to maintain the wall under slight tension. The posterior row of the anastomosis between the bile duct and jejunum is completed (FIGURE 38). A series of interrupted 4-0 or 5-0 absorbable sutures is used to accurately approximate the mucosa of the jejunum to the common duct (FIGURE 38). The fixed angle sutures are allowed to remain for traction (FIGURE 38). Placement of the interrupted sutures in the closure of the anterior layer is then performed (FIGURE 39). The peritoneum, which tends to be thickened over the region of the common duct, is anchored with interrupted sutures to the serosa of the jejunum, starting beyond the angles of the anastomosis and extending anteriorly parallel with the anastomosis (FIGURE 40), which holds the divided end of the pancreas.

The gastrojejunal anastomosis may be made over the entire length of the gastric outlet, or the outlet may be partly closed and the stoma limited in size. The full thickness of the gastric wall, including the staples, is excised to provide a stoma three to four fingers wide (FIGURE 41). Any retained gastric contents are aspirated, and all bleeding points in the mucosa of the gastric wall are controlled. The serosa of the jejunum near the mesenteric border then is anchored to the posterior wall of the stomach from one curvature to the other with 000 silk. The jejunum should be approximated loosely so that there is some laxity between the anastomosis of the pancreas and the gastric wall in the region of the lesser curvature. An opening about two fingers wide is made in the jejunum, and the gastrojejunal mucosa is approximated with interrupted 0000 absorbable sutures (FIGURE 42). The gastrojejunal anastomosis is then completed with a layer of interrupted 0000 nonabsorbable sutures, with the knots buried on the inside. The second layer of the gastrojejunal anastomosis is then completed with a layer of interrupted 000 sutures from one curvature to the other. The opening in the mesocolon should be approximated to the jejunal wall (FIGURE 43) to prevent prolapse of small bowel up through this opening. The opening about the region of the ligament of Treitz should be closed with 000 silk. A gastrostomy tube and feeding jejunostomy may be indicated in the malnourished patient. Closed-suction drains are placed adjacent to the cholechojejunostomy and pancreaticojejunostomy.

CLOSURE The abdominal wall is closed in the routine manner, recognizing the potential for poor wound healing in an emaciated patient.

POSTOPERATIVE CARE It is of paramount importance, especially in the jaundiced patient, to make certain that the blood volume is restored at all times. Fluid balance is sustained by administration of 5% Ringer's lactate solution. Blood sugar levels should be tightly regulated, often requiring insulin in the early postoperative period. The hourly urine output should be watched carefully and should be maintained at 30 to 40 mL/h. The administration of intravenous fluids should be balanced throughout the 24-hour period. Urinary output and the replacement of gastric drainage will determine the amount of fluids required.

The patient's weight must be watched carefully, and an adequate daily caloric and vitamin intake assured. If a feeding jejunostomy tube has been inserted, tube feedings by continuous infusion may be started 24 to 48 hours after surgery. Initial infusion rate should be slow and gradually increased. The output from the closed suction drains should be monitored and may be removed early after surgery if there is no bile in the drain fluid and if the amylase is similar to that of serum. ∎

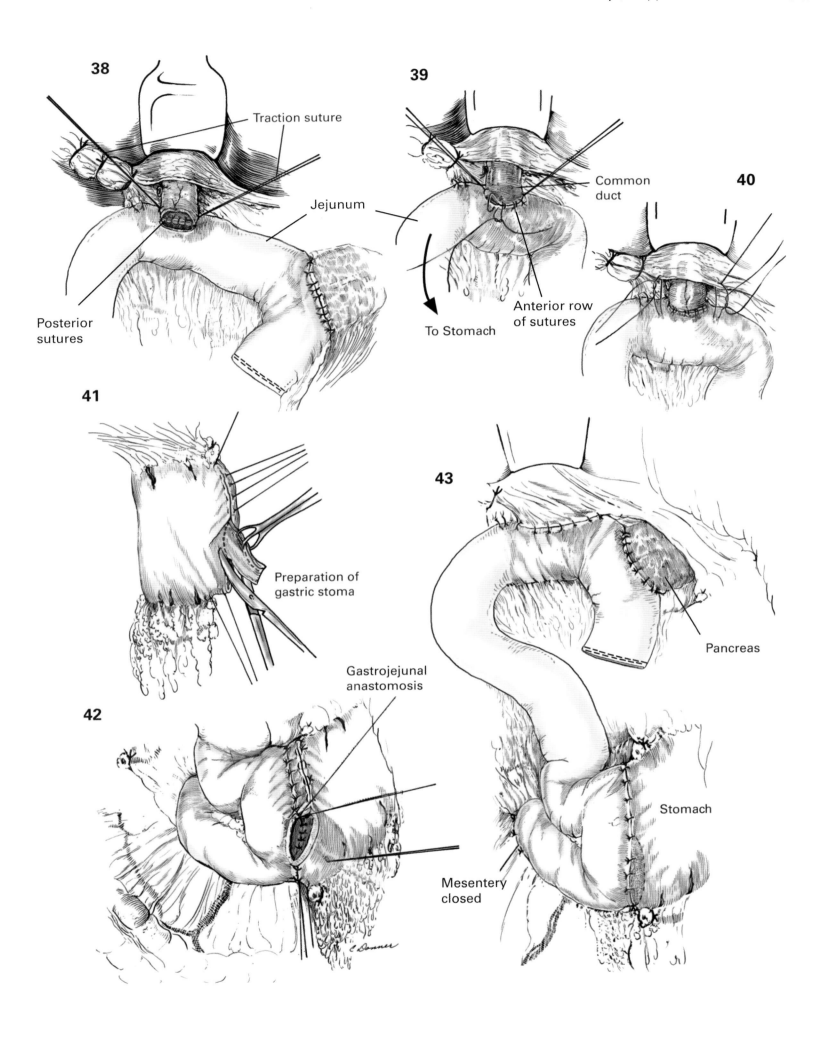

38

Traction suture

Jejunum

Posterior sutures

39

Common duct

Anterior row of sutures

To Stomach

40

41

Preparation of gastric stoma

43

Pancreas

Gastrojejunal anastomosis

42

Mesentery closed

Stomach

TOTAL PANCREATECTOMY

INDICATIONS Total pancreatectomy may be indicated in the treatment of neoplasms of the pancreas as well as for incapacitating, chronic, recurrent pancreatitis. Excision of the entire gland ensures more complete removal of neoplasms but adds little to the average long-term survival. Multicentric tumor locations are excised and cellular implantations are obliterated within the remaining ductal system, and intimately attached lymph nodes are excised. Removal of the pancreas simplifies the reconstruction of the upper gastrointestinal tract and minimizes the complications from pancreatic duct implantation, postoperative pancreatitis, hemorrhage, and sepsis.

The diabetes associated with total pancreatectomy is difficult to manage because of hypoglycemia and requires careful and frequent evaluation of insulin requirements. The indications for this procedure are related not only to the clinical history but also to the findings at the time of the surgical exploration.

PREOPERATIVE PREPARATION These patients are frequently poor surgical risks who have lost considerable weight and may be diabetic. The blood volume should be restored and blood sugar levels monitored. In the presence of deep jaundice, the biliary tree is decompressed by percutaneous transhepatic intubation or stenting at the time of endoscopic retrograde cholangiopancreatography. Vitamins are given along with pancreatic replacement if floating stools are present. Several units of blood should be available. Systemic antibiotics are given. Constant gastric suction is instituted.

ANESTHESIA General anesthesia combined with endotracheal intubation is satisfactory.

POSITION The patient is placed in a comfortable supine position.

OPERATIVE PREPARATION The skin of the lower thorax as well as of the entire abdomen is prepared in a routine manner.

INCISION AND EXPOSURE A liberal midline incision extending from over the xiphoid process down to or below the left of the umbilicus is made (FIGURE 1). Some prefer an inverted U incision that parallels the costal margins and crosses the midline near the top of the xiphoid process. All bleeding points are carefully controlled. The first decision involves establishing the diagnosis, ascertaining the presence or absence of metastases, and finally, establishing the mobility of the pancreas with special reference to the portal vein. Any evidence of distant metastasis to the omentum, the base of the mesentery of the transverse colon, or to the liver or adjacent lymph nodes makes any procedure palliative. In the absence of metastasis, and in the presence of a freely movable pancreas, further exploration is warranted. The removal of the entire pancreas does simplify the reconstruction of the gastrointestinal tract by a variety of methods (FIGURES 2 and 3). Only the common duct and the remaining hemigastrectomy remain to be anastomosed to the jejunum.

DETAILS OF PROCEDURE The omentum is detached from the transverse colon and the lesser sac inspected after the right gastroepiploic vessels are divided. A Kocher maneuver is carried out to mobilize the duodenum and head of the pancreas (FIGURE 4).

The duodenum and head of the pancreas can be mobilized as for the Whipple procedure (Chapter 88). When it has been decided to remove the body and tail of the pancreas as well as the head, the peritoneum along the inferior border of the pancreas is incised in preparation for mobilization by blunt finger dissection (FIGURE 5). The splenic artery is ligated near its point of origin. After the peritoneum over the portal vein has been incised, it is possible to insert the finger between the pancreas and the portal vein (FIGURE 6). There should be no communicating veins anteriorly. The pancreas can be divided with electrocautery in this area, and the two segments of the pancreas resected separately if preferred. CONTINUES ▶

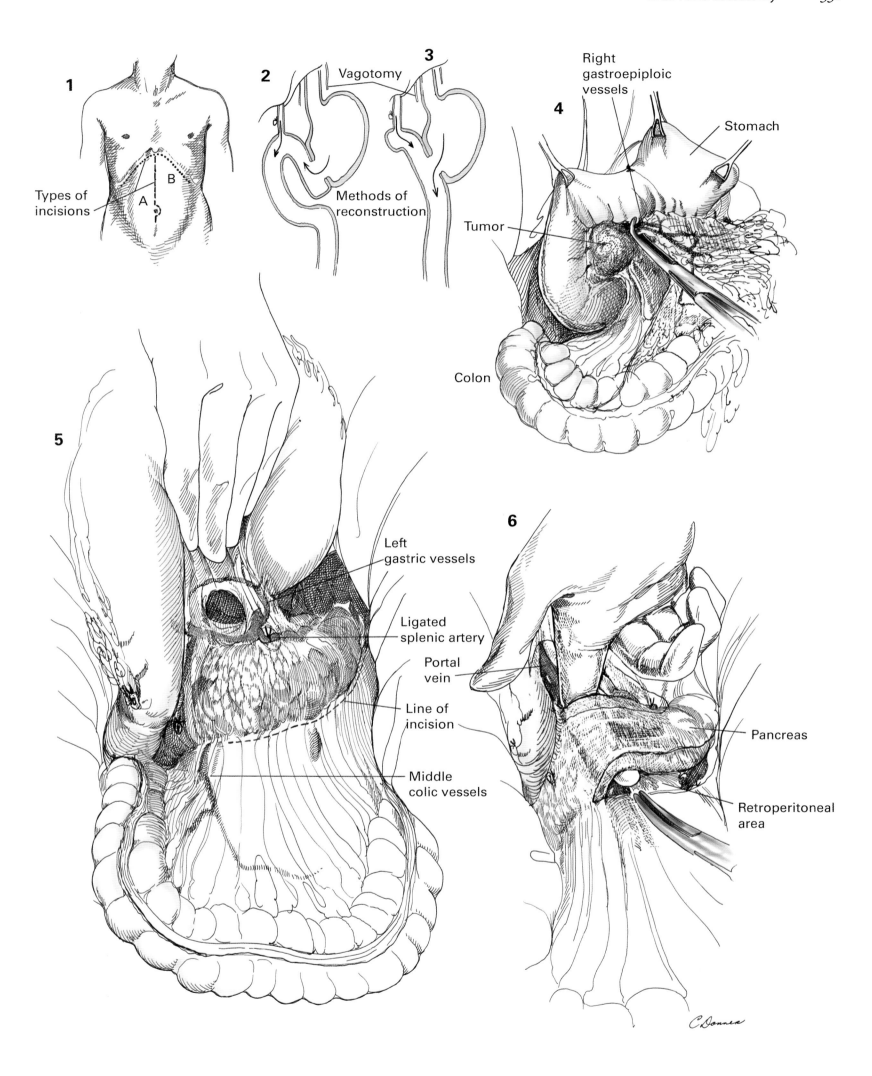

1

Types of incisions

A B

2

Vagotomy

Methods of reconstruction

3

4

Right gastroepiploic vessels

Stomach

Tumor

Colon

5

Left gastric vessels

Ligated splenic artery

Line of incision

Middle colic vessels

6

Portal vein

Pancreas

Retroperitoneal area

DETAILS OF PROCEDURE ⟨**CONTINUED**⟩ Although antrectomy with gastroje-junostomy is the usual technique for reconstruction, some preserve the entire stomach and pylorus plus several centimeters of duodenal bulb for end-to-side anastomosis to the jejunal limb according to the method of Longmire. In the usual reconstruction, however, better exposure is obtained for the subsequent steps of the procedure if the stomach is divided at a level that ensures complete removal of the antrum (FIGURE 7). Truncal vagotomy (Chapter 23) also is performed to decrease the incidence of late postoperative gastrojejunal stomal ulceration, unless lifetime treatment with proton pump inhibitors or other acid suppressing medication is determined to be preferable.

The spleen is freed up and all gastrosplenic vessels are divided and ligated. The spleen and left half of the pancreas are reflected to the right, providing good exposure for maximal ligation and division of the splenic artery and vein at their origins (FIGURE 8). Any arterial branches to the superior mesenteric artery are carefully isolated and ligated (FIGURE 9). The most difficult part of the procedure may be the isolation and ligation of the several short veins entering between the portal vein and the pancreas (FIGURE 10). The ligated right gastric artery and the pancreaticoduodenal artery are shown in FIGURE 10. CONTINUES⟩

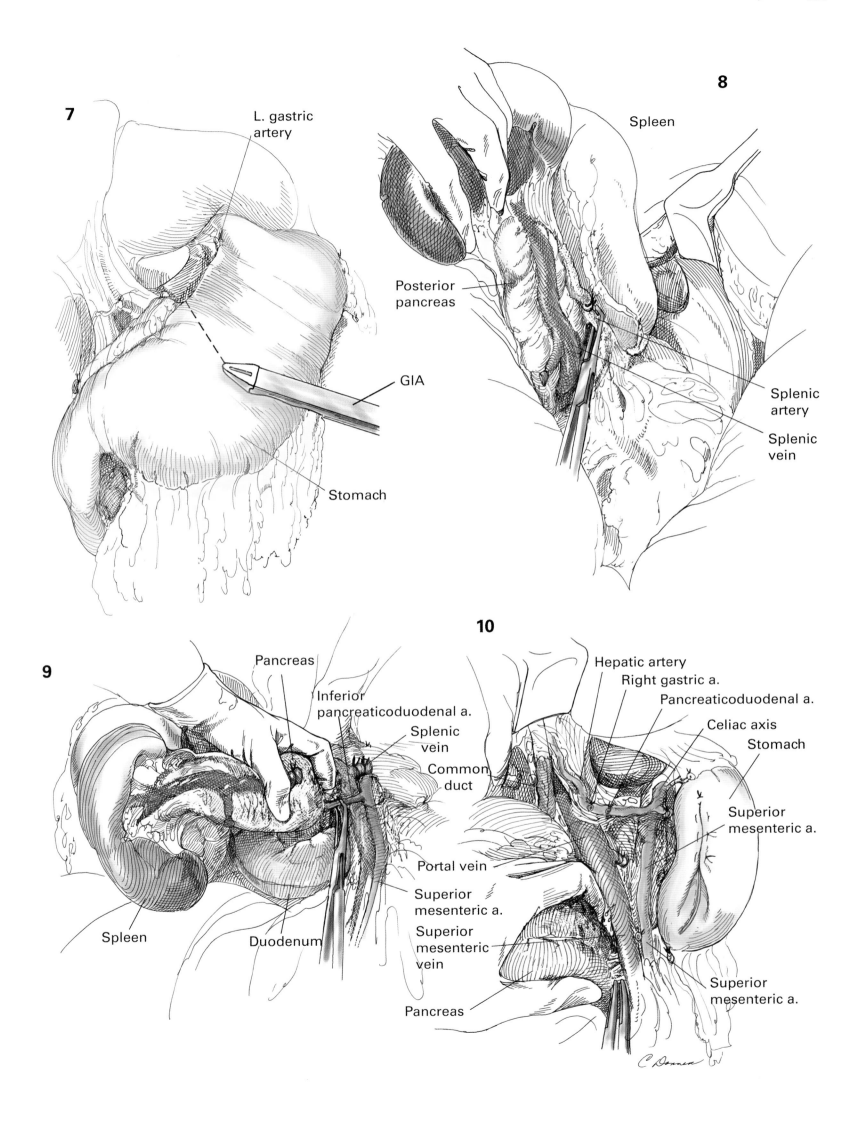

7

L. gastric artery

GIA

Stomach

8

Spleen

Posterior pancreas

Splenic artery

Splenic vein

9

Pancreas

Inferior pancreaticoduodenal a.

Splenic vein

Common duct

Portal vein

Superior mesenteric a.

Superior mesenteric vein

Pancreas

Spleen

Duodenum

10

Hepatic artery

Right gastric a.

Pancreaticoduodenal a.

Celiac axis

Stomach

Superior mesenteric a.

Superior mesenteric a.

DETAILS OF PROCEDURE CONTINUED The gallbladder is removed in a routine manner and the common duct is divided (FIGURE 11). The next step is to excise the rest of the duodenum down to and slightly beyond the ligament of Treitz (Chapter 88, FIGURES 27 and 28).

A long arm of the jejunum is prepared by dividing several vascular arcades (FIGURE 12). The mobilized jejunum is brought through an opening made in the mesentery of the transverse colon (FIGURE 12). This opening is made at either side of the middle colic vessels, depending upon how easily the jejunal loop can be brought up to the region of the common duct. The jejunum is closed with a running oo absorbable suture or a stapler, and this layer is inverted with a layer of oo silk mattress or interrupted sutures. Following a gastrojejunal anastomosis, the jejunal loop is anastomosed without tension to the common duct (FIGURE 2). Alternatively, some prefer to anastomose the biliary duct to the jejunum, followed by an anastomosis with the gastric pouch (FIGURE 3). It is not necessary to make the stoma the full width of the stomach. A stoma of 3 to 5 cm can be made at the greater curvature end (FIGURE 13). The jejunum should be anchored to the entire gastric outlet, regardless of how much has been closed off by sutures. The jejunum between the stomach and the common duct should be quite loose and free of tension (FIGURE 14). All openings in the mesocolon about the arm of the jejunum should be closed with interrupted sutures to avoid angulation of the arm of jejunum or the possibility of an internal hernia. Closed-system suction catheters are commonly used.

CLOSURE The incision is closed in the routine manner. A subcuticular closure of the skin may be used, or the skin may be approximated with interrupted sutures or clips.

POSTOPERATIVE CARE Constant gastric suction is maintained but may be discontinued in the early postoperative period. Blood sugar levels are monitored closely. The amount of insulin may not exceed 25 to 30 units daily in some patients. An insulin drip may be necessary in the initial days after surgery. Blood losses must be replaced. Oral pancreatic replacement therapy is started as soon as tolerated. Frequent nutritional evaluation is essential in postoperative care. ■

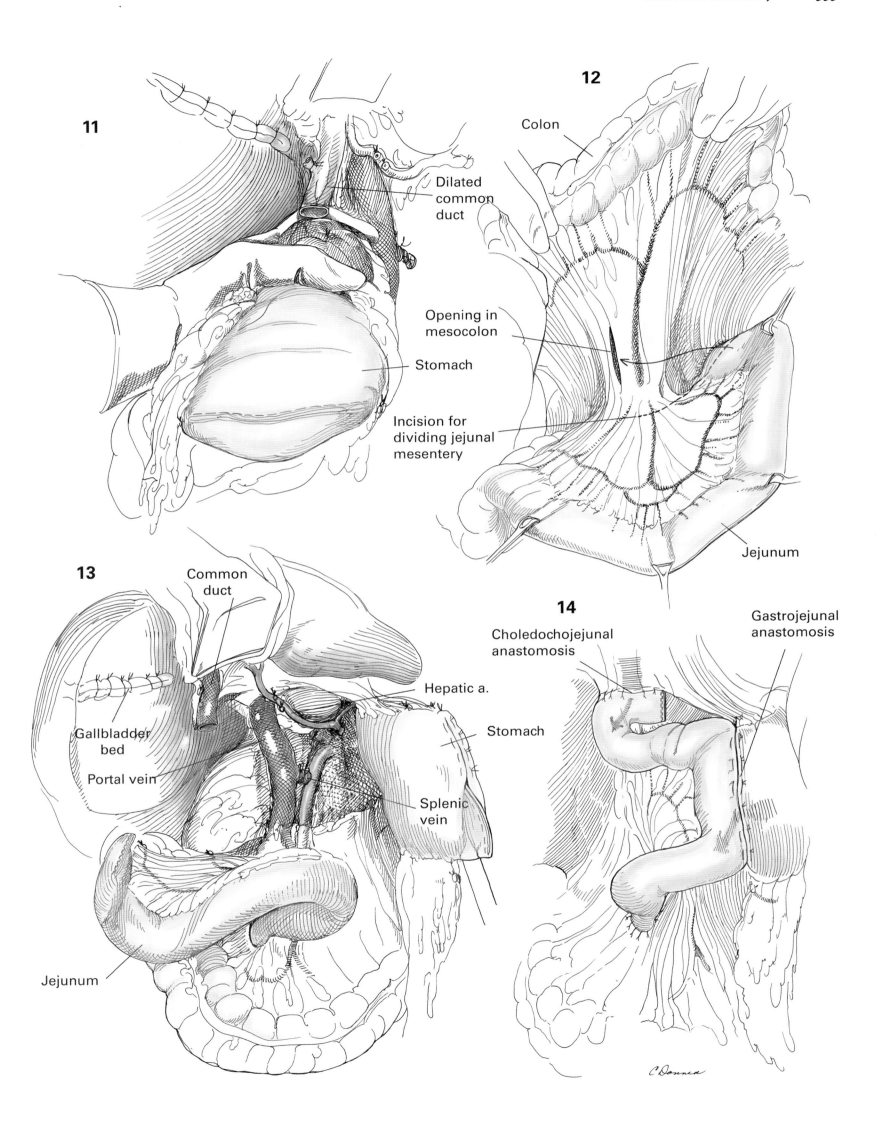

11

Dilated common duct

Opening in mesocolon

Stomach

Incision for dividing jejunal mesentery

12

Colon

Jejunum

13

Common duct

Gallbladder bed

Portal vein

Jejunum

Hepatic a.

Stomach

Splenic vein

14

Choledochojejunal anastomosis

Gastrojejunal anastomosis

INDICATIONS The most common indications for splenectomy are irreparable traumatic rupture and hematologic disorders. In splenic injury, nonoperative protocols result in a significant improvement in splenic salvage in both children and adults. However, in severe splenic injury, particularly in severe multisystem trauma, splenectomy is indicated. In some cases, splenic salvage is warranted. The most common hematologic disorders requiring splenectomy include immune (idiopathic) thrombocytopenic purpura, thrombotic thrombocytopenic purpura, and hereditary spherocytosis. Prior to splenectomy, clinical evaluation should be performed by an experienced hematologist and a bone marrow biopsy may be necessary to exclude unexpected bone marrow disorders not improved by splenectomy. Whereas in the past emergency splenectomy may have been occasionally needed in severe thrombocytopenia associated with hemorrhagic complications, today this is almost never needed, as nearly all patients will have improvement in platelet counts in response to steroids, intravenous immune globulin or Rho D immune globulin (winrho). Splenectomy may be indicated in cysts and tumors. Symptomatic benefit may follow splenectomy in certain other conditions, such as secondary hypersplenism, Felty's syndrome, Banti's syndrome, Boeck's sarcoid, or Gaucher's disease. In these latter patients, the surgeon should work in consultation with an experienced hematologist and medical specialists. In the past either total or partial splenectomy was indicated as part of the procedure of "staging" to determine the extent of Hodgkin's disease. Historically stage I and II Hodgkin's disease, traditionally, those patients who are considered candidates for primary radiation therapy, would undergo staging laparotomy (pathologic staging) to rule out definitively the presence of occult subdiaphragmatic disease. An appreciation of the risks of laparotomy and a recognition of the effectiveness of salvage chemotherapy in patients who fail primary radiation therapy have permitted the increased use of clinical staging as the basis for treatment of these patients.

Laparoscopic splenectomy is clearly the procedure of choice when technically feasible for elective splenectomy. It should be considered in all elective splenectomy cases. Relative contraindications may be considered in certain cases of previous surgery or a large spleen. Coagulopathy is not a contraindication and may actually do better with the laparoscopic approach.

PREOPERATIVE PREPARATION It is necessary to consider the nature of the disease for which splenectomy is indicated in order to give the proper preoperative treatment. In congenital hemolytic icterus, preoperative transfusion is contraindicated, even in the presence of the most severe anemia, because of the likelihood of precipitating a hemolytic crisis. In cases of thrombocytopenic purpura, platelet transfusions may be given the morning of operation if indicated. The patient with primary splenic neutropenia, pancytopenia, or other types of hypersplenism is transfused as indicated by his general condition and the information gained from the clinical studies. Antibiotic therapy is given in the presence of neutropenia. Large amounts of blood should be available in cases of suspected traumatic rupture of the spleen, and the patient should be operated on as soon as his condition permits. Prompt splenectomy may be a lifesaving procedure in some patients with a blood dyscrasia, especially those with primary thrombocytopenic purpura. Previous steroid therapy should be continued preoperatively and during the early postoperative period.

ANESTHESIA General anesthesia is usually satisfactory and may be supplemented with muscle relaxants. Patients who have severe anemia should receive little premedication, and ample oxygen should be administered with the anesthetic. In the presence of a low platelet count, great care is taken to avoid trauma to the mouth and upper respiratory passages, since hemorrhage may occur.

POSITION The patient is placed in a supine position. The spleen is made more accessible by tilting the table to lower the feet.

OPERATIVE PREPARATION The skin is prepared in the routine manner. Gastric intubation is avoided in portal hypertension or in the presence of a low platelet count, that is, thrombocytopenic purpura, in order to avoid initiating hemorrhage. However, in other indications it can be used to ensure a collapsed stomach and an improved exposure.

INCISION AND EXPOSURE Two types of incision are commonly used: a liberal incision midline from the xiphoid down to the level of the umbilicus (FIGURE 1A), or a left oblique subcostal incision (FIGURE 1B). The vertical incision is usually employed as it avoids division of muscle fibers in a patient who may have compromised coagulation profile.

If a bleeding tendency exists in the presence of blood dyscrasias, it is necessary to exercise rigid control of all bleeding points. In the very ill and anemic patient the general oozing may be controlled by pressure with warm, moist gauze pads, so that the abdomen may be opened and the splenic artery ligated as soon as possible. This will often affect a marked decrease in the bleeding tendency as soon as the artery is clamped. In the absence of acute intra-abdominal hemorrhage or an acute hemolytic blood crisis, the abdomen is explored. The gallbladder should be carefully palpated if the splenectomy has been indicated for hemolytic jaundice, since gallstones frequently occur in such patients and can be addressed at the conclusion of splenectomy if the patient's status permits. The pelvic organs in the female are palpated carefully for evidence of other pathology that might be responsible for excessive blood loss from the reproductive system. Enlarged lymph nodes should be biopsied and any accessory spleens removed.

The colon is packed downward out of the field of operation by warm, moist gauze, and the first assistant maintains downward traction with a large S retractor. A Babcock forceps is applied to the stomach, and a retractor is placed under the rib margin on the left to facilitate the exposure of the spleen.

DETAILS OF PROCEDURE The exact procedure depends upon many factors: the size and mobility of the spleen, the presence of extensive adhesions between the spleen and the parietal peritoneum, the length of the splenic pedicle, the presence of active bleeding from a ruptured spleen, or the patient's poor general condition as a result of blood dyscrasia. The approach to the immobilization and control of the blood supply of the spleen must be individualized in each case. A thorough understanding of the attachments and blood supply of the spleen is essential (FIGURE 2). In general, it is best to devascularize the spleen prior to mobilizing to minimize capsular trauma.

When splenectomy is indicated for blood dyscrasias, a careful search should be made for an accessory spleen both before and after the spleen is removed and hemostasis is effected. A routine search is made in the following order: the hilar region, the splenorenal ligament, the greater omentum, the retroperitoneal region surrounding the tail of the pancreas, the splenocolic ligament, and the mesentery of the large and small intestines. If accessory spleens are found in two or more locations, one is usually in the hilus. In some cases of blood dyscrasias the clinical course of the patient may suggest recurrence of the disease because of a retained accessory spleen. In such instances not only should the sites mentioned above be searched but the search should also be extended to the adnexa in the pelvis. The spleen must not be lacerated, nor should remnants be left within the abdomen because of the danger of seeding, which may result in splenosis. CONTINUES ▸

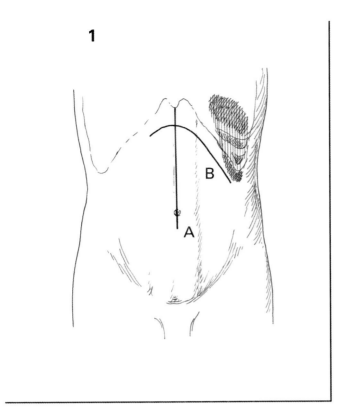

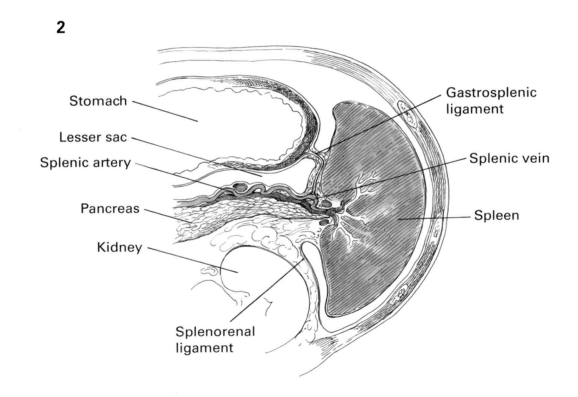

DETAILS OF PROCEDURE ◀ **CONTINUED** The diagram in FIGURE 2 illustrates the anatomic relationships of the spleen. As traction is exerted on the stomach medially, an avascular area in the gastrosplenic ligament may be incised, giving direct entrance to the lesser sac. Several blood vessels in the gastrosplenic ligament are divided and ligated to provide adequate exposure of the splenic artery. Along the upper margin of the pancreas, the tortuous course of the splenic artery can be palpated. The peritoneum over the vessel is incised carefully, and a long right-angle clamp is introduced beneath the artery to isolate it and to facilitate its ligation. The splenic vein is immediately beneath the artery. One or more 00 silk sutures are drawn beneath the artery and carefully tied (FIGURE 3). Alternatively it may be divided with a vascular stapler at this point. Preliminary ligation of the splenic artery has many advantages. It allows blood to drain from the spleen, providing an autotransfusion. The spleen tends to shrink, making its removal easier and with less blood loss. Finally, blood transfusions can be given immediately to the patient with hemolytic anemia. This preliminary step does not prolong the procedure and tends to ensure a safer splenectomy with minimal blood loss.

After the splenic artery has been secured, the remainder of the gastrosplenic ligament is divided between small curved clamps or with an energy device (FIGURE 4). Great care is exercised, especially toward the upper margin of the spleen, to avoid injuring the gastric wall during the application of clamps, for in this area the gastrosplenic ligament is sometimes extremely short. This is especially true when the spleen is very large or in the presence of portal hypertension. Failure to secure the uppermost vein in the gastrosplenic ligament can result in serious blood loss. Because of the danger of postoperative bleeding following gastric dilatation, the vessels along the greater curvature should be ligated with a transfixing suture that includes a bite of the gastric wall. In addition, in this area several vessels commonly extend from

the hilus of the spleen over to the posterior wall near the greater curvature high on the fundus. At the inferior margin of the spleen, fairly sizable vessels, the left gastroepiploic artery and vein, commonly will be encountered in the gastrosplenic ligament (FIGURE 4). The contents of the clamps are ligated on both the gastric and splenic sides, since the division of the gastrosplenic ligament will leave a large opening directly into the lesser sac.

The early ligation of the major splenic artery makes mobilization of the spleen easier and safer. The surgeon passes the left hand over the spleen in an effort to deliver it into the wound (FIGURE 5). Dense adhesions may be present between the spleen and the peritoneum of the abdominal wall or the left diaphragm; however, the spleen can usually be mobilized after a few avascular adhesions and the gastrosplenic ligament have been divided.

As the spleen is mobilized, the surgeon passes the fingers over its margin to expose the splenorenal ligament, which should be incised carefully (FIGURE 6). The peritoneal reflection in this area is usually rather avascular; however, it is necessary to ligate many bleeding points in the presence of portal hypertension. Usually, the index finger can be inserted into the peritoneal opening, and by blunt dissection with the index finger of the left hand, which extends over the surface of the spleen, the margin of the spleen can be freed easily (FIGURE 7). This must be done gently since the capsule may be torn, resulting in troublesome bleeding or seeding of splenic tissue.

After the posterior margin of the spleen has been mobilized, the spleen may be brought well outside the abdomen; however, if dense adhesions between the spleen and the parietal peritoneum are encountered, it is easier to incise the overlying peritoneum and carry out a subperitoneal resection, which leaves a large, raw space. This may be safer than attempting to free the spleen with sharp dissection. Warm, moist packs may be introduced into the splenic bed to control oozing. Active bleeding points should be controlled with electrocautery. **CONTINUES** ▶

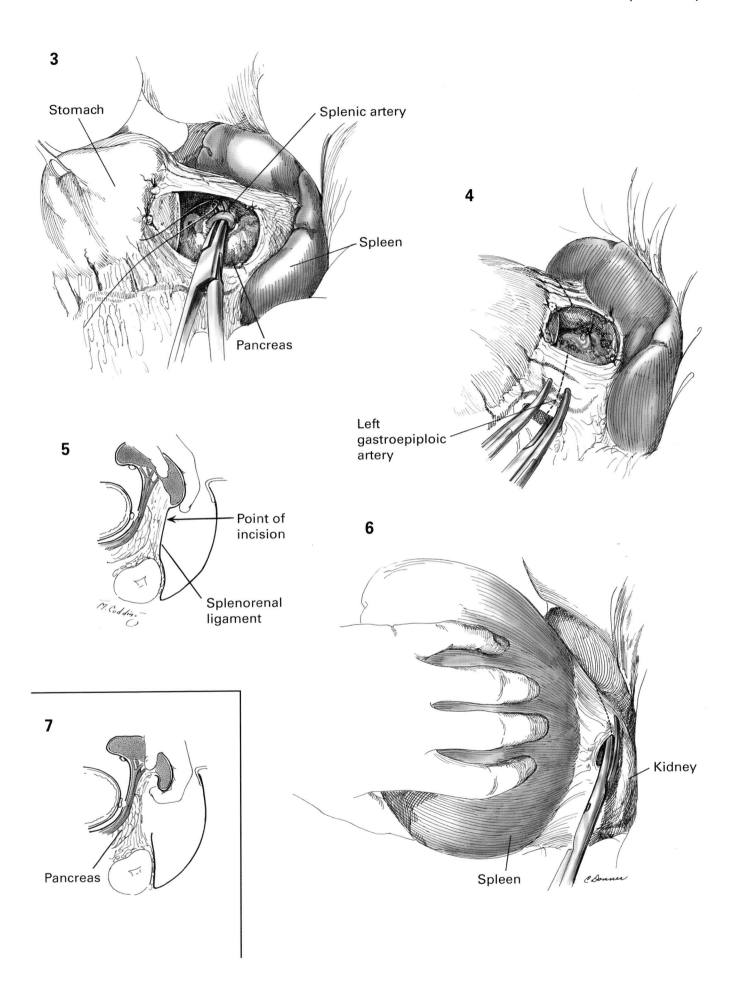

3

Stomach

Splenic artery

Spleen

Pancreas

4

Left
gastroepiploic
artery

5

Point of
incision

Splenorenal
ligament

6

Kidney

Spleen

7

Pancreas

DETAILS OF PROCEDURE ◂CONTINUED▸ When the spleen is mobilized outside the wound, the splenocolic ligament is divided between curved clamps (FIGURE 8). This procedure is carried out carefully in order to avoid any possibility of damage to the colon. The contents of these clamps are ligated with a transfixing suture of oo silk or absorbable suture. In the presence of portal hypertension, many large veins may be present in this area. The spleen is then retracted medially by the surgeon's left hand, while the tail of the pancreas, if it extends up to the splenic hilus, is separated by blunt dissection from the splenic vessels in order to avoid damage to it by the subsequent ligation of the pedicle (FIGURES 9 and 10). The surgeon should keep in mind the possibility of accessory spleens in this location. The spleen is held upward and laterally by an assistant, while the large vessels in the pedicle are separated from the adjacent tissues to permit the application of several curved clamps to the individual vessels (FIGURE 11). These vessels should be ligated at the base of the pedicle proximal to the bifurcation of the splenic vessels. Despite the fact that the splenic artery has been ligated previously, it is tied again proximally and transfixed distally (FIGURE 12). The same principle of double ligature for the splenic vein is also carried out. Alternatively, vascular stapler may be liberally applied in this region. In those instances where preoperative transfusions have been contraindicated, they may be started as soon as the splenic artery has been divided. The operative site is searched for evidence of persistent oozing. Warm, moist packs or a coagulant matrix may be introduced to control the small bleeding points. Following this, a final careful search is made for any existing accessory spleens that must be resected.

ALTERNATIVE METHOD When the spleen is quite mobile and the pedicle is long, which is apt to be the case in the presence of long-standing splenomegaly, splenectomy may be facilitated if the splenorenal ligament is incised first without an attempt to divide the gastrosplenic ligament (FIGURE 13). The spleen is pulled gently upward and medially, providing exposure of the vessels in the pedicle from the lateral side (FIGURE 14). It may be necessary to divide the splenocolic ligament first in order to better expose the contents of the splenic pedicle. In the presence of a ruptured spleen the urgency of the situation may require mass clamping or stapling of the splenic pedicle; however, individual ligation of the major vessels is safer and more desirable. This may be accomplished by ascertaining the position of the splenic artery by palpation followed by blunt dissection, in an effort to isolate the splenic artery (FIGURE 14). When the splenic artery has been divided, the spleen should be compressed to ensure an autotransfusion through the intact splenic vein. Since the gastrosplenic ligament has not been previously divided, it may be included in the clamps applied to the splenic pedicle, thereby sealing off the lesser omental sac (FIGURE 15). If the gastrosplenic ligament is to be included in these clamps, great care is necessary to avoid including a portion of the greater curvature of the stomach, especially when the gastrosplenic ligament is very short. This is more likely to occur high in the region of the fundus of the stomach. The inclusion of the gastrosplenic ligament in the clamps applied to the splenic pedicle should not be attempted unless the pedicle is long and all structures may be identified easily and clearly (FIGURE 16). The contents of the clamps applied to the splenic pedicle are doubly ligated. The most superficial of these ligatures should be of the transfixing type. Deep transfixing sutures should not be taken, since troublesome hemorrhage may result, especially from the splenic vein.

In good-risk patients cholecystectomy is performed if gallstones are found, especially in association with congenital hemolytic anemia. A routine cholangiogram also is carried out if choledocholithiasis is suggested. In the younger age groups with primary hypersplenism the appendix may be removed if the cecum is easily mobilized.

SPLENIC PRESERVATION Recognition that splenectomy increases susceptibility to infection by encapsulated bacterial organisms necessitates a conservative approach to splenic injuries. Special effort should be made to conserve spleen tissue with its attached blood supply, especially in the very young. Every effort is made to avoid splenectomy in children by following a conservative routine of close observation, nasogastric suction, frequent recordings of pulse and blood pressure, repeated blood counts and radionuclide, or computed tomography (CT) scans. If the scan shows only a single linear laceration, a non-operative regimen is followed. When the scan shows a fragmented spleen or evidence of devascularization, surgical repair is required.

Tears of the splenic capsule during upper abdominal operations are minimized by avoiding undue traction on the greater omentum of the stomach or the left transverse colon, or by dividing peritoneal strands attached to the splenic capsule. Mobilization of the spleen with temporary control of the major blood supply permits evaluation of the feasibility of repair of the capsule or, alternatively, segmental resection with ligation of the segmental vasculature in the hilum, as well as in the small intrahepatic vessels, combined with liberal use of a hemostatic agent and possible fixation of the omentum to the area of repair. Locally applied hemostatic agents, compression of splenic tissue by mattress sutures on atraumatic needles, or ligation of one or more major vessels in the splenic hilum may control the bleeding and avoid splenectomy.

CLOSURE The wound edges can be approximated more easily by returning the table to its original horizontal position, thus facilitating return of the abdominal contents to their anatomic location. A routine closure is done without drainage. On occasion, a closed-suction Silastic drain may be placed near the tail of the pancreas if there has been extensive dissection in this region.

POSTOPERATIVE CARE This will vary, depending upon the requirement for whole blood replacement. Within a short time after splenectomy for a blood dyscrasia involving a bleeding tendency, it is usually noted that the platelet count rises rapidly; thus, transfusion may be unnecessary for this purpose. It is good practice to monitor platelet counts postoperatively, even in elective procedures, because of the marked thrombocytosis that is occasionally seen. In patients with markedly elevated platelet counts or abnormal platelet function, anticoagulants, such as acetylsalicylic acid and dipyridamole, may be indicated. Anticoagulants are rarely necessary in routine splenectomy. A marked leukocytosis commonly follows splenectomy and should not be interpreted as indicative of infection. Constant gastric suction for a day or so is often advisable. The patient is permitted out of bed on the first postoperative day. Fluid balance is carefully maintained according to the patient's general condition. Any steroid therapy given preoperatively is continued during the postoperative period. Further steroid therapy will be regulated by the hematologist, who will be guided by the response of the patient's blood picture to splenectomy. In patients with secondary hypersplenism, their primary disease will not be altered, although the patient's life has been saved or prolonged by removal of the overactive spleen. The incidence of venous thrombosis is increased when the splenectomy is performed for myeloproliferative disorders or lymphomas. Anticoagulant prophylaxis should be considered in such patients. Atelectasis of the left basal lobe is one of the common complications after splenectomy. When complete splenectomy has been performed, patients should be informed and urged to seek immediate medical attention at the first sign or symptom of infection. Polyvalent vaccines for pneumococcus, *Haemophilus influenzae,* and *Neisseria meningitidis* are also suggested except for pregnant women. ■

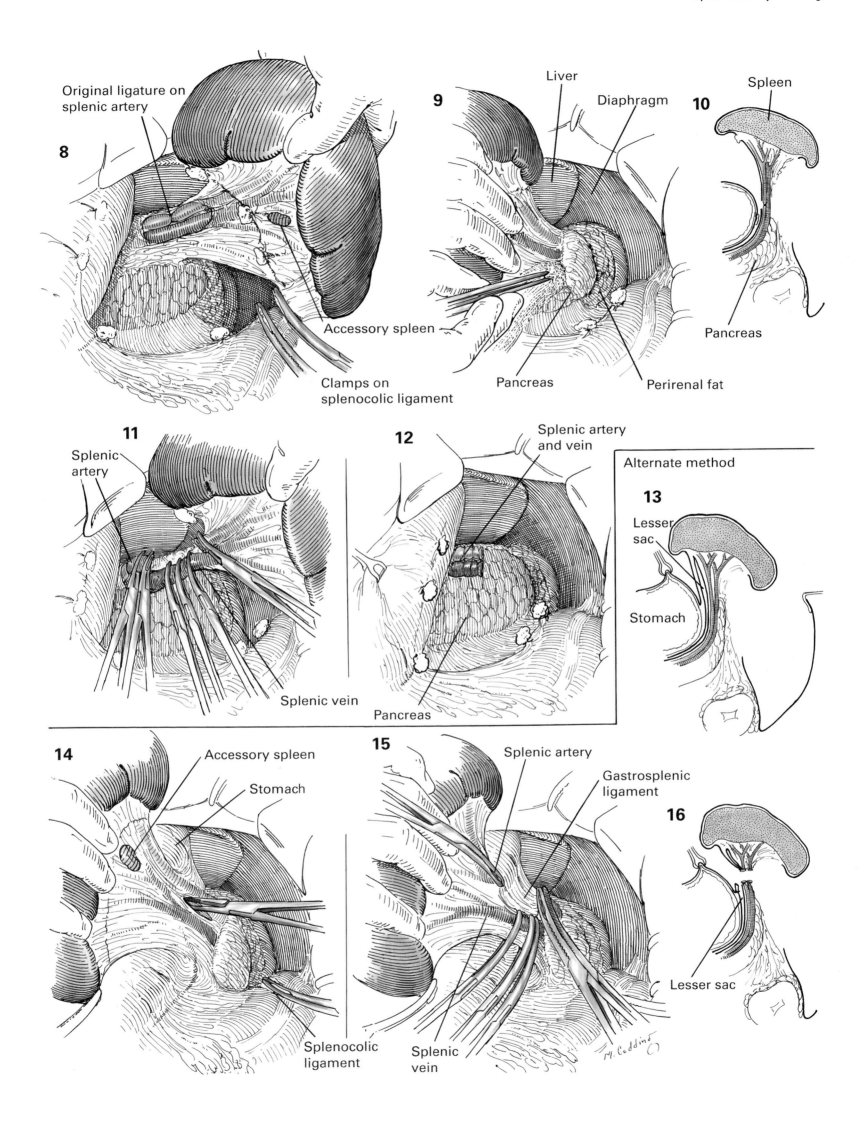

8 Original ligature on splenic artery

Accessory spleen

Clamps on splenocolic ligament

9 Liver   Diaphragm

Pancreas   Perirenal fat

10 Spleen

Pancreas

11 Splenic artery

Splenic vein

12 Splenic artery and vein

Pancreas

Alternate method

13 Lesser sac

Stomach

14 Accessory spleen

Stomach

Splenocolic ligament

15 Splenic artery

Gastrosplenic ligament

Splenic vein

16 Lesser sac

M. Codding

CHAPTER 91

SPLENECTOMY, LAPAROSCOPIC

INDICATIONS Laparoscopic splenectomy is most commonly performed for immune (idiopathic) thrombocytopenic purpura (ITP) or other splenic conditions causing anemia or neutropenia. Massive trauma to the spleen as well as overly large spleens are still best approached with an open laparotomy. However, virtually all other indications for splenectomy listed in Chapter 90 apply for laparoscopic splenectomy. A complete hematologic evaluation, including bone marrow studies, is essential. The patient must be informed of the lifelong consequences of increased susceptibility to bacterial infection. Ideally, the patient should receive polyvalent pneumococcal, *Haemophilus influenzae*, and *Neisseria meningitidis* vaccination prior to surgery.

PREOPERATIVE PREPARATION Patients for elective splenectomy are usually referred to the surgeon by hematologists or oncologists, because their treatment with blood products, corticosteroids, plasmaphoresis, gamma globulins, or chemotherapy can no longer safely control the primary disease. Accordingly, the patient may require transfusion of blood products to raise the hematocrit or platelet counts to safe levels for general anesthesia and coagulation during surgery. Packed red cells may be given in advance of planned surgery, whereas platelets, with their short life span, may be infused just prior to and during the procedure. When platelet transfusions are contraindicated, endogenous platelet counts are often temporarily boosted with a few days of increased corticosteroid therapy, immune globulin or Rho D immune globulin (winrho) prior to surgery. If steroids are used, then they must be continued during and immediately after surgery. The patient should have a type and screening blood test, and blood products must be available for infusion. The size of the spleen should be determined by physical examination or imaging studies, as massive spleens are usually more safely approached by open splenectomy.

ANESTHESIA General anesthesia with endotracheal intubation is required. Two large, well-secured intravenous catheters are placed for easy access by the anesthesiologist. The intravenous sites and any finger pulse oximeters should not be positioned distal to an arm blood pressure cuff. A Foley catheter and an orogastric (OG) tube are passed and pneumatic sequential compression stockings are applied to the lower legs. Care must be taken in the placement of the endotracheal, OG, and Foley tubes in patients with marked thrombocytopenia lest bleeding occur.

POSITION The patient is placed in a lateral position with the left arm crossing the chest and lying on top of the right arm. Liberal padding is used between and around both arms. The left hip and chest are elevated with pillows, leaving the flank area open and the left knee flexed, with a padding of blankets between the legs. The patient is secured across the chest and hips to the table with wide adhesive tape, as the operating room table will be tilted.

OPERATIVE PREPARATION The skin is prepared from the lower chest to the pubis in a routine manner.

INCISION AND EXPOSURE A 5-mm videoscope port is placed either through the umbilicus or in the lateral midsubcostal position using the open technique of Hasson as described in Chapter 11. The videoscope is introduced and all four quadrants of the abdomen are examined. The size and location of the spleen and the presence of accessory spleens are noted. A second 10-mm port is placed in the left lateral subcostal position and a 12-mm port is placed just to the left of the midline. These ports are in a line about two fingerbreadths or so below the edge of the costal margin for a normal-sized spleen. Additional locations or ports may be placed according to the preference of the surgeon, the size of the spleen, and the shape of the patient's body. In general, larger spleens require a lower (more caudal) and more medial placement of ports. The patient is positioned with the left side up and then placed in a reversed Trendelenburg position.

DETAILS OF PROCEDURE The general anatomy of the spleen, stomach, colon, and omentum is shown in FIGURE 1, which complements the cross-sectional anatomy of this region shown in Chapter 90. The splenocolic ligament is visualized along with the greater omentum in its attachment to the transverse colon is visualized. The splenic end of this ligament is elevated with traction (FIGURE 2) and a suitable zone just above the splenic flexure of the colon is entered with the energy device. This elevation is done with grasping and gentle traction using a dissecting instrument. The dissection proceeds medially around the tip of the spleen, where the gastrosplenic ligament containing the short gastric vessels is identified. Using blunt dissection, the lesser sac is entered and the short gastric vessels are sequentially divided about 1 cm away from the gastric wall (FIGURE 3). This cuff minimizes potential thermal damage to the stomach. As the dissection proceeds toward the gastroesophageal junction, care is taken to visualize each short gastric vessel within the jaws of the energy device before it is activated. Partial transection of the next short gastric vessel will result in bleeding that is difficult to control. Exposure for this dissection within the gastrosplenic ligament is improved by gentle retraction of the greater curvature of the stomach, using the dissecting instrument to lift the greater curvature forward and medially. The pancreas, with the splenic artery and vein running along its superior or cephalad border, is seen in the base of the lesser sac. The short gastrics are divided almost to the gastroesophageal junction (FIGURE 4).

The splenorenal ligament is opened by gently elevating the spleen medially with the dissecting instrument (FIGURE 5). This thin peritoneal layer is easily seen in the left gutter behind the spleen. The ligament has few vessels, but it must be transected with coagulation in a cephalad direction until the top of the spleen is free. The splenic pedicle is inspected in all areas by lifting the spleen from side to side to make certain that no ligamentous attachments remain. The spleen should be completely mobile on its vascular pedicle (FIGURE 6). **CONTINUES** ▶

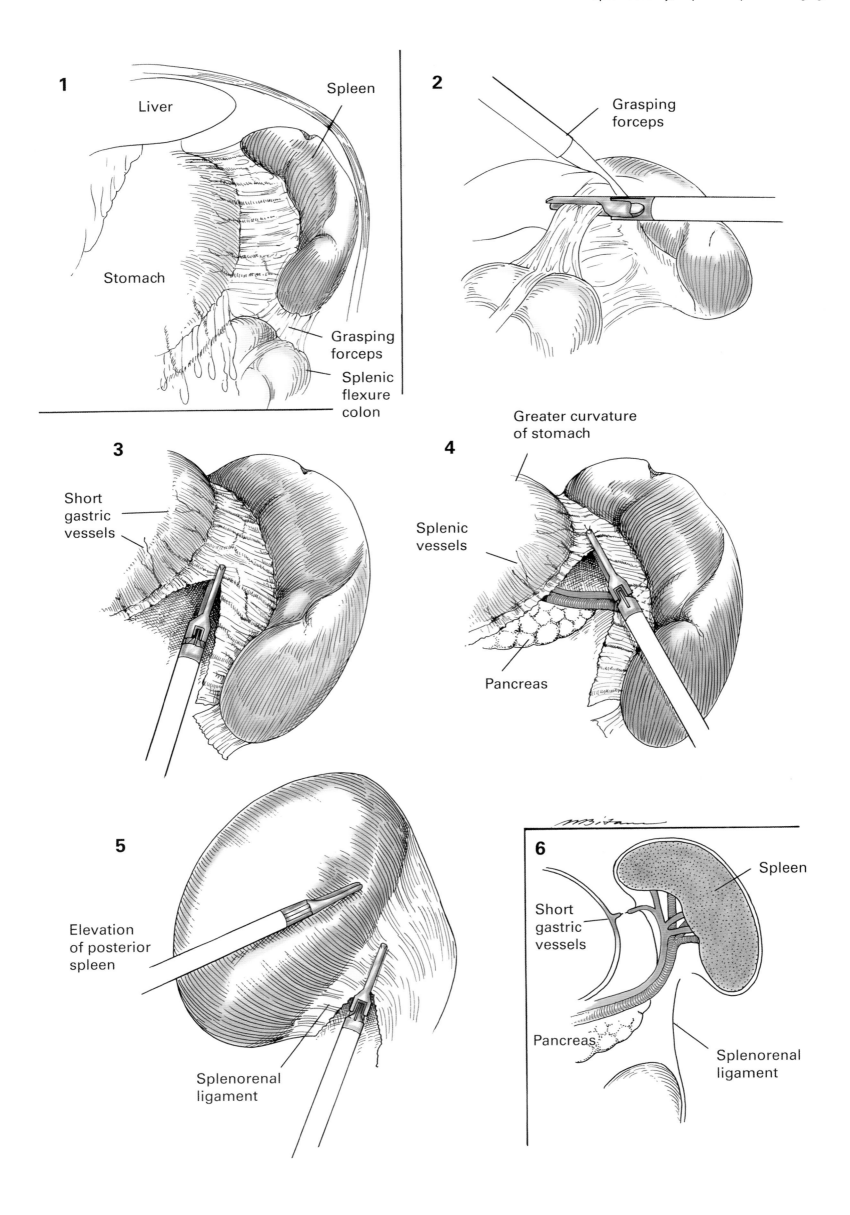

1

Liver

Spleen

Stomach

Grasping
forceps

Splenic
flexure
colon

2

Grasping
forceps

3

Short
gastric
vessels

4

Greater curvature
of stomach

Splenic
vessels

Pancreas

5

Elevation
of posterior
spleen

Splenorenal
ligament

6

Spleen

Short
gastric
vessels

Pancreas

Splenorenal
ligament

DETAILS OF PROCEDURE [CONTINUED] The area chosen should be distal to the tail of the pancreas but proximal to the trifurcation of the splenic vessels. Dissection is performed until the vessels can be safely encompassed within the jaws of an endoscopic vascular stapler. This instrument currently requires a 12-mm port. It is common practice to use a vascular stapling device to occlude and divide the entire splenic pedicle together. In some cases it is preferable to individually ligate the splenic artery and vein using the endovascular stapler. When this technique is employed the artery should be divided first. If either splenic vessel is entered during the dissection, emergency control of the hemorrhage is obtained by cross-clamping both the splenic artery and vein with the dissecting instrument (FIGURE 7). As all collateral vessels to the spleen have been transected, only temporary back bleeding should occur. This maneuver allows the surgeon to place another operating port for further proximal dissection and stapling of the splenic artery and vein or to control the hemorrhage during conversion to an open procedure.

When the tail of the pancreatic tissue extends into the hilum of the spleen, the zone for transection of the splenic vessels is quite short. Dissection is more difficult, as the vessels may have divided into their branches. In this case, the pedicle may be taken in serial transections, as opposed to stapling of the vascular pedicle en bloc (FIGURE 8). In reality, the splenic artery and vein are rarely skeletonized as cleanly as shown in these illustrations, but the general principle is that the tissue to be stapled must be contained well within the span of the stapling instrument's jaws. A useful maneuver is a 180-degree rotation of the stapler to ensure that no tissue or vessels extend beyond the staple zone within the instrument's jaws.

A reinforced oversized plastic bag is placed through a large port site. This special bag comes in an extra-large instrument that usually requires removal of a 10-mm port and finger dilation of this site to approximately 12 mm. The videoscope is used for visualization as the collapsed bag and instrument are passed through the abdominal wall. The bag is opened, noting the arrow orientation on its rim. The spleen is placed into the bag (FIGURE 9), which is closed. This reinforced bag is then partially withdrawn through the abdominal wall until the open rim of the bag is under control outside of the abdomen. The bag is cut free from the carrier using the drawstring in the end of the instrument handle. The spleen is morcellized with either finger fracture within the bag or, most often, with a ringed forceps, which then extracts the spleen in pieces (FIGURE 10). Care must be taken not to pinch or tear the bag with the ringed forceps.

Following complete extraction of the spleen and bag, the right upper quadrant of the abdomen is lavaged with the suction irrigator and a careful inspection is made of all cut surfaces and vessels. The tail of the pancreas is examined for possible injury that might necessitate placement of a closed-suction Silastic catheter drain. A final search for accessory spleens is made in the usual locations and they are simply excised using the ultrasonic dissector.

CLOSURE Each of the ports is removed under direct vision of the videoscope and the enlarged Hasson and 10-mm port sites are closed with interrupted delayed absorbable oo sutures. The skin is approximated with ooooo absorbable subcuticular sutures. Adhesive skin strips and dry sterile dressings complete the procedure.

POSTOPERATIVE CARE The OG tube is removed before the patient awakens and the Foley catheter is discontinued when the patient is alert enough to void. Intake of clear liquid is begun within a day and the diet is advanced as tolerated. Corticosteroid coverage is tapered to the preoperative basal levels and serial blood counts are performed. Additional medical consultation may be needed with the hematologist or oncologist to regulate medications in complex cases. Recurrence of left-upper-quadrant and shoulder pain along with the appearance of a left pleural effusion may signal either a pancreatic leak or an abscess if signs of infection are present. Either may require placement of a subdiaphragmatic closed drain using imaging study guidance. Prolonged follow-up by the hematologist or oncologist is necessary. ■

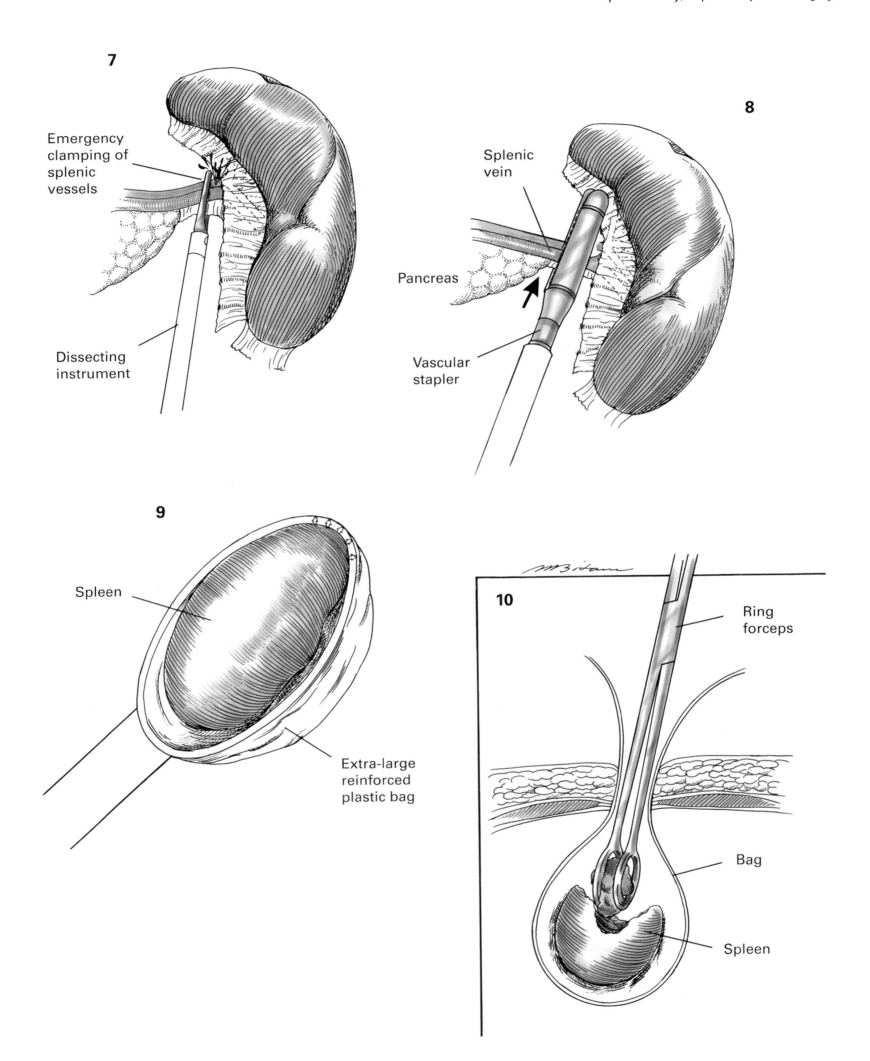

7

Emergency
clamping of
splenic
vessels

Dissecting
instrument

8

Splenic
vein

Pancreas

Vascular
stapler

9

Spleen

Extra-large
reinforced
plastic bag

10

Ring
forceps

Bag

Spleen

SPLENIC CONSERVATION

INDICATIONS Injury to the spleen is one of the more serious problems associated with trauma. Emergently there is the possibility of exsanguination. However, for the remainder of the patient's life after splenectomy, there is the possibility of catastrophic bacterial infection with encapsulated organisms, such as pneumococci, especially in the very young. This has stimulated clinicians to conserve the spleen with or without operation. Nonoperative treatment in children is often successful if careful monitoring is provided in-hospital and thereafter at home until full healing is documented. In addition, in adults as well as in children, splenorrhaphy is often possible, as it is desirable to salvage as much of the traumatized spleen as possible. It is uncertain how much retained spleen is essential to provide normal protection for the patient, but many recommend preservation of half or more if possible. The surgeon must appreciate that it is essential to control exsanguination and that total splenectomy should be performed for splenic fractures that are massive or that cannot be easily controlled in the presence of continued major hemorrhage.

Rib fractures (especially those in the left lower and posterior region) and an elevated left diaphragm on roentgenograms of the chest are suggestive of splenic injury. Abdominal CT scans are invaluable in demonstrating splenic injury and their findings may support a decision for or against immediate splenectomy. Early operation should be considered when the scan shows a fracture that extends into the hilum of the spleen. The patient with splenic injury who is managed with observation must be evaluated frequently as occult hemorrhage may result in sudden hypotension and shock. The decision for or against nonsurgical treatment of a splenic injury should be based upon clinical judgment rather than solely on radiographic findings. If the diagnosis is not clear, a peritoneal tap or lavage yielding an obviously bloody return can be helpful in supporting surgical intervention as this indicates a free or noncontained rupture of the spleen.

Familiarity with the major blood supply of the spleen is required if salvage of the portion of the spleen is to be successful (FIGURE 1). The major splenic artery and vein run just under the peritoneum along the top of the pancreas. The easiest accessibility to the vessels occurs through an opening in the gastrocolic omentum (Chapter 90). A bulldog clamp can be applied temporarily to the splenic artery and this will lessen the massive bleeding as the surgeon mobilizes up the extensively damaged spleen. The clamp is applied proximally as the splenic artery within the hilum divides into three terminal vessels, each supplying approximately one-third of the spleen. It is important to remember that the spleen has a dual blood supply—namely, the short gastric vessels from the greater curve of the stomach in the gastrosplenic ligament as well as the retroperitoneal splenic artery and vein.

PREOPERATIVE PREPARATION Evidence of shock associated with a falling hematocrit or hemoglobin should be viewed with alarm and result in early surgical intervention. The patient with a potential splenic injury should be typed and cross-matched while reserving several units of packed red cells or blood at all times. The importance of sustained observation day and night in a patient treated nonsurgically cannot be overemphasized, since the decision for surgical intervention can come at any time!

Hypotension and shock must be treated with adequate volumes of fluid and blood. A tendency to recurrent hypotension after resuscitation should be viewed with alarm and early surgical intervention undertaken. CT scans of the spleen in a stable patient can provide significant help in establishing the location, extent, and progress of the injury.

ANESTHESIA A general anesthesia is required. Large-bore venous access catheters are placed in both arms for rapid administration of blood, fluids, and medications.

POSITION Because of associated injury, the supine position may need to be altered. The patient is usually placed flat upon the table, thus preserving the option to accomplish a Trendelenburg position if shock develops.

OPERATIVE PREPARATION Nasogastric intubation is useful in improving exposure by lessening gastric dilatation. Antibiotics are given, and a routine preparation of the skin of the upper abdomen and left side of the lower chest is rapidly performed.

INCISION AND EXPOSURE A midline or left subcostal incision is made. The latter may provide a better exposure when the splenic trauma is severe, whereas the midline incision may be useful if other associated intraabdominal injuries are suspect.

One of the more common minor injuries to the spleen may occur during an upper abdominal procedure when traction is placed upon adjacent structures which have attachments to the surface of the spleen. The resultant tear in the capsule of the spleen can lead to a slow loss of blood (FIGURE 2). Such superficial injuries should be recognized early. Compression with a gauze sponge is applied to the denuded area for several minutes, remembering that clotting times are usually in the range of 6 to 8 minutes. If the bleeding persists, microfibrillar collagen is applied directly to the spleen and further gauze compression is given.

In the presence of major fracture of the spleen, a large gauze pad or towel is placed over the spleen to enable medial traction by the surgeon's left hand (FIGURE 3). This left hand also compresses the spleen so as to provide some control over the bleeding. Blood in the left lumbar gutter is aspirated by suction and an incision is made in the splenorenal ligament several centimeters away from the capsule of the spleen (FIGURE 4). This incision is extended upward to free the spleen from the base of the diaphragm. The spleen and tail of the pancreas are mobilized and lifted anteriorly and medially, as shown in Chapter 90. If splenic preservation rather than splenectomy is to be attempted, temporary control of the splenic artery is obtained with a bulldog or vascular clamp. Finger compression of the splenic pedicle may be utilized until the clamp is applied through either an anterior or posterior (Chapter 90) approach. Salvage of the spleen that appears to be badly injured may become feasible after control of the arterial inflow slows the bleeding such that a more thorough evaluation of the spleen and its vascular pedicle can be made. **CONTINUES** ▶

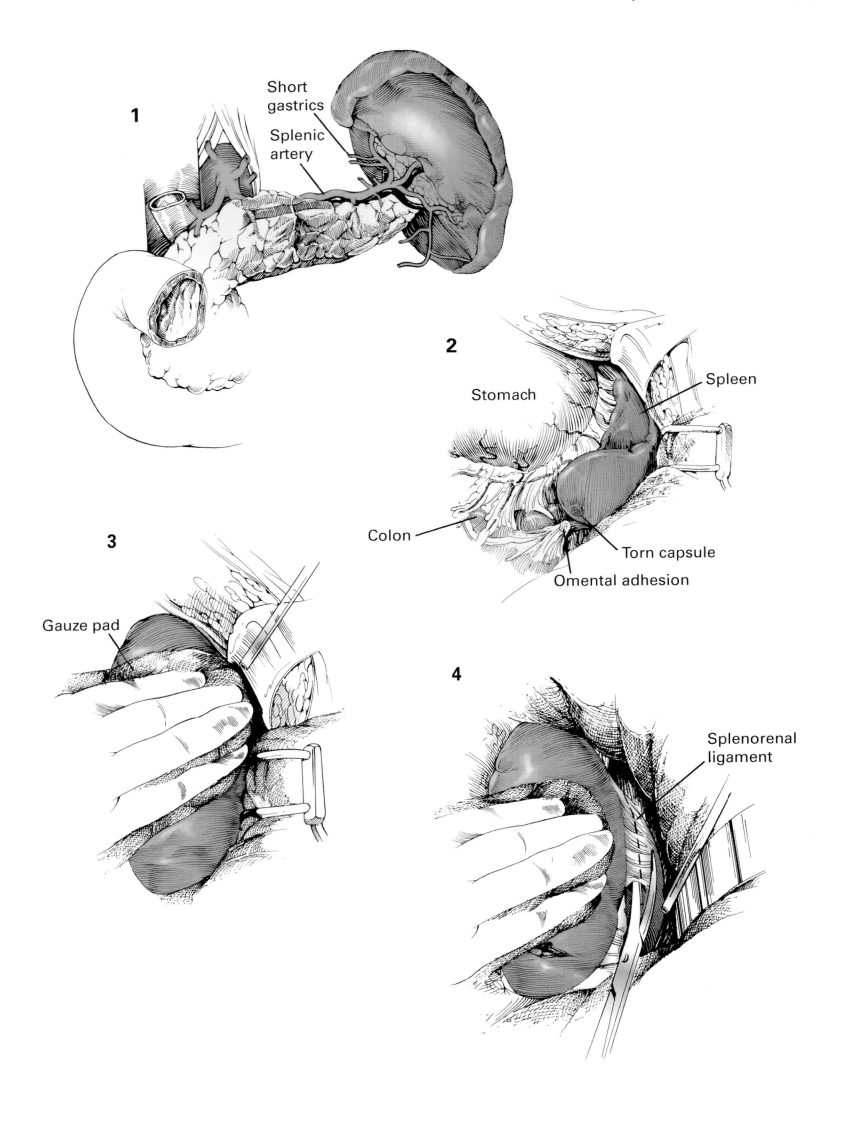

INCISION AND EXPOSURE <CONTINUED> The success of saving the spleen depends first upon the extent of damage from the trauma and second upon the effective compression of the lacerated splenic tissue with interrupted sutures. The splenic tissue is quite friable and some prefer to fill the crevice of the injury with hemostatic material such as microfibrillar collagen and then hold the cavity material in place with a series of carefully placed interrupted sutures which gently compress the spleen (FIGURE 5). Alternatively, the adjacent omentum may be mobilized on a viable vascular pedicle so as to fill the cavity created by the laceration. Again mattress sutures are used to hold the omentum in place so as to approximate the margins of the laceration and minimize further bleeding.

Laceration of the midportion of the spleen with extension into the hilum is usually considered an indication against splenic conservation. However, laceration involving either pole of the spleen may be controlled by isolating the appropriate artery and vein within the hilus that supplies the polar region of the organ. After dividing the gastrosplenic ligament and securely ligating the short gastric blood vessels, control of bleeding is enhanced by freeing up a segment of the splenic artery for the application of a bulldog clamp. The major arterial and venous vessels heading to the lower pole of the spleen are dissected free, ligated, and divided (FIGURE 6).

The devascularized section of the lower pole of the spleen is demarcated by its change in color and this ischemic damaged section is excised using cautery (FIGURE 7). The bulldog clamp on the splenic artery can be released after the polar splenic artery and vein branches of the major splenic vessels are divided and ligated. Active bleeding points are ligated by fine absorbable or silk sutures. Mattress sutures tied over Gelfoam pledgets may be required to control the bleeding (FIGURE 8). Additional hemostasis can be obtained using the argon-beam electrocoagulation system. It is desirable to have the raw splenic surface as dry as possible before microfibrillar collagen is applied.

The surface is compressed with a dry gauze sponge. If no active bleeding occurs after 5 to 10 minutes, the spleen is returned to the left upper quadrant after inspecting the cut edge of the splenorenal ligament for hemostasis.

CLOSURE Closure is delayed if there is any uncertainty about continued slow bleeding. Accessory spleens need not be excised, but all free splenic tissue should be removed to avoid subsequent splenosis. The tail of the pancreas is inspected to determine if pancreatic tissue has been injured. If disruption of the pancreatic tail is found, the pancreatic duct should be ligated if it is visible. Mattress sutures may be placed through the anterior and posterior capsules of the pancreas so as to compress the cut end. Alternatively, the pancreas may be divided with a stapling instrument. A Silastic closed-suction catheter may be placed in this region although, in general, catheter drainage in a splenectomy site is to be avoided as it may increase the hazard of subphrenic abscess.

It is important to evaluate the liver and other intra-abdominal organs that also may have been injured. After a final look at the spleen to verify viability and hemostasis, the abdominal incision is closed. This is done in a routine manner after all bleeding points have been ligated. Skin staples or subcuticular closure may be used for skin approximation.

POSTOPERATIVE CARE Frequent monitoring is required for several days and additional transfusions may be needed. Many surgeons maintain nasogastric decompression for a few days until gastrointestinal function resumes. This lessens the chance of gastric dilation, which may dislodge ligatures on the short gastric vessels along the greater curvature of the stomach. Vigorous pulmonary toilet may be necessary to avoid atelectasis and pneumonia, especially if rib fractures are present. The patient should be observed for signs and symptoms of a subphrenic abscess or an unrecognized pancreatic leak. If the injured spleen is removed, polyvalent vaccines for *pneumococcus, Haemophilus influenzae,* and *Neisseria meningitidis* are given except to pregnant patients and children below 2 years of age. Antibiotics may be given prophylactically to the very young patient after splenectomy. Both children and adults should be advised to seek medical attention without delay if signs of infection develop at any time for the remainder of their lives. ■

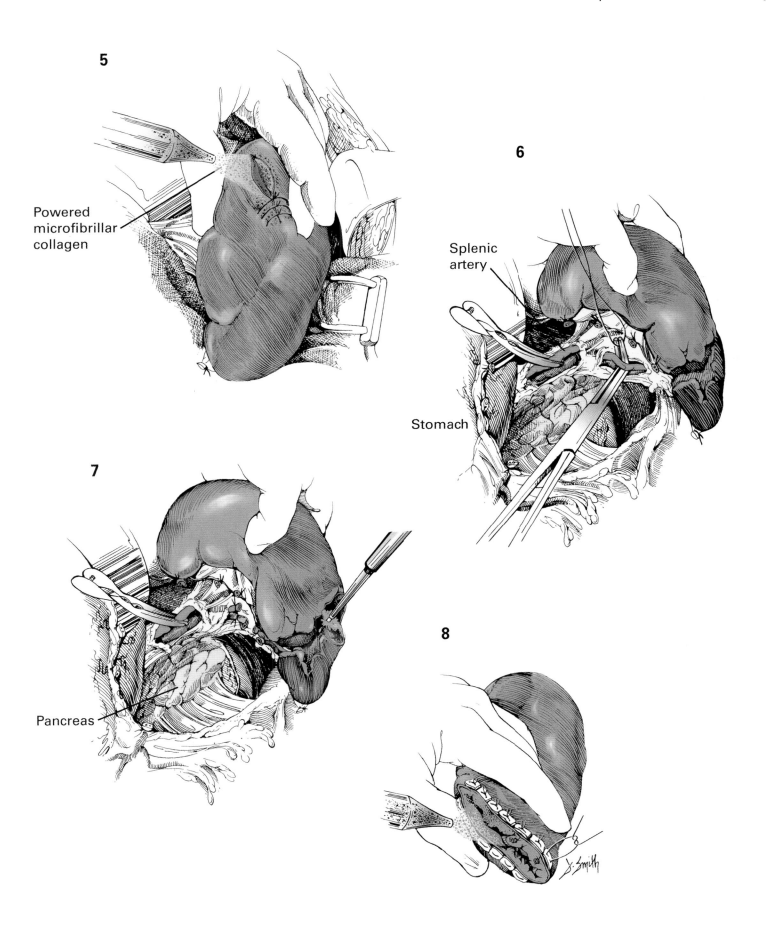

5

Powered
microfibrillar
collagen

6

Splenic
artery

Stomach

7

Pancreas

8

GENITOURINARY

A Gynecologic Procedures Overview

GYNECOLOGIC SYSTEM—ROUTINE FOR OPEN ABDOMINAL PROCEDURES Gynecologic procedures, in general, carry less risk than other abdominal surgical procedures because of the minimal amount of manipulative trauma to the alimentary tract and the patient's generally good condition. However, the same general principles apply here as in any major surgical operation, and the patient's condition must be appraised carefully.

PREOPERATIVE PREPARATION The obese patient should diet sufficiently to obtain a more normal weight before elective procedures are done. Secondary anemia is corrected preoperatively. Urinary complaints are investigated by analysis of the catheterized specimen of urine and endoscopic and roentgenographic studies when indicated. Bowel preparation, including enemas, is individualized. Antibiotics are given when sepsis is suspected. A cleansing enema is given and may be followed by an antiseptic vaginal douche. Prophylactic antibiotics are indicated for major vaginal and abdominal procedures.

ANESTHESIA A general anesthetic is satisfactory. Spinal or continuous spinal anesthesia may be used if desired.

INCISION AND EXPOSURE Many major gynecologic procedures can now be performed via minimally invasive techniques, which include laparoscopic and robotic approaches. A lower midline incision is made, and the lower angle of the wound is held open with a superficial retractor to permit a free dissection of the fascia until the location of the midline is absolutely ascertained.

Some operators prefer the transverse incision (Pfannenstiel), which is a convex incision following the lines of skin cleavage just above the symphysis. The upper skin flap may be dissected from the underlying rectus muscles, and the usual midline incision of the muscles and peritoneum is made. When an extensive exposure is required, it is better to use a Mallard incision which cuts across the recti muscles or a Cherney incision which detaches these muscles from the symphysis. An increased number of blood vessels require ligation by this approach in comparison to the midline incision, most notably, the inferior epigastric vessels.

The fascia is incised, scissors being employed at the lower angle of the wound to open the fascia down to the symphysis. The medial edge of presenting rectus muscles is freed and pushed laterally with the scalpel handle. Although few bleeding points are encountered in the midline, all must be clamped and tied or controlled by electrocoagulation. As the incision progresses, its margins are protected with gauze pads. The peritoneum, before being incised, is picked up to one side of the urachus with toothed forceps alternately by the operator and first assistant as in any abdominal procedure. The urachus, which can be seen through the peritoneum as a thickened cord, should be left intact, since it is not only vascular but also exerts traction on the bladder, inviting its accidental opening.

A self-retaining retractor is substituted for the superficial ones, although deep individual retractors may be used if a shifting of the retraction is desired to procure the maximum exposure as the operation progresses. Careful inspection is made to ensure that no intestine is caught in the retractor. When a self-retaining retractor is used, the smooth blade is inserted and the whole apparatus is adjusted.

Unless contraindicated by infection in the pelvis, a general abdominal exploration is carried out. The surgeon moistens his or her hands in saline and systematically explores the abdomen and finally the pelvis. The surgeon's operative note should contain a description of the findings, especially the presence or absence of gallstones. If a large uterus with extensive involvement by fibromyomata is encountered, it may be advantageous to deliver the uterus through the abdominal opening before the introduction of the self-retaining retractor. Large ovarian cysts, if benign and not grossly adherent, may be reduced in size by aspirating their contents through a trocar, great caution being used to avoid contamination from their contents. If the surgeon suspects ovarian malignancy, the organ is removed intact and a frozen section is performed. In addition, the surgeon should perform a saline peritoneal lavage for cytology and biopsy of the pelvic, lateral abdominal, and diaphragmatic peritoneal surface. Comprehensive staging of ovarian cancer also includes a pelvic periaortic lymph node dissection, infracolic node removal, and sampling of the iliac and preaortic lymph nodes. A tenaculum is applied to the fundus of the uterus to maintain traction while the intestines are walled off completely with several moist gauze pads. To accomplish this, the intestines are retracted upward by the left hand as the gauze pads are directed inward and upward by long, smooth dressing forceps, the packing being continued until the pelvis is free of small intestine. The pouch of Douglas is emptied of intestines, other than the rectosigmoid, and is likewise protected by a gauze pack. To maintain these packs in position, a moderate-sized smooth retractor is sometimes placed in the midline at the umbilical end of the wound.

CLOSURE Before the abdominal closure is started, the site of operation is finally inspected for evidence of bleeding, and the appendix may be removed. A search is made for needles, instruments, and sponges, and a correct count is reported before closure is started. The sigmoid and omentum are returned to the pelvis. After the peritoneum has been closed, the patient is gradually returned from the Trendelenburg position to horizontal to release tension on the wound and to permit stabilization of the blood pressure while the patient is under the surgeon's direct supervision. A routine abdominal wall closure is done (Chapter 10). The surgeon inspects as well as palpates the fascial suture line to ensure a secure closure.

POSTOPERATIVE CARE When conscious, the patient is placed in a comfortable position. The fluid balance is maintained with 2 L of glucose in lactated Ringer's solution the day of operation and each day thereafter until fluids and food are tolerated by mouth. If constant gastric suction is necessary, saline and potassium are added after the first day to accurately replace the losses by gastric intubation. The measured blood loss during surgery may be replaced if it exceeds 700 mL and the patient is hemodynamically unstable. Significant anemia can be tolerated in a healthy patient given the additional support of supplemental oxygen, colloid expansion (Hespan), and bed rest. In addition to surgical site infection prophylaxis, additional antibiotics are not routinely administered.

The patient should be ambulated at the earliest possible time. Ambulation in contrast to dangling is advisable. The inlying Foley catheter is removed in 24 to 72 hours, depending upon the extent of the surgical procedure and the patient's general condition. If repeated catheterizations are necessary, the amount of residual urine should be recorded and the catheterized specimens examined for evidence of infection. If infection is found, the appropriate antibiotics are given. Sterile perineal care is observed. Elastic stockings may be worn, especially if varicose veins are prominent or there has been a history of phlebitis. ∎

TOTAL ABDOMINAL HYSTERECTOMY

INDICATIONS A total abdominal hysterectomy is most commonly performed for benign conditions of the uterus including leiomyoma, adenomyosis, endometriosis, pelvic inflammatory disease, and dysfunctional uterine bleeding. Other indications include malignancies of the cervix, uterus, and ovaries.

POSITION See Chapter 93.

OPERATIVE PREPARATION Routine vaginal and abdominal preparation is given. The patient is catheterized, and an indwelling Foley catheter, No. 16–18 French, is inserted with inflation of the balloon and then anchored to the inner thigh. If access to the vagina and or anus is required, then the patient should be places in the low lithotomy position.

INCISION AND EXPOSURE See Chapter 93.

DETAILS OF PROCEDURE Whenever conditions will permit, the uterus is retracted upward toward the umbilicus, exposing the anterior uterine surface and allowing incision of the peritoneum at the cervicovesical fold (FIGURE 1). The surgeon should anticipate the course of the ureters. The round ligaments are ligated or incised with an electrosurgical unit (ESU) which enhances the surgeon's ability to dissect the retroperitoneal tissue planes. The loose layer of peritoneum is picked up with atraumatic forceps and incised transversely with scissors, or the ESU, close to its attachment to the uterus (FIGURE 2). If there are indications to remove the tubes and ovaries, the ovarian vessels are clamped proximal to the ovaries with a Heaney or curved Zeppelin clamp and doubly ligated with 2-0 delayed absorbable suture. Prior to applying the clamp the surgeon should insure that the ureter is out of the field of dissection. The ureters are identified along the medial leaf of the broad ligament to insure that they are out of the field of dissection. The adnexa is mobilized away from the pelvic sidewall structures (FIGURE 3). If the adnexa are to be spared, the uterine-ovarian ligament

is clamped and ligated (FIGURE 3). The operator uses sharp dissection to open the cervicovesical space and to dissect the areolar tissue between the bladder and the lower uterine segment. Blunt dissection should be used.

After the ovarian vessels have been ligated, the surgeon can palpate the region of the cervix with two fingers to determine its length and the position of the bladder. The bladder is sharply dissected off of the lower uterine segment and cervix (FIGURE 4). It is advantageous to divide the tissue over the cervix with sharp dissection until a definite avascular cleavage plane is established. Blunt dissection should be used sparingly and only in the midline directly over the cervix, or troublesome bleeding will be induced from tearing vessels in the broad ligament. Sharp dissection will permit the bladder to be directed forward and downward until the operator's thumb and index finger can compress the vaginal wall below the cervix (FIGURE 5).

SUPRAVAGINAL HYSTERECTOMY

DETAILS OF PROCEDURE For supravaginal hysterectomy, the operation proceeds as in total abdominal hysterectomy except that the uterine arteries may be ligated higher on the cervix. This procedure is shown in FIGURE 6. Technically, this is an easier and safer operation to perform, as the uterine artery suture ligatures are placed further away from the ureters. It requires, however, that the patient be compliant with lifelong gynecologic examinations that include cervical Pap tests. The posterior leaf of the broad ligament is incised down the level of the lower uterine segment and then the uterine vessels are skeletonized. The cervix is kept in position by Teale or similar forceps at the lateral margins and is divided at the level of the internal os, or lower uterine segment (FIGURE 6). The cervical stump then is closed transversely by placing several figure-of-eight sutures of 0 absorbable suture, one in each lateral angle and one or more in the central portion. These sutures must be placed sufficiently deep to secure complete hemostasis. **CONTINUES**

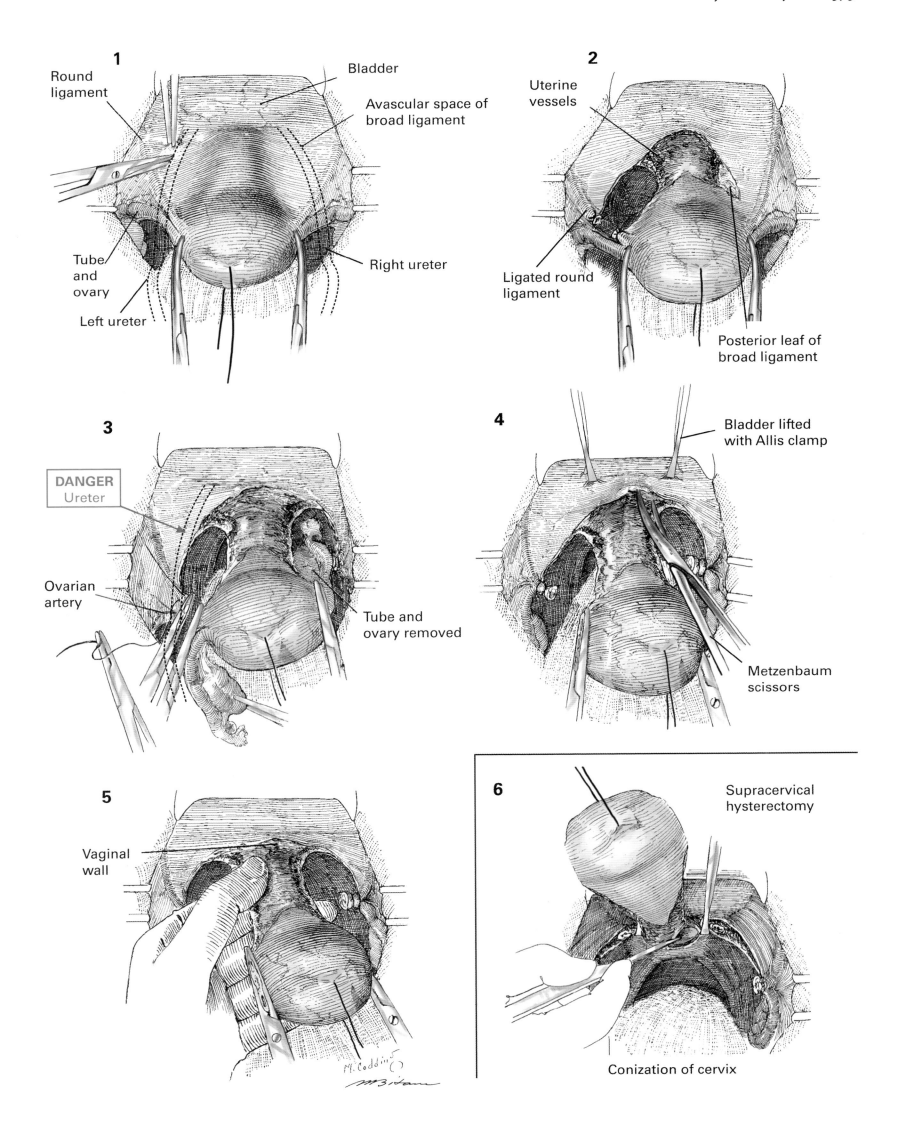

1

Round ligament

Bladder

Avascular space of broad ligament

Tube and ovary

Left ureter

Right ureter

2

Uterine vessels

Ligated round ligament

Posterior leaf of broad ligament

3

DANGER Ureter

Ovarian artery

Tube and ovary removed

4

Bladder lifted with Allis clamp

Metzenbaum scissors

5

Vaginal wall

M. Codding

6

Supracervical hysterectomy

Conization of cervix

DETAILS OF PROCEDURE ◀CONTINUED▶ The surgeon then holds the uterus forward and makes certain that the rectum is not adherent to the upper portion of the vagina. Should the rectum be adherent to the vagina, it is sharply dissected free to avoid possible injury. A moist gauze sponge or malleable retractor is loosely introduced into the pouch of Douglas to prevent any intestine from coming into the field of operation. The uterus is rotated slightly to the right in preparation for the application of a Heaney or Zeppelin clamp (FIGURE 7). The ureter is mobilized out of the field of dissection by mobilizing the bladder off of the lower uterine segment and cervix, and skeletonizing the uterine vessels. The surgeon can also skeletonize the anterior bladder pillars when necessary. Once the relative position of the ureter is established, the slightly curved clamp is applied from the side at a 90-degree angle to the cervix (FIGURE 7A). It is not necessary to include cervical tissue in the clamp. Now the uterine vessels are divided with curved scissors (FIGURE 7). If the uterus is quite large, a half-length clamp may be affixed to the vessels higher up along its wall to prevent troublesome backbleeding as the uterine vessels are divided. The paracervical tissue is divided with scissors to a point just below the level of the clamp to develop a free pedicle that can be tied easily (FIGURE 8). Failure to carry the incision beyond the tip of the distal clamp hinders accurate ligation of the uterine vessel pedicle, and troublesome bleeding results. A transfixing suture, a, of 2-0 delayed absorbable suture is tied as the clamp is slowly withdrawn (FIGURE 8). The development of an easily tied pedicle that includes the uterine artery is one of the most important steps in abdominal hysterectomy.

After a similar procedure has been concluded on the opposite side, a series of straight clamps are applied to the paracervical tissue and the uterosacral ligaments between the cervix and the uterine vessels (FIGURE 9). Modest-sized pedicles are taken with the straight clamps until the surgeon reaches the lower portion of the cervix which can be confirmed by palpation. At this point curved clamps are placed at each angle of the vagina just below the level of the cervix and then the tissue is cut with curved scissors. Any remaining attachments of the vagina to the cervix are incised with the scissors. (FIGURE 10). As the cervix is freed from the vaginal vault, the anterior and posterior vaginal walls are approximated with Teale forceps to include the full thickness of the vaginal wall as well as its posterior peritoneal surface (FIGURE 11). The lateral angles of the vaginal vault are first closed with transfixing sutures of 2-0 absorbable suture (FIGURE 12), following which one or more sutures are placed at the middle portion to ensure complete closure and hemostasis. The most likely place for troublesome bleeding is at the outer angles of the vagina near the ligated uterine vessels. Accurate and firm closure of the angles is imperative (FIGURE 12). Upward traction on the vaginal vault is released to determine whether any bleeding occurs.

CLOSURE The sigmoid and omentum are returned to the pouch of Douglas. It is not necessary to close the peritoneum. The patient is returned to the horizontal position while the fascia and skin are being closed. Only in rare instances is drainage instituted either through the vagina or abdominal wall.

POSTOPERATIVE CARE See Chapter 93. ■

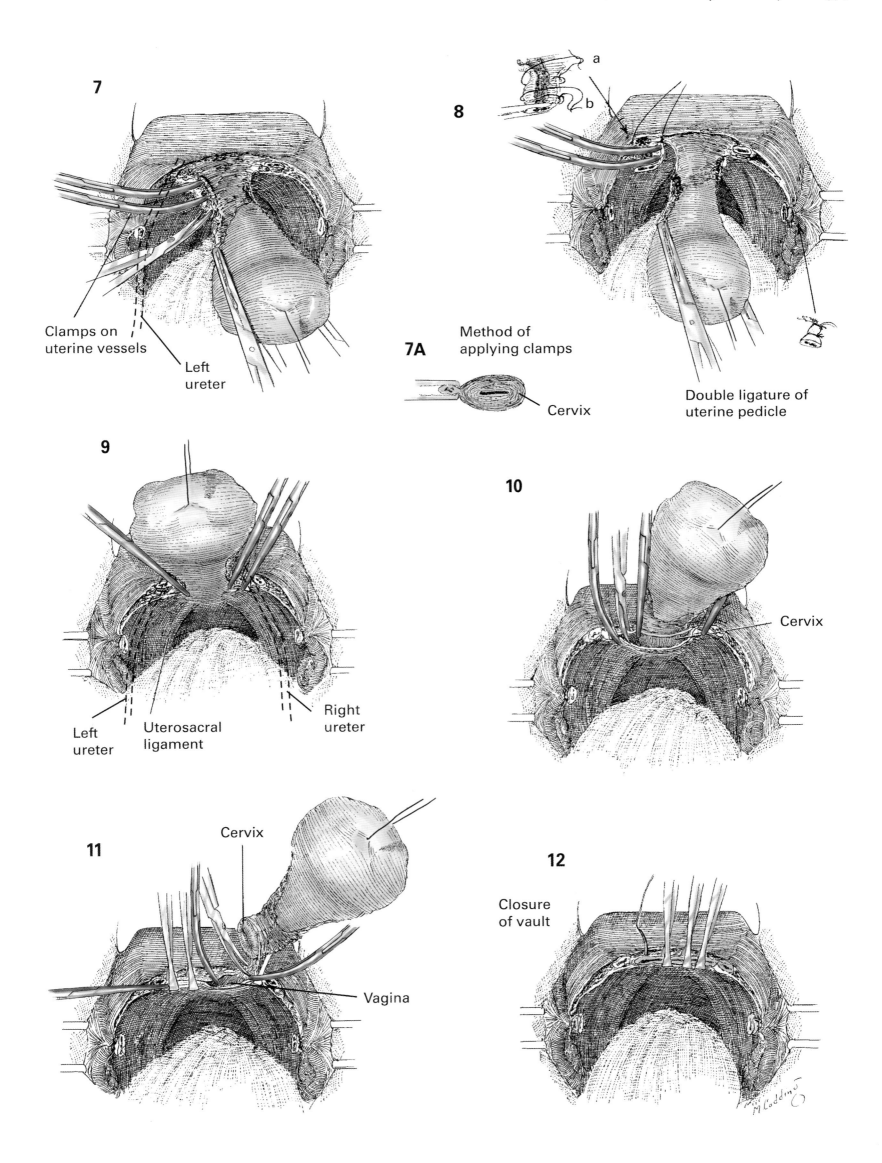

7

Clamps on
uterine vessels

Left
ureter

7A Method of
applying clamps

Cervix

8

a

b

Double ligature of
uterine pedicle

9

Left
ureter

Uterosacral
ligament

Right
ureter

10

Cervix

11

Cervix

Vagina

12

Closure
of vault

SALPINGECTOMY—OOPHORECTOMY

INDICATIONS Removal of the fallopian tubes and/or ovaries is indicated for inflammatory involvement of the adnexa that cannot be relieved by the use of conservative measures including antibiotics, for ovarian cysts, neoplasms, ectopic pregnancies, and endometriosis. Bilateral oophorectomy is advised by some as a desirable procedure in extensive carcinoma of the rectum because of the susceptibility of the ovaries to tumor transplantation from lesions of the gastrointestinal tract. In the absence of malignancy every effort should be made to conserve even remnants of functioning ovarian tissue especially in the younger patients, but recently conservation has also been recommended for menopausal patients without other indications for ovarian removal.

PREOPERATIVE PREPARATION See Chapter 93.

OPERATIVE PREPARATION The skin is prepared in the routine manner.

INCISION AND EXPOSURE See Chapter 93. In the presence of extensive pelvic inflammation, the intestines are often attached to the adnexa by adhesions that must be separated by sharp dissection. Meticulous dissection and careful handling of the tissue is important in order to avoid unintentional injury to the bowel. By placing the adhesions on tension as they are cut, the cautious surgeon can almost always develop a cleavage plane between the diseased adnexa and the other structures. In minimally invasive surgery, the bowel (except for the pelvic sigmoid colon) will usually fall out of the pelvis secondary to placing the patient in Trendelenburg position, but loops of small bowel may be needed to be carefully flipped into the upper abdomen with blunt atraumatic instruments. During a laparotomy, the intestines are carefully packed away with warm, moist gauze pads, or placed in a plastic bag and moistened with warm saline. The free adnexa are then held upward with a half-length clamp (FIGURE 1).

A. SALPINGECTOMY

DETAILS OF PROCEDURE The uterus is held forward by placing a Kelly clamp to the round ligament adjacent to the uterus (FIGURE 1).

The mesosalpinx is clamped with a sufficient number of half-length clamps, usually three pairs, to include its entire length (FIGURES 1 and 2). To avoid possible interference with the blood supply of the ovary, the line of incision is kept near the fallopian tube (FIGURE 1). The clamps are then ligated with transfixing sutures using 2-0 absorbable suture. Alternatively, a bipolar electrosurgical unit (ESU) can be applied in sequential bites along the mesosalpinx to the level of the cornu of the uterus (FIGURE 3). The proximal aspect of the fallopian tube is then excised from the cornu (FIGURE 4) and ligated at the level of the uterine fundus with a transfixing suture (FIGURE 5) or with the bipolar ESU.

B. SALPINGECTOMY AND OOPHORECTOMY

DETAILS OF PROCEDURE When both the tube and ovary are to be removed, a peritoneal incision is made parallel and lateral to the fallopian tube and the ovarian vessels as shown in FIGURE 6. Prior to ligating the ovarian vessels the pararectal space should be opened and the ureter identified at the level of the bifurcation of the common iliac artery (FIGURE 6). After establishing that the ureter is out of the field of dissection, curved Heaney clamps are applied to the infundibulopelvic ligament, which includes the ovarian vessels (FIGURE 6). The vessels are divided and doubly tied with 2-0 delayed-absorbable sutures. The medial leaf of the broad ligament is then incised with scissors or the ESU down to the level of the uterine vessels while staying above the level of the ureter. Next the proximal portion of the fallopian tube is ligated as shown in FIGURE 5. The peritoneal surfaces may be approximated (FIGURE 7) and a possible, but not necessary, partial suspension is shown (FIGURE 8). Anti-adhesive barriers may be applied, when indicated, in cases where fertility preservation is a concern.

CLOSURE See Chapter 93.

POSTOPERATIVE CARE See Chapter 93. ∎

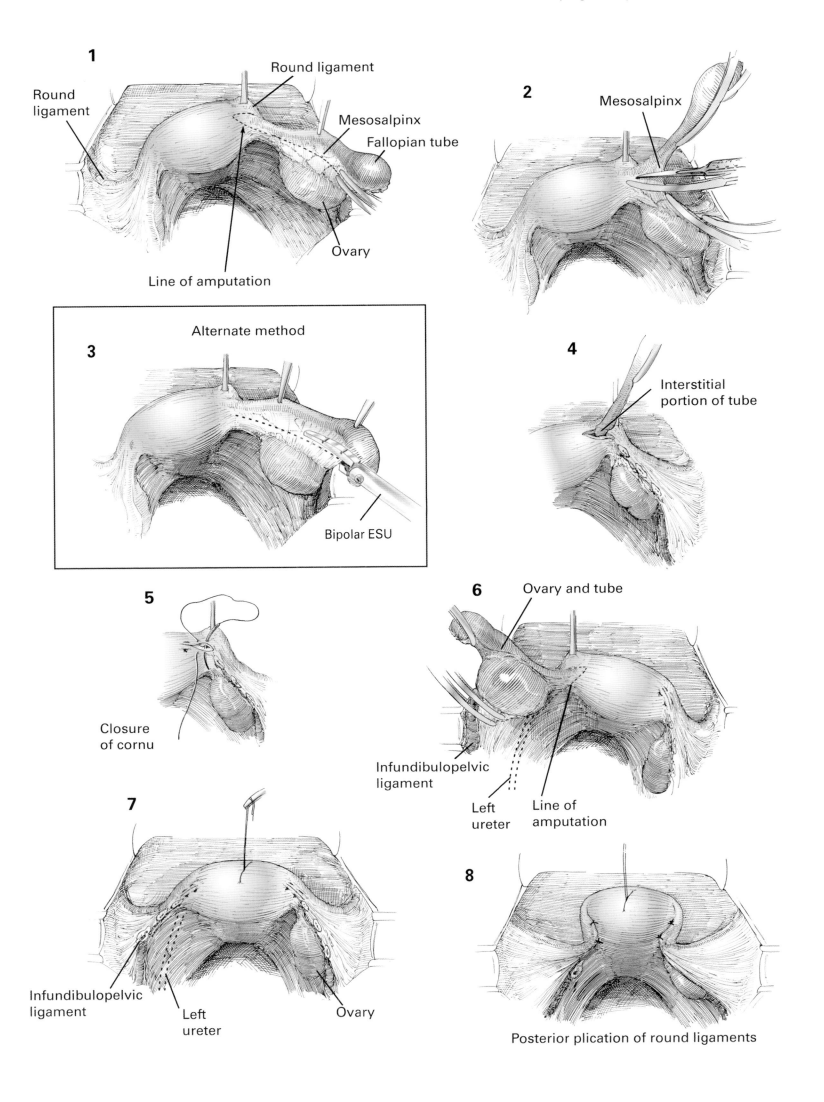

1

Round ligament

Round ligament

Line of amputation

Mesosalpinx

Fallopian tube

Ovary

2

Mesosalpinx

Alternate method

3

Bipolar ESU

4

Interstitial portion of tube

5

Closure of cornu

6

Ovary and tube

Infundibulopelvic ligament

Left ureter

Line of amputation

7

Infundibulopelvic ligament

Left ureter

Ovary

8

Posterior plication of round ligaments

CHAPTER 96

GYNECOLOGIC SYSTEM—ROUTINE FOR VAGINAL PROCEDURES

PREOPERATIVE PREPARATION In the majority of instances, no preoperative douches are used. The symphysis, perineum, and adjacent surfaces are not shaved but may be clipped carefully before operation. A preoperative cleansing enema is optional. Prophylactic antibiotics are administered.

ANESTHESIA General or regional anesthesia is satisfactory.

POSITION Vaginal procedures are carried out in the lithotomy position. After the induction of anesthesia, the patient's buttocks are brought to the edge of the table. The legs are raised simultaneously to avoid straining the sacroiliac joints and are fixed in stirrups with the knees flexed. Whenever possible, the legs are elevated upward and backward to permit the assistant to be nearer the field of operation. Excessive hip flexion, abduction, and external rotation should be avoided. The buttocks are brought to the edge of the table. The operating table is turned so that the light falls on the field and is focused on the introitus.

OPERATIVE PREPARATION The vulva and adjacent skin areas are scrubbed from above downward with pairs of prepping sponges held in gloved hands. The sponges are saturated with a solution of water and a detergent with germicidal action, such as a povidone-iodine–containing scrub. In all, approximately five pairs of sponges are used, each being discarded as it comes in contact with the anus. The vaginal vault is cleaned with approximately five saturated sponges which are attached to a prepping stick. Dry sponges are used to remove excess solution from the vaginal vault and the cleaned skin is blotted dry with a sterile towel. The anus may be excluded from the operative area by the use of a spray-on adhesive compound and the application of a piece of sterile, transparent plastic film. The footboard of the operating table can be raised to a convenient level and serves as an instrument table for the surgeon. A sterile, fenestrated perineal drape is applied, and the bladder is emptied by catheterization.

EXPOSURE Adequate exposure is obtained by introducing into the vagina either a weighted vaginal speculum, hand held retractors or a self-retaining retractor, depending on the type and location of the operation to follow. A thorough pelvic examination is made as a preliminary to the technical procedures.

POSTOPERATIVE CARE After the completion of the operation, the vagina and perineum are cleaned with sponges moistened with saline or a mild antiseptic solution. A sterile perineal pad is then applied and held in position by a T binder. When constant bladder drainage is desired, a Foley catheter is inserted and held by adhesive tape anchored to the thigh. The drapes are removed, and the legs are withdrawn slowly and simultaneously from the stirrups to prevent disturbances in blood pressure and straining of the sacroiliac joints.

The immediate postoperative care is similar to that following abdominal procedures, with certain added perineal precautions. Indwelling catheters are not necessary. The patient may be catheterized every 4 to 6 hours, depending on the fluid intake, until she voids voluntarily. Postvoiding residuals should be checked. Values less than 50 mL usually indicate satisfactory emptying. These patients should take in extra oral liquids to ensure a liberal urine output. Antibiotics may be given if a urinary tract infection occurs. The daily intake and output are recorded during the hospital admission.

The perineum is kept clean and dry with a peri-pad and is rinsed with clean water after urination and defecation. Warm, moist applications or dry heat to the perineum may be used to relieve pain. Sitz baths promote comfort and stimulate voiding. A stool-softening preparation is given starting either on the evening of surgery or the first postoperative morning. After procedures requiring extensive tissue dissection, bowel movements are often delayed for 3 to 5 days. The principle of early ambulation is followed. ∎

DIAGNOSTIC TECHNIQUES FOR CERVICAL LESIONS—DILATATION AND CURETTAGE

INDICATIONS Cervical conization is indicated for suspicious lesions of the uterine cervix to confirm or exclude the diagnosis of cervical cancer. It is also a therapeutic procedure for preinvasive lesions of the cervix. Certain outpatient procedures, such as colposcopy, usually precede conization and are useful in the investigation of cervical lesions and/or an abnormal pap smear. A grossly apparent lesion that is suspicious for neoplasia should be biopsied regardless of Pap smear results. A punch biopsy is the usual approach in this situation (FIGURE 1). After exposure of the cervix, the punch biopsy forceps is introduced, and a piece of cervical tissue is removed with inclusion of a small bite of surrounding healthy tissue. Alternatively, many surgeons now stain the cervix with acetic acid and perform the biopsies via colposcopic guidance.

A suspicious or positive Papanicolaou smear and/or positive punch biopsy may necessitate operation with cold knife conization, the definitive diagnostic procedure for malignant lesions of the cervix. Alternatively, a loop electrical excisional procedure (LEEP) can be performed in the office setting.

PREOPERATIVE PREPARATION See Chapter 96. Douches are omitted.

ANESTHESIA Either general or spinal anesthesia is given.

POSITION The patient is placed in a dorsal lithotomy position.

OPERATIVE PROCEDURE The usual preparation of the perineum and vagina is carried out. Following a pelvic examination under anesthesia, a speculum is inserted into the vagina and the anterior lip of the cervix is grasped with a single-toothed tenaculum. Dilatation and curettage is not performed before conization because it interferes with the lining of the endocervical canal and the squamocolumnar junction, making a pathologic diagnosis more difficult.

DETAILS OF PROCEDURE The cervix may be sprayed with a 7% iodine solution for evidence of possible carcinoma. The cervix is circumferentially injected with a vasoconstrictive solution such as diluted Pitressin or lidocaine with epinephrine. The surgeon maintains traction on the tenaculum as an incision is made with a No. 11 triangular-shaped blade at a 45-degree angle toward the endocervical canal. The involved portion of the cervix is excised (FIGURE 3A). The proximal 1.5 to 2.5 cm of the endocervix

is also removed (FIGURE 4). The removed tissue, which appears as a cone, is immediately placed in a fixative to avoid loss of diagnostic epithelium through contact with gauze and so forth. The length and width of the conization procedure can be tailored to the size and location of the lesion, and to the age of the patient. Alternatively, a CO_2 laser or electrocautery wire (LEEP) may be used in place of the cold knife (FIGURE 2 and 3).

After the cone is removed, the conization bed may be coagulated with the electrosurgical unit to maintain hemostasis. Individual points of hemorrhage are coagulated if necessary (FIGURE 4). The patency of the canal is verified with a dilator (FIGURE 5) and usually figure of eight sutures are placed on each lateral aspect of the cervix to achieve hemostasis (FIGURE 6). Occasionally, additional anterior and posterior figure-of-eight sutures are required.

The patency and direction of the cervical canal are determined by the passage of a uterine sound. The cervix is dilated gently with a series of lubricated, graduated Hegar dilators, and a systematic curettage is carried out (FIGURES 7 and 8). For diagnostic curettage dilatation up to a No. 8 or 10 Hegar dilator is adequate. The largest sharp curette than can pass through the dilated cervix is gently inserted and passed to the fundus. It is important to maintain counter-traction on the cervix with a tenaculum while placing dilators and performing the curettage. The anterior wall is scraped until all endometrium is removed, then the posterior wall. Curettage is then repeated on the right and left walls, the fundus, and finally the uterine cornu. Following curettage of the uterus, persistent bleeding from the cold-knife conization is controlled with figure-of-eight sutures.

POSTOPERATIVE CARE Postoperative care in a cervical conization is most important. Wide and deep conizations of the internal os may be the source of cervical stenosis. Postconization stenosis may be associated with the development of dysmenorrhea as well as sterility, early pregnancy loss and/or pre-term labor. Postconization patients should be seen in the office in 6 weeks for dilatation of the cervix if necessary. Under no circumstances should a stem pessary be left in the cervix at the time of conization, since infection may supervene in the presence of a foreign body. On occasion, patients develop a perimetritis. This usually responds very well to antibiotics. ∎

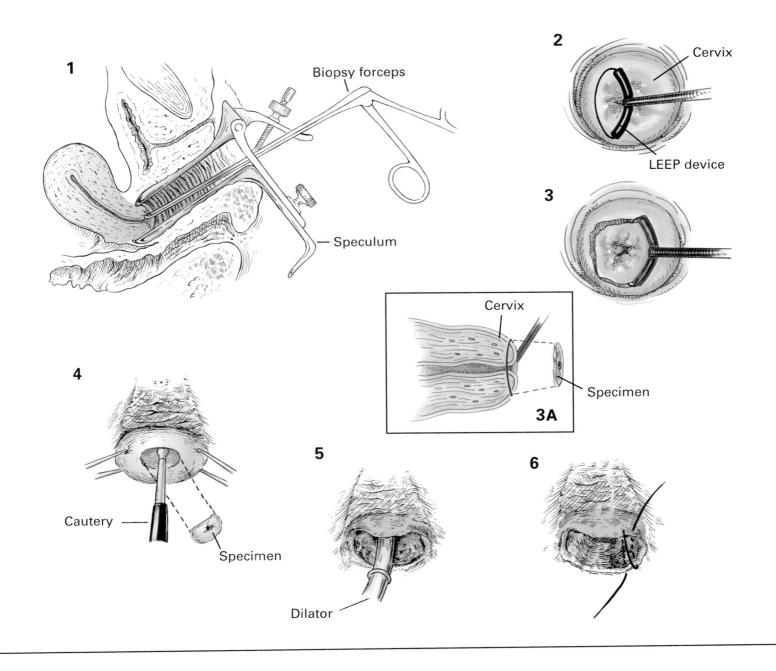

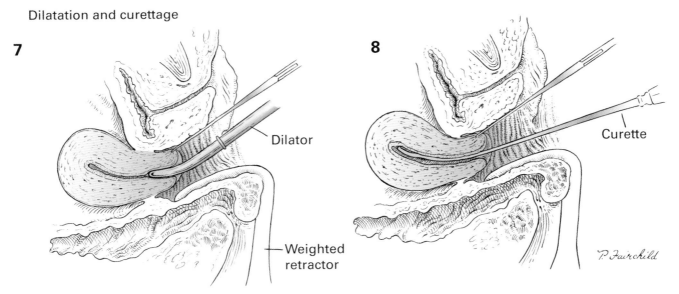

Dilatation and curettage

URETERAL INJURY REPAIR

INDICATIONS The left ureter is at risk for injury during hysterectomy, hemicolectomy, and any procedure performed in the pelvis. Recognition and repair of the injury limits post-operative morbidity. Once the injury is recognized, a number of repairs are possible. In all repairs, a water-tight closure and mucosa-to-mucosa apposition of the anastomosis is necessary. The location of the injury often determines the type of repair utilized.

More commonly, injuries occur outside the pelvis. In these cases, a ureteroureterostomy can be performed to restore continuity of the urinary tract. For injuries in the pelvis, commonly a simple ureteral reimplantation into the bladder is the most effective option. The ureter is spatulated and a new opening created in the bladder wall. The ureter is anastomosed to the bladder mucosa with 4-0 or 5-0 absorbable suture, and potential tension on the anastomoses is lessened with a psoas hitch.

DETAILS OF PROCEDURE Injuries in the middle to proximal third of the ureter are often repaired with ureteroureterostomy (FIGURE 1). The proximal ureter around the injury is mobilized for a short segment. This can often be performed with blunt dissection that preserves the periureteral vascular supply. The same is then completed for the distal segment. The two ends should meet, excluding the injured portion, without tension. A healthy portion of the ureter needs to be identified and used for the anastomosis on each end. The injured portion of the ureter can often be removed. Once the two ends are able to reach without tension, spatulation longitudinally is performed to widen the region of anastomosis (FIGURE 2A and B). This will allow minor contraction without narrowing the lumen. A stay stitch may be used in each end to minimize tissue handling. The mucosa should not be manipulated with forceps. Using a 4-0 or 5-0 synthetic absorbable suture, the apex of one end is anastomosed to the spatulated portion of the other (FIGURE 2C). A full thickness suture is placed with the knot on the outside of the mucosal apposition. Interrupted sutures are placed approximately every 2 to 3 mm to ensure a water tight closure. Once half the anastomosis is completed, a ureteral stent may be placed to facilitate drainage while the injury heals. The ureteral anastomosis is then completed. Post-operatively, a closed suction drain should not be left adjacent to the repair as this may promote further urine leak and fistula formation. If a ureteral stent is placed, it should be removed in 4 to 6 weeks (FIGURE 3).

Injuries occurring in the lower third of the ureter can be repaired with primary ureteral reimplantation with or without a psoas hitch. To prepare the proximal ureteral segment, gentle mobilization of the peritoneum medially is accomplished using a vessel loop around the ureter and bluntly dissecting proximally. The ureteral segment is transected at 90 degrees, followed by a longitudinal spatulation of approximately 5 mm (FIGURE 4). A stay stitch is placed in the apex to allow manipulation of the ureter. The bladder is then filled with saline through a sterile Foley catheter. This allows the surgeon to assess overall bladder volume and if the ureter will reach without tension. If it does not, a psoas hitch (FIGURE 4) is performed to gain additional length to reach the proximal ureter.

A psoas hitch brings the bladder to the ureter and anchors it to the psoas muscle. The peritoneum over the dome of the bladder is reflected. In men,

the vas may need to be ligated and the round ligament may need to be divided in women. The bladder is opened horizontally in the middle of the anterior bladder wall (FIGURE 5). This can be made with the cutting cautery current and stay sutures placed on either side of the incision facilitate a clean incision. This incision will ultimately be closed vertically and can be opened to approximately half of the bladder equator for maximal length. The superior portion of the bladder is then elevated toward the psoas tendon. This often allows elevation above the iliac vessels. An overlap of the ureter and bladder dome ensures there is no tension on the closure. If further distance is needed, the contralateral superior vesical artery and vein may be ligated. This may be done with a vascular stapler or suture ligation. In additiona, the contralateral endopelvic fascia can be incised to allow a few extra centimeters elevation. Once the necessary distance is attained, the psoas muscle and tendon are exposed. The bladder is held along this region and two 0 or 2-0 nonabsorbable sutures are placed into the detrusor muscle and tied to the psoas tendon (FIGURE 4). More sutures can be placed if needed. Care should be taken to place the sutures in the psoas tendon in a longitudinal fashion to ensure the genitofemoral nerve is not entrapped. The anastomosis is ready at this point. A small opening is created in the bladder wall with cutting current electrocautery and a small hemostat creates a direct entrance into the bladder lumen at 90 degrees (FIGURE 6A). From within the bladder a narrow hemostat is passed in an inferior direction to create a submucosal tunnel from opening A to B as in FIGURE 6B. The previously placed stay suture on the ureter is used to pass the ureter through the superior/posterior bladder wall into opening A (FIGURE 6A) and the stay suture is used to bring the ureter through the submucosal tunnel exiting through opening B into the bladder lumen (FIGURE 6C). The ureter is then sewn to the bladder mucosa with visualization through the previously created cystotomy incision. A full thickness 4-0 or 5-0 synthetic absorbable suture is placed through the ureteral wall and placed deep into the bladder wall so the mucosa is approximated. Intermittent sutures are placed in this fashion until the ureter anastomosis is completed (FIGURE 6D). This creates a flap valve to lessen reflux as shown in FIGURE 6E. It is generally recommended a ureteral stent be left in place. The ureteral stent is placed prior to closing the bladder wall. The mucosal opening A is closed with absorbable sutures. The anterior bladder incision is closed with 3-0 chromic suture in a running layer incorporating mainly mucosa. A second layer is closed with 3-0 synthetic absorbable suture to include the muscularis and serosal layers (FIGURE 7). If possible, a third layer can be closed with 3-0 suture along the serosa. The previous created flap of peritoneum is then replaced. A drain may be left in place; however, a closed suction drain should not be placed over the anastomosis or bladder closure. A Foley catheter should be left in place to straight drain.

POSTOPERATIVE CARE Post-operatively the bladder is drained with the Foley catheter for 1 week. A cystogram is performed to ensure no urine leak exists prior to catheter removal. If a leak exists, the catheter should be left another two weeks prior to the next cystogram. The ureteral stent is removed after 4 to 6 weeks. ■

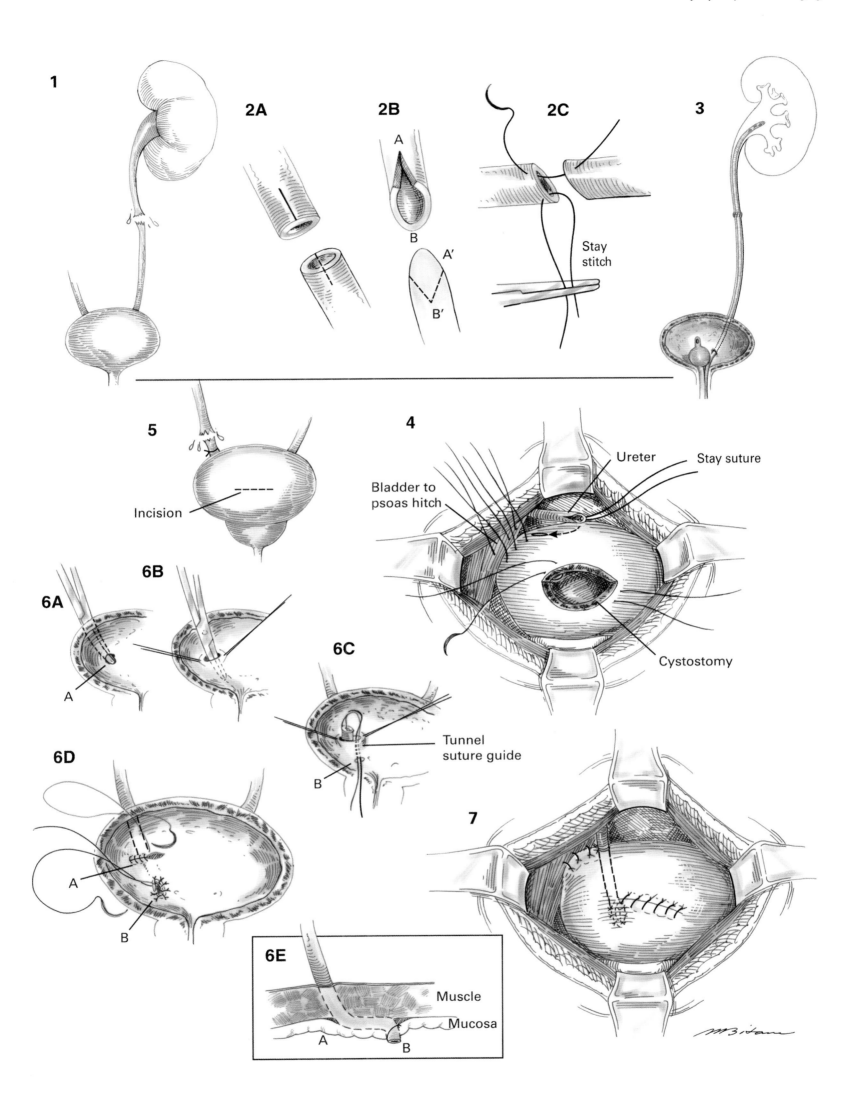

1

2A

2B

A

B

A'

B'

2C

Stay
stitch

3

5

Incision

4

Ureter   Stay suture

Bladder to
psoas hitch

Cystostomy

6A

A

6B

6C

Tunnel
suture guide

B

6D

A

B

7

6E

Muscle

Mucosa

A   B

DONOR NEPHRECTOMY, LAPAROSCOPIC

INDICATIONS Only persons who have voluntarily referred themselves as willing kidney donors are considered for this operation. Donor candidates undergo psychosocial and medical evaluation to determine their suitability for donation. In general these donor candidates must be of sound mind and in good health, nondiabetic, normotensive, nonobese, and with preserved renal function.

PREOPERATIVE PREPARATION Candidates that have been deemed suitable for donation undergo abdominal imaging with CAT scan angiography, magnetic resonant angiography, or less commonly bilateral renal artery arteriography. Imaging must verify the presence of two kidneys. In patients with multiple renal arteries, determination of kidney suitability for donation is based upon the experience and comfort of the donor, as well as the recipient and surgeon.

Intravenous access is obtained prior to administration of general anesthesia and endotracheal intubation. Antibiotics are administered intravenously within 1 hour prior to procedure commencement. Intravenous volume loading with crystalloid (25–50 cc/kg) is given prior to incision. This obviates compromised renal blood flow during abdominal insufflation which can result in acute tubular necrosis of the donated kidney after reperfusion in the recipient. Following intubation a urinary catheter is placed for bladder decompression and continuous urine output monitoring. An oral gastric tube is placed and kept on suction to evacuate and decompress the stomach. Deep venous thrombosis prophylaxis should be employed.

ANESTHESIA General and endotracheal anesthesia is required.

POSITION The patient is placed in the lateral decubitus position with the left side up for left-sided nephrectomy and right side up for right donor nephrectomy. A kidney rest is centered under the patient's flank and axillary roll under the dependent axilla. A bean bag may be used for holding the patient in place. The lower arm is placed on an arm board and the upper arm is supported on stacked padding or an elevated arm rest. The dependent leg is flexed at the knee and hip while the upper leg is kept straight. Padding is placed between the legs. The trunk is kept at right angle to the table and the pelvis and chest are strapped to the table to prevent movement during the procedure. The table is flexed 20 degrees and placed in slight Trendelenburg. The head should be supported to avoid lateral cervical flexion (FIGURE 1A).

OPERATIVE PREPARATION Hair within the surgical field is removed with clippers immediately prior to positioning the patient in the lateral decubitus position. The midline of the lower abdomen is also marked prior to lateral decubitus positioning, especially for obese patients. The abdomen is prepped from the xiphoid process to symphysis pubis and laterally from the table dependently to the midaxillary line. The surgeon and assistant stand facing the patient's abdomen with video monitors placed behind the patient facing the surgeon and behind the surgeon and the surgeon's assistant.

INCISION AND EXPOSURE A 10-mm port site incision is placed in the skin at the anterior axillary line below the costal margin on the left or right side ipsilateral to the kidney which is being removed (FIGURE 1B). A Veress needle is used to inflate the abdomen up to a pressure of 15 cm of water that will be maintained during the operation. The Veress needle is replaced with the 10-mm port that will serve as the port for the camera. The laparoscope can be inserted to examine the abdomen for adhesions, especially for patients with previous abdominal operations. Another 10-mm camera port is placed below the costal margin just lateral to the midline. For hand-assisted procedures an 8-cm hand port is generally placed either as an infraumbilical midline incision or a transverse Pfannenstiel incision (FIGURE 2). For the totally laparoscopic approach the extraction incision is created at the end of the procedure and can be placed either as described for the hand port site or as a muscle splitting incision lateral to the rectus muscle on the left or right side. The camera operator will stand towards the head of the patient and the surgeon towards the patient's feet. Additional ports are placed as needed.

DETAILS OF PROCEDURE The descending colon is mobilized from the spleen to its transition to the sigmoid colon (left-sided nephrectomy) or ascending colon from the hepatic flexure down to and including the cecum (right-sided nephrectomy). On the left side, the surgeon or assistant's hand pulls the colon gently away from its attachments which are divided along the white line of Toldt with an ultrasonic shears or alternate energy device. The superficial peritoneal attachments are released. The lateral renal attachments are not released in order to prevent medial rotation of the kidney. Gravity will allow the colon to remain deep or medial to the operative

region. This will expose the kidney surrounded by Gerota's fascia and caudal to this the psoas muscle (FIGURE 3).

The ureter is next identified. The ureter will be found 8 to 10 cm caudal to the tip of the inferior pole of the kidney anterior to the psoas muscle and lateral to the aorta (left side) or vena cava (right side) in close proximity and posterior to the gonadal vein (FIGURE 4). The gonadal vein is a good anatomic landmark to help identify the ureter. The ureter is mobilized away from the gonadal vein leaving adequate soft tissue around the ureter to avoid stripping of its blood supply, resulting in ureteral ischemia which could lead to urine leakage in the recipient. Alternatively, the gonadal vein and ureter can be mobilized and removed together to ensure integrity of the ureteral blood supply. Dissection proceeds in a cephalad direction along the gonadal vein until reaching the renal vein (left side) or the vena cava (right side).

On the left side, the gonadal vein is secured with titanium vascular clips adjacent to the renal vein and sharply divided (FIGURE 6). A bipolar energy device may also be used to transect the gonadal vein. If the gonadal vein is removed with the ureter, the vein will be similarly clipped more caudally, at the same level that the ureter is eventually divided. On the right side, the gonadal vein is kept intact unless it is removed with the ureter, in which case it is secured with vascular clips and sharply divided adjacent to its termination at the vena cava as well as at the level that the ureter is eventually divided.

The kidney is next mobilized. Mobilization may begin inferiorly, as shown in the accompanying figures or superiorly. Gerota's fascia is entered along the anterior aspect of the lower pole of the kidney (FIGURE 4). Then the upper pole of the kidney is dissected (FIGURE 5) and the adrenal gland is retracted medially and dissected away with a bipolar energy device from the upper pole as shown in Chapter 118 (FIGURE 7). In this dissection renal artery branches to the upper pole may be identified and care should be taken not to injure them. After the upper pole of the kidney is released then the lateral and posterior attachments are divided. The kidney may be rotated in the medial direction to facilitate dissection and identify any posterior attachments to the renal artery and vein.

It is preferable to divide all the branches of the left renal vein prior to complete mobilization of the kidney for ease of exposure during their dissection. On the left side, the adrenal vein is dissected at its insertion into the renal vein. It is divided with clips or a bipolar energy device. The left renal lumbar vein should be identified. If present it should enter the renal vein on its posterior aspect. The left renal lumbar vein is found joining the inferior/posterior aspect of the left renal vein anterior to the renal artery. It then courses posteriorly and just lateral to the aorta, inferior to the renal artery, and posterior to the gonadal vein (FIGURE 6). This vein must be divided in order to identify the renal artery that lies immediately posterior. The left renal lumbar vein is carefully dissected, clipped, and sharply divided (FIGURE 6). Occasionally the lumbar vein will be absent and occasionally the predominant venous drainage to the vena cava will be the via lumbar vein posterior to the aorta (retroaortic renal vein). Note that there are no lumbar branches arising from the the right renal vein if the right kidney is being donated. In order to provide adequate length for the anastomosis the renal vein is dissected from all surrounding perivascular attachments to a point medial to the adrenal vein.

The renal artery is identified posterior to the renal vein and bluntly dissected from the surrounding tissues using an ultrasonic device to minimize blood loss. On the left side, an adrenal artery originating from the cephalad aspect of the renal artery is usually encountered and must be clipped and divided or divided with a bipolar vessel sealing device (FIGURE 6). The renal artery is dissected proximately to the aorta (left side) or well posterior of the inferior vena cava (right side). The renal vein should be dissected about 2 cm proximal to the adrenal vein (left side) or to the vena cava (right side) to allow adequate length for the anastomosis. During the renal vessel dissection it is important to maintain the soft tissue lying between the ureter and the inferior pole of the kidney to avoid disrupting ureteral blood supply in this area. Once the artery is circumferentially dissected, the renal vessels are the only intact structures within the renal hilum.

On the right side, the artery is best approached by reflecting the kidney medially and dissecting directly over the renal artery behind the inferior vena cava. There are no renal vein branches to divide. Once the renal artery is dissected, the remaining tissue lying between the artery and the vena cava is dissected. Upon completion the renal vessels are the only intact structures within the renal hilum.

After the kidney is mobilized the patient is administered intravenous furosemide and mannitol. One should avoid administration of these diuretics before the kidney is mobilized as the kidney swells, making the dissection more difficult. **CONTINUES ▶**

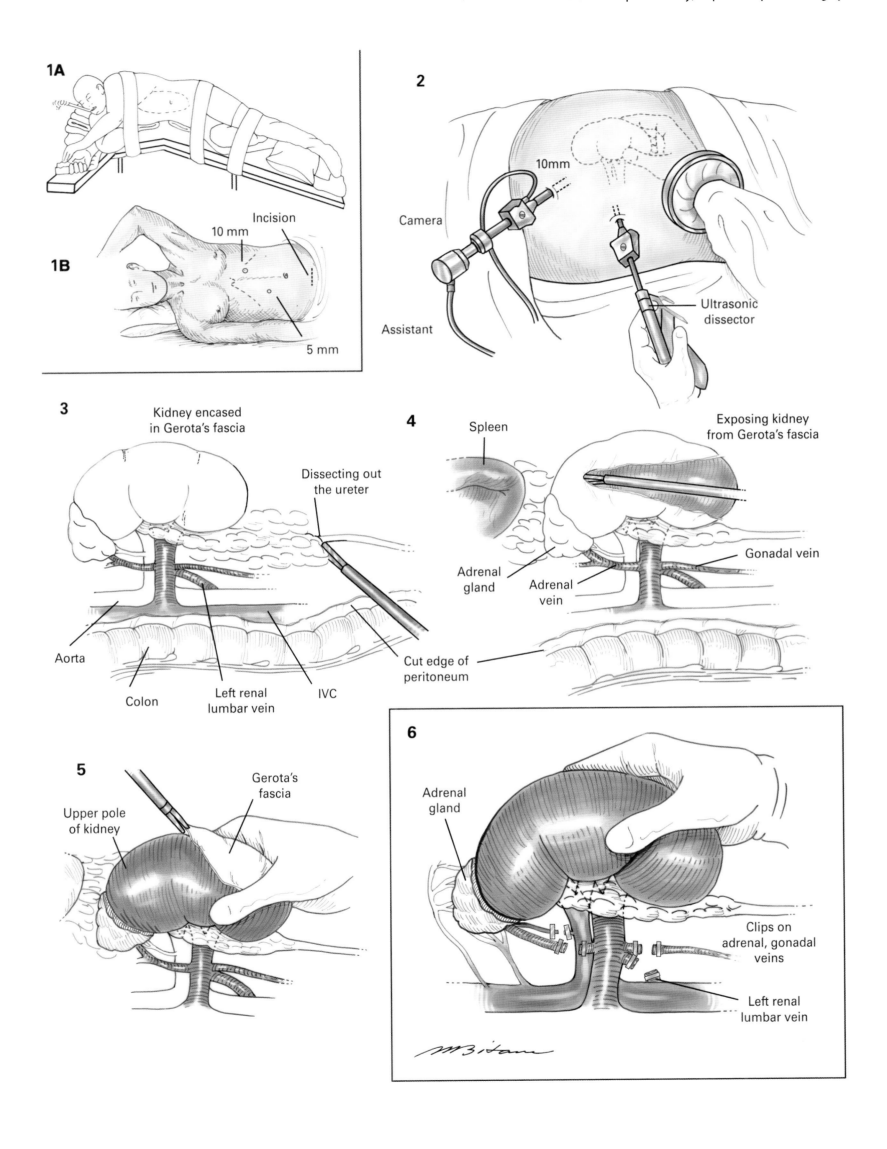

1A

1B
10 mm
Incision
5 mm

2
10mm
Camera
Assistant
Ultrasonic
dissector

3
Kidney encased
in Gerota's fascia
Dissecting out
the ureter
Aorta
Colon
Left renal
lumbar vein
IVC
Cut edge of
peritoneum

4
Spleen
Exposing kidney
from Gerota's fascia
Adrenal
gland
Adrenal
vein
Gonadal vein
Cut edge of
peritoneum

5
Upper pole
of kidney
Gerota's
fascia

6
Adrenal
gland
Clips on
adrenal, gonadal
veins
Left renal
lumbar vein

DETAILS OF PROCEDURE CONTINUED Finally the ureter, with or without the gonadal vein, is dissected caudally until the common iliac vessels are encountered deep to the ureter. The kidney is now ready for removal. The patient is systemically heparinized as the ureter is clipped with vascular clips at the caudal limit of the dissection and sharply divided leaving the proximal ureter open. This preserves adequate length of the ureter (FIGURE 7A and B). The renal artery is stapled close to the aorta (left side) or behind the inferior vena cava (right side) (FIGURE 8). The renal vein is stapled ≥2 cm proximal to the adrenal vein stump (left side, FIGURE 9) or at the vena cava (right side). The kidney is extracted through the hand port. The heparin is reversed with protamine.

The surgical site is inspected to assure hemostasis (FIGURE 10). The previously mobilized colon is placed back in its in situ position and port sites are closed in standard fashion and sterile dressing applied.

POSTOPERATIVE CARE The oral gastric tube is removed by the anesthesiologist. Oral fluids are begun the day of surgery and the diet is advanced as tolerated. Cough and deep breathing are encouraged immediately. The patient is ambulated on the first day after surgery, and the sterile dressing is changed on the second day. ■

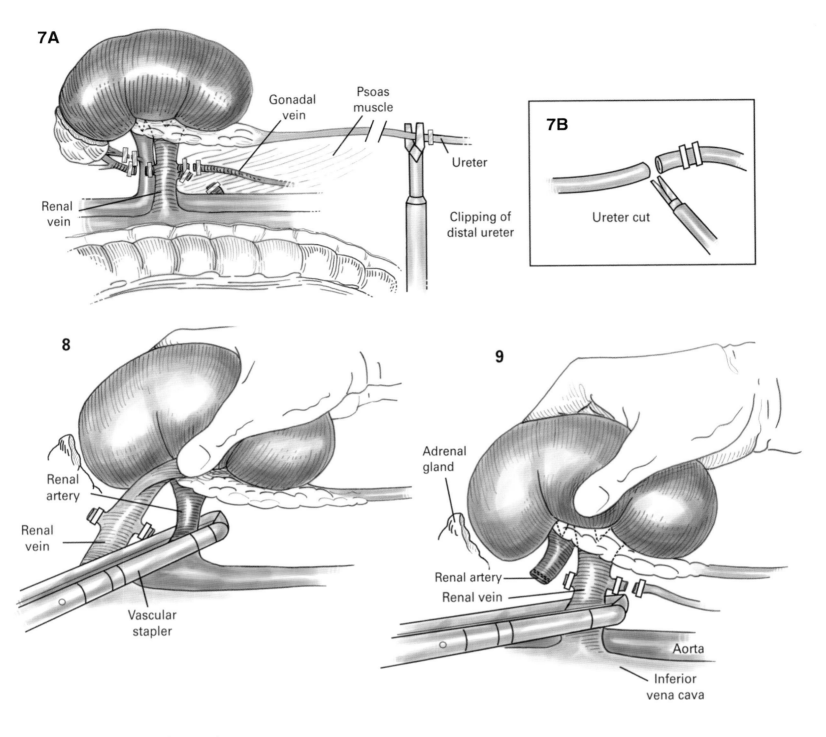

7A

Gonadal vein

Psoas muscle

Ureter

Clipping of distal ureter

Renal vein

7B

Ureter cut

8

Renal artery

Renal vein

Vascular stapler

9

Adrenal gland

Renal artery

Renal vein

Aorta

Inferior vena cava

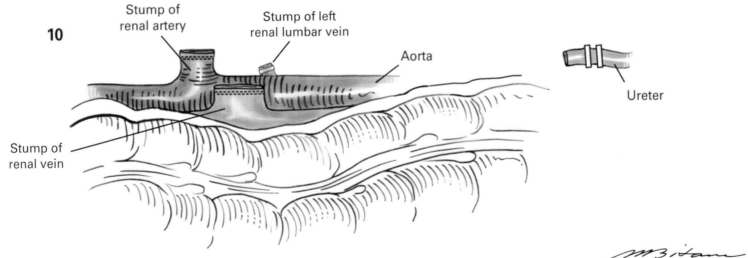

Stump of renal artery

Stump of left renal lumbar vein

Aorta

10

Stump of renal vein

Ureter

KIDNEY TRANSPLANT

INDICATIONS This procedure is for patients with end-stage chronic kidney disease with a glomerular filtration rate ≤20 mL/min who possess adequate cardiopulmonary reserve to undergo surgery. In addition, the patient cannot have an active infection or malignancy that would be exacerbated after the transplant due to the necessity of ongoing immunosuppression therapy following engraftment.

PREOPERATIVE PREPARATION Candidates are evaluated prior to transplantation for suitability based on the above indications as well as other psychosocial factors. Candidates found to have pre-existing comorbidities will receive additional evaluation and testing at this time as needed to aid in determining suitability. Once the candidate has been deemed suitable, the patient is ready for transplantation with a living donor kidney, if available, or listed for a deceased donor kidney.

Intravenous access is obtained prior to administration of general anesthesia and endotracheal intubation. Central venous access is preferable as it allows for intravascular volume assessment during the procedure. Antibiotics are administered intravenously within 1 hour prior to procedure commencement. Following intubation, a urinary catheter is placed and the bladder is irrigated with antibiotic-containing saline. If the patient is oliguric or anuric saline is left in the bladder after irrigation to distend it, aiding intraoperative identification. The Foley drainage bag is clamped to keep the bladder distended until the neoureterocystostomy is performed. An oral gastric tube is placed and kept on suction to evacuate and decompress the stomach. Deep venous thrombosis prophylaxis should be employed.

ANESTHESIA General and endotracheal anesthesia is required.

POSITION The patient is placed in the supine position. The legs are secured to the table with a strap with slight laxity. The lower extremities should be exposed enough to allow surgical access to the infrainguinal femoral vessels for the rare case where arterial reconstruction is necessary. If the patient has a peritoneal dialysis catheter every attempt should be made to position and drape it out of the surgical field. The ipsilateral femoral artery is palpated to verify iliac artery patency.

OPERATIVE PREPARATION The hair overlying the surgical field is removed with hair clippers. The abdomen is prepped from the midaxillary line on the side chosen for implantation to well beyond the midline, or if desired to the opposite midaxillary line. Caudally the abdomen is prepped below the symphysis pubis, and includes the femoral region on the implantation side. The prep extends cephalad to at least 5 cm above the umbilicus.

INCISION AND EXPOSURE The straight or curvilinear skin incision is made on the left or right side of the lower abdomen from the symphysis pubis at the midline laterally and cephalad far enough to provide adequate exposure of the external iliac vessels and to perform the vascular anastomoses (FIGURE 1). The external and internal oblique aponeuroses are divided just lateral to the rectus muscle, exposing the superficial inferior epigastric artery and vein. These vessels are ligated and divided. The round ligament (females) or spermatic cord is encountered as the peritoneum is swept medially exposing the contents of the iliac fossa. The round ligament is ligated and divided. The spermatic cord is encircled with a vessel loop and retracted medially and inferiorly to aid in exposure of the iliac fossa. Exposure is maintained with a Balfour self-retaining retractor.

DETAILS OF PROCEDURE The external iliac artery and vein are dissected free from surrounding tissues from the inguinal ligament distally to its origin proximately and encircled with vessel loops (FIGURE 2). The genitofemoral nerve is found lateral to the artery and can lie quite close to it. This nerve should be identified and spared. Lymphatics are ligated with permanent 2-0 suture to prevent postoperative lymph leakage. The donor kidney is now prepared on a back table for implantation.

The donor kidney is placed in a bowl filled with iced saline. The configuration of right and left deceased donor kidneys is shown in FIGURE 3A and B. The configuration of the right and left living related kidneys is shown in

FIGURE 3C and D. Deceased donor kidneys will have a cuff of aorta and on the right side a segment of inferior vena cava.

The renal artery and vein are dissected free from surrounding tissues, without over dissecting too close to the renal hilum. The gonadal, adrenal, and lumbar veins need to be ligated with 2-0 permanent suture and divided for a left kidney. For the right kidney the inferior vena cava is stapled (or over sewn with 4-0 nonabsorbable monofilament suture) both cephalad and caudal to the renal vein orifice and the left lateral edge of the inferior vena cava is opened, thereby creating a longer vein. Thus the cava and renal vein are dissected free from surrounding tissues with ligation of any venous branches, including lumbar veins, with 2-0 and 4-0 silk sutures. The extra cava is then removed. For deceased donor kidneys a cuff of aorta is included with the renal artery (FIGURE 3 A and B). For living donor kidneys this cannot be done. If multiple arteries exist they can be anastomosed together on the back table to reduce the number of anastomoses needed during implantation or they can be implanted separately, depending on surgeon preference. Any extra tissue adherent to the kidney capsule is removed as well as extra retroperitoneal tissue associated with the ureter. The triangle of soft tissue between the ureter and inferior pole of the kidney is left in place to assure adequate blood supply to the ureter. The kidney is brought to the operative field.

A left living related donor kidney transplant is illustrated. The external iliac artery and vein are clamped with vascular clamps proximal and distal to the intended anastomotic site. The patient is heparinized prior to clamping if not yet dialyzing. A venotomy is created in the external iliac vein, appropriately sized to the renal vein orifice (left kidney) or inferior vena cava orifice (right kidney). Four 5-0 nonabsorbable double-armed monofilament sutures are placed one each at the proximal and distal ends of the external iliac vein venotomy and one each at the midpoint of the medial and lateral sides, and then brought through the appropriate, corresponding area on the renal vein (or inferior vena cava) (FIGURE 4). The proximal and distal "corner" sutures are tied and the medial and lateral sutures are clamped with nontraumatic clamps and placed on tension to hold the walls of the external iliac vein apart. One of the two ends of a "corner" suture is then run down one side of the anastomosis to the opposing "corner" proceeding outside to inside the renal vein and inside to outside of the external iliac vein, approximating the renal vein (or inferior vena cava) to the external iliac vein, then tied to one of the ends of the opposite "corner" suture. This maneuver is then repeated on the opposite side, completing the anastomosis. An arteriotomy is created in the external iliac artery either with mucosal scissors or an #11 scalpel blade followed by an appropriately sized aortic punch. The arteriotomy site is selected to avoid kinking of the renal artery once the kidney is placed into the iliac fossa and to avoid (as much as feasible) areas involving severe atherosclerotic disease or calcification. Four 5-0 nonabsorbable double-armed monofilament sutures are placed as was done for the venous anastomosis (FIGURE 5). The medial and lateral sutures are clamped and placed under tension and the "corner" sutures are tied with one arm of the suture run to the opposite "corner" proceeding outside to inside the renal artery and inside to outside of the external iliac artery, as was done for the venous anastomosis. If accessory arteries are present and require implantation then the arterial anastomosis is repeated as necessary.

The renal artery and vein are then clamped with bulldog clamps prior to sequentially removing the iliac vessel clamps; proximal iliac vein, distal vein, distal iliac artery, and proximal iliac artery. Clamping the renal vessels allows for inspection of the vascular anastomoses and placement of repair stitches if necessary prior to reperfusion of the kidney. When the anastomoses are hemostatic, sponges are placed adjacent to the anastomoses to promote sealing of the suture line with platelet thrombi, and the renal vessel bulldogs are removed and the kidney reperfused. A small bulldog clamp is placed near the end of the ureter so it will distend with urine. The kidney will become pink, firm, and often pulsatile to palpation. Bleeding from the kidney surface and small vessels is controlled with vascular clips and electrocautery. The sponges are removed and the kidney is positioned in the iliac fossa and the renal vessels are inspected to assure they are not kinked or twisted. **CONTINUES**

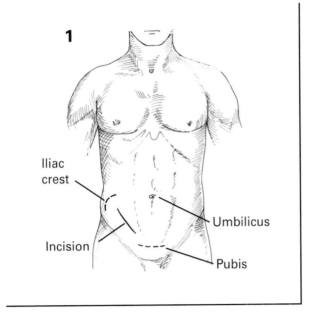

1

Iliac crest

Umbilicus

Incision

Pubis

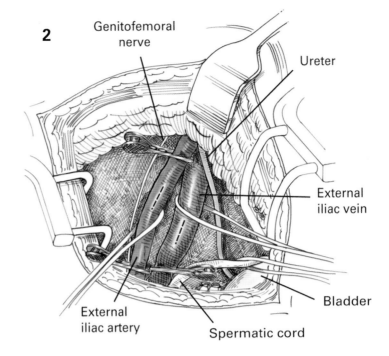

2

Genitofemoral nerve

Ureter

External iliac vein

External iliac artery

Bladder

Spermatic cord

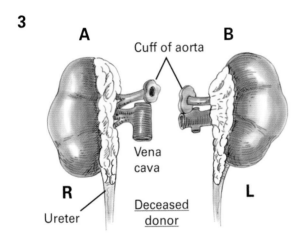

3

A **B**

Cuff of aorta

Vena cava

R

Ureter

Deceased donor

L

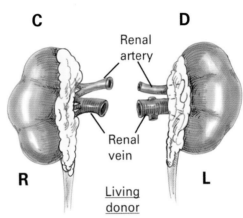

C **D**

Renal artery

Renal vein

R

Living donor

L

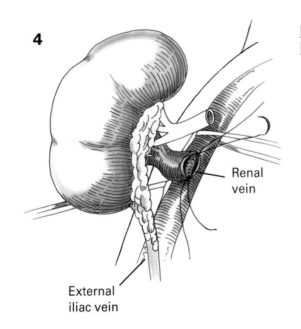

4

Renal vein

External iliac vein

Living donor left kidney

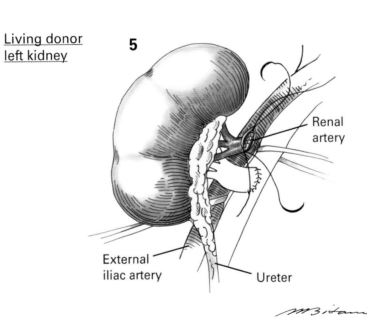

5

Renal artery

External iliac artery

Ureter

DETAILS OF PROCEDURE ◀ CONTINUED ▶ The Balfour self-retaining retractor is removed and an Adson–Beckman self-retaining retractor is placed at the medial-caudal end of the incision to expose the bladder. A 1.5- to 2.0- cm incision is made in the bladder using electrocautery, oriented parallel to the long axis of the ureter (FIGURE 6A). Three 4-0 absorbable retention sutures are placed full thickness into the bladder, clamped and placed on tension. The ureter is passed underneath the spermatic cord in male patients assuring it is not kinked or twisted. The ureter is spatulated an appropriate length and an 8-French red rubber catheter placed into it to divert urine away from the operative field and to stent the ureter during the creation of the anastomosis. A ureter that is too long will result in unwanted redundancy and too short will not allow the kidney to rest in the intended location within the iliac fossa. The ureter-to-bladder anastomosis is begun using a 5-0 double-armed absorbable monofilament suture placing one arm inside out in the end of the bladder incision closest to the kidney and the other arm inside out in the proximal corner of the spatulated ureter (FIGURE 6B). This suture is tied. Each arm of the suture is used to run the two sides of the anastomosis, proceeding from outside to inside on the bladder wall and inside to outside on the ureter. Prior to completing the anastomosis the red rubber catheter is removed and any extra length of ureter is removed with mucosal scissors. The anastomosis is completed and the two arms of the suture tied together (FIGURE 6C). An indwelling 6-French, 12-cm double-J stent (not shown) may be placed into the ureter based on surgeon preference. If used, this stent is placed in the ureter instead of the red rubber catheter and the bladder end of the catheter is "dunked" into the bladder prior to completing the anastomosis. Once the anastomosis is completed the retention sutures are removed. The bladder muscularis is imbricated over the anastomosis with two or three 4-0 absorbable sutures to create a tunnel for the ureter to prevent urine reflux into the ureter (FIGURE 6D). These sutures must be carefully placed to avoid constricting the ureter, causing obstruction.

The kidney, renal vessels, and iliac vessels proximal and distal to the vascular anastomoses are inspected to assure adequate blood flow and no thrombosis (FIGURE 7). The anesthesia team is queried to determine the quantity of urine output. If the kidney appears adequately perfused and the urine output is satisfactory the retractor and sponges, if present, are removed. The iliac fossa is irrigated with antibiotic-containing saline. The fascia and skin are reapproximated. An ipsilateral femoral pulse is palpated and confirmed.

POSTOPERATIVE CARE Hourly urine output should be measured for the first postoperative 24-hour period. Any sudden and unexpected decrease in output should be immediately investigated. An ipsilateral femoral pulse is confirmed. Loss of a femoral pulse indicates arterial thrombosis or dissection, requiring immediate reoperation. The bladder can be gently flushed through the Foley catheter to dislodge any obstructing clots that may be present. Recipient intravascular volume status is assessed and postoperative hemorrhage considered. A renal ultrasound can be performed to verify blood flow to the kidney. If concern persists, a timely return to the operating room is warranted for visual inspection of the transplanted kidney. Laboratory studies are obtained every 6 hours to monitor renal function and blood loss. Electrolyte values are obtained and abnormalities that may develop due to renal insufficiency or large volume diuresis are corrected. ■

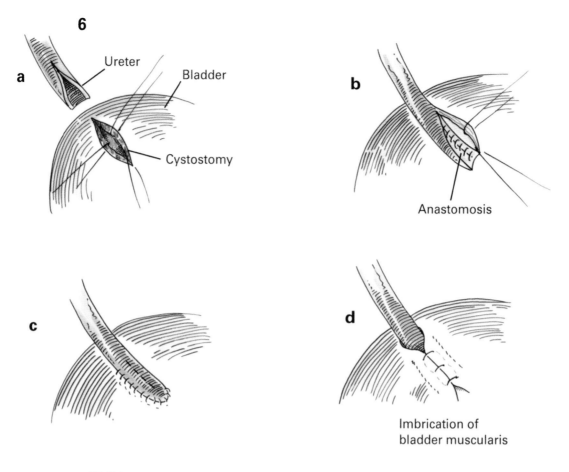

6

a Ureter Bladder

Cystostomy

b Anastomosis

c

d Imbrication of
bladder muscularis

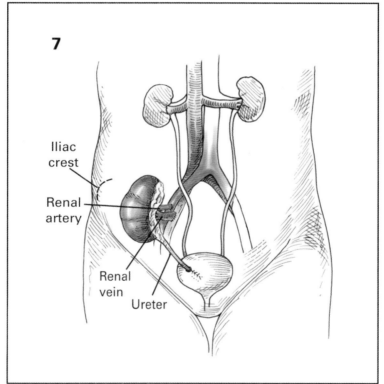

7

Iliac
crest

Renal
artery

Renal
vein

Ureter

SECTION IX
HERNIA

REPAIR OF VENTRAL HERNIA, LAPAROSCOPIC

INDICATIONS Ventral hernias in the anterior abdominal wall include both spontaneous or primary hernias (e.g., umbilical, epigastric, and spigelian) and, most commonly, incisional hernias after an abdominal operation. Small primary ventral hernias less than 2½ cm in diameter are often successfully closed with primary tissue repairs. However, larger ones have a recurrence rate of up to 30% or 40% when a tissue repair alone is performed. It is estimated that 2% to 10% of all abdominal operations result in an incisional hernia. This explains the predominance of such hernias. Fortunately, the use of mesh has revolutionized the repair of abdominal wall hernias. Anterior placement of polypropylene mesh as an onlay to the primary repair is helpful and a retrorectus muscle placement is even better. However, the development of dual-sided mesh has allowed for an improved placement of mesh behind the abdominal wall and hernial defect. These meshes present an intraperitoneal nonadherent surface to the bowel and an open synthetic mesh grid or screen for adherence and incorporation into the peritoneum and posterior abdominal wall fascia. The dual-sided meshes can be placed laparoscopically for almost any ventral hernia, but extremely large hernias with loss of abdominal domain or those associated with extensive, dense intra-abdominal adhesions (e.g., peritoneal dialysis, prior peritonitis) are relative contraindications. The meshes are very expensive; however, operating room time and hospital length of stay are shortened. The laparoscopic incisions cause less pain and there is a faster return to normal activities or work. Finally, laparoscopic repair enables the detection and repair of multiple defects—a common finding in midline incisional hernias.

PREOPERATIVE PREPARATION The patient must be free of infections, especially in the skin. Respiratory function should be optimized with cessation of smoking and appropriate pulmonary function evaluation. If bowel is contained with the hernia, endoscopic visualization, contrast studies, or imaging may be performed and the patient may be given a bowel preparation with a liquid diet and cathartics for 1 or 2 days prior to surgery. The major factors in the occurrence of this hernia, as well as the preceding operative note, should be reviewed.

ANESTHESIA General anesthesia with an endotracheal tube is required.

POSITION The patient is placed in a supine position with a pillow placed to produce mild flexion of the hips and knees. This helps to relax the abdominal wall. For ventral hernias that are not midline, the patient may be positioned with pillows for some lateral elevation of the chest, flank, and hips.

OPERATIVE PREPARATION The patient is given perioperative antibiotics. An orogastric tube is passed for gastric decompression. A Foley catheter is placed and pneumatic sequential stockings are applied. The skin is prepared in the routine manner.

INCISION AND EXPOSURE The 10-mm videoscope port (o) and the 5-mm operating ports (X) are a function of the position of the hernial defect and the preference of the surgeon (FIGURE 1A). The general principle is that of triangulation. The ports should be about a hand's breadth or more apart from each other and the two operating ports should be placed as widely apart as possible. Typical hernias and the placement of ports are shown (FIGURE 1B to E). One of the operating ports should be 10 mm in size if a 5-mm videoscope is not available.

The videoscope port is placed first, using the open Hasson technique (Chapter 11) or an optical trocar may be used after preinsufflation of the abdomen using a Veress needle when accessing the abdominal cavity laterally. After the abdomen is entered safely and the port secured with stay sutures, the intraperitoneal space is inflated with carbon dioxide. The surgeon sets the gas flow rate and the maximum pressure (≤15 mm Hg). The rising intra-abdominal pressure and total volume of gas infused is observed as the abdomen and hernia distend. The videoscope is white-balanced and focused. The optical end, usually a 30-degree angle, is coated with antifog solution and the scope is advanced down the port into the abdomen under direct vision. All four quadrants of the abdomen are explored visually. The hernia and its contents are evaluated and additional unrecognized incisional hernial defects may be found, especially in long midline incisions. Omental and other adhesions to the abdominal and anterior abdominal

wall about the hernial defect are visualized. A zone of about 4 to 6 cm must be made clear about the rim of the hernial defect for the wide attachment of the mesh beyond the borders of the actual defect.

Placement of the operating ports begins with the infiltration of the skin with a long-acting local anesthetic. The local needle may be passed perpendicularly full thickness through the abdominal wall and its entry site verified with the videoscope. The skin is incised and the subcutaneous tissues are dilated with a small hemostat. The abdominal wall is transilluminated with the videoscope to show any regional vessels within the abdominal musculature. The 5-mm operating ports are placed, with visualization of their clean entry into the intraperitoneal space.

DETAILS OF PROCEDURE In the typical ventral or incisional hernia, the omentum will have formed some adhesions to the sac of the hernia. The omentum is grasped near the abdominal wall with the forceps or the dissecting instrument and gentle traction is applied. Using laparoscopic scissors, the surgeon sharply incises the junction of the omentum with the peritoneum of the abdominal wall (FIGURE 2). After each cut, a sweeping motion in the same area will open up the next zone for cutting. Minimal bleeding occurs. Electrocautery or other heat-generating coagulating systems should be used sparingly and only with full visualization so as to minimize the chance of thermal injury to the bowel. Extensive dense adhesions, inability to reduce the hernial contents from the sac, or an enterotomy that is not easily repaired all require conversion to an open laparotomy and repair. After the abdominal wall adhesions are taken down, the omentum is removed from the hernial sac, which is left intact. A useful maneuver is the inversion of the hernial sac using several fingers externally (FIGURE 3). This allows the sharp cutting to continue with the best visualization of the junction of the omentum with the peritoneal sac. Again, gentle traction is applied to the omentum while the surgeon spreads, cuts, and sweeps. Throughout this dissection, the surgeon must be vigilant for the appearance of a loop of bowel hidden within these adhesions. Small and large bowel may also be cautiously cut away from the abdominal wall and hernia sac, but less sweeping and traction is applied lest an enterostomy occur. The appearance of bile or succus demands a search for the source, which may be repaired laparoscopically or after conversion to and open laparotomy. Some surgeons regard this complication as a contraindication to the placement of mesh, which is porous and may harbor a chronic infection, requiring eventual removal of the mesh.

After careful inspection of the omentum and other adhesions that have been removed from the abdominal wall, the surgeon makes a visual measurement about the perimeter of the defect to be certain there is an adequately clear zone for attachment of the mesh and its sutures. In general, 4 to 6 cm is sufficient. An important next step is to lower the intra-abdominal CO_2 gas pressure to about 6 or 8 mm Hg, which minimizes the stretching of the abdominal wall and hernia. If measurements of the defect are made with the abdomen fully inflated at 15 mm Hg, the mesh will be too large. It will become very wrinkled and loose when the CO_2 is removed at the end of the operation. The size of the defect is measured. Some surgeons use an internal measurement based upon a 2-cm spread, tip to tip, of the opened dissecting instrument. Most perform an external measurement and marking maneuver (FIGURE 4). A long needle is passed perpendicularly at the edge of the fascial defect in each of the four quadrants. The entrance site at the internal edge of the hernial defect is verified with the videoscope and the external sites are marked with indelible ink. The pattern of the defect is outlined so as to determine the size and shape of the mesh. A 3- to 4-cm margin is drawn out from this defect. This is marked and measured for choosing the mesh's size and shape (FIGURE 4). The dual-sided mesh is prepared with placement of four sutures, one in each quadrant (FIGURE 5). The sutures are nonabsorbable 00 in size and may be placed with parallel or perpendicular to the edge of the mesh. A useful maneuver is to use a pair of parallel sutures in one axis (12 and 6 o'clock) and perpendicular sutures in the other axis (3 and 9 o'clock). In this manner, the axis for internal attachment is identified when the mesh is not round in shape. Each suture is tied in its midpoint and the long tails are left intact. The mesh is rolled snugly with the nonadherent surface inside and synthetic mesh outside, so as not to create tension that may peel the two layers apart (FIGURE 6). **CONTINUES** ▶

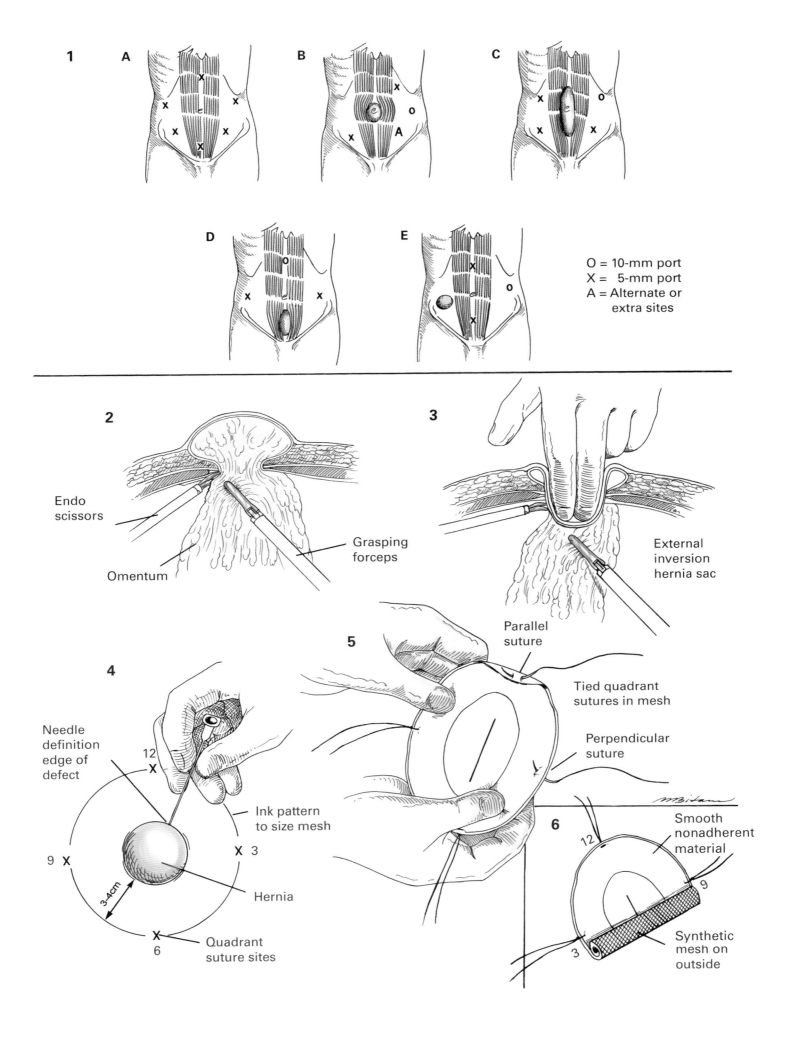

O = 10-mm port
X = 5-mm port
A = Alternate or
    extra sites

2
Endo
scissors

Omentum

Grasping
forceps

3
External
inversion
hernia sac

Parallel
suture

Tied quadrant
sutures in mesh

Perpendicular
suture

4
Needle
definition
edge of
defect

12
X

Ink pattern
to size mesh

9 X

X 3

3-4cm

Hernia

X
6

Quadrant
suture sites

5

6
12

9

3

Smooth
nonadherent
material

Synthetic
mesh on
outside

DETAILS OF PROCEDURE ◄CONTINUED► In the hernia illustrated, the 10-mm Hasson port for the videoscope was placed in the left lateral abdominal position. This large port site is needed for the difficult passage of the rolled up mesh through the abdominal wall. A useful technique is to pass a grasping forceps through an operating port and then out through the Hasson port (FIGURE 7). The port tube is removed and the rolled up mesh is grasped with the forceps (FIGURE 8) and drawn back into the abdomen. The mesh is unrolled and oriented with the smooth nonadherent surface down toward the bowel. Getting the mesh into the abdomen and unrolling it in the correct orientation can be quite tedious. The mesh is first secured with one of the preattached sutures at the four quadrants. Most surgeons begin with the 12 or 6 o'clock sutures. The four previously marked skin sites are incised with a No. 11 scalpel blade, which makes a 3-mm skin opening (FIGURE 9). A special suturing needle is passed perpendicularly through the abdominal wall. The needle tip is opened and one of the suture ends is grasped as it closes. The loose suture end is brought out through the abdominal wall and secured with a hemostat. A special suturing needle is passed again through the abdominal incision, but this time it is aimed to enter the abdominal space about 1 cm away from the first site. The other half of the tied suture is grasped and brought out. The suture is tied down through the skin incision, setting the knot deeply. This secures the mesh to the abdominal wall fascia (FIGURE 10). This transabdominal suturing continues with placement of the two lateral sutures and then, last, the opposite (6 o'clock) suture. A minimum of four transfascial sutures should be placed to secure the mesh to the anterior abdominal wall. Larger pieces of mesh may require eight transfascial sutures to appropriately fix the mesh to the anterior abdominal wall. In general, the mesh should be slightly loose but not wrinkled rather than precisely tight. The exposed perimeter of the mesh is now secured with an endoscopic stapling device. Spiral screws or tacks are preferred.

These are placed 1 cm apart. It is important that the perimeter be securely attached with closely spaced tacks such that no bowel or omentum can get under the edge of the mesh. Placement of the tacks is facilitated by having the surgeon apply external counterpressure with the hand while the tacking instrument spreads out the mesh in a radial manner (FIGURE 11). These two actions provide a little lip to the edge of the mesh, thus allowing a more precise placement of each tack. Upon completion of the procedure, the abdomen is lavaged with the suction irrigator. Careful inspection is made for any bleeding sites and bile or succus. Each of the operating ports is removed under direct vision to be certain that there are no bleeding sites in the abdominal wall. As intra-abdominal gas is vented, the final view of the loosely applied mesh is seen (FIGURE 12). The fascia of any 10-mm port site is closed with 00 delayed absorbable sutures. The skin is approximated with fine subcuticular sutures. Adhesive skin strips and dry sterile dressings are applied.

POSTOPERATIVE CARE The orogastric tube is removed before the patient awakens and the Foley catheter is discontinued when the patient is alert enough to void. He or she may experience a moderate amount of pain for a day or so. Clear liquids are resumed within 1 day and the diet is advanced as tolerated. Some surgeons recommend the use of an abdominal binder for 1 month after surgery. Hematomas and surgical-site infections can occur. The latter may require eventual removal of the mesh if the infection becomes chronic. Accumulation of serum in the old hernial sac occurs frequently and may require aspiration. Finally, some patients may experience chronic pain at the sites of transfascial suture fixation. ■

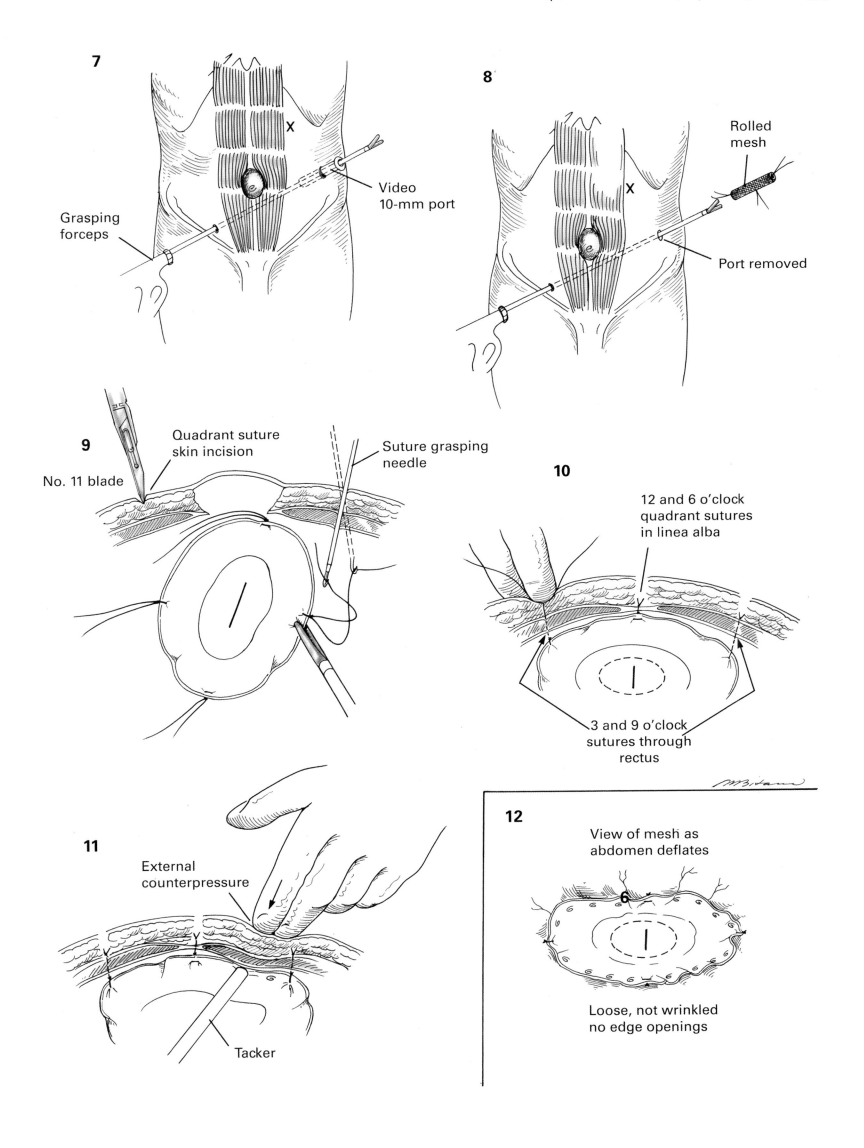

7

Grasping forceps

Video 10-mm port

8

Rolled mesh

Port removed

9

No. 11 blade

Quadrant suture skin incision

Suture grasping needle

10

12 and 6 o'clock quadrant sutures in linea alba

3 and 9 o'clock sutures through rectus

11

External counterpressure

Tacker

12

View of mesh as abdomen deflates

Loose, not wrinkled no edge openings

REPAIR OF VENTRAL HERNIA, OPEN COMPONENT PARTS SEPARATION

INDICATIONS Ventral hernias in the anterior abdominal wall include both spontaneous or primary hernias (e.g., umbilical, epigastric, and spigelian) and, most commonly, incisional hernias that occur after an abdominal operation. It is estimated that 2% to 13% of all abdominal operations result in an incisional hernia. Risk factors for the development of an incisional hernia include obesity, multiple abdominal procedures, diabetes, wound infections, and the use of immunosuppressive medication(s). Small primary ventral hernias are often successfully closed with primary tissue repairs. Repair of incisional hernias often utilizes synthetic or biologic mesh to decrease recurrence rates. In some patients, the use of mesh is contraindicated or not desired and the hernia defect is too large or extensive to allow for appropriate primary closure. In the event of real or potential contamination, the use of synthetic mesh may be contraindicated. In addition, patients may request or require a more cosmetic repair of their abdominal wall as part of their treatment with "medialization" of their abdominal wall musculature that was previously displaced due to the ventral/incisional hernia. In patients whom synthetic mesh cannot be utilized, native abdominal wall fascia and musculature must be used to close the hernia defect and reapproximate the abdominal wall components while minimizing the potential for hernia recurrence. Open component separation is used almost exclusively for midline ventral hernia defects, whether they are single or multiple, when the use of synthetic or biologic mesh is not an option for repair. Component separation enables the detection and repair of multiple defects—a common finding in midline incisional hernias.

PREOPERATIVE PREPARATION The patient must be free of active infections, especially in the skin. Respiratory function should be optimized with cessation of smoking and appropriate pulmonary function evaluation. If bowel is contained with the hernia, endoscopic visualization, contrast studies, or imaging may be performed preoperatively and the patient may be given a bowel preparation with a liquid diet and cathartics for 1 or 2 days prior to surgery. The major factors in the occurrence of this hernia, as well as the preceding operative note(s), should be reviewed.

ANESTHESIA General anesthesia with an endotracheal tube is required.

POSITION The patient is placed in a supine position with a pillow placed to produce mild flexion of the hips and knees. This helps to relax the abdominal wall and take some tension off of any repair performed.

OPERATIVE PREPARATION The patient is given perioperative antibiotics. An orogastric tube is passed for gastric decompression. If significant dissection is anticipated, a nasogastric tube may be placed for postoperative decompression of the stomach in the event of an ileus. A Foley catheter may be placed and pneumatic sequential stockings are applied. The skin is prepared in the routine manner with attention to prepping the patient's abdominal wall laterally as this may be accessed as part of the operative procedure.

INCISION AND EXPOSURE A component separation technique is most effectively utilized for midline abdominal hernias when synthetic or biologic mesh is unavailable or contraindicated and a midline primary closure is desired but unattainable due to the "space" created in the midline by the fascial defect. This technique may also be used in conjunction with a retromuscular piece of synthetic or biologic mesh to "bolster" the repair. For this reason, typically a midline abdominal incision is made overlying the hernia (FIGURE 1). The incision may extend from the xiphoid to the pubis or be shorter and tailored to the size of the defect undergoing repair. Adequate length of the incision is necessary to insure appropriate exposure of the abdominal wall musculature above and below the hernia. The incision is carried down through the subcutaneous tissue onto the hernia sac in the midline and the unadulterated fascia. Exposure is facilitated by elevation of subcutaneous flaps laterally overlying the abdominal wall musculature. These flaps extend to the anterior axillary line just lateral to the insertion of the external oblique fascia onto the more medial rectus sheath (FIGURE 2).

DETAILS OF PROCEDURE Once the incision and subcutaneous flaps are complete exposing the insertion of the external oblique on the rectus sheath, the external oblique fascia is incised on its anterior border just laterally to its insertion on the rectus sheath (FIGURE 3). The length of the incision may be tailored to the hernia defect but can extend the entire length of the abdominal wall. Once the external oblique is incised a plane is created laterally between the external oblique aponeurosis and internal oblique aponeurosis effectively lifting the external oblique musculature off of the internal oblique aponeurosis and allowing for advancement or "medialization" of the rectus sheath into the midline for primary closure. Release of the external oblique fully along its course from xiphoid to pubis may allow for primary closure of small to moderate sized defects. Tension on closure should be evaluated by the surgeon after mobilization of both sides. If tension is considered to be too high, consideration of further mobilization is undertaken. Incision of the posterior rectus sheath along its course (FIGURE 4) and dissection of the posterior rectus sheath off of the posterior elements of the rectus abdominis muscle further mobilize the abdominal wall musculature to allow for midline closure. Full mobilization of the external oblique aponeurosis and the posterior rectus sheath can be expected to allow for 3 to 5 cm advancement in the upper and lower abdomen and 8 to 10 cm of advancement at the waist (FIGURE 5). This technique insures at least two layers of abdominal wall envelope the intra-abdominal organs except in the midline which is closed in a single layer. Primary closure of the midline wound is often performed with interrupted nonabsorbable sutures (FIGURE 6). **CONTINUES**

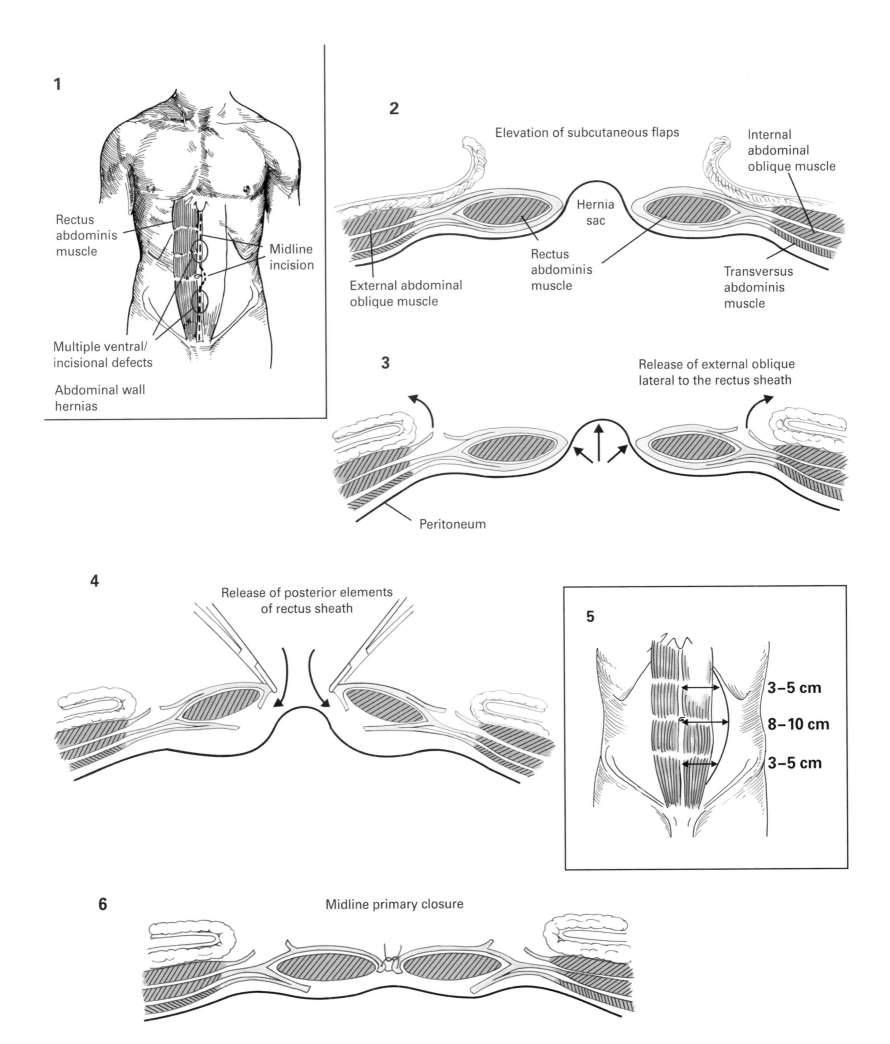

1

Rectus abdominis muscle

Midline incision

Multiple ventral/ incisional defects

Abdominal wall hernias

2   Elevation of subcutaneous flaps

Internal abdominal oblique muscle

Hernia sac

Rectus abdominis muscle

Transversus abdominis muscle

External abdominal oblique muscle

3   Release of external oblique lateral to the rectus sheath

Peritoneum

4   Release of posterior elements of rectus sheath

5

3–5 cm

8–10 cm

3–5 cm

6   Midline primary closure

DETAILS OF PROCEDURE CONTINUED **‹CONTINUED›** In an effort to prevent midline recurrences, many surgeons place an underlay of synthetic or biologic mesh to prevent a recurrence in the suture line (FIGURE 7). The mesh should overlap the fascial edges by 4 to 5 cm. Heavy number 0 or 1 nonabsorbable sutures are placed laterally about 2 to 4 cm from the fascial edge with the knots on top (FIGURE 7). If the posterior rectus sheath is missing (as in inferior to the level of the semilunaris line in the suprapubic region) then the sutures are passed through the confluence of the fascia of the oblique muscles. If the mesh will be in contact with the intra-abdominal organs, a mesh coated with an antiadhesive surface should be employed to prevent adhesions from forming between the mesh and intra-abdominal organs/bowel. With the fascia closed, attempts should be made to reapproximate the subcutaneous tissue elevated off of the abdominal wall musculature in an attempt to eliminate the "dead-space." The use of 2-0 absorbable interrupted suture is desired. Often, the subcutaneous flaps create an opportunity for blood and/or fluid to accumulate and placement of two closed suction drains within the flaps collect fluid/blood and prevent a postoperative seroma or hematoma from developing (FIGURE 8). These drains are not in contact with and must be excluded from mesh that may be placed retromuscularly so as to pose no additional risk to "seeding" or infecting mesh. The skin may be close with staples or an absorbable running suture. A sterile dressing is applied. Overtop the dressing, many surgeons will wrap the abdominal wall in a binder in an effort to provide additional support to the abdominal wall in the postoperative period.

If the surgeon does not believe mesh should be used because of patient factors, then it may be possible to achieve closure with the extended separation shown in FIGURE 9. The anterior rectus sheath from points A to C is freed (FIGURE 9A) and the insertion of the internal oblique and transversus fascia along with remaining posterior rectus sheath (FIGURE 9B) is secured anteriorly to the lateral edge of the anterior rectus sheath at point C (FIGURE 9C). The external oblique muscle with fascial cuts (**point C**) is allowed to retract laterally and thus provide the needed slack for the points B to C closure in front of the rectus muscle.

POSTOPERATIVE CARE The orogastric tube is removed before the patient awakens if it is anticipated that the patient will not have a significant ileus. If an ileus is anticipated due to bowel manipulation or extensive dissection, a nasogastric tube should remain until return of bowel function. The Foley catheter is discontinued when the patient is alert enough to void. He or she may experience a moderate amount of pain for a few days. Clear liquids are resumed within 1 day and the diet is advanced as tolerated. Some surgeons recommend the use of an abdominal binder for up to 6 weeks after surgery. Hematomas and surgical-site infections can occur. Accumulation of serum in the old hernia sac may occur and require aspiration. If a subcutaneous drain was placed in the subcutaneous flaps, it is removed once the drainage is serous and minimal to prevent accumulation of fluid in this space. The patient is asked to refrain from strenuous physical activity and lifting heavy weight for 6 weeks postoperatively in an attempt to allow fascial healing until the wound strength is such that strenuous activity will not compromise the repair. An abdominal binder is continued at home for several weeks and the patient is asked to wear the binder as much as possible. Removal of the binder during sleep is necessary in some patients. ∎

7

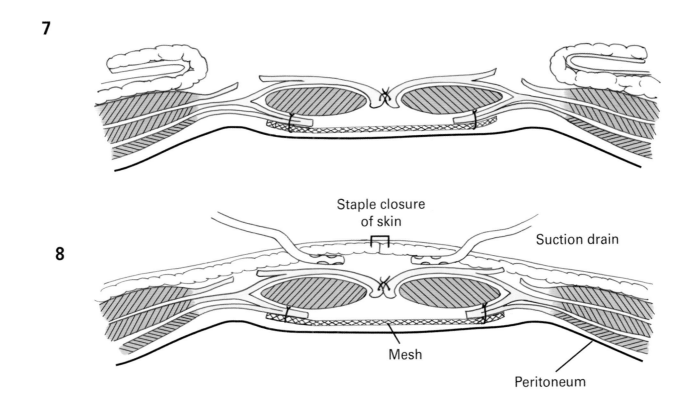

8

Staple closure
of skin

Suction drain

Mesh

Peritoneum

9A

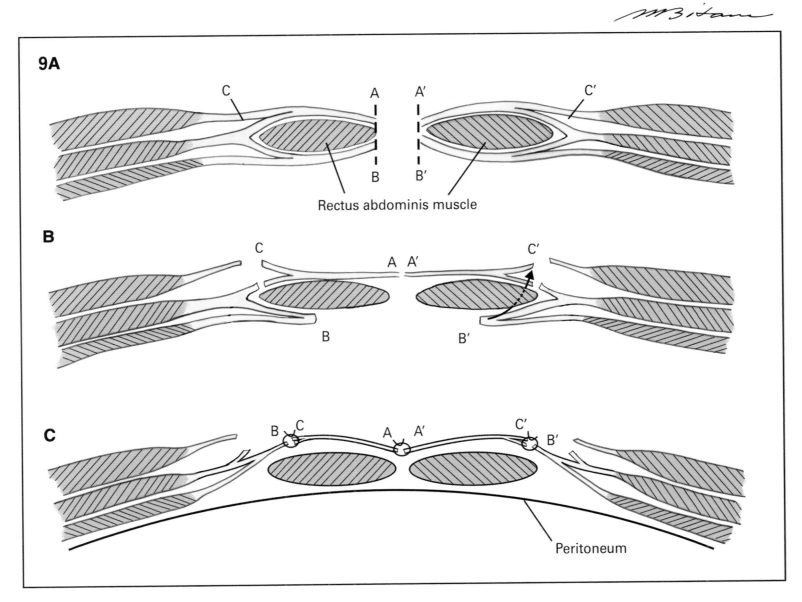

C   A   A'   C'

B   B'

Rectus abdominis muscle

B

C   A   A'   C'

B   B'

C

B C   A A'   C' B'

Peritoneum

REPAIR OF UMBILICAL HERNIA

INDICATIONS An umbilical hernia is usually a congenital defect, although a variation may follow surgery such as the placement of an incision or laparoscopic port in this region. The increased susceptibility to strangulation of an umbilical hernia in an adult necessitates repair as the patient's condition permits.

Repair of an umbilical hernia in the very young child is rarely indicated, since 80% of these fascial defects will close by the age of 2 years. In addition, the incidence of incarceration and strangulation within an umbilical hernia in this age group is extremely low. However, if supportive measures such as the "keystone" type of strapping during infancy have failed and the fascial ring is sufficiently large to admit the index finger, the hernia should be repaired before school age.

PREOPERATIVE PREPARATION This defect is usually seen in either children or obese adults, and the preoperative preparation depends entirely upon the patient's general condition and age. Obese patients are placed on a diet. A general medical assessment is indicated. The patient may be placed on a low-residue diet for a day or two and the bowels emptied with a mild cathartic. Repair is delayed in the presence of acute respiratory infection, chronic cough, or infection about the navel. Special attention is given to cleaning of the navel.

ANESTHESIA Spinal anesthesia may be preferred in large hernias because of the excellent relaxation it provides; however, inhalation anesthesia can be used if not contraindicated. Inhalation anesthesia is the method of choice for children.

POSITION The patient is placed in a comfortable supine position.

OPERATIVE PREPARATION The skin is prepared in the usual manner after the umbilicus has been carefully cleaned. This may require cotton applicators saturated with antiseptic to reach any deep crevices.

INCISION AND EXPOSURE A curved incision placed superiorly or inferiorly about the umbilicus is most commonly used (FIGURE 1). A vertical incision that curves around the umbilicus may be necessary for very large hernias. The umbilicus proper should be retained in the skin flap. The incision is made to the hernia sac. The sac is easily mobilized except for its attachment to the back of the umbilical skin. This is dissected carefully so as not to create a buttonhole that may put the repair at risk for infection. The neck of the herniated sac is then dissected from adjacent tissues by a combination of blunt and sharp dissection, which is carried down to the level of the linea alba and anterior sheaths of the rectus muscle.

ADULTS

DETAILS OF PROCEDURE Most commonly, omentum is contained within the sac, but small and large bowel may also be present. Frequently the omentum will have formed adhesions to various areas of the sac, thus preventing reduction of the hernia. Sharp dissection is required to detach hernial contents from the sac as well as from the peritoneum around the neck of the sac as it joins the peritoneum. When there is a strong suspicion of gangrenous intestine within the sac, the abdominal cavity should be entered through an extended midline incision that enters either above or below the umbilicus. This incision is extended to the fascial defect and up the side of the sac so as to allow complete mobilization of the incarcerated bowel. The intestine is either reduced or resected as indicated. In the majority of cases, omentum is incarcerated within the sac.

In these patients, the sac may be opened (FIGURE 2). If the omentum cannot easily be freed and/or reduced, it is wise to resect it with sequential clamping and suture ligature placement. When the contents of the sac have been reduced and its neck has been well defined, a decision is made as to how to repair the fascial defect.

In general, when the defect is less than 2 cm in diameter, the peritoneum is closed and the excess sac excised. The perimeter of the fascial defect is cleaned of fat both anteriorly and posteriorly, and a primary repair is performed using interrupted oo sutures that may be of a delayed absorbable or nonabsorbable nature (FIGURE 3). This primary repair is performed only for small defects of 2.5 cm or less.

If an intermediate-sized defect in the range of 2 to 4 cm is found, many surgeons prefer to repair it with the two-layer "vest-over-trousers" (Mayo)

technique (FIGURES 4 to 6). The upper fascia is imbricated over the lower fascia with a row of interrupted oo sutures. These begin and end high on the vest, while the trousers are secured in a horizontal manner at the belt line (FIGURE 4). When these sutures are secured, the free superior edge (vest) overhangs the inferior fascia (trousers) and a second layer of interrupted oo sutures is used to secure the free edge (FIGURE 5 and 5A). The technique is illustrated schematically in the cross-sectional view illustrated in FIGURE 6.

Many surgeons believe that a medium to large defect should be repaired with mesh, as primary tissue repairs in large hernias have a significant recurrence rate. The preferred site for placement of the mesh is posterior to the defect and posterior rectus sheath. If the zone between the peritoneum and posterior rectus sheath can be freely dissected, some surgeons use a synthetic mesh after first being certain that the omentum is directly behind this region when the umbilical hernia sac is closed. Alternatively, if this plane cannot be developed and the mesh must be placed in an intraperitoneal position, a dual-sided mesh is used wherein the smooth, nonadherent surface is posterior toward the omentum and bowel, while the unprotected screen-like synthetic mesh is anterior against the peritoneum and posterior fascia (FIGURE 6). The mesh should be sized to extend 3 to 5 cm beyond the anticipated edges of the closed defect. This mesh is secured with nonabsorbable oo mattress sutures that are placed full thickness through the linea alba at the 12 and 6 o'clock positions and through the rectus sheaths and muscle at the 3 and 9 o'clock positions (FIGURE 6A). These sutures should secure only the unprotected side of the synthetic mesh and should not go full thickness as this may create a free intra-abdominal loop that may catch a loop of bowel. The anchoring sutures are tied and the defect is closed either vertically or transversely using interrupted oo sutures.

CLOSURE After careful hemostasis is obtained, the apex of the subcutaneous tissue beneath the umbilicus is sutured down to the linea alba with oo absorbable sutures. This produces the desirable ingoing bellybutton. Further absorbable sutures are used to obliterate the subcutaneous dead space. A triple-bite suture that secures Scarpa's fascia to the deep fascia and then the Scarpa's fascia on the other side of the incision minimizes the space for a potential accumulation of serum or a hematoma. When the hernia is quite large, a closed-system Silastic suction catheter may be placed through an adjacent stab wound such that it does not communicate or come in contact with the mesh placed as part of the hernia repair.

POSTOPERATIVE CARE Special attention is given to the avoidance of abdominal distention. An adhesive tape strip 3-in wide is liberally applied across the abdomen, and the patient may use an abdominal binder for approximately 1 month. The patient is warned to avoid overly heavy lifting and straining for a minimum of 6 weeks.

CHILDREN

DETAILS OF PROCEDURE A curved incision around the superior half of the umbilical depression is made and the hernia sac is freed down to the linea alba. This dissection extends laterally onto either rectus sheath. The hernia sac is dissected free from the back of the umbilical skin, using countertraction with skin hooks. The fascia is cleaned for a few centimeters in all directions. In most patients, the sac can be reduced without being opened. The edges of the fascial ring are grasped with Kocher clamps and the posterior aspect of the fascia is cleaned for 1 or 2 cm. As most of these fascial defects are small, a primary repair using oo interrupted sutures can be performed in either a vertical or horizontal manner, depending upon the shape of the defect.

CLOSURE The skin margins are approximated with interrupted subcuticular ooooo absorbable suture. Skin strips are applied and the umbilicus is packed with a small wad of gauze. A dry sterile dressing is applied.

POSTOPERATIVE CARE The routine postoperative care is performed. Most patients are able to tolerate fluid within a few hours and are discharged home within a day on a soft diet. The skin of the umbilicus should be observed for viability if an extensive dissection has been performed. In most patients, the curved periumbilical incision becomes minimally visible as the area heals. ■

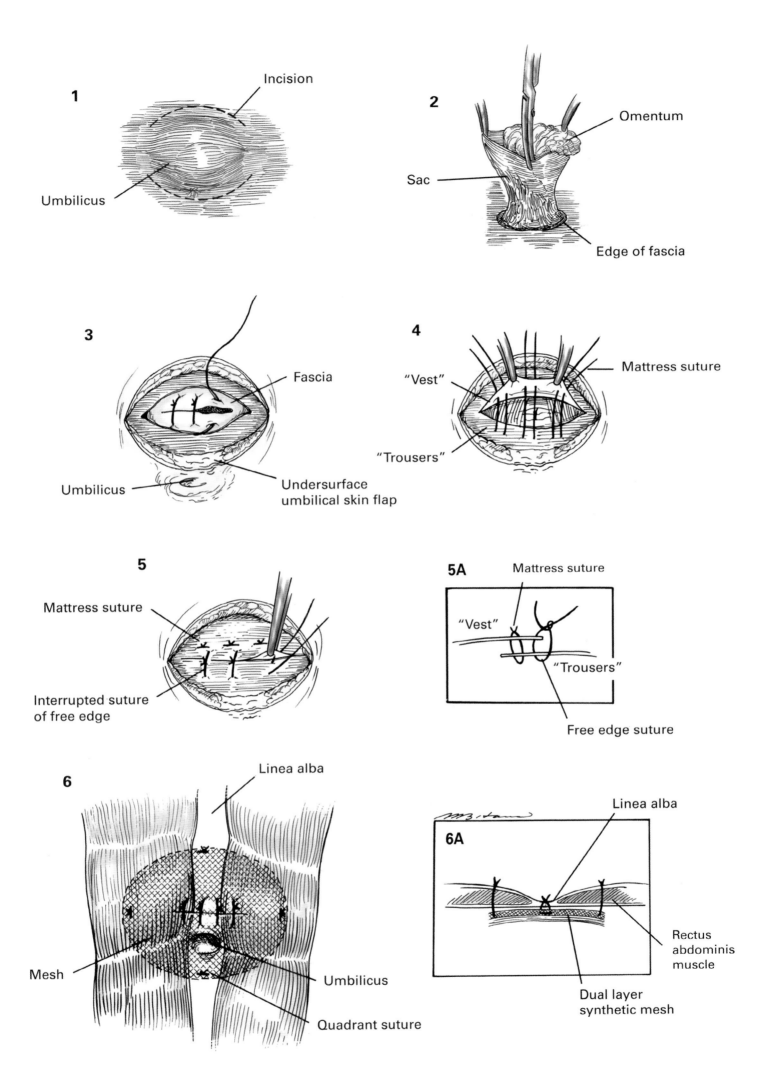

1   Incision
Umbilicus

2   Omentum
Sac
Edge of fascia

3   Fascia
Umbilicus
Undersurface umbilical skin flap

4   "Vest"
"Trousers"
Mattress suture

5   Mattress suture
Interrupted suture of free edge

5A   Mattress suture
"Vest"
"Trousers"
Free edge suture

6   Linea alba
Mesh
Umbilicus
Quadrant suture

6A   Linea alba
Rectus abdominis muscle
Dual layer synthetic mesh

REPAIR OF INDIRECT INGUINAL HERNIA

INDICATIONS Any indirect inguinal hernia should be repaired electively unless contraindicated by the large size of the hernia or by the age or poor physical condition of the patient. The appearance of indirect inguinal hernia in middle-aged or elderly patients requires thorough medical investigation. Before repair is advised, it is wise to rule out any other source of pathology as a cause for the patient's complaint rather than ascribe it to the presence of an indirect inguinal hernia. Patients who have straining from symptomatic gastrointestinal tract obstruction, chronic pulmonary disease, or prostatism need appropriate diagnostic studies.

Repair of an inguinal hernia in an infant or child is indicated as soon as practical after the diagnosis is made. In the presence of an undescended testicle, the repair, which includes an orchiopexy, should be delayed until 3 to 5 years of age to permit maximum spontaneous descent. The orchiopexy is indicated at any age if there is strong indication for repairing the hernia due to incarceration.

PREOPERATIVE PREPARATION Obese persons should be refused repair until their weight has been substantially reduced to a point within the range of their calculated ideal weight in order to ensure a low recurrence rate. Repair should also be delayed in patients with acute upper respiratory infections or a chronic cough until these conditions have been remedied. Smoking is curtailed or stopped and frequent intermittent positive pressure breathing, with appropriate drugs added, should be instituted several days before surgery.

In the presence of strangulation, the operation is delayed only long enough for fluid and electrolyte balance to be established by the intravenous administration of Ringer's lactate solution. Systemic antibiotic therapy is instituted. Colloid solutions or blood products may be needed, especially if gangrenous bowel is suspected. A small nasogastric tube is passed, and constant gastric suction is maintained before, during, and for several days after operation. Sufficient time must be taken to ensure a satisfactory urine output of at least 30 to 50 mL per hour, a pulse under 100 per minute, and an appropriate blood pressure with a normal central venous pressure. Repeated electrolyte values should be approaching normal. Adequate resuscitation may require from several hours to a much longer period for the administration of several liters of fluids and electrolytes, especially potassium and blood, in the patient who has had intestinal obstruction for several days. Operative intervention before stabilization may have disastrous results.

A child 2 years or older should be prepared psychologically in advance for the hospital experience. Booklets that describe in simple narrative style the various details of hospitalization and operation can be read to the child before operation. Such preparation undoubtedly serves to diminish the incidence of emotional trauma as a complication of elective surgery.

Uncomplicated inguinal hernias in patients of any age may be repaired as ambulatory surgical procedures using local, regional, or general anesthesia.

ANESTHESIA Intravenous sedation plus local infiltration should be considered in low risk patients who are suitable for repair in an ambulatory surgical setting. Local anesthesia allows approximation of the tissues at a more normal tension and also makes it possible for the patient to increase the intra-abdominal pressure by coughing, which will aid in identifying the sac and in testing the adequacy of the repair. Note the position of the nerves for local anesthesia (FIGURE 1). If obstruction is present, general anesthesia with an endotracheal tube and cuff is recommended to avoid the ever-present threat of tracheal aspiration.

Inhalation anesthesia is the method of choice in children and anxious adults.

POSITION The patient is placed in a supine position with a pillow beneath the knees so that slight relaxation at the groin is achieved. The table is tilted with the head down slightly to aid in reducing the contents of the hernia sac and in retracting a thick abdominal wall by gravity.

OPERATIVE PREPARATION The skin preparation is routine after clipping of the hair.

TRADITIONAL EXPOSURE

INCISION AND EXPOSURE A skin incision, extending from just below and medial to the anterosuperior iliac spine to the pubic spine, is made 2 to 3 cm above and parallel to Poupart's ligament (FIGURE 1A). A more comfortable and cosmetic incision results if the major crease in the lines of skin cleavage is followed (FIGURE 1B). This may be defined by gentle downward traction on the abdominal wall, which demarcates the natural crease in the skin beneath the plastic drape. Either incision is carried down to the external oblique fascia. Several blood vessels, especially the superficial epigastric vein and the external pudendal vein, are usually encountered in the subcutaneous tissue in the lower portion of the incision. These must be clamped and tied (FIGURE 2).

DETAILS OF PROCEDURE The external oblique is carefully cleaned of all fat by sharp dissection throughout the length of the wound, and the external ring is visualized (FIGURE 2). After the margins of the wound have been covered with gauze moistened in isotonic saline, a small incision is made in the direction of the fibers of the external oblique, which extend into the medial side of the external inguinal ring (FIGURE 2). The edges of the external oblique are held away from the internal oblique muscle to avoid injury to the underlying nerves as the incision is continued through the medial side of the external ring (FIGURE 3). The nerves are most commonly injured at the external ring. The lower side of the external oblique is freed by blunt dissection down to include Poupart's ligament. The upper margin is similarly freed for some distance. As the ilioinguinal nerve is dissected free from the adjacent structures, a bleeding point is commonly encountered as it passes over the internal oblique (FIGURE 4). This bleeding vessel, if encountered, must be tied carefully; otherwise a hematoma may develop in the wound. When the ilioinguinal nerve has been carefully dissected free, it is pulled to one side over a hemostat placed at the edge of the incision (FIGURE 5). The cremasteric fibers are grasped with toothed forceps and divided in order to approach the sac (FIGURE 6). The sac itself is seen as a definite white membrane that lies in front and toward the inner side of the cord; it is usually easily differentiated from surrounding tissues. If the hernia is small, the sac lies high in the canal. The vas deferens can be recognized by palpation because it is firmer than the other structures of the cord. The wall of the sac is lifted up gently and opened with care to avoid possible injury to its contents (FIGURE 7). While the margins of the opened sac are grasped with hemostats, the contents are replaced within the peritoneal cavity. With the index finger of the left hand introduced into the sac to give counter-resistance, the surgeon frees the sac with the right hand by either blunt or sharp dissection (FIGURE 8). If the dissection is kept close to the sac, an avascular cleavage plane will be found. Sharp dissection is advisable to separate the vas deferens and adjacent vessels from the sac (FIGURE 9). If this is done carefully, fewer bleeding points will be encountered than if an effort is made to sweep these structures away from the sac by means of blunt dissection with gauze. The dissection is then continued until the properitoneal fat is displaced and the peritoneum beyond the narrow neck of the sac is visualized. **CONTINUES ▶**

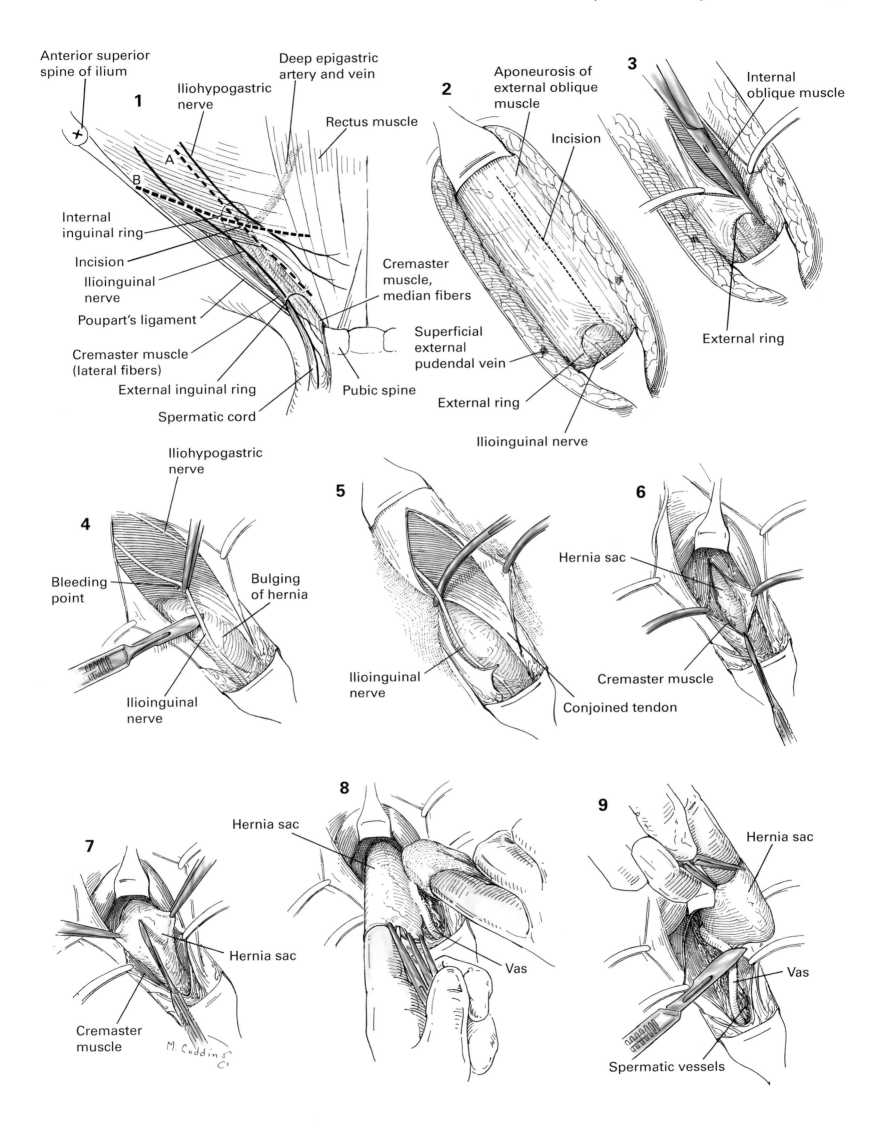

1

Anterior superior spine of ilium

Iliohypogastric nerve

Deep epigastric artery and vein

Rectus muscle

A

B

Internal inguinal ring

Incision

Ilioinguinal nerve

Poupart's ligament

Cremaster muscle (lateral fibers)

External inguinal ring

Spermatic cord

Cremaster muscle, median fibers

Superficial external pudendal vein

Pubic spine

2

Aponeurosis of external oblique muscle

Incision

External ring

Ilioinguinal nerve

3

Internal oblique muscle

External ring

4

Iliohypogastric nerve

Bleeding point

Bulging of hernia

Ilioinguinal nerve

5

Ilioinguinal nerve

Conjoined tendon

6

Hernia sac

Cremaster muscle

7

Hernia sac

Hernia sac

Cremaster muscle

M. Codding C¹

8

Hernia sac

Vas

9

Hernia sac

Vas

Spermatic vessels

DETAILS OF PROCEDURE ◄ **CONTINUED** The sac is opened within 2 to 3 cm of its neck, and exploration is carried out with the index finger to rule out the presence of a "pantaloon" or secondary direct or femoral hernia (FIGURE 10). To ensure obliteration of the sac, a purse-string suture is placed at the inner side of the neck (FIGURE 11), or several transfixing sutures may be used if preferred. The lumen of the neck of the sac must be visualized as sutures are placed or tied to avoid possible injury to omentum or intestine. This suture should include the transversalis fascia with the peritoneum. The neck of the sac can sometimes be identified as a slightly thickened white ring. The sac should be ligated proximal to this ring. After the purse-string suture is tied, the excess sac is amputated with scissors (FIGURE 12).

If desired, the ligated sac may be anchored to the overlying muscle. In this instance the long ends of the suture used to close the neck of the sac are rethreaded. The needle is inserted beneath the transversalis fascia and brought up in the edge of the internal oblique muscle, the two ends being brought through separately and tied (FIGURE 13). Care should be taken to avoid injuring the inferior deep epigastric vessels.

ALTERNATE TECHNIQUES FOR SAC Although the classic inguinal hernia operations utilize high ligation with division of the hernia sac, two alternate methods have gained popularity with mesh repair. In small to medium-sized indirect hernias, the sac is left intact as it is dissected from the posterior cord structures. Electrocautery is used along the edge of the sac while gentle traction is applied. This minimizes bleedsing and ecchymosis after surgery. Any entry into the sac is used for finger exploration and guidance of further dissection well up into the internal ring. Any opening in the sac is closed using oo absorbable suture, and the entire sac, along with any lipoma of the cord, is returned to the preperitoneal space behind the abdominal muscular wall.

In very large inguinoscrotal hernias, the indirect sac is transected and suture ligated near the internal ring. Only the proximal sac is dissected free into the internal ring. The distal very large sac is left untouched, as the extensive dissection from the cord vessels and the mobilization of the testicle up and out of the scrotum may result in venous thrombosis or possible ischemic orchiditis. A residual hydrocele rarely occurs.

CLOSURE There are various methods of repair after the sac has been removed. Large or recurrent hernias in older persons or hernias in patients doing very heavy work may be corrected by a method that either partially or completely transplants the cord or narrows the internal ring.

NONTRANSPLANTATION OF CORD (FERGUSON REPAIR) The cremasteric fibers, which may or may not be well developed, are approximated with interrupted oo silk sutures (FIGURE 14). This covers the raw surface remaining after removal of the sac and restores the structures to a normal appearance. The cremaster muscle is pulled beneath the conjoined tendon to relieve strain on the next layer of sutures and to increase the efficiency of the repair (FIGURE 15). Sutures are then placed to approximate the conjoined tendon and internal oblique muscle to Poupart's ligament, the sutures being tied anterior to the cord (FIGURE 16). The sutures in Poupart's ligament are placed from below upward, unequal portions of the ligament being taken to avoid fraying. The first suture should be tied loosely enough so that the cord is not constricted and there is sufficient space about the cord to permit an instrument tip to pass; moreover, care should be taken to avoid injury or inclusion of the ilioinguinal nerve by the sutures. The external oblique fascia is approximated with interrupted sutures (FIGURE 17). Here again, the external ring should not constrict the cord (FIGURE 18). The subcutaneous tissue is carefully approximated with interrupted oooo absorbable sutures to (FIGURE 19). Alternatively a continuous subcutaneous closure with absorbable suture may be used, followed by adhesive skin strips and a dry sterile dressing. **CONTINUES** ►

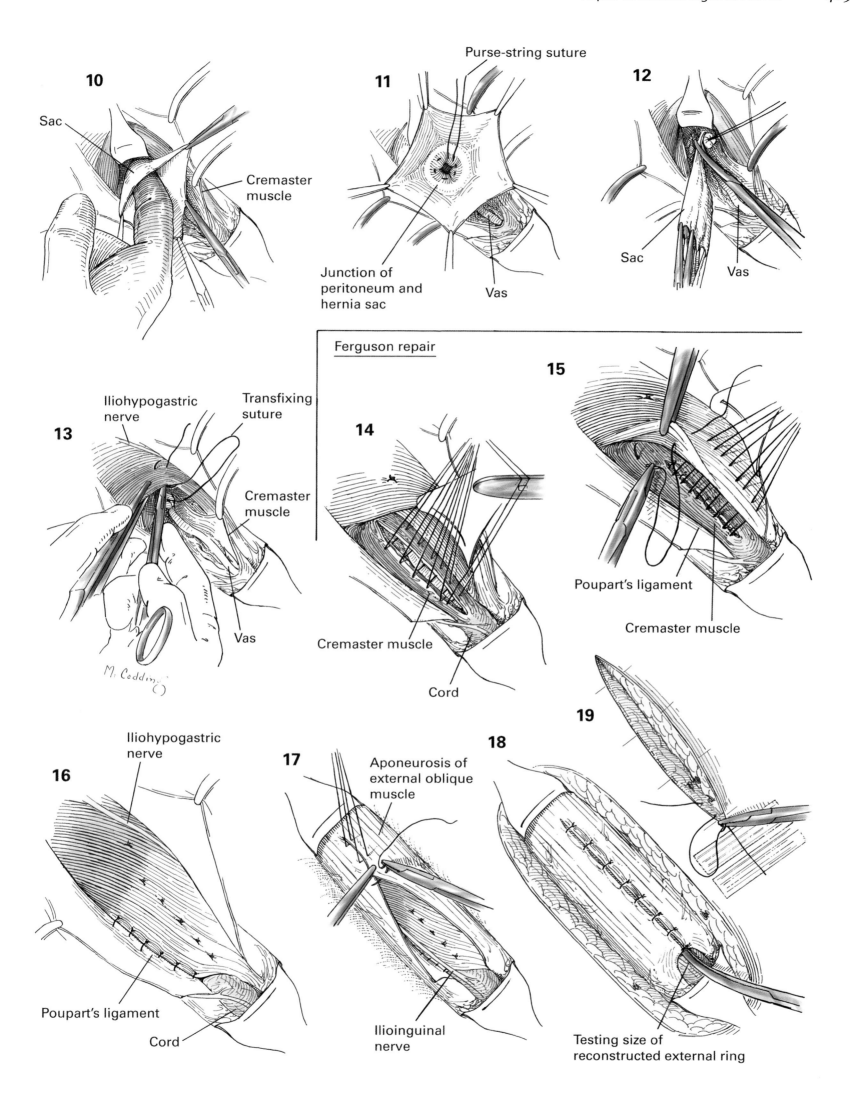

10

Sac

Cremaster muscle

11

Purse-string suture

Junction of peritoneum and hernia sac

Vas

12

Sac

Vas

13

Iliohypogastric nerve

Transfixing suture

Cremaster muscle

Vas

M. Codding

Ferguson repair

14

Cremaster muscle

Cord

15

Poupart's ligament

Cremaster muscle

16

Iliohypogastric nerve

Poupart's ligament

Cord

17

Aponeurosis of external oblique muscle

Ilioinguinal nerve

18

19

Testing size of reconstructed external ring

REPAIR IN CHILDREN ◄ CONTINUED A short (3 cm) skin incision is made in the suprapubic crease above the inguinal ligament and centered over the internal inguinal ring.

After the incision has been made through the skin, a small curved mosquito hemostat is placed in the subcutaneous tissue on either side of the midportion of the incision for traction. Scarpa's fascia is exposed and divided. The underlying aponeurosis of the external oblique is cleared down to the external inguinal ring. The aponeurosis of the external oblique is then opened upward from the external inguinal ring. If there is no associated scrotal hydrocele, the incision through the external oblique aponeurosis may be placed just above rather than through the external ring. Superior and inferior flaps of the aponeurosis of the external oblique are developed with the scalpel handle, and a small right angle retractor is placed under the superior flap to expose the inguinal canal. The cremasteric muscle fibers are separated by blunt dissection. The hernia sac is identified on the anteromedial aspect of the cord structures, lifted up, and gently separated in the midportion of the inguinal canal from the vas and vessels. The cord structures themselves should not be mobilized from the inguinal canal. The sac is divided between two straight mosquito hemostats in the midportion of the inguinal canal, and the proximal portion is freed well above the level of the internal ring. The neck of the sac then is closed with a suture ligature of fine silk and the sac amputated. Ordinarily, it is not necessary to open the sac during this process. However, if omentum or a loop of intestine is within the sac, the sac is opened, and these structures are returned to the peritoneal cavity before the neck of the hernia sac is closed. The distal portion of the sac is freed below the level of the external ring and excised.

The testis and cord structures are repositioned into their normal anatomic bed if they have been disturbed, and an anatomic closure is performed. The aponeurosis of the external oblique and Scarpa's fascia are closed with interrupted sutures of fine silk. A subcuticular closure with fine absorbable suture is used in children. Because of the high incidence of a patent processus vaginalis on the opposite side in instances of a clinical inguinal hernia in infants, it is common practice to perform an inguinal exploration on the opposite side in infants but not older children.

In female children, the incision and initial stages of the procedure are as described above. However, in a high proportion of cases a congenital indirect hernia in a female is a sliding type of hernia, with the fallopian tube and its mesenteric attachments making up a portion of the hernia sac. In such instances the hernia sac and round ligament are closed with a suture ligature of fine silk distal to the attachment of the mesosalpinx. The remainder of the procedure is identical with that done in the male.

REPAIR IN ADULT FEMALES The round ligament is usually closely attached to the sac, making sharp dissection necessary for separation. After the neck of the sac is freed and ligated, the repair proceeds as in the operation on the male, except that the round ligament may be included in the sutures that bring the conjoined tendon to Poupart's ligament. If the round ligament is divided, it must be ligated, since it contains a small artery, and the proximal end must be anchored in order to give support to the uterus.

POSTOPERATIVE CARE *Adult* The patient is placed flat in bed with the thighs somewhat flexed either by a pillow beneath the knees or, if in an adjustable bed, with the lower part of the bed somewhat elevated in order to prevent undue tension upon the sutures in the wound. Support to the scrotum may be furnished by suspensory. An ice pack may be applied to the scrotum. Coughing must be controlled by sedation. Laxatives are given in sufficient dosage to avoid undue straining at stool. Patients should ambulate and void as soon as possible. Normal activities are resumed as tolerated. However, several weeks should elapse before the patient is permitted to perform heavy physical work. Special abdominal supports usually are not necessary.

Child The infant or child is fed 4 to 6 hours after operation and, by the evening of operation, should be taking a normal diet.

MODIFIED BASSINI REPAIR

DETAILS OF PROCEDURE The cord is visualized by the approach described earlier in this Chapter. Since the structures of the cord are to be transplanted, it may be easier to separate the cord from the surrounding structures before the hernia sac is identified and opened. The index finger may be inserted beneath the cord from the medial side just above the pubic tubercle in order to assist in the blunt dissection and freeing of the cord from the underlying Poupart's ligament (FIGURE 20). A curved half-length clamp directed over Poupart's ligament and toward the pubic spine is then passed beneath the cord and guided by the index finger (FIGURE 21). A tube of soft rubber (Penrose drain) is drawn through beneath the cord for traction (FIGURE 22). Many times blood vessels that course downward beneath the cord must be clamped and tied to ensure a dry field. The cremaster muscle is divided, and the hernial sac is grasped with toothed forceps preliminary to opening it (FIGURE 23). Some prefer to completely divide the cremaster muscle near the internal oblique muscle, leaving the vas and its accompanying vessels exposed. The sacrifice of the cremaster muscle at this level permits a more accurate closure of the internal ring. The hernia sac is opened, and traction is maintained by curved or straight hemostats applied to its margin. With the surgeon's index finger in the hernia sac, the vas deferens and accompanying vessels are dissected free by sharp and blunt dissection (FIGURE 24). With the surgeon's finger in the neck of the hernia sac to ensure that all abdominal contents are completely reduced, a purse-string suture is placed at the inner side proximal to the neck of the sac or several transfixing mattress sutures are used, as preferred (FIGURE 25). Care must be taken that the adjacent epigastric vessels are not injured.

CLOSURE (TRANSPLANTATION OF CORD, BASSINI) The first step in the closure is to provide adequate retraction of the cord as well as the internal oblique muscle, so that the deep-lying aponeurosis of the transversus abdominis and transversalis fascia can be identified (FIGURE 26). It is important to reinforce the weakened area over the ligated hernia sac by approximating the thickened fascia just below the free edge of Poupart's ligament, the so-called iliopubic tract, and the edge of the aponeurosis of the transverse abdominal muscle (FIGURE 26, Suture X). The remaining opening in the cremaster muscle is closed with interrupted sutures unless it has been completely divided adjacent to the internal oblique muscle. The transversalis fascia may appear to be very thinned out adjacent to Poupart's ligament, but an aponeurosis, the strong white membrane forming the inferior margin of the transversus abdominis, is exposed (FIGURE 26) by retracting the internal oblique sharply upward. The hernial repair is strengthened if an effort is made to approximate the latter structure to the iliopubic tract beyond the margins of Poupart's ligament. The conjoined tendon is retracted upward so that each bite of the needle includes a good portion of the aponeurosis of the transversus muscle (FIGURE 27) and the thickened fascia adjacent to the margin of Poupart's ligament. Several sutures between the iliopubic tract and the aponeurosis of the transversus muscle are taken lateral to the cord to close the redundancy of the internal ring (FIGURE 28). CONTINUES ►

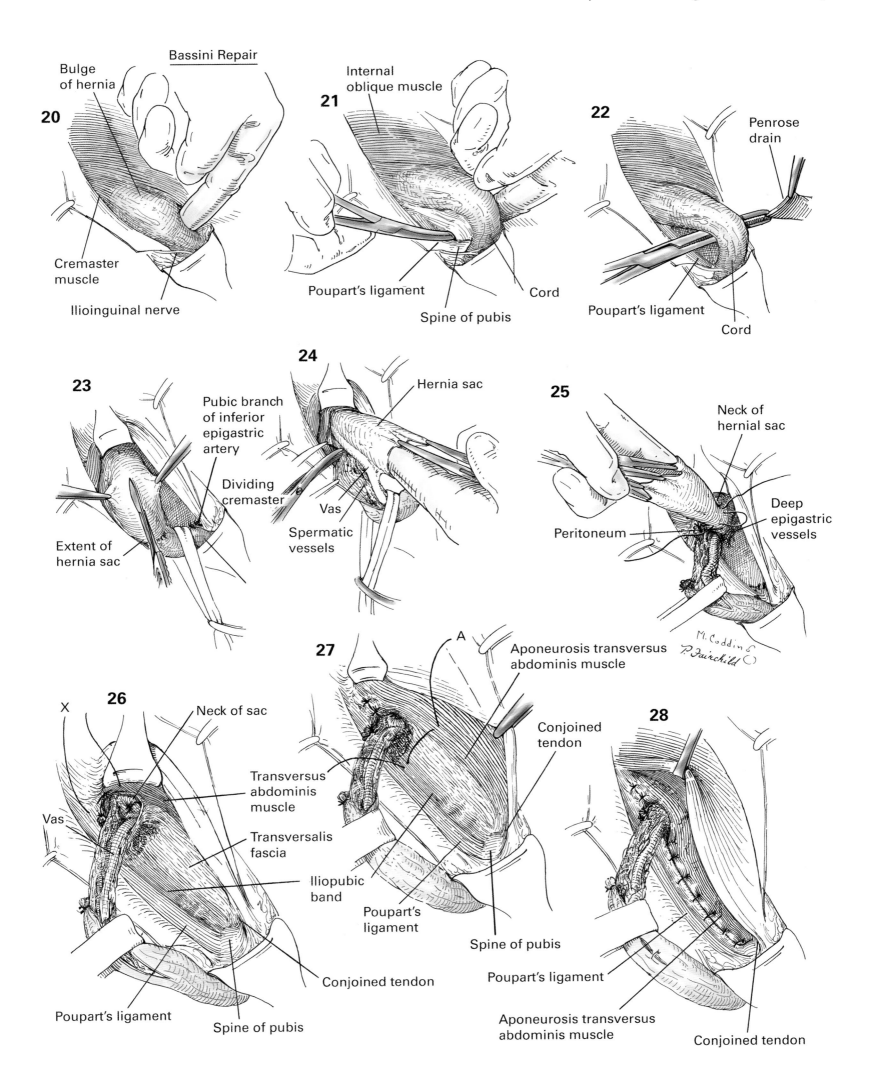

Bassini Repair

20 Bulge of hernia — Cremaster muscle — Ilioinguinal nerve

21 Internal oblique muscle — Poupart's ligament — Spine of pubis — Cord

22 Penrose drain — Poupart's ligament — Cord

23 Pubic branch of inferior epigastric artery — Dividing cremaster — Extent of hernia sac

24 Hernia sac — Vas — Spermatic vessels

25 Neck of hernial sac — Deep epigastric vessels — Peritoneum

M. Coddins
P. Fairchild

26 X — Vas — Neck of sac — Transversus abdominis muscle — Transversalis fascia — Iliopubic band — Conjoined tendon — Poupart's ligament — Spine of pubis

27 A — Aponeurosis transversus abdominis muscle — Conjoined tendon — Poupart's ligament — Spine of pubis

28 Poupart's ligament — Aponeurosis transversus abdominis muscle — Conjoined tendon

CLOSURE (TRANSPLANTATION OF CORD, BASSINI) ◄ CONTINUED ▶ A second layer of oo nonabsorbable sutures includes unequal portions of the shelving edge of Poupart's ligament and a bite of the conjoined tendon. This suture line extends from the pubic tubercle outward over the deep epigastric vessels until the cord appears to be angulated laterally. Before these sutures are placed, the mobility and composition of the tendon should be determined. In many instances the conjoined tendon cannot be brought down to Poupart's ligament except under a great deal of tension. A preliminary trial should be carried out by attempting to approximate the conjoined tendon to Poupart's ligament at the proposed suture line to determine the amount of tension that will be present (FIGURE 29). The medial leaf of the external oblique fascia is retracted medially, and by blunt dissection the underlying sheath of the rectus is exposed (FIGURE 30). If the tension appears to be excessive, relaxation of the fascia with retained support of the underlying rectus muscle is achieved by multiple incisions in the rectus sheath (FIGURE 31). The relaxing incisions can be made about 1 cm apart and 1 cm in length. Eight or ten or even more may be required to produce the desired relaxation (FIGURES 31 and 32). The number required can be judged by the spread of the tissues as the incisions are made and as traction on the fascia is maintained. The conjoined tendon is sutured to the lower edge of Poupart's ligament adjacent to the suture line that has approximated the aponeurosis of the transverse abdominal muscle to the iliopubic tract. The initial suture should include the periosteum of the pubic spine and the medial portion of the conjoined tendon. Several sutures are taken to approximate the muscle to Poupart's ligament above the point of exit of the cord, but these must not constrict the cord, especially if its size has been decreased markedly by the excision of some of the dilated veins and the cremaster muscle (FIGURE 33). The ilioinguinal nerve is replaced, and the external oblique aponeurosis is closed over the cord, either by imbricating the mesial flap of the external oblique muscle over the lower flap by two rows of mattress sutures (FIGURES 34 and 35) or by a simple approximation of the edges of the external oblique with a running oo suture. The newly constructed external ring should be tested to make certain that the cord is not unduly constricted.

TRANSPLANTATION OF CORD (HALSTED) Some surgeons prefer the method of transplanting the cord to the subcutaneous fatty layer (FIGURE 36). Here, the cord is brought out through the upper third of the incision in the external oblique fascia (FIGURE 36) and the fascia is closed beneath the cord, leaving it entirely in the superficial fatty tissue (FIGURE 37). The size of the cord is usually decreased by the excision of many of the spermatic veins as well as the cremaster muscle; however, sufficient blood supply to the testicle must be retained. The cord must not be constricted, or atrophy of the testicle may occur. The size of the external ring is tested with a curved clamp, and, if necessary, a small incision is made just through the margin to release the constriction about the cord (FIGURE 36).

POSTOPERATIVE CARE The usual postoperative care is given, as described in Chapter 105. ■

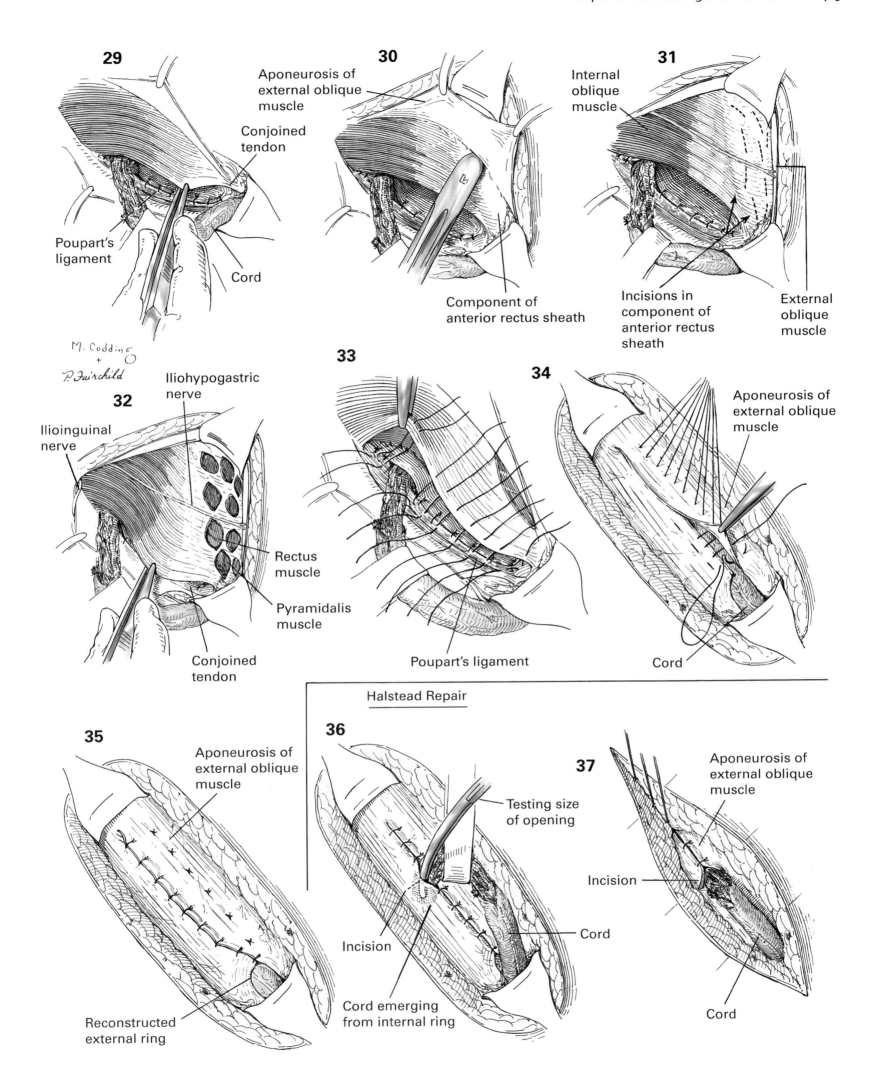

29

Aponeurosis of
external oblique
muscle

Conjoined
tendon

Poupart's
ligament

Cord

M. Codding
+
P. Fairchild

30

Aponeurosis of
external oblique
muscle

Component of
anterior rectus sheath

31

Internal
oblique
muscle

Incisions in
component of
anterior rectus
sheath

External
oblique
muscle

32

Ilioinguinal
nerve

Iliohypogastric
nerve

Rectus
muscle

Pyramidalis
muscle

Conjoined
tendon

33

Poupart's ligament

34

Aponeurosis of
external oblique
muscle

Cord

35

Aponeurosis of
external oblique
muscle

Reconstructed
external ring

Halstead Repair

36

Testing size
of opening

Incision

Cord emerging
from internal ring

37

Aponeurosis of
external oblique
muscle

Incision

Cord

Cord

REPAIR OF INDIRECT INGUINAL HERNIA (SHOULDICE)

INDICATIONS Herniorrhaphy has become an outpatient surgical procedure, regardless of the age of the patient. The Shouldice repair has been advocated for some years as the procedure of choice for adults with inguinal hernias.

PREOPERATIVE PREPARATION The obese patient should be required to lose weight, preferably to within 10% of calculated ideal weight. This may delay the operation for a considerable time. Any infections of the skin should be cleared up before operation. A productive cough or an upper respiratory infection delays the procedure. Chronic smokers should be encouraged to curtail their smoking. Evidence of prostatic obstruction should be sought in older men. All patients should be taught how to get out of bed with a minimum of discomfort and advised to practice this. Sensitivity to drugs, including local anesthetics, should be ascertained. A mild cathartic should be given a day before the operation to ensure an empty colon. A mild laxative or mineral oil may be given to ensure bowel action without excessive straining after operation. A thorough medical evaluation is essential in older patients. A hernia should be relatively asymptomatic unless it becomes incarcerated. Any other symptoms must be evaluated, because they may be due to causes other than hernia.

ANESTHESIA Deep sedation plus local anesthesia is commonly used. The type of sedation will vary, but may include midazolam, fentanyl or meperidine, and propofol. Local anesthesia is limited to 30 mL of 1% lidocaine without epinephrine (total lidocaine dose <300 mg). The amount is reduced in elderly patients.

SKIN PREPARATION The skin is carefully inspected for any evidence of localized infection. All hair of the lower abdomen and pubis is removed with an electric hair clipper. In patients with scrotal hernias, the skin of the scrotum should be included in the usual skin preparation with topical antiseptics.

POSITION The legs should be slightly flexed, with pillows under the knees, and the patient placed in a modified Trendelenburg position to assist in the reduction of the hernia sac. Following the draping of the patient, the local anesthetic is injected. Keeping in mind the location of the ilioinguinal and iliohypogastric nerves, the original injection of a few milliliters of anesthetic agent is made, using a fine needle (No. 25), just medial to the anterosuperior spine. Approximately 10 mL of (lidocaine) anesthetic solution is injected subcutaneously with a No. 25 needle above and parallel to the inguinal ligament. About 5 mL is injected medial to the anterosuperior spine deep into the external oblique aponeurosis to anesthetize the ilioinguinal nerve. Another 5 mL is injected about the internal ring to eliminate painful impulses from the peritoneum and from the genital branch of the genitofemoral nerve. In elderly patients, less anesthetic solution is used. Epinephrine is not used in the elderly or in patients with cardiovascular disease.

INCISION AND EXPOSURE A 10-cm incision is made parallel to the inguinal ligament, although some prefer a more transverse or skinfold incision. The external pudendal vessels are spared, especially in bilateral repairs, in an effort to minimize postoperative edema.

DETAILS OF PROCEDURE The external oblique aponeurosis is divided along the line of its fibers. Great care is exercised to avoid possible injury to the underlying ilioinguinal nerve. The aponeurosis of the external oblique is divided from the level of the internal ring down through the external ring, and both flaps are mobilized (FIGURE 1). Mobilization of the lower flap should involve some division in the superficial fascia of the thigh to allow inspection of the femoral area for evidence of a femoral hernia. The cremaster muscle is carefully divided longitudinally, with the lateral side being made the larger, since it contains the cremaster vessels and the genital branch of the genitofemoral nerve in its base.

The internal ring is freed from attachments, and evidence of a hernial sac is sought. If no indirect hernial sac is found, a small crescent reflection of peritoneum (processus vaginalis) is visible proximally. When an obvious hernial sac is found, it is freed by blunt and sharp dissection. When the sac is large, it can be filled with gauze sponge to provide counterpressure, which simplifies the pushing away of other tissues. The sac is opened and the index finger inserted medially under the inferior epigastric vessels in an

effort to determine the presence or absence of a direct hernial defect. The neck of the hernial sac is freed from the surrounding tissue. Following this, the sac is ligated (FIGURE 2). Some believe an effort for a high ligation of the sac is unnecessary. If a lipoma of the cord is found, it is carefully excised, but the cord is not stripped of interstitial fat. Even large sliding hernia sacs can be freed and reduced without opening the sac.

The two cremaster muscles are excised with double ligation of the stumps. The posterior inguinal wall should now be fully visible. The posterior inguinal wall is palpated for an area of weakness or general bulge. The transversalis fascia is divided starting on the medial aspect of the internal ring but avoiding the inferior epigastric vessels and proceeding to the pubic tubercle (FIGURE 2). The femoral ring is evaluated for evidence of a femoral hernia.

If the transversalis fascia has been stretched by the diffuse bulge of a direct hernia, the excess from each flap is excised. The upper flap (A) is usually narrower than the lower flap (B). It is extremely important to develop an adequate lower flap if the repair is to have the best chance of success. The latter tends to be 1 to 2 cm wide and somewhat stronger. The lower flap is completely freed by careful dissection. The development of the flaps of the transversalis is very important in the subsequent steps of the Shouldice repair (FIGURE 2). The subsequent repair involves the development of a four-layered closure, using either two different continuous sutures of 34-gauge monofilament stainless steel wire or a nonabsorbable suture material. Absorbable suture or mesh is not used. Continuous sutures are preferred for distributing the stresses evenly.

The repair of the posterior inguinal wall must be carefully performed, using small, even bites without tension on the suture. Retaining sutures are not used. The first suture anchors the free edge of the lower flap (B) of the transversalis to the posterior aspect of the lateral edge of the rectus close to its insertion (FIGURE 2A). The placement of the suture must be accurate, and the knot securely tied without leaving a defect in this area. Only a short distance from the edge of the rectus sheath is included before the suture is continued laterally to include the deep underneath surface of the upper flap (A) of the transversalis and the internal oblique (FIGURE 3). The inferior epigastric vessels are carefully avoided as the suture line is extended to include the upper lateral cremasteric stump. The suture is now reversed at the internal inguinal ring (FIGURE 4), extending medially as it unites the free edge of the upper transversus flap (A) to the edge of Poupart's ligament. The suture is continued down to the pubic bone and tied. The space medial to the femoral vein may be obliterated by including the lacunar ligament if necessary.

Another continuous suture line is used to reinforce the second suture line just completed. The third suture line starts at the internal ring and includes bites of the internal oblique and transversalis muscles as well as the deep surface of the inguinal ligament as it continues medially to the pubic bone (FIGURE 5). The fourth suture line returns from the pubic bone, bringing together the same structures at a slightly more superficial plane up to the internal ring, where it is tied (FIGURE 6).

The spermatic cord is tested to determine that it can be freely moved and the veins are not engorged. The cord is returned to its normal position and the external oblique fascia approximated without constricting the vein in the region of the external inguinal ring (FIGURE 7).

The subcutaneous tissues are carefully approximated with interrupted sutures. The skin can be closed with interrupted or a continuous subcutaneous suture of absorbable material reinforced with skin tapes of a "butterfly" nature. Some prefer metal staples. A small dressing is applied to cover the wound.

POSTOPERATIVE CARE The patient may return home several hours after the operation with full written instructions concerning activities, signs of bleeding or infection, or any other unusual reaction. Oral narcotic is supplied, and an ice pack may be applied locally for several hours. The patient should rest in bed except for voiding in the bathroom on the day of surgery. A suspensory for men is optional. Physical activity is restricted for an additional few days. Many experience improvement after 3 days, and some may drive or return to light duty work after 7 to 10 days. Vigorous exertion, as in sports, is limited for 4 weeks, and extreme exertion should be avoided. See also Chapter 104. ∎

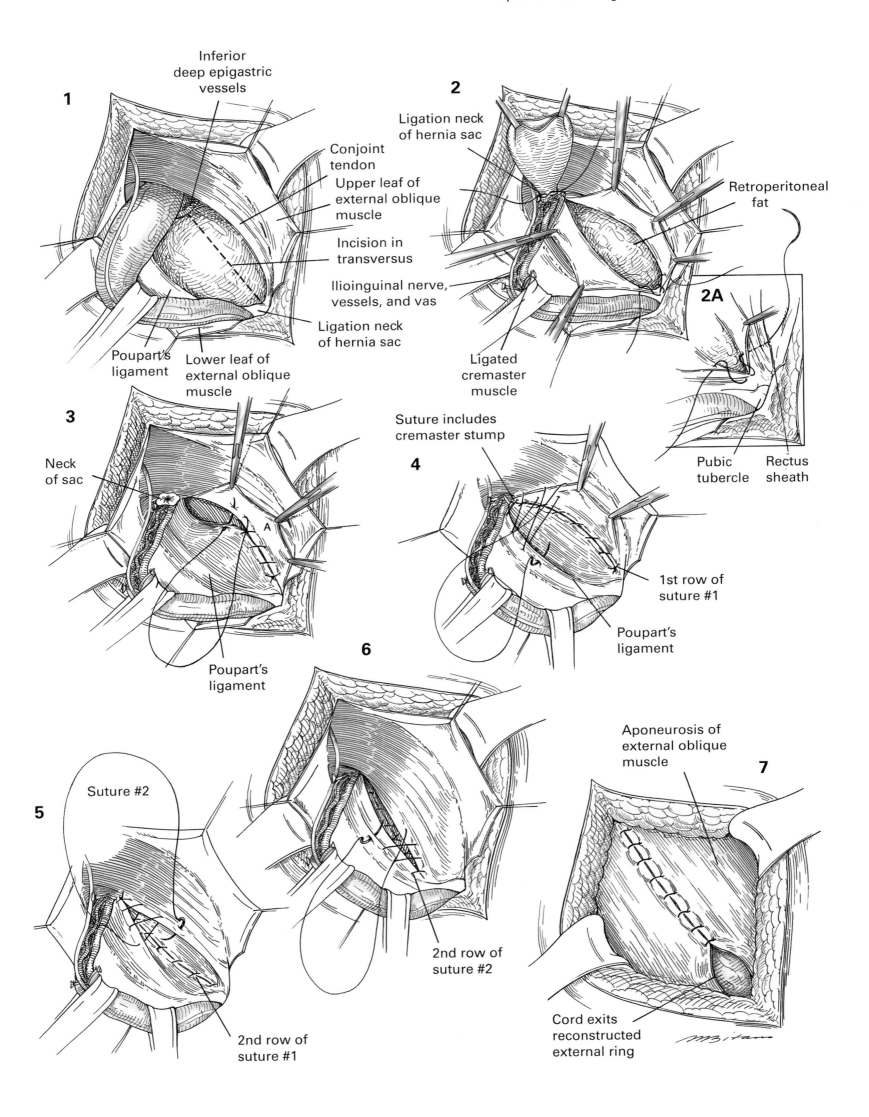

1
Inferior deep epigastric vessels
Conjoint tendon
Upper leaf of external oblique muscle
Incision in transversus
Ilioinguinal nerve, vessels, and vas
Ligation neck of hernia sac
Poupart's ligament
Lower leaf of external oblique muscle

2
Ligation neck of hernia sac
Retroperitoneal fat
Ligated cremaster muscle

2A
Pubic tubercle
Rectus sheath

3
Neck of sac
Poupart's ligament

4
Suture includes cremaster stump
1st row of suture #1
Poupart's ligament

5
Suture #2
2nd row of suture #1

6
2nd row of suture #2

7
Aponeurosis of external oblique muscle
Cord exits reconstructed external ring

REPAIR OF DIRECT INGUINAL HERNIA (McVay)

INDICATIONS A McVay primary tissue repair is infrequently performed as an initial herniorrhaphy, as it is associated with a high rate of recurrence. However in patients where mesh from a previous operation must be removed (e.g., chronic infection), some form of primary tissue repair is needed. The McVay procedure may be useful in these cases, especially when the femoral space must also be obliterated.

DETAILS OF PROCEDURE Instead of approximating the transversalis fascia and the aponeurotic margin of the transverse abdominal muscle to the iliopubic tract and to Poupart's ligament to repair either a direct or indirect hernia, the McVay repair attaches these musculotendinous structures to Cooper's ligament and the lacunar ligament medially and the inguinal ligament laterally. To accomplish this, it is necessary to retract the conjoined tendon upward and the cord downward, while the transversalis fascia adjacent to the pubic spine is freed from Cooper's ligament (FIGURE 1). In FIGURE 1 a direct inguinal hernia sac has been reduced and the floor of traversalis fascia has been reconstituted with interrupted non absorbable sutures.

By blunt dissection and the use of a curved retractor (FIGURE 2), the region of Cooper's ligament can be visualized, and the external iliac vessels can be identified. As the conjoined tendon or internal oblique muscle is held upward, a firm aponeurotic margin of transverse abdominal muscle is exposed in order to facilitate the placement of interrupted sutures. As the bulge in this region is retracted upward and medially by an appropriate retractor, Cooper's ligament is clearly visualized as a white, fibrous ridge, deep in the wound at the innermost portion of the concavity and closely

applied to the horizontal ramus of the pubis (FIGURE 2). Interrupted oo silk sutures approximate the aponeurotic margin of the transverse abdominal muscle and the transversalis fascia to Cooper's ligament. The iliac vessels may be protected by the surgeon's left index finger or a narrow S retractor as the innermost suture is placed. The sutures are continued downward until the region of the pubic spine is included in the last one (FIGURE 3). Three to five interrupted sutures are usually required. In obese individuals it may be difficult to obtain an easy exposure in this location, and constant care must be exercised to avoid injury to the iliac vessels and to effect a complete and solid repair (FIGURE 4). Some operators prefer to make an incision in Cooper's ligament before placing the sutures in order to ensure a better fascial approximation. After the aponeurotic margin of the transverse abdominal muscle has been anchored as far medially to Cooper's ligament as can be done safely, more superficial sutures may be taken to approximate it to the iliopubic tract (FIGURES 4 and 5). Some surgeons prefer to reinforce the repair to Cooper's ligament by another row of sutures approximating Poupart's ligament to the aponeurosis of the transverse abdominal muscle (FIGURE 6). The suturing of the internal oblique muscle to Poupart's ligament is not considered worthwhile. The type of repair should be varied to suit the anatomic conditions encountered. A combination of the technique described may be advantageous to ensure a solid repair without tension upon the suture lines and an accurate approximation of fascia to fascia.

POSTOPERATIVE CARE Care is routine. (See Chapter 105.) ■

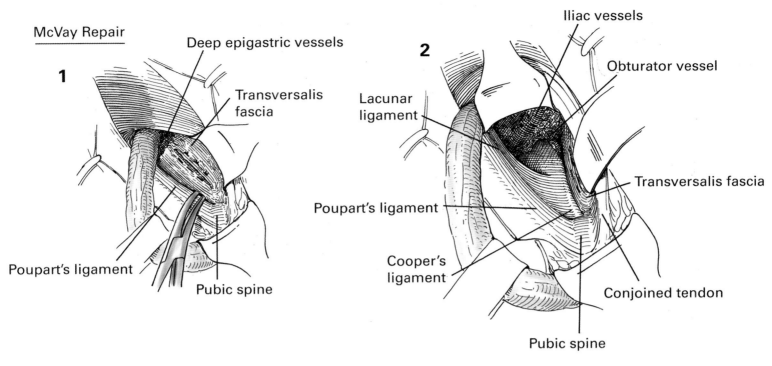

McVay Repair

1

Deep epigastric vessels

Transversalis fascia

Poupart's ligament

Pubic spine

2

Iliac vessels

Obturator vessel

Lacunar ligament

Poupart's ligament

Cooper's ligament

Transversalis fascia

Conjoined tendon

Pubic spine

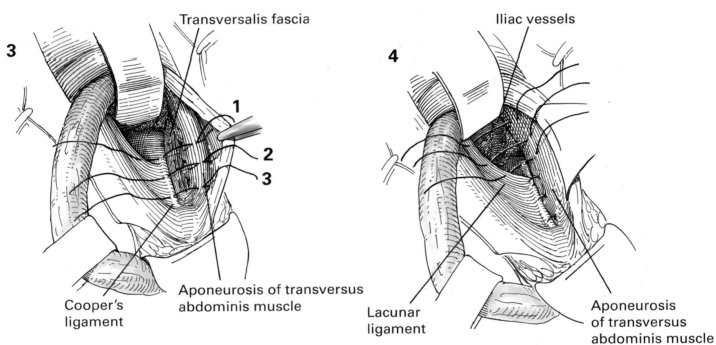

3

Transversalis fascia

1

2

3

Cooper's ligament

Aponeurosis of transversus abdominis muscle

4

Iliac vessels

Lacunar ligament

Aponeurosis of transversus abdominis muscle

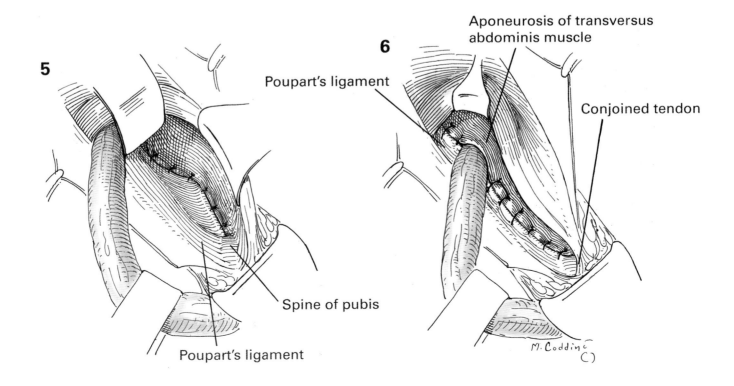

5

Poupart's ligament

Spine of pubis

Poupart's ligament

6

Aponeurosis of transversus abdominis muscle

Conjoined tendon

M. Codding

CHAPTER 107 · REPAIR OF INGUINAL HERNIA WITH MESH (LICHTENSTEIN)

INDICATIONS Adult inguinal hernias are usually repaired in an ambulatory surgery setting unless coexisting medical conditions merit hospitalization for specialized monitoring or care. The use of synthetic mesh has become increasingly popular as it may be used for both direct and indirect hernias and it results in a lower rate of recurrence.

PREOPERATIVE PREPARATION The obese patient should be required to lose weight, preferably to within 10% of calculated ideal weight, which may delay the operation for a considerable time. Any open-skin infections must be healed prior to operation. Systemic causes of increased intra-abdominal pressure or straining should be reviewed. A productive cough or an upper respiratory infection will delay the procedure until resolution. Chronic smokers should be encouraged to curtail their smoking. Evidence of prostatic obstruction should be evaluated in older men and the possibility of new colon lesions should be evaluated in older men and women. All patients should be taught how to get out of bed with a minimum of discomfort and advised to practice this. Sensitivity to drugs, including local anesthetics, should be ascertained. A mild cathartic may be given a day before the operation to ensure an empty colon. Mineral oil may be given to ensure bowel action without excessive straining after operation. A thorough medical evaluation is essential in older patients. A hernia should be relatively asymptomatic unless it becomes incarcerated. Any other symptoms must be evaluated, because they may be due to causes other than hernia.

ANESTHESIA Deep sedation with an anxiolytic, narcotic, and hypnotic (commonly midazolam, fentanyl, and propofol) is combined with a field block of local anesthesia. Lidocaine 1% or ½% without adrenaline is preferred and the total dose is limited to less than 300 mg (30 mL of 1% lidocaine). This amount may be reduced in elderly patients. No adrenalin is used during the opening as this may obscure small bleeding vessels that should be ligated or cauterized thus lessening ecchymosis or hematoma formation. However, during the closure, when hemostasis is secured, many surgeons reinfiltrate the operative field with a long-acting local anesthetic such as bupivacaine. Adrenalin is often added except in patients with heart disease so as to extend the duration of the local anesthetic.

POSITIONING The patient is placed in a supine position with a pillow under the knees to lessen tension in the inguinal region.

OPERATIVE PREPARATION The hair in the planned operative field is clipped and the skin prepared in a routine manner. In men, the penis and scrotum should be prepared, especially if the hernia extends into the scrotum or if a hydrocele is present.

INCISION AND EXPOSURE After a sterile draping of the region, the local anesthetic is injected. The surgeon may perform a selective nerve block of the ilioinguinal and iliohypogastric nerves, which are just medial to the anterior superior spine (FIGURE 1). The incision may be made either parallel to the inguinal ligament (FIGURE 2A) or more transversely along a skinfold line (FIGURE 2B). Most surgeons prefer a field block with multiple injections along the incision (FIGURE 3) followed by further injections at each new level of fascial dissection.

DIRECT INGUINAL HERNIA

DETAILS OF PROCEDURE The incision is carried down through Scarpa's fascia to the external oblique aponeurosis. Additional local is infiltrated beneath this fascia, especially laterally (FIGURE 4). The external oblique is opened in a direction parallel to its fibers down through the external ring. Care is taken to lift this fascia away from the cord and ilioinguinal nerve during the opening so as to lessen the chance of transection of the nerve.

The free edges of the external oblique fascia are grasped with a pair of hemostats medially and laterally. Using blunt dissection, the fascia is separated from the internal oblique muscle superiorly and the cord inferiorly. The cord is encircled with a soft rubber Penrose drain. Additional local anesthesia is injected along the inguinal ligament and about the pubic tubercle. The direct hernial sac is carefully separated from the cord, which is cleaned back to the level of its exit at the internal ring. It is verified that this is a direct herniation rather than a medial protrusion of an indirect herniation. The cremaster muscle about the cord is opened anteriorly. The cord structures are identified and the region of the internal ring inspected for evidence of an indirect hernia and sac. A direct hernia only is shown (FIGURE 5). The direct hernial sac is cleaned with blunt and sharp dissection around to its neck. This protrudes through a defect in the transversalis fascia of the canal floor. These defects may be discrete, with a finger-sized punched out hole, or may involve the entire floor as a diffuse blowout from the inguinal ligament below to the conjoint tendon above. Some surgeons prefer to open the direct sac, reduce the properitoneal fat, and excise the residual sac, as is done with indirect hernias. Almost always, however, the sac and fat are easily reduced (FIGURE 5) and then kept reduced with an instrument as the floor is reconstructed.

A continuous nonabsorbable 00 suture is placed for reconstruction of the canal floor. This begins at the pubic tubercle and approximates the residual transversalis fascia just above the inguinal ligament to the transversalis fascia or muscle just below the conjoint tendon so as to imbricate the herniation (FIGURE 6). This suture continues laterally to the level of the internal ring. Care is taken to avoid the inferior epigastric vessels. After this suture is tied, the internal ring should be snug about the cord (FIGURE 7). The floor of the canal is now solid and the conjoint tendon lies in its normal position. The conjoint tendon is not artificially pulled down under tension to the inguinal ligament as in the classic Bassini repair. **CONTINUES▶**

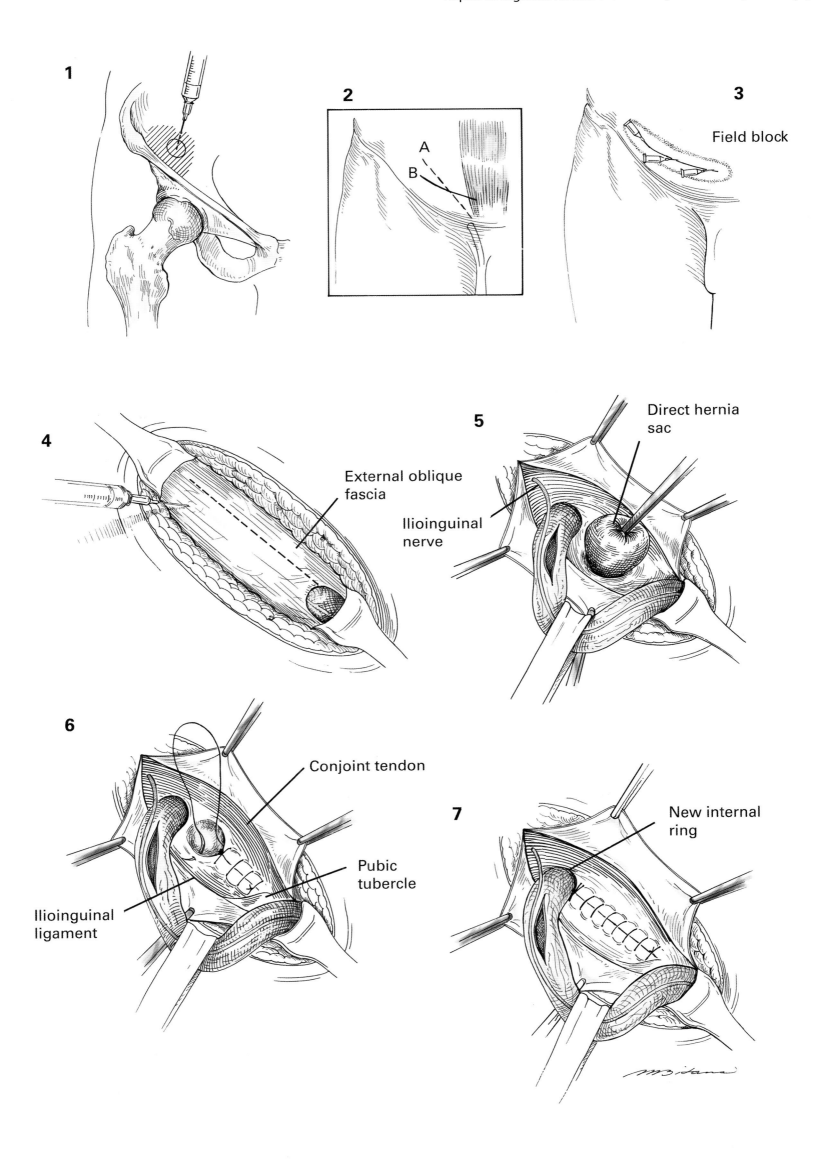

1

2

A

B

3

Field block

4

External oblique
fascia

5

Direct hernia
sac

Ilioinguinal
nerve

6

Conjoint tendon

Pubic
tubercle

Ilioinguinal
ligament

7

New internal
ring

DETAILS OF PROCEDURE ◄CONTINUED Once the continuity of the direct floor is restored, the repair continues in the same manner as that for an indirect inguinal herniorrhaphy for a Lichtenstein indirect inguinal herniorrhaphy. The cremaster muscle is opened anteriorly. The vital cord structures are identified and a concurrent indirect hernia sac is found. This sac is freed from the cord using electrocautery and gentle traction. The key landmark is the vas, which is directly posterior to the sac. After the sac is opened and examined, a transfixing nonabsorbable suture is placed through its neck and ligated (FIGURE 8). The excess sac is then excised, as is any significant lateral lipoma of the cord. Alternatively some surgeons do not open the hernia sac and merely return it to the preoperational space.

A rectangular piece of synthetic mesh approximately 2½ to 3 cm by 8 to 10 cm in size is cut with a lateral slit for the cord and a medial blunt oval for the pubis (FIGURE 9). The mesh is positioned on the floor of the canal with the tails overlapping lateral to the internal ring and cord. A nonabsorbable 00 suture anchors the mesh to the pubic tubercle. This continuous suture secures the inferior edge of the mesh to the inguinal ligament while interrupted absorbable sutures anchor the superior edge to the internal oblique muscle (FIGURE 10). Care is taken in the placement of the superior suture so as to avoid any nerve branches. Additional care is needed in the placement of interrupted sutures laterally so as to avoid the ilioinguinal nerve, which lies upon the internal oblique muscle just lateral to the cord. The two tails of the mesh are overlapped and then sewn together. It is important that the mesh not be stretched tightly. The superior suture placements are chosen such that the mesh is not stretched but rather is loose and almost wrinkles longitudinally. The importance of this maneuver becomes apparent when the patient is asked to cough or strain (an advantage possible with the use of local anesthesia). The wrinkles disappear as the abdominal wall tightens. If the mesh had been placed without slack, the suture lines would now be under tension. A few interrupted sutures are placed to further close the lateral slit and create an appropriate size for the internal ring opening. Currently, only a few (4 or 5) loops of each continuous suture are placed on the inferior and superior edges of the mesh by Lichtenstein surgeons.

An alternate pattern for the mesh may be used where the slit is placed inferior to the cord (FIGURE 11). The mesh is sewn in place with the same continuous nonabsorbable suture, which begins at the pubic tubercle. Additional interrupted sutures are used to anchor the superior edge of the mesh to the internal oblique muscle and to close the inferior slit about the cord (FIGURE 12). A modification described in the classic Lichtenstein repair is shown for males in this illustration where the spermatic cord has been thinned and partitioned. The superior bundle of cremasteric muscle has been transected and ligated at the internal ring. The cord is then partitioned into a major portion containing ilioinguinal nerve, vas, and major vessels and a minor portion containing the intact inferior cremaster muscle bundle with the external spermatic vessels and the genital branch of the genitofemoral nerve. The major cord exits through the internal ring and is shown encircled with a soft rubber Penrose drain. The minor portion is left undisturbed, with minimal dissection or disruption in the floor of the canal near the internal ring. This minor portion now exits through a separate opening left between the inferior edge of the mesh and the inguinal ligament. It is important to use a double loop or locking stitch on either side of this opening such that the minor portion of the cord will not be compressed.

The external oblique fascia is reapproximated with a running suture, which may begin at either end of the incision and which creates a snug-defined external ring (FIGURE 13). Scarpa's fascia is approximated with interrupted absorbable sutures and the skin is approximated with subcutaneous absorbable sutures reinforced with skin paper tapes. A small dressing is applied to cover the incision.

POSTOPERATIVE CARE The patient may return home several hours after the operation with written instructions concerning activities, signs of bleeding or infection, or any other unusual reaction. Oral narcotic is supplied, and an ice pack may be applied locally for several hours. The patient should rest in bed except for voiding in the bathroom on the day of surgery. A suspensory for men is optional. Physical activity is restricted for an additional few days. Many experience improvement after 3 days, and some may drive or return to light duty work after 5 to 7 days. Vigorous exertion, as in sports, is limited for a few weeks, and extreme exertion should be avoided. ■

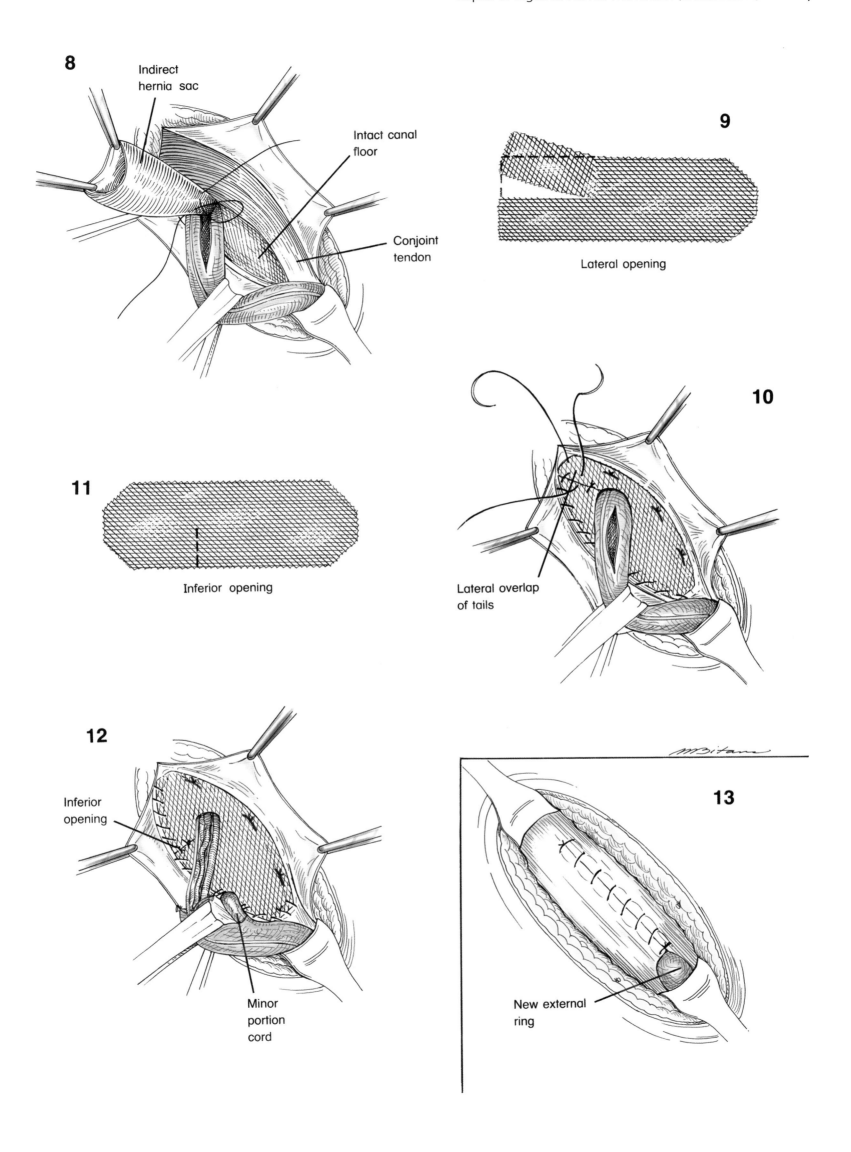

8

Indirect hernia sac

Intact canal floor

Conjoint tendon

9

Lateral opening

11

Inferior opening

10

Lateral overlap of tails

12

Inferior opening

Minor portion cord

13

New external ring

REPAIR OF INGUINAL HERNIA WITH MESH (RUTKOW AND ROBBINS)

INDICATIONS The repair of inguinal hernias in adults has shifted from pure tissue repairs (e.g., Bassini) to "tension-free" repairs using synthetic mesh. The Lichtenstein repair, shown in Chapter 107, represents the first widely accepted method for repair of an inguinal hernia using mesh. Since 1990, however, multiple new configurations of mesh have been invented. A frequently used variation is the "plug and patch," popularized by Drs. Rutkow and Robbins. This technique has results equivalent to those of the Lichtenstein method. The mesh cone or "plug" brings a new approach to the correction of the actual hernial defect. This technique may be used for recurrent as well as primary inguinal hernias.

PREOPERATIVE PREPARATION The patient is evaluated for general medical and anesthesia risks, as discussed in Chapter 4, Ambulatory Surgery, and in the preceding chapters concerning hernia repair. As most operations are elective and performed in an ambulatory setting, sufficient time should be available to optimize the management of any medical diseases. Chronic coughing, new constipation with straining, and symptoms of prostatism require a specialty evaluation prior to surgery. Any active infections, including intertrigo, must be controlled. Although synthetic mesh and sutures do not harbor bacteria, an infection may become established or chronic in the presence of mesh, thus requiring its removal.

ANESTHESIA Most patients can be managed effectively with deep sedation plus local anesthesia. The use of anxiolytic drugs followed by a narcotic and hypnotic (typically midazolam, fentanyl, and propofol) allows a pleasant induction. Dilute 0.5% lidocaine without adrenaline is placed by intradermal infiltration. This produces instant skin anesthesia, which lessens the discomfort of deeper injections. At the same time, the swelling serves as a marker for the skin incision. Adrenaline is not used with the entry local anesthetic as it may obscure bleeding points. Later during the closure, when hemostasis has been fully secured, adrenaline may be added to the long-acting local anesthetic to prolong its duration of action. Adrenaline is not used in older patients or in those with cardiovascular disease. Alternatively, some surgeons prefer epidural anesthesia for their patients, as they believe there is a significant interval of hyperesthesia during recovery. Finally, general anesthesia may be required for the very anxious patient.

POSITIONING The patient is placed in a comfortable supine position. A pillow is often put under the knees to lessen tension in the inguinal region, and some older patients may require an additional pillow under the head and neck.

OPERATIVE PREPARATION The skin hair is clipped and the skin is prepared in the usual manner. In men, the penis and scrotum should be prepared, especially if the hernia extends into the scrotum or if a hydrocele is present.

INCISION AND EXPOSURE The area is draped in a sterile manner and local anesthesia is injected along the planned 5-cm incision. The incision is placed directly over the inguinal canal and extends obliquely and laterally from the external ring. In very obese patients, a more transverse incision may be required because of a major skinfold crease. In general, these incisions are placed below and parallel to the crease. Alternatively, a recurrent hernia may be approached through the old or original incision. It may be prudent to make a longer incision that extends laterally into an area that has not been scarred from the previous operation, as recurrences are best approached laterally through new tissue planes. After the skin is opened, the dissection proceeds down through Scarpa's fascia to the level of the external oblique fascia. More local anesthetic is injected deeply beneath the fascia, especially laterally toward the origin of the nerves. The external oblique fascia is opened in a direction parallel to its fibers from laterally to the midportion of the external ring (FIGURE 1). Some surgeons prefer to make a small lateral opening and lift the external oblique fascia away from the cord and ilioinguinal nerve. Scissors are inserted into the opening and the fascia is cut under direct vision from lateral to medial with avoidance of the nerve.

INDIRECT INGUINAL HERNIA

DETAILS OF PROCEDURE The inferior leaf of the external oblique fascia is grasped with two hemostats, one lateral and the other at the external ring. Using blunt dissection with the peanut on a Kelly, the wispy attachments between the cord and inguinal ligament are swept from lateral to medial, exposing the clean shelving edge of the inguinal ligament and the pubic tubercle. Additional local anesthetic is injected along the ligament and at the pubic tubercle. The superior leaf of the external oblique fascia is grasped by two hemostats. The cord is dissected free, again beginning laterally. The pubic tubercle is cleaned. Further extension of this dissection from above, out along the first centimeter or so of inguinal ligament lateral to the pubic tubercle, ensures an easy mobilization of the cord. The surgeon's finger is placed around the cord and a soft-rubber Penrose drain is placed around it for inferior retraction (FIGURE 2). The cremaster muscle is opened anteriorly and longitudinally for a few centimeters in its proximal region. The sac is identified anterior to the vas deferens and is carefully dissected away from the vas and blood vessels. This dissection is performed using electrocautery at the edge of the sac while gentle traction is applied to the fat and vessels. Historically, this dissection was done bluntly with smooth forceps or with a sweeping motion using a gauze sponge; however, careful dissection with electrocautery along the edge of the sac minimizes bleeding. The sac is freed up well into the internal ring (FIGURE 2). If the sac is entered, the opening is closed with a 00 absorbable suture. When an extremely large sac associated with an inguinoscrotal hernia is present, it may be prudent to perform a high transection and ligation of the proximal sac. This leaves the distal sac intact and minimizes potential trauma of the cord veins, with consequent testicular complications.

The hernia sac in this example of an indirect hernia is not divided but rather is invaginated back up through the internal ring with an instrument (FIGURE 3). The internal ring may be sized with the surgeon's finger, which then guides the polypropylene cone or "plug" into the opening. The cone is secured to the conjoint tendon (internal oblique muscle) with one or more 00 absorbable sutures. It is important that the cone be positioned behind the muscle and that a sufficient number of sutures be placed such that the sac or preperitoneal fat cannot get out around the perimeter of the cone (FIGURE 4).

The onlay "patch" of synthetic mesh is placed with the pointed or shield end overlapping the pubic tubercle. The cord is passed through the lateral slit and the two tails are joined together with 00 absorbable suture (FIGURE 5). A suture is placed near the cord, thus determining the diameter of the new internal ring. Traditionally, this opening has been sized for easy passage of the cord plus an instrument tip. It is important that the onlay patch be of sufficient size to overlap the inguinal ligament inferiorly, the pubic tubercle medially, and the entire floor centrally, as shown in the cross section (FIGURE 5A). In addition, the mesh should reach well lateral to the internal ring. This may require the custom cutting of a sheet of synthetic mesh for large indirect hernias.

The perimeter of the incision, both deep and superficial, is infiltrated with a long-acting local anesthetic. The external oblique fascia is reapproximated above the level of the cord using a 00 absorbable suture. The closure begins at the external ring with observation of the cord, the ilioinguinal nerve, and the path of each edge of the oblique fascia. Starting the closure here allows the surgeon to size the external ring. The closure is continued laterally as a running suture (FIGURE 6). Scarpa's fascia is approximated with a few 00 or 000 absorbable sutures and the skin is closed in a subcuticular manner with a fine absorbable suture. Adhesive skin strips and a dry sterile dressing are applied.

POSTOPERATIVE CARE Patients operated upon in an ambulatory surgery setting are observed for about an hour until discharge criteria are met. They may take liquids by mouth and are encouraged to void. The homegoing instructions detailing activities and the signs of bleeding or infection are reviewed with the patient and caregiver. Most patients require pain medications for a day or two. Normal activities are resumed as tolerated. CONTINUES ▶

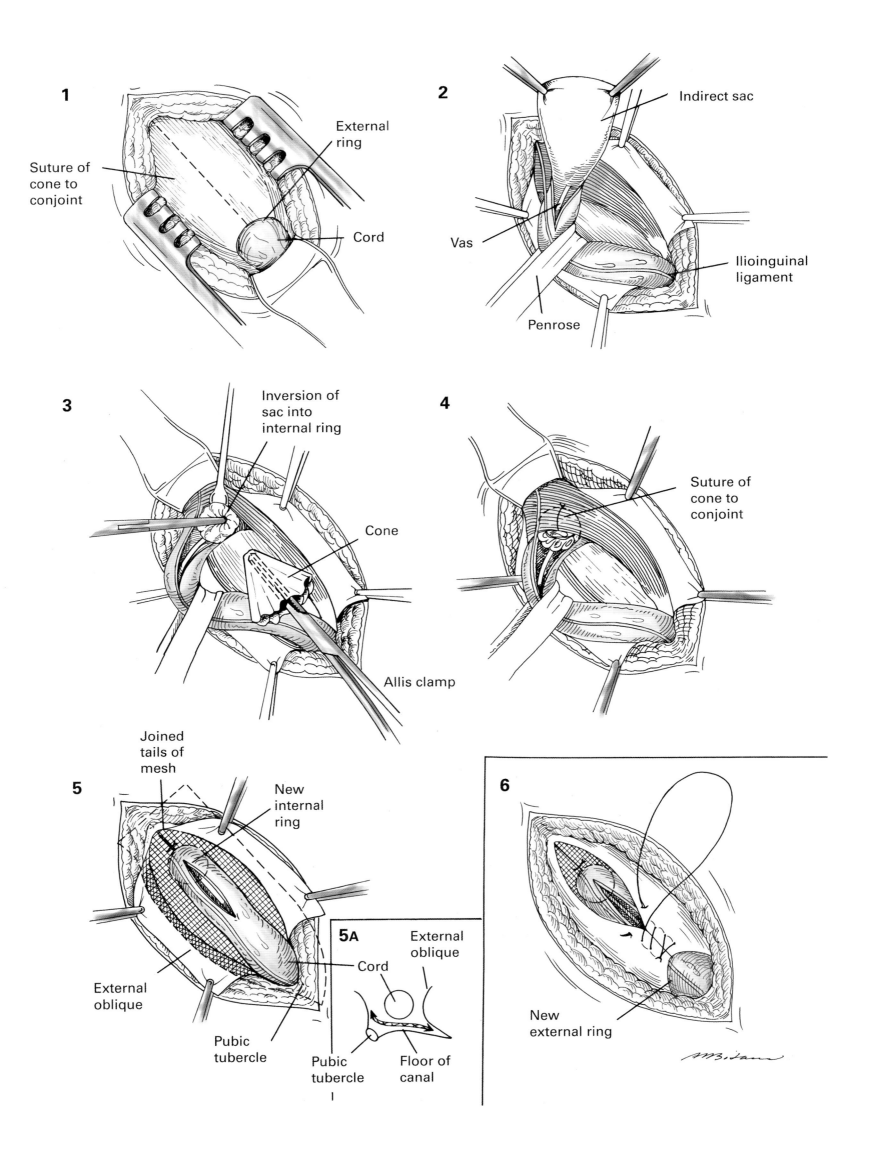

1 Suture of cone to conjoint — External ring — Cord

2 Indirect sac — Vas — Penrose — Ilioinguinal ligament

3 Inversion of sac into internal ring — Cone — Allis clamp

4 Suture of cone to conjoint

5 Joined tails of mesh — New internal ring — External oblique — Cord — Pubic tubercle

5A External oblique — Cord — Pubic tubercle — Floor of canal

6 New external ring

DIRECT INGUINAL HERNIA CONTINUED

DETAILS OF PROCEDURE The incision and exposure is the same as that utilized for the indirect hernia. The external oblique fascia is opened and the superior and inferior edges are grasped with pairs of hemostats. The shelving edge of the inguinal ligament is cleared first with blunt dissection using a peanut on a Kelly. However, as the surgeon begins the superior exposure, the direct floor is not apparent as a structure separate from the cord. It appears as though the cord and hernial process covered both areas (FIGURE 7). As the cremaster is opened anteriorly, the cord is identified as separate from the direct herniation. The cord is dissected free and isolated for retraction with a soft-rubber Penrose drain. The direct hernial sac, which is often quite large compared to its defect in the floor, is cleaned carefully back to its junction with the floor or transversalis fascia and muscle. A suitable zone approximately 1 cm above the junction of the direct sac with the floor is chosen for incision with the electrocautery. As the sac is cut, the preperitoneal fat literally pops into view (FIGURE 8). This circumscription is carried for 360 degrees about the entire neck of the sac. This allows the tethered sac and its content of preperitoneal fat to be easily returned into the preperitoneal space. The actual size of the direct defect is often smaller than anticipated. On palpation of the defect, there is usually a clear-cut rim of transversalis fascia and muscle that persists, although these layers are often quite thin. The synthetic mesh cone or "plug" is placed into the direct opening such that its rim is directly flush with the transversalis floor. Multiple interrupted 00 absorbable sutures are used to secure the perimeter of cone to the transversalis tissues (FIGURE 9).

Usually eight or more sutures are placed such that none of the preperitoneal fat can protrude between the edge of the cone and the rim of the transversalis. The cremaster is opened anteriorly (FIGURE 10) and a search is made for any indirect hernia, which may require a second cone for repair. The cord structures including the vas are identified and the cremasteric opening is not closed. The onlay "patch" of synthetic mesh is placed over the entire direct floor in the same manner as described in the preceding chapter for indirect hernia. The two tails of mesh are joined together producing the new internal ring (FIGURE 11). The same precautions apply— namely, the mesh must clearly overlap the inguinal ligament inferiorly, the pubic tubercle medially, the entire direct floor and cone centrally, and the internal ring laterally. If this coverage is in doubt, a custom-cut piece of synthetic mesh is prepared. In their original description, Rutkow and Robbins do not suture down the perimeter of the onlay mesh "patch," as in the Lichtenstein repair. However, some surgeons prefer to suture the inferior edge of the patch to the inguinal ligament and the superior edge to the internal oblique muscle, thus creating a hybrid procedure that Rutkow has humorously named the "plugstein."

POSTOPERATIVE CARE The perimeter of the incision is infiltrated with long-acting local anesthetic and the external oblique is reapproximated above the level of the cord using a running 00 absorbable suture that begins at the external ring. Scarpa's fascia may be approximated with absorbable sutures. The skin is approximated with a fine absorbable subcuticular suture. Adhesive skin strips and a dry sterile dressing are applied. The postoperative care is the same as that described earlier for the indirect hernia in Chapter 104. ■

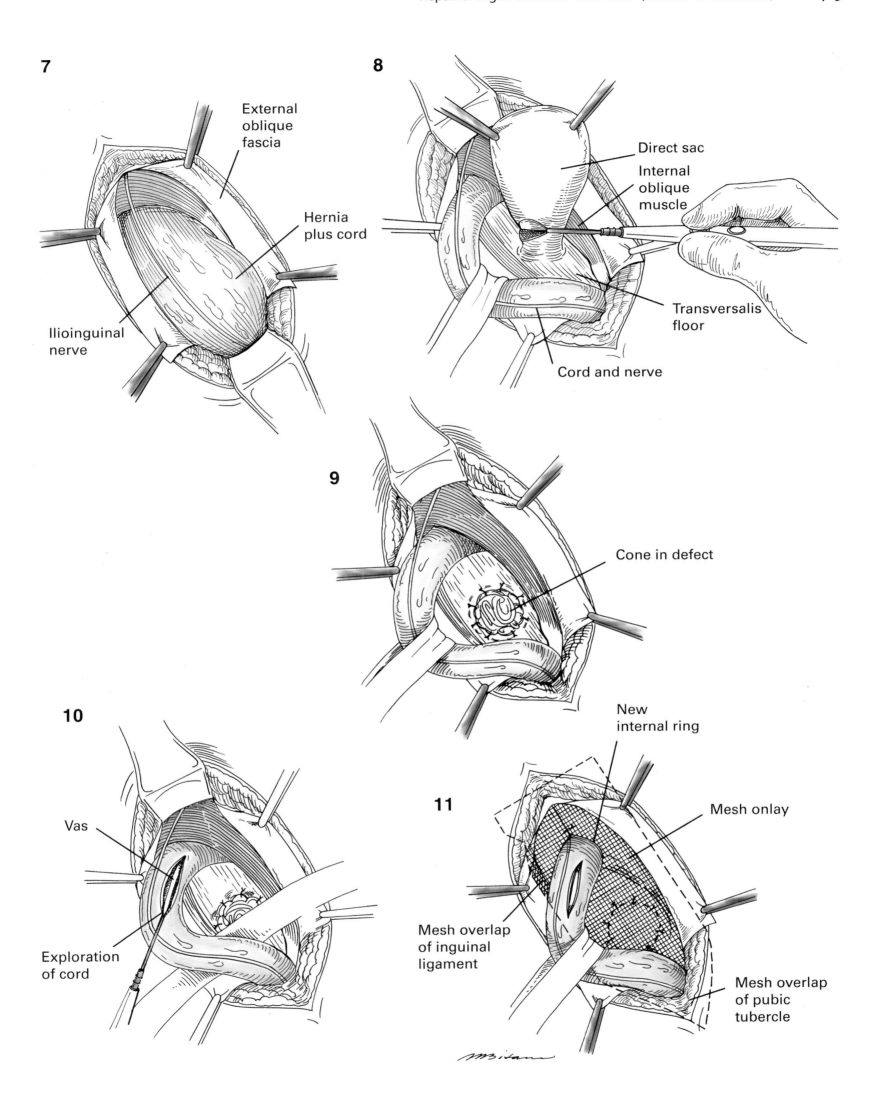

7

External
oblique
fascia

Hernia
plus cord

Ilioinguinal
nerve

8

Direct sac

Internal
oblique
muscle

Transversalis
floor

Cord and nerve

9

Cone in defect

10

Vas

Exploration
of cord

11

New
internal ring

Mesh onlay

Mesh overlap
of inguinal
ligament

Mesh overlap
of pubic
tubercle

REPAIR OF FEMORAL HERNIA

INDICATIONS All femoral hernias should be repaired unless contraindicated by the patient's condition.

PREOPERATIVE PREPARATION The preoperative preparation is directed by the patient's general condition. When the contents of the hernia sac are strangulated, the fluid and electrolyte balance is restored by Ringer's lactate solution administered intravenously. Antibiotics are instituted if the examination indicates the possibility of nonviability of the bowel and consequent necessity for resection of intestine. Sufficient time is taken to fully resuscitate the patient. Constant gastric suction is instituted. A slowing of the pulse and a good output of urine are signs favorable to early surgical intervention. Uncomplicated femoral hernias may be repaired as ambulatory surgical procedures.

ANESTHESIA (See Chapter 104, page 406)

POSITION The patient is placed in a supine position with the knees slightly flexed to lessen the tension in the groin. The entire table is tilted slightly with the patient's head down.

OPERATIVE PREPARATION The skin is prepared in the routine manner. A sterile transparent plastic drape may be used to cover the operative area.

INCISION AND EXPOSURE The surgeon should have in mind the relationship of the hernia sac to the deep femoral vessels and Poupart's ligament (FIGURE 1). The usual incision for inguinal hernia is made just above Poupart's ligament in the line of skin cleavage (FIGURE 2). The incision above Poupart's ligament is preferred because it gives the best exposure of the neck of the sac and provides better exposure if bowel resection and anastomosis are necessary. The incision is made and carried down to the external oblique fascia. After the fascia has been dissected free of the subcutaneous fat, retractors are inserted in the wound. The external oblique fascia is divided in the direction of its fibers, as in the incision for inguinal hernia (Chapter 104). The round ligament or spermatic cord is retracted upward along with the margin of the conjoined tendon (FIGURE 3). The peritoneum, covered by transversalis fascia, now bulges in the wound. The neck of the hernia sac is freed from the surrounding tissues.

DETAILS OF PROCEDURE The operator must now choose one of two procedures. If the sac can be pulled upward through the femoral canal to the surface, it may be unnecessary to open the abdominal cavity until the sac itself is opened. This is facilitated by retracting the neck of the sac upward with forceps, while the operator applies counterpressure below Poupart's

ligament through the hernial mass (FIGURE 4). If the sac cannot be reduced from beneath Poupart's ligament by this maneuver, it becomes necessary to dissect the subcutaneous tissue from the lower leaf of the external oblique until the hernial sac is exposed as it appears in the femoral canal beneath Poupart's ligament (FIGURE 5). Following this procedure, it is frequently possible to withdraw the hernial sac from the femoral canal, converting the femoral hernia to a diverticular type of direct hernia (FIGURE 6).

If the contents of the hernial sac appear to be reduced so that it can be opened without possible injury to incarcerated bowel, the sac is opened (FIGURE 7). A purse-string suture, which should include transversalis fascia as well as peritoneum, is placed at the junction of the sac and the peritoneal cavity so that when it is tied, no residual peritoneal pouch remains (FIGURES 8 and 9). Great care is taken that the suture closing the neck of the sac does not include intestine or omentum.

CLOSURE There are several methods of preventing recurrence of the hernia. The transversalis fascia and the aponeurotic margin of the transverse abdominal muscle may be approximated from the spine of the pubis upward along Cooper's ligament (FIGURE 10), as in the repair of a direct inguinal hernia by the McVay technique (Chapter 106, page 416). It is essential to have adequate exposure of the iliac vessels such that they are not injured when these interrupted sutures (FIGURES 11 and 12) are placed. Several sutures are taken in Cooper's ligament and the lacunar ligament on the inferior edge of Poupart's ligament in order to close the femoral canal (FIGURE 11). The iliac vessels should not be constricted as the transition suture is placed near the medial wall of the femoral vein. The repair then proceeds laterally in the McVay manner, with interrupted sutures securing the conjoint tendon (internal oblique muscle) to the shelving edge of the inguinal ligament (FIGURE 12). The round ligament in the female or the cord in the male is returned to normal position or transplanted as in other types of hernia repair. The external oblique is closed without constriction about the cord or round ligament, followed by the usual approximation of the subcutaneous tissue and skin. A continuous subcutaneous absorbable suture is used to approximate the skin. Adhesive strips and a dry sterile dressing are then applied.

POSTOPERATIVE CARE It is wise to keep the thigh slightly flexed during the immediate postoperative period. The patient is encouraged to ambulate as soon as possible. Heavy manual labor, especially such as which greatly increases intra-abdominal tension, should be avoided for about 1 month. ∎

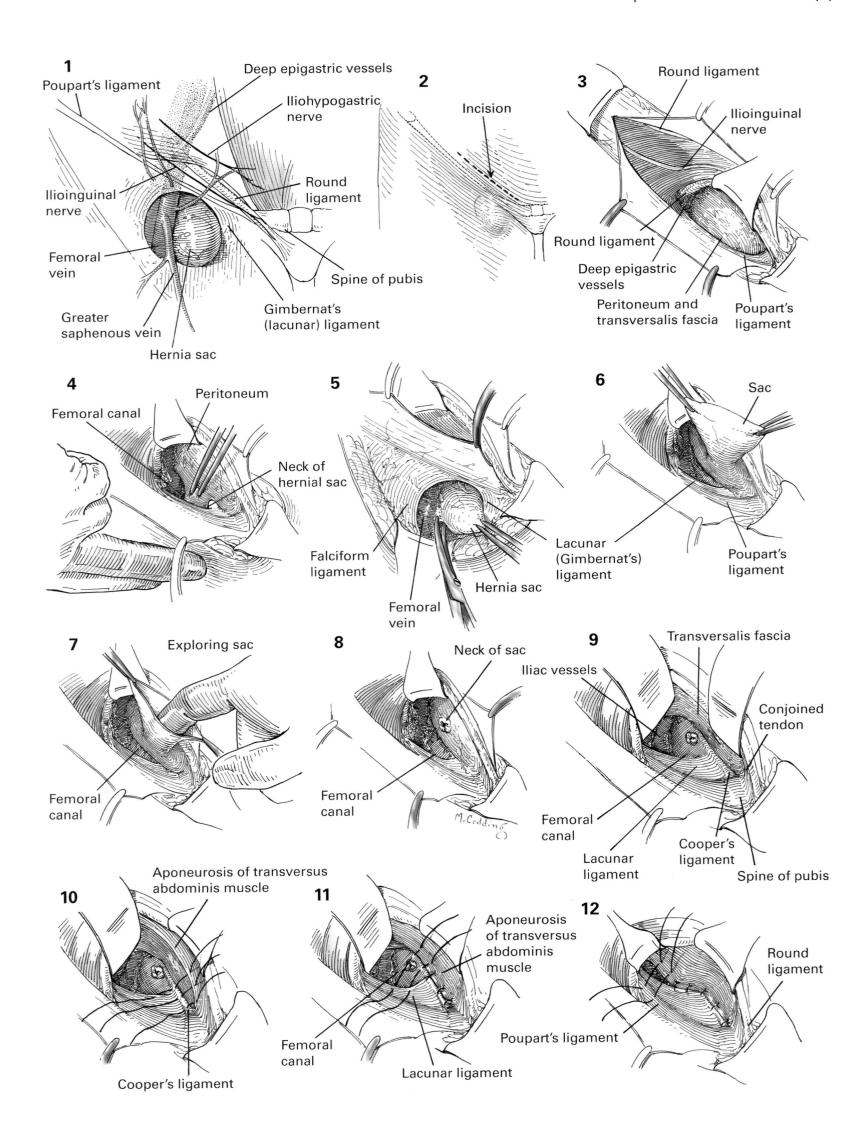

1
Poupart's ligament
Deep epigastric vessels
Iliohypogastric nerve
Round ligament
Ilioinguinal nerve
Femoral vein
Spine of pubis
Greater saphenous vein
Gimbernat's (lacunar) ligament
Hernia sac

2
Incision

3
Round ligament
Ilioinguinal nerve
Round ligament
Deep epigastric vessels
Peritoneum and transversalis fascia
Poupart's ligament

4
Femoral canal
Peritoneum
Neck of hernial sac

5
Falciform ligament
Femoral vein
Hernia sac
Lacunar (Gimbernat's) ligament

6
Sac
Lacunar (Gimbernat's) ligament
Poupart's ligament

7
Exploring sac
Femoral canal

8
Neck of sac
Femoral canal

9
Transversalis fascia
Iliac vessels
Conjoined tendon
Femoral canal
Lacunar ligament
Cooper's ligament
Spine of pubis

10
Aponeurosis of transversus abdominis muscle
Cooper's ligament

11
Aponeurosis of transversus abdominis muscle
Femoral canal
Lacunar ligament

12
Round ligament
Poupart's ligament

M. Cedding

REPAIR OF FEMORAL HERNIA WITH MESH

INDICATIONS All femoral hernias should be repaired unless contraindicated by the physical or medical condition of the patient. Incarceration with possible strangulation is a concern, as the femoral opening is small and its boundaries are unyielding. Ultrasound imaging studies may be useful when the diagnosis is difficult.

PREOPERATIVE PREPARATION The preoperative preparation is determined by the general condition of the patient. Uncomplicated femoral hernias may be repaired in an ambulatory surgery setting. Incarcerated femoral hernias without gastrointestinal signs or symptoms should be repaired expeditiously, while symptomatic hernias are treated urgently. Strangulation requires hospitalization and resuscitation of the patient with nasogastric tube decompression, intravenous rehydration, and parenteral antibiotics. Any general medical conditions are evaluated and sufficient time is allowed for volume and electrolyte stabilization. Improved vital signs and a good urine output indicate readiness for surgery.

ANESTHESIA Deep sedation with infiltration of a local anesthetic as a field block may be used in elective cases, as can spinal or epidural anesthetic techniques. Patients with strangulation and obstruction should have general anesthesia with an endotracheal tube and cuff to lessen the threat of tracheal aspiration.

POSITION The patient is placed in a supine position with the knees slightly flexed by a pillow so as to lessen the tension in the groin.

OPERATIVE PREPARATION The hair in the planned operative site is clipped and the skin prepared in the routine manner. Parenteral antibiotics appropriate for prophylaxis against the usual skin bacteria are given immediately prior to the start of the procedure and in sufficient time to reach therapeutic tissue levels.

INCISION AND EXPOSURE It is important that the surgeon understand the regional anatomy of the femoral space. This opening is approximately 1 to 1½ cm in diameter and lies directly lateral to the pubic tubercle but inferior to the inguinal ligament (FIGURE 1). The fascia overlying the pectineus muscle forms the posterior wall, whereas the lateral aspect is bounded by the slightly compressible femoral vein as it emerges under the inguinal ligament. Clinically, the femoral herniation presents as a mass that may be confused with superficial inguinal lymphadenopathy. In thin patients, the line of the inguinal ligament from the anterior superior spine to the pubic tubercle can be projected and the femoral herniation will clearly present below this, being immediately lateral to the pubic tubercle and medial to the pulsation of the femoral vessels. If the surgeon is certain of this diagnosis, which may be aided by the use of ultrasonography, then the lower limited oblique incision directly over the mass may be made (FIGURE 2B). If the diagnosis is in doubt, the patient is obese, or the possibility of strangulation exists, then the upper incision (FIGURE 2A) is made so as to provide maximum exposure and flexibility. This incision is slightly lower than that made for the usual inguinal hernia. It is above and parallel in general to the inguinal ligament with a more transverse medial extension. The incision is made and carried down to the external oblique fascia. The fascia over the canal is cleaned so as to expose the external ring. The external oblique fascia is divided in the direction of its fibers in the manner used for exposure in inguinal hernias. A pair of hemostats are placed on the superior and inferior leaves of the external oblique, which is then cleaned by blunt dissection down to the internal oblique muscle superiorly and the shelving edge of the inguinal ligament inferiorly. The round ligament or spermatic cord with attached ilioinguinal nerve is dissected free and retracted superiorly either with a rubber Penrose drain or a Richardson retractor (FIGURE 3). The transversalis fascia constituting the floor of the canal is explored to rule out any direct herniation, and thereafter the region of the internal ring is explored to rule out the presence of an indirect herniation.

DETAILS OF PROCEDURE The inferior leaf of the external oblique is retracted superiorly and the femoral herniation becomes apparent as it emerges just under the inguinal ligament lateral to the pubic tubercle. This same exposure is obtained if the lower incision is made directly over the hernia. The sac is grasped and, using a combination of sharp and blunt dissection, it is freed from the surrounding fat of the upper thigh (FIGURE 4). As the dissection proceeds, the herniation is found to occur through a narrow opening that is approximately the size of the surgeon's fifth finger. Most often the sac contains preperitoneal fat or omentum, which can be reduced; however, should strangulated gangrenous bowel be encountered, the surgeon must plan for resection with a synchronous laparotomy.

After successful reduction in an uncomplicated case, it is not necessary to open the sac. This is usually invaginated back through the femoral opening, which now presents as a defined hole (FIGURE 5). A synthetic plug is made according to the method of Lichtenstein by rolling up a piece of synthetic mesh approximately 2 by 15 cm in length. This spiral winding creates a cylinder of mesh that is grasped with a Babcock clamp (FIGURE 6) and then inserted into the femoral opening such that a few millimeters protrude externally. Three quadrants of the cylinder are secured with interrupted nonabsorbable sutures of polypropylene or nylon. Each is anchored to the adjacent fascia with the suture extending well into the center of the rolled cylinder so as to prevent an intussusception of the mesh. The superior suture attaches to the inguinal ligament, the medial one to the lacunar ligament and fascia investing the pubic tubercle, and the inferior one to the fascia over the pectineus muscle. No suture is placed laterally, as this wall is the femoral vein (FIGURE 7). The external oblique fascia is reapproximated with either interrupted or running nonabsorbable sutures and then routine closure of Scarpa's fascia and the skin is performed. A small dressing is applied to cover the incision.

POSTOPERATIVE CARE In the uncomplicated case, the patient is quickly discharged home with written instructions concerning activities, signs of bleeding or infection, or any other unusual reaction. Most are able to resume normal activities within a few days. ∎

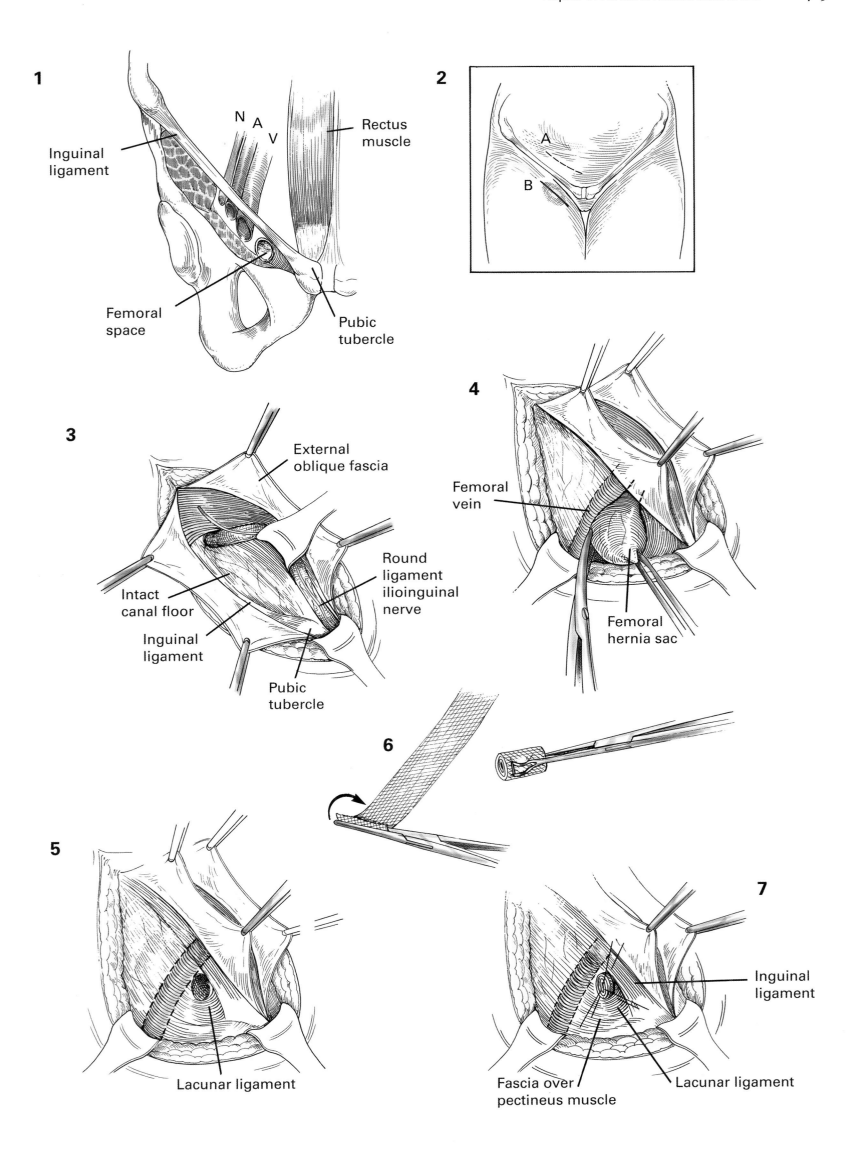

1

Inguinal ligament

N A V

Rectus muscle

Femoral space

Pubic tubercle

2

A

B

3

External oblique fascia

Intact canal floor

Inguinal ligament

Pubic tubercle

Round ligament ilioinguinal nerve

4

Femoral vein

Femoral hernia sac

6

5

Lacunar ligament

7

Inguinal ligament

Fascia over pectineus muscle

Lacunar ligament

LAPAROSCOPIC ANATOMY OF THE INGUINAL REGION

This chapter shows the key anatomic features of importance that the skilled surgeon must know thoroughly during any type of laparoscopic operation for inguinal and femoral hernia repair.

The first concept is to recognize that the parietal peritoneum covers certain structures forming five ligaments that are useful landmarks in identifying the hernia spaces when approaching the groin from the intraperitoneal route as in the TAPP repair. These ligaments include the median umbilical ligament (1) running from the bladder to the umbilicus, the medial umbilical ligaments (3), which are the remnants of the obliterated umbilical arteries, and the lateral umbilical ligaments (4) formed by the peritoneum covering the inferior epigastric vessels (13). The spatial relationships of these ligaments allow recognition of the various types of hernias. A direct inguinal hernia (19) occurs in the medial space bounded by the inferior epigastric vessels or lateral umbilical ligament, the iliopubic tract (21), the pubic tubercle (23) (the medial end of the muscular conjoined tendon [internal oblique muscle]). An indirect inguinal hernia presents through the internal ring (18) above the iliopubic tract and is lateral to the lateral umbilical ligament containing the epigastric vessels (13) on the posterior surface of the rectus muscle (2). A view of the femoral hernia space (20) can be seen below the iliopubic tract (21) and medial to the femoral vessels exiting through the femoral canal. During the laparoscopic repair, the direct, indirect, and femoral spaces should all be covered with mesh.

The second important concept concerns the spaces that occur beneath the peritoneal covering (17). The preperitoneal space is the space bounded by the peritoneum posteriorly and the transversalis fascia anteriorly. The space of Retzius is that space between the pubis and the bladder. The lateral extent of this space is named Bogros' space. The transversalis fascia forms the floor of the inguinal canal and the iliopectineal arch, iliopubic tract, and crura of the deep inguinal ring. The iliopectineal arch divides the vascular compartment (iliac vessels) from the neuromuscular compartment (iliopsoas muscle, femoral nerve, and the lateral femoral cutaneous nerve). The iliopubic tract is an aponeurotic band that begins near the anterior superior iliac spine and inserts on the pubic tubercle (23) medially. In its medial extent, it contributes to the formation of Cooper's ligament (22). It forms the inferior margin of the deep musculoaponeurotic layer made up of the transversus abdominis muscle and aponeurosis and the transversalis fascia. Laterally, it extends to the iliacus and psoas fascia. It forms with fibers of the transversalis fascia, the anterior margin of the femoral sheath and the medial border of the femoral ring and canal. Its lower margin is attached to the inguinal ligament. The iliopubic tract is an important landmark. Dissection or tacking of preperitoneal mesh should not take place inferior to the iliopubic tract except in the limited region of Cooper's ligament. Dissection or tack placement centrally beneath the iliopubic tract will injure the femoral vein, artery, and nerve, whereas placement laterally may damage the lumbar nerve branches. The superior and inferior crura of the deep inguinal ring are formed by the transversalis fascia. Cooper's ligament is formed by the periosteum of the superior pubic ramus and the iliopubic tract.

The inferior epigastric vessels give off two branches: the external spermatic vessel that travels in the spermatic cord and the iliopubic branch. The latter may form a corona mortis. This vascular anomaly presents as a branch of either the inferior epigastric or the external iliac that passes over the pubic tubercle en route to the obturator system. Either the arterial or the venous system may be involved in this "triangle of death," which may cause significant hemorrhage during dissection and exposure of Cooper's ligament or mesh fixation with penetrating tacks.

Finally, there are two zones that must be avoided during preperitoneal dissection and fixation of mesh. The first is the lateral zone that is bounded on the medial side by the spermatic cord, superiorly by the iliopubic tract and by the iliac crest laterally. This is known as the "triangle of pain." (the next Chapter 112, FIGURE 2) This area contains the femoral (10), lateral femoral cutaneous (8), anterior femoral cutaneous, and the femoral branch of the genitofemoral nerves. Injury to these nerves may cause chronic neuralgia. The second is the inferior zone bounded by the vas deferens (24) medially, the gonadal vessels (15) laterally, and posteriorly by the peritoneal edge. This zone is known as the "triangle of doom," as it contains the external iliac vein (12), the deep circumflex iliac vein, and the external iliac artery (11). (Chapter 112, FIGURE 2, page 433) ■

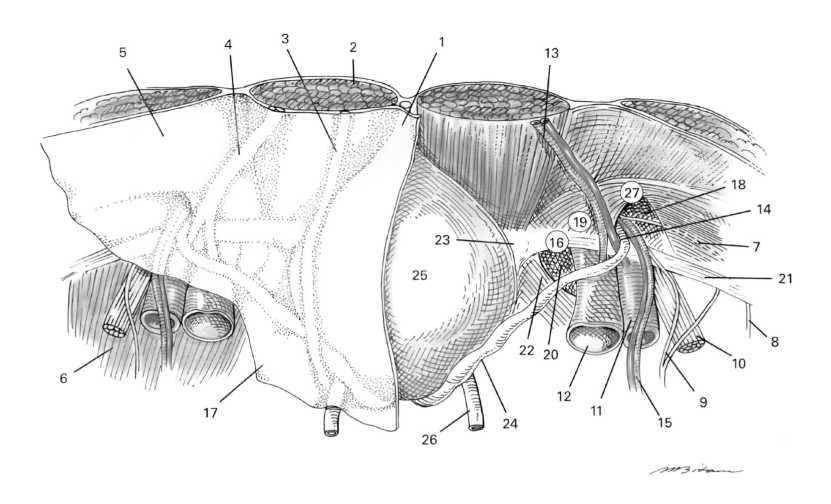

1 Median umbilical ligament	14 Spermatic cord
2 Rectus muscle	15 Spermatic A & V
3 Medial umbilical ligament	16 Corona mortis area
4 Lateral umbilical ligament	17 Peritoneum
5 Lateral abdominal wall muscles	18 Indirect area
6 Iliopsoas muscle	19 Direct area
7 Ilioinguinal nerve	20 Femoral area
8 Lateral femoral cutaneous nerve	21 Iliopubic tract
9 Genitofemoral nerve	22 Cooper's ligament
10 Femoral nerve	23 Pubic tubercle
11 External iliac artery	24 Vas deferens
12 External iliac vein	25 Bladder
13 Inferior epigastric A & V	26 Ureter
	27 Conjoint tendon

REPAIR OF INGUINAL HERNIA, LAPAROSCOPIC TRANSABDOMINAL PREPERITONEAL (TAPP)

INDICATIONS The indications for inguinal hernia repair have been described in the preceding chapters. The techniques that will be described include the transabdominal preperitoneal (TAPP) and the totally extraperitoneal (TEP). Laparoscopic repair may be applied to indirect, direct, or femoral hernias. Laparoscopic inguinal herniorrhaphy is contraindicated in the presence of intraperitoneal infection, irreversible coagulopathy, and in patients who are poor risks for general anesthesia. Relative contraindications include large sliding hernias that contain colon, long-standing irreducible scrotal hernias, ascites, and previous suprapubic surgery. For TEP repairs, specific relative contraindications include incarceration and bowel ischemia. A thorough knowledge of the anatomy of the inguinal region is essential when it is approached posteriorly using a laparoscope. The view of this area as seen from the intraperitoneal perspective in the TAPP repair, as well as the one from the preperitoneal perspective in TEP, is shown on the preceding Chapter 111, entitled Laparoscopic Anatomy of the Inguinal Region. In addition, proficiency with laparoscopic skills or mentored experience with this type of hernia repair is strongly recommended.

TRANSABDOMINAL PREPERITONEAL (TAPP)

PREOPERATIVE PREPARATION The patient must be a suitable candidate for general anesthesia. Anticoagulation, aspirin, and antiplatelet drugs such as Clopidogrel Bisulfate (Plavix) must be discontinued in advance of the procedure in order to avoid postoperative hematoma formation. Preoperative antibiotics should be administered intravenously within one hour of the incision.

EQUIPMENT AND SUPPLIES All laparoscopic repairs use some form of prosthetic material. These include synthetic mesh created from polypropylene (Marlex or Prolene), Dacron (Mersilene), or polyester (Parietex). Expanded polytetrafluoroethylene (e-PTFE) (Gortex) is supplied as an extruded sheet. Mesh is generally preferred to e-PTFE because the structure allows fibrous in growth and hence greater fixation to the surrounding tissues. E-PTFE, composite mesh, or biologic materials are preferred in situations in which the prosthetic would be in touch with the intestine or other intra-abdominal organs, as it promotes less of a fibrous response and lessens adhesions to these structures. In this regard, e-PTFE has been modified to have polypropylene on one side. This so-called "dual mesh" might be useful in cases in which the mesh cannot be completely covered by peritoneum.

Fixation of the mesh is necessary to prevent migration and the tendency for the mesh to shrink overtime. There are a variety of tacking devices that may be used including helical coils, shaped like a key ring, and anchors. They may be absorbable or nonabsorbable metal. Most are delivered with 5-mm disposable instruments.

ANESTHESIA General endotracheal anesthesia is required.

POSITION The patient is placed in the supine position, and the arms are tucked. The operating room setup and port placements are shown in FIGURE 1.

OPERATIVE PREPARATION Skin hair is removed with a clipper. A catheter is placed in the bladder and removed at the end of the case.

INCISION AND EXPOSURE FIGURE 1 shows the typical room setup for a left inguinal hernia repair by either TAPP or TEP. The surgeon stands contralateral to the hernia. The camera operator is next to the surgeon and the assistant directly across. One or two monitors may be positioned at the foot of the operating table. In this chapter, a left indirect inguinal TAPP is shown with the surgeon on the patient's right side, whereas the TEP repair shown in Chapter 113 demonstrates a right direct inguinal repair where the surgeon would be positioned on the patient's left side.

FIGURES 3 to 7 illustrate a TAPP for a left indirect inguinal hernia. The Hasson technique as described in Chapter 11 is used to gain access to the peritoneal cavity. A supraumbilical incision is made for placement of the Hasson trocar. The patient is placed in a gentle Trendelenburg position.

A 10-mm 30-degree laparoscope is passed. Two 5-mm trocars are placed under direct laparoscopic vision in the right and left midabdomen at the level of the umbilicus (FIGURE 1). A diagnostic laparoscopy is performed and the hernia spaces inspected for additional hernias. Utilizing the two lateral trocars, a peritoneal flap is created using laparoscopic scissors and electrocautery. The incision is begun lateral to the medial umbilical ligament, which should not be divided, as this may cause bleeding from a vestigial umbilical artery. An incision is made in the peritoneum 2 to 3 cm above the hernia sac and carried laterally to the anterior iliac spine. The preperitoneal space is entered and blunt dissection is carried out with a laparoscopic Kittner dissector in the avascular plane between the peritoneum and the transversalis fascia. For a direct hernia, the dissection is begun laterally to expose the cord structures and epigastric vessels. As the flap is dissected, the critical anatomic landmarks from medial to lateral include Cooper's ligament, the inferior epigastric vessels, the vas deferens, and the lateral zone or fossa (FIGURE 2). The sites of an indirect and direct hernia are shown. Care should be to avoid dissection in the area labeled the Triangle of Pain which contains sensory nerves (FIGURE 2), injury to which may cause chronic pain in the inguinal region, testicle, or thigh. Likewise care is exercised to avoid dissection in the Triangle of Doom (FIGURE 2), the area which contains the major vascular structures. A corona mortis, a branch of the inferior epigastric may be seen on the lateral edge of Cooper's ligament in 30% of patients (Chapter 111). This must be avoided when dissecting Cooper's ligament or tacking the mesh in order to prevent troublesome bleeding. The left indirect sac is carefully teased and dissected away from the cord structures as it is brought back into the preperitoneal space. A small indirect sac may be completely reduced, but a larger sac that extends into the scrotum may need to be divided. Downward traction on the cord structures facilitates dissection of fatty tissue in the spermatic cord (cord lipoma). The iliopubic tract is identified (FIGURE 3). The peritoneal flap is developed inferiorly. Care is taken to avoid injury to the genital branch of the genitofemoral nerve and the lateral femoral cutaneous nerve (Chapter 111). After an inferior flap is created, the following structures are identified: the inferior epigastric vessels, the symphysis pubis, and the rectus abdominis. Dissection is then carried medially to the contralateral pubic tubercle to allow sufficient overlap for the mesh placement to cover all of the potential hernia spaces. FIGURE 3 demonstrates the final peritoneal flap and space.

For bilateral hernias, the space of Retzius is dissected through two lateral incisions avoiding division of the urachus. This creates a large common space connecting the two sides.

The mesh is introduced through the 10-mm trocar (FIGURE 4). For a unilateral repair, the mesh can either be a preformed one or a sheet that is at least 15 × 10 cm in size. Although not shown in the illustrations for a bilateral repair, two similar sheets of mesh or one large (30 × 15 cm) may be employed. For the unilateral repair, the mesh is placed over the peritoneal opening so that it covers all of the hernia spaces (direct, indirect, and femoral). A wide overlap is necessary and extends from the contralateral pubic tubercle medially to the ipsilateral anterior iliac spine. The mesh is unrolled and positioned with generous overlap in all directions. A slit may be made for the cord structures. Tacking devices are applied medially to the superior edge and inferior one edge. This is facilitated by direct counter-pressure by the surgeon's nondominant hand. The lateral edge aspect of the mesh is usually not tacked into place because of potential nerve injury (lateral femoral cutaneous and the femoral branch of the genitofemoral nerve). The mesh is secured medially to the tissues immediately adjacent to the contralateral and the ipsilateral pubic tubercle and Cooper's ligament (FIGURE 6). Any redundancy in the inferior edge of the mesh should be trimmed in order to avoid rolling up.

The next step is to close the redundant peritoneum over the mesh. The mesh needs to be completely covered. Once the mesh is in place, the patient is taken out of the reverse Trendelenburg position. Desufflation to 10 mm Hg is accomplished. The peritoneal flap is then tacked to the anterior abdominal wall or sutured closed (FIGURE 7). ■

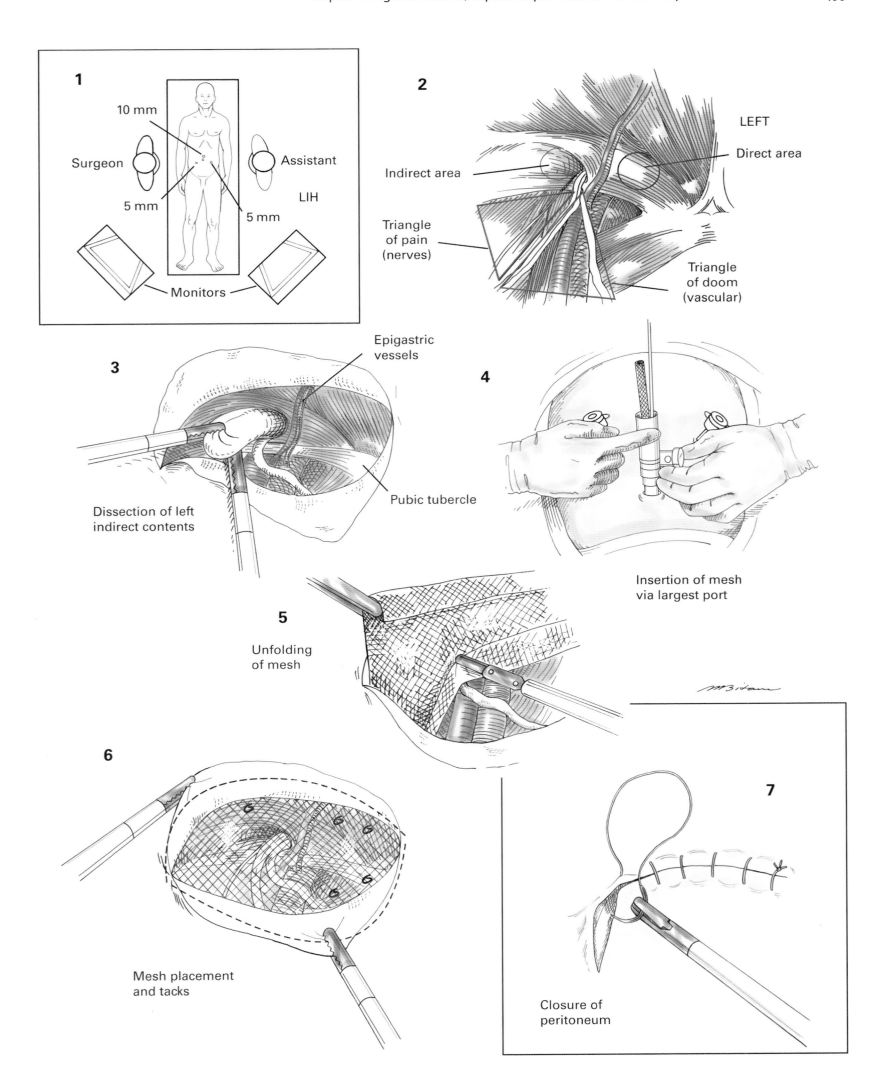

1

10 mm

Surgeon

Assistant

5 mm

5 mm

LIH

Monitors

2

LEFT

Indirect area

Direct area

Triangle
of pain
(nerves)

Triangle
of doom
(vascular)

3

Epigastric
vessels

Dissection of left
indirect contents

Pubic tubercle

4

Insertion of mesh
via largest port

5

Unfolding
of mesh

6

Mesh placement
and tacks

7

Closure of
peritoneum

CHAPTER 113 REPAIR OF INGUINAL HERNIA, LAPAROSCOPIC TOTALLY EXTRAPERITONEAL (TEP)

Total extraperitoneal (TEP) approach avoids entering the peritoneal cavity; hence, there is the theoretical advantage of less probability for visceral injury or incisional hernias. In addition, it avoids the problem of closure of the peritoneal flap. It is more difficult than TAPP because the operative space is tight. The preoperative preparation, anesthesia considerations, patient position, and operating room setup are the same as those for TAPP.

EQUIPMENT AND SUPPLIES A one- or three-component dissecting balloon should be used to do the initial dissection of the preperitoneal space (FIGURE 1A, B, and C).

INCISION AND EXPOSURE A 2-cm incision is made just lateral and inferior to the umbilicus on the same side as the hernia. The muscle is retracted laterally so as to expose the posterior rectus fascia. Blunt dissection with the s-retractors or finger opens the preperitoneal space (FIGURE 2B). The dissection of this space is facilitated by the use of a single- or three-component dissecting balloon. This is inserted into the space via the umbilical incision. The bulb insufflator device is used to expand the balloon. During the insufflation, the surgeon monitors the dissection process with the laparoscope which lies within the dissecting balloon (FIGURES 1A, B). The expansion is gradual. It is important to have all the creases in the dissecting balloon flatten out. The balloon is desufflated and removed. The smaller stay balloon is then inserted (FIGURE 1C) and filled with 40 mL of air. It is used to hold traction on the fascia by being retracted back and locked. This is attached to the CO_2 insufflator, which is set to a pressure of 15 mm Hg. The patient is placed in a slight Trendelenburg position to avoid external compression of the preperitoneal space by the abdominal viscera. The hernia spaces are examined. Two 5-mm trocars are placed in the midline inferior to the umbilicus (FIGURE 2A) The first is two fingerbreadths above the pubic tubercle and the second five fingerbreadths above the pubic tubercle just below the camera port. FIGURE 3 shows the anatomy of the region which is explained in detail in Chapter 111. A right direct inguinal is identified and the area is cleared (FIGURE 4). The pubic tubercle is identified and slight lateral dissection is continued until the obturator vein is visualized. Blunt dissection with laparoscopic Kittner is used to open the preperitoneal space. Small tears in the peritoneum should be repaired in order to prevent competing pneumoperitoneum. If this becomes problematic, a Veress needle or 5-mm trocar can be placed in the peritoneal cavity to release the CO_2 pressure. The spermatic cord is then skeletonized and the preperitoneal space dissected to the same extent as the TAPP. Although the orientation is different, the dissection and the mesh placement are similar to the TAPP. The mesh is cut to the size and shape shown in FIGURE 5. It is then rolled and inserted under direct vision through the 10-mm trocar used for the camera (FIGURE 6). The mesh is unrolled and positioned in order to cover all three hernia areas—indirect, direct, and femoral (FIGURE 7A). It may be tacked medially in place, as described in the TAPP section, avoiding the danger points previously discussed (FIGURE 7A). Alternatively, some surgeons prefer to use a fibrin-based glue to secure fixation, while others use no fixation while relying upon the deflated peritoneum to anchor the mesh. The trocars are removed under direct vision. The CO_2 is slowly vented such that the mesh does not move. The mesh and collapsing peritoneum are observed as the videoscope is removed. The final position of the mesh in the preperitoneal space is shown in the cross-sectional FIGURE 7B.

CLOSURE The fascia is closed with absorbable interrupted suture. The skin is closed with subcuticular absorbable suture. The bladder catheter is removed prior to leaving the operating room.

POSTOPERATIVE CONSIDERATIONS Local anesthetic may be injected into the incision sites or instilled into the preperitoneal space to facilitate pain management. If the patient is able to void urine, then he is discharged the day of the surgery if there are no immediate complications. The patient is also advised not lift greater than 15 lb (about two gallons of milk) for the first week. Return to work is dictated by pain tolerance. Many patients are back to work in 5 to 7 days. ■

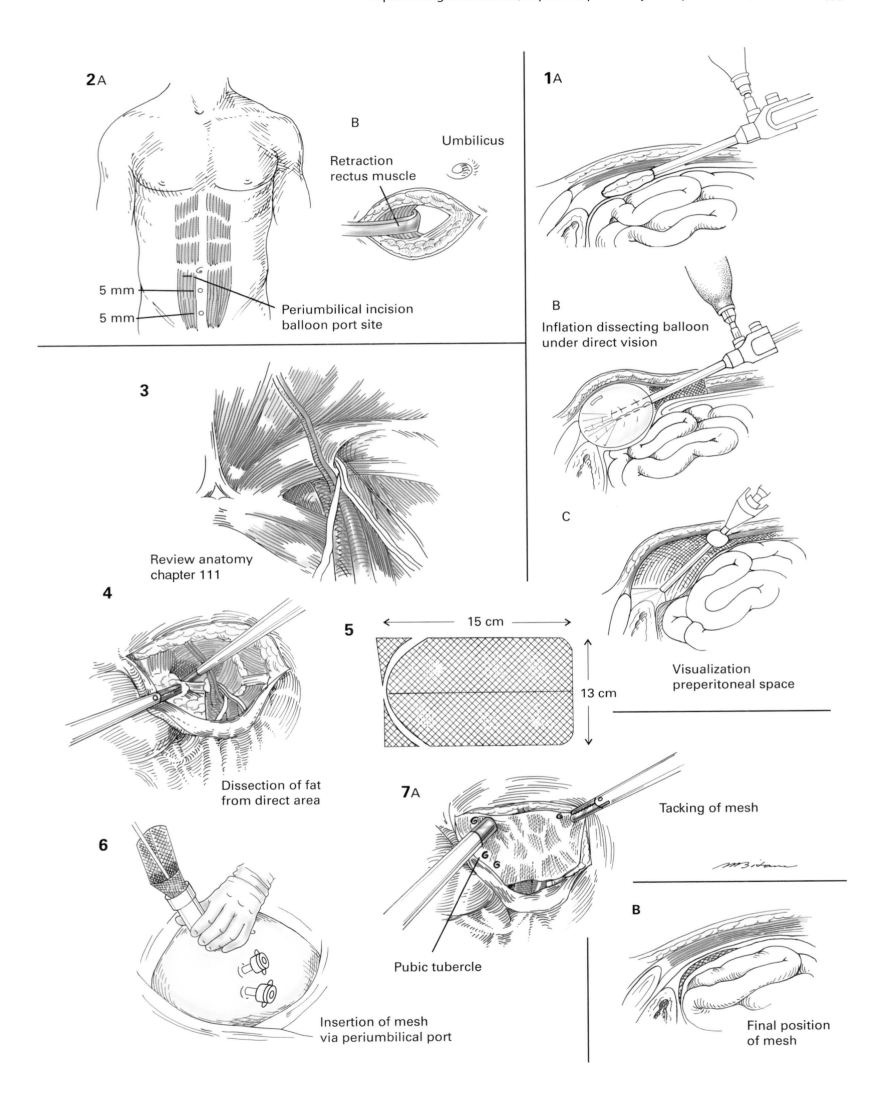

2 A

B

Umbilicus

Retraction
rectus muscle

5 mm

5 mm

Periumbilical incision
balloon port site

3

Review anatomy
chapter 111

4

Dissection of fat
from direct area

6

Insertion of mesh
via periumbilical port

5

15 cm

13 cm

7 A

Pubic tubercle

Tacking of mesh

B

Final position
of mesh

1 A

B

Inflation dissecting balloon
under direct vision

C

Visualization
preperitoneal space

HYDROCELE REPAIR

INDICATIONS A hydrocele of the tunica vaginalis occurring within the first year of life seldom requires operation, since it will often disappear without treatment. Hydroceles that persist after the first year or appear later in life usually require treatment, since they show little tendency toward spontaneous regression. All symptomatic hydroceles in adults or in children older than 2 years should be removed. Most hydroceles are painless, and symptoms arise only from the inconvenience caused by their size or weight. The long-continued presence of a hydrocele infrequently causes atrophy of the testicle. Open operation is the method of choice for removing the hydrocele. Aspiration of the hydrocele contents and injection with sclerosing agents are generally regarded as unsatisfactory treatment because of the high incidence of recurrences and the frequent necessity for repetition of the procedure. Occasionally, severe infection can be introduced by aspiration. Simple aspiration, however, often may be used as a temporary measure in those cases where surgery is contraindicated or must be postponed.

The accuracy of the diagnosis must be ascertained. Great care must be taken to differentiate a hydrocele from a scrotal hernia or tumor of the testicle. Ultrasound imaging can be very useful in these cases. A hernia usually can be reduced, transmits a cough impulse, and is not translucent. A hydrocele cannot be reduced into the inguinal canal and gives no impulse on coughing unless a hernia is also present. In young children, a hydrocele is often associated with a complete congenital type of hernial sac.

ANESTHESIA Either spinal or general anesthesia is satisfactory in adults. General anesthesia is the choice in children. Local infiltration anesthesia is generally unsatisfactory because it fails to abolish abdominal pain produced by traction on the spermatic cord. Uncomplicated hydroceles may be excised as an ambulatory surgical procedure.

POSITION The patient is placed on his back on a level table with his legs slightly separated. The surgeon stands on the side of the table nearest the operative site.

OPERATIVE PREPARATION The skin is prepared routinely, with particular care given to scrubbing the scrotal area. Iodine should be avoided for preparation of the scrotal skin, since it will cause severe excoriation. The area is draped as for any other operation on the scrotum.

INCISION AND EXPOSURE The relationship of the hydrocele of the tunica vaginalis testis to the testicle, epididymis, spermatic cord, and covering layers of the scrotum is shown in FIGURE 1. If the hydrocele is associated with an inguinal hernia, separate incisions are made. If just a hydrocele is present, then after the mass is grasped firmly in one hand so as to stretch the scrotal skin and to fix the hydrocele, an incision 6 to 10 cm long is made on the anterior surface of the scrotum, over the most prominent part of the hydrocele, well away from the testicle that lies inferiorly and posteriorly (FIGURE 2). The skin, dartos muscle, and thin cremasteric fascia are incised and reflected back together as a single layer from the underlying parietal layer of the tunica vaginalis, which is the outer wall of the hydrocele (FIGURES 3 and 4).

DETAILS OF PROCEDURE When the hydrocele is well separated laterally and medially from the overlying layers, its wall is grasped with two Allis forceps, and a trocar attached to a suction tube is thrust into it to evacuate the fluid (FIGURE 5). With a finger in the opening of the sac acting as a guide and providing traction, the surgeon completely separates the wall of the hydrocele from the scrotum so that the spermatic cord and testicle with attached hydrocele sac lie entirely free in the operative field (FIGURES 6, 7, and 8). The hydrocele sac then is opened completely (FIGURE 9). Some surgeons prefer to delay emptying the hydrocele until it has been dissected completely free from the surrounding tissues and delivered outside the scrotum.

In younger men particularly, the testicle is carefully inspected and palpated, since hydrocele has been known to occur in the presence of testicular neoplasm.

The relationship of the testicle to the tunica vaginalis is shown in FIGURE 10. With the walls of the hydrocele sac completely freed and completely opened, the redundant sac wall is trimmed with scissors, leaving only a margin of about 2 cm around the testicle, epididymis, and spermatic cord (FIGURE 10A and B). Great care must be taken to obtain absolute hemostasis, since the smallest bleeding point left uncontrolled is likely to ooze slowly into the loose scrotal tissues, producing a massive scrotal hematoma. Large and painful hematomas that are slowly absorbed after surgery may occur if there is not careful and complete hemostasis.

When the redundant portions of the sac have been excised, the edges are sewed behind the testicle and spermatic cord with interrupted fine suture, thus everting the retained portion of the old hydrocele sac (FIGURES 11 and 12). Some surgeons prefer not to evert the sac but to place a continuous fine absorbable hemostatic suture along its margin. In children especially, the contents of the upper portion of the cord should be inspected for a possible hernia sac.

CLOSURE The testicle and spermatic cord are replaced carefully in the scrotum, care being taken that no abnormal rotation of the cord has occurred. The testicle may be anchored to the bottom of the wall of the scrotum with one or two absorbable sutures to prevent torsion of the cord (FIGURE 13). The dartos fascia is closed with interrupted absorbable sutures (FIGURE 14). A small Penrose drain may be brought out through a small stab wound at the most dependent portion of the scrotum. This allows escape of blood and prevents hematoma. The skin is closed with a subcutaneous absorbable suture.

POSTOPERATIVE CARE The scrotum should be supported by a suspensory for 1 to 2 weeks postoperatively. Ice bags should be placed under the scrotum for the first 24 hours. The dressing should be changed daily. The drain is removed in 24 to 48 hours, depending on the amount of drainage. Significant pain or swelling may signal a hematoma or torsion, which can be differentiated with duplex ultrasound scanning. Plain absorbable skin sutures will fall out as they disintegrate. The patient may be ambulatory immediately after surgery. ■

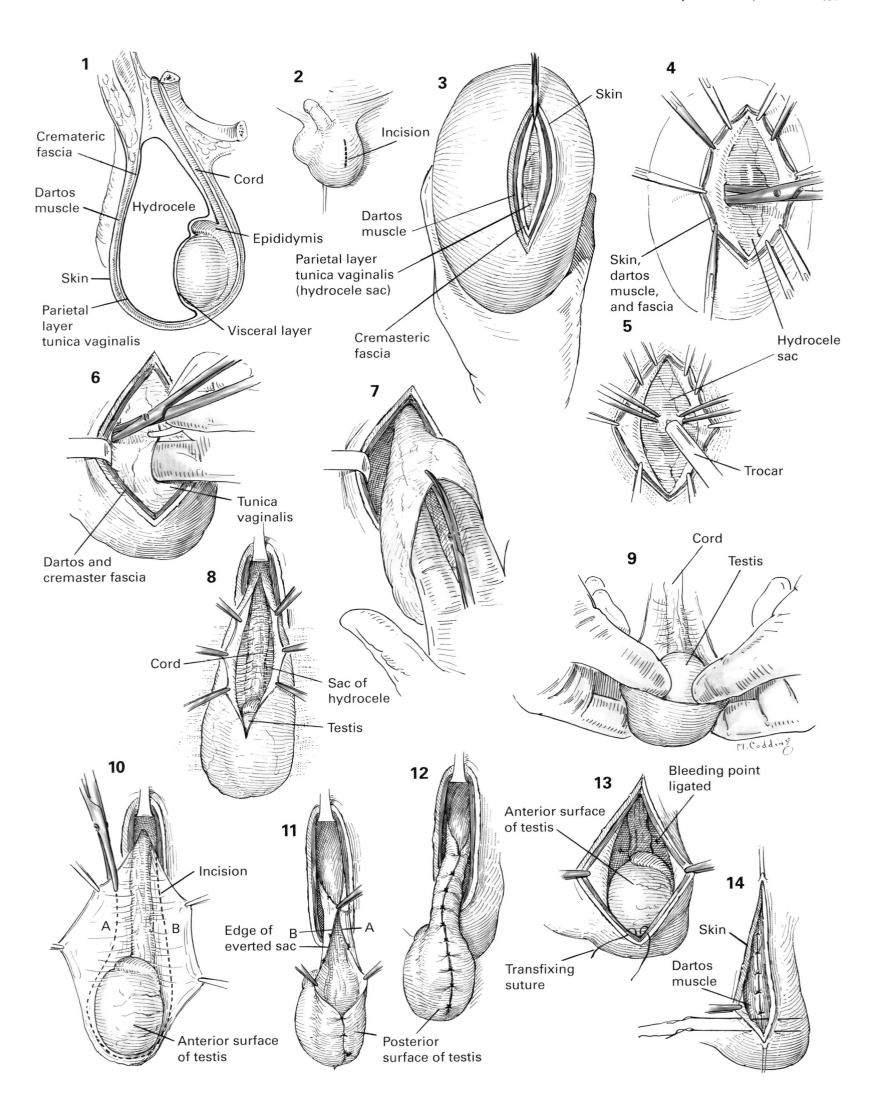

1 Cremateric fascia · Cord · Dartos muscle · Hydrocele · Skin · Epididymis · Parietal layer tunica vaginalis · Visceral layer

2 Incision

3 Skin · Dartos muscle · Parietal layer tunica vaginalis (hydrocele sac) · Cremasteric fascia

4 Skin, dartos muscle, and fascia · Hydrocele sac

5 Trocar

6 Dartos and cremaster fascia · Tunica vaginalis

7

8 Cord · Sac of hydrocele · Testis

9 Cord · Testis

10 Incision · A · B · Anterior surface of testis

11 Edge of everted sac · B · A · Posterior surface of testis

12

13 Bleeding point ligated · Anterior surface of testis · Transfixing suture

14 Skin · Dartos muscle

SECTION X
ENDOCRINE

CHAPTER 115

THYROIDECTOMY, SUBTOTAL

INDICATIONS The indications for subtotal thyroidectomy are decreasing because of the lower incidence of endemic goiters, both colloid and nodular, and the increasing effectiveness of medical therapy in patients who present with thyrotoxicosis, whether this is due to Graves' disease or to nodular toxic goiter.

A definite indication for subtotal thyroidectomy is the removal of a solitary nodule in a young person, especially female, when the mass does not take up radioiodide on thyroid scan and hence is suspected of being malignant. A simple fine needle aspiration may yield a suspicious cytology. Total lobectomy ensures a better margin and allows pathologic examination of the excised thyroid lobe for multicentric foci should a malignant tumor be found. Many surgeons combine a total lobectomy on the involved side with a subtotal lobectomy on the alternate side.

The controversy as to whether surgical or medical treatment for thyrotoxicosis is desirable in patients younger than 35 to 40 years and in pregnant patients has yet to be resolved, but it is generally agreed that the use of radioactive iodine is contraindicated. Surgical removal should be considered if antithyroid drugs are tolerated poorly or required in large, prolonged doses and if thyrotoxicosis recurs after an apparently successful medication regimen. In the poor-risk patient or one who has had a recurrence of toxicity following previous thyroid surgery, medical therapy is usually the treatment of choice. Also, some pregnant patients may be best treated with antithyroid drugs in order to defer surgery until after the patient has delivered. However, thyroid replacement is given daily once the patient is euthyroid to prevent the development of a goiter in the fetus.

Subtotal thyroidectomy or total thyroidectomy is performed for an enlarged thyroid gland that produced pressure symptoms or an undesirable cosmetic effect (endemic goiter), for toxic goiters, and occasionally for inflammatory conditions such as Riedel's struma and Hashimoto's disease.

PREOPERATIVE PREPARATION The only indication for emergency thyroidectomy is in that exceedingly rare situation where pressure symptoms develop rapidly due to intrathyroid hemorrhage. In all other situations thyroidectomy should be considered an elective procedure performed when the patient is in optimal physical health. This is true particularly in thyrotoxicosis.

Patients with thyrotoxicosis should be treated with antithyroid drugs preferentially until they are euthyroid. Because the (thiourea) compounds block the synthesis of thyroxine but do not inhibit the release of the hormone from existing colloid stores, the time required for symptomatic improvement may vary widely from 2 weeks to as long as 3 months. The variability is in part related to the size of the gland, since large goiters usually contain more colloid. When the patient has become euthyroid, iodine—given as Lugol's solution, potassium iodide solution, or tablets or syrup of hydriodic acid—can be administered for 10 days before surgery (optional). If this procedure is followed, almost any thyroidectomy can be performed under optimal conditions. If significant tachycardia due to an increased intraoperative or postoperative release of thyroid hormone is encountered, propranolol should be used to control it.

ANESTHESIA Endotracheal intubation is preferred, particularly if there has been long-standing pressure against the trachea, substernal extension, or severe thyrotoxicosis. For the severely toxic or apprehensive patient, a short-acting intravenous barbiturate may be given in the patient's room to avoid undue excitement. General inhalation anesthetic agents are used.

POSITION The patient is placed in a semierect position with a folded sheet or shoulder roll underneath the shoulders so that the head is sharply angulated backward (FIGURE 1). The head rest of the table can be lowered to hyperextend the neck further. The anesthetist should make certain that the head is perfectly aligned with the body before the line of incision is marked. Any deviation to the side may cause the surgeon to make an inaccurately placed incision.

OPERATIVE PREPARATION The patient's hair may be covered with a mesh cap to avoid contamination of the field. The skin is prepared routinely. Before the incision is made, it may be accurately outlined by compressing a heavy silk thread against the skin. The incision should be made about two fingers above the sternal notch and should be almost exactly transverse, extending well onto the borders of the sternocleidomastoid muscles (FIGURE 2). In the presence of a large goiter, it should be made a little higher so that the final scar will not lie in the suprasternal notch. A short midline crosshatch may be made across the outlined incision to provide a guide to accurate approximation of the skin at closure (FIGURE 2). The site for the incision is then draped with sterile towels secured with towel clips at the four corners, similar to a routine abdominal draping. Transfixing sutures or staples may be placed through the towel into the skin in the middle of the incision on either side. This secures the towel at the center of the incision and avoids contamination when the flaps are reflected upward and downward. Skin towels sutured or clipped to the field may be eliminated by the use of a sterile transparent plastic drape that is made adherent to the skin with an adhesive spray. A large sterile sheet with an oval opening completes the draping.

INCISION AND EXPOSURE The surgeon stands at the patient's right side, since it is customary to commence the procedure at the right upper pole. He or she should be thoroughly familiar with the anatomy of the neck, especially with the blood supply and anatomic relationships of the thyroid gland (FIGURES 3 to 5). A thorough understanding of the anatomy of this region should lessen the complications of hemorrhage or injury to the recurrent laryngeal nerve, which may course through the bifurcation of the inferior thyroid artery, and injury to the parathyroids. A dry field is maintained if the various fascial planes are carefully considered during the procedure (FIGURE 3). The locations of the major blood vessels, the parathyroids, and recurrent laryngeal nerve are shown in FIGURES 3 and 5.

The surgeon applies firm pressure over gauze sponges to one margin of the wound, while the first assistant applies similar pressure to the opposite margin. In this manner the active bleeding from subcutaneous tissue is controlled and the margins of the wound are evenly separated. The skin incision is made with a deliberate sweep of the scalpel, dividing the skin and subcutaneous tissue simultaneously if the panniculus is not too thick. The belly of the scalpel should be swept across the tissues but not pressed into them. Bleeding vessels in the subcutaneous tissues are seized with hemostats; the large vessels are ligated, while small vessels are merely clamped and released or cauterized. Hemostats with finely tapered jaws that can be applied to the vessel alone are the best type to use, because they permit ligation without strangulation of a tab of surrounding fat. One or two mass ligatures may do no harm, but many strangulated bits of tissue cause induration and inflammation during healing since the avascular tabs must be absorbed. Electrocautery is preferred to control bleeding.

The incision is deepened to the areolar tissue plane just below the platysma muscle where an avascular space is reached. All active bleeding points are grasped with curved, pointed hemostats that are reflected upward or downward depending upon to which side of the incision they have been applied (FIGURE 6). Active bleeding and danger of air embolus may occur from accidental openings made into the anterior jugular vein if too deep an incision is made. Sharp dissection may be used alternately with blunt gauze dissection to facilitate the freeing of the upper flap (FIGURES 7 and 8). Usually, a small blood vessel will be encountered, high up beneath the flap on either side, which will produce troublesome bleeding unless it is ligated (FIGURES 8 and 9). The dissection goes up to the thyroid cartilage, as well as down to the suprasternal notch. Outward and downward traction is then applied to the lower skin flap as it is freed from the adjacent tissue down to the suprasternal notch (FIGURE 9). **CONTINUES** ▶

440

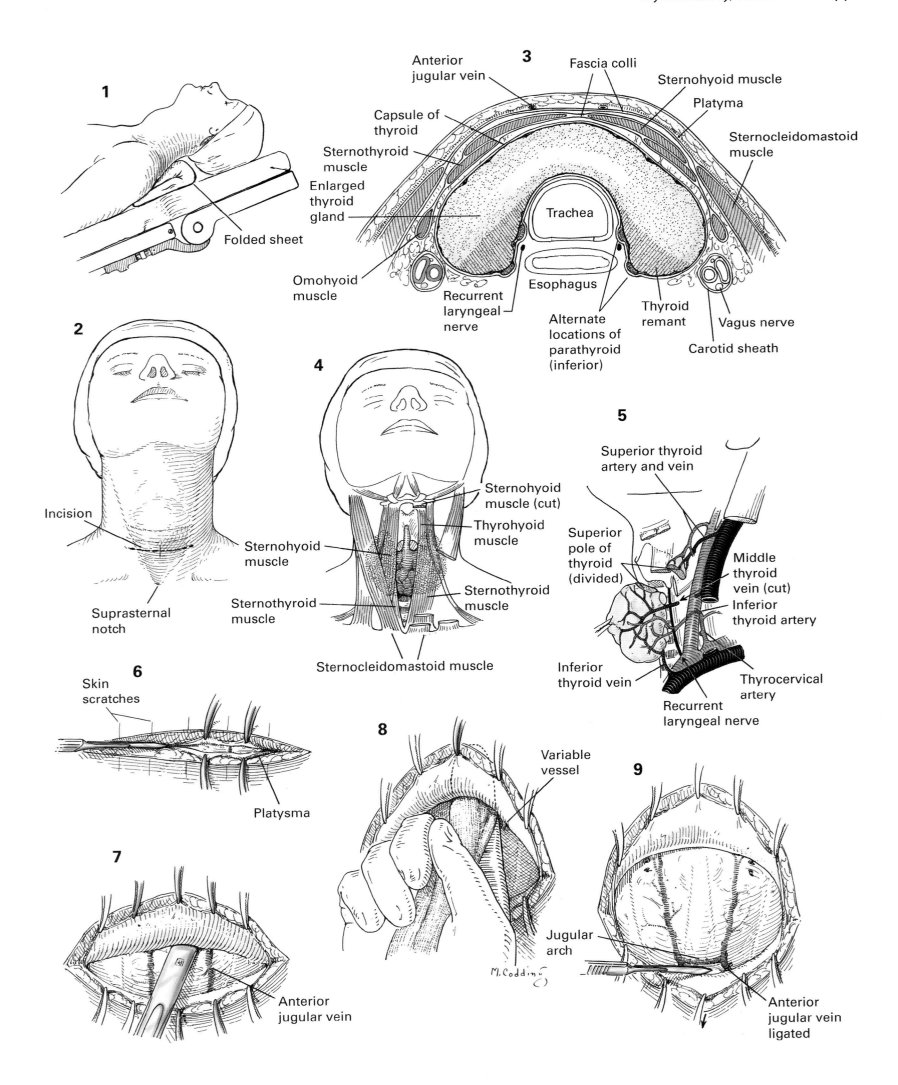

3

Anterior jugular vein

Fascia colli

Sternohyoid muscle

Capsule of thyroid

Platyma

Sternothyroid muscle

Sternocleidomastoid muscle

Enlarged thyroid gland

Trachea

Folded sheet

Omohyoid muscle

Esophagus

Thyroid remant

Vagus nerve

Recurrent laryngeal nerve

Alternate locations of parathyroid (inferior)

Carotid sheath

1

2

Incision

Suprasternal notch

4

Sternohyoid muscle (cut)

Thyrohyoid muscle

Sternohyoid muscle

Sternothyroid muscle

Sternothyroid muscle

Sternocleidomastoid muscle

5

Superior thyroid artery and vein

Superior pole of thyroid (divided)

Middle thyroid vein (cut)

Inferior thyroid artery

Inferior thyroid vein

Thyrocervical artery

Recurrent laryngeal nerve

6

Skin scratches

Platysma

7

Anterior jugular vein

8

Variable vessel

M. Codding

9

Jugular arch

Anterior jugular vein ligated

DETAILS OF PROCEDURE `CONTINUED` This operation is based on careful dissection of various tissue planes between the muscles, vessels, and thyroid gland. Some type of self-retaining retractor is inserted to hold apart the skin flaps. In the presence of a large thyroid gland division of sternohyoid and sternothyroid muscles may be needed. In these cases, the anterior margins of the sternocleidomastoid muscles can be freed. (FIGURE 10). The handle of the scalpel can be used as a dissecting tool to develop the correct plane of cleavage between the sternocleidomastoid muscle and the outer boundaries of the sternothyroid muscle (FIGURES 11 and 12).

To avoid bleeding, a vertical incision is placed exactly in the midline of the neck between the sternohyoid muscles, extending from the thyroid notch to the level of the sternal notch (FIGURE 13). All bleeding points are controlled by the application of clips or hemostats. The tissues on either side of the incision are lifted up so that the incision is not carried directly through into the thyroid gland. Electrocautery or the blunt handle of the knife can be inserted beneath the exposed sternohyoid muscles (FIGURES 14 and 15). At this point the loose fascia over the thyroid gland should be picked up with forceps and incised with the scalpel in order to develop a cleavage plane between the thyroid gland and the sternothyroid muscle (FIGURES 16 to 18). This is one of the most important steps in a thyroidectomy. Many difficulties may be encountered unless the proper cleavage plane is entered at this time. When the fascia of the sternothyroid muscle has been completely incised and reflected, the blood vessels in the capsule of the thyroid gland are clearly visible (FIGURE 18). After the proper cleavage plane is developed, the sternohyoid and sternothyroid muscles are pulled outward from the thyroid gland by means of a retractor, so that any unusual blood vessel communication between the sternothyroid muscle and the thyroid gland can be clamped and ligated (FIGURE 18). Once the surgeon is working in the proper cleavage plane, the delivery of the gland may be facilitated by inserting the two forefingers side by side to the outer edge of the thyroid gland and separating them, thus freeing the gland without injuring blood vessels (FIGURES 19 and 20). If an effort is made to free the entire lateral surface of the gland by finger dissection, it must be remembered that in some instances the middle thyroid vein is quite large and may be torn accidentally by this maneuver, resulting in troublesome bleeding.

If the thyroid is only moderately enlarged, retraction of the prethyroid muscles forward and laterally by narrow retractors will give adequate exposure for the subsequent procedure. However, if the mass of thyroid tissue is large, it may be wiser to divide the strap (prethyroid) muscles. There is no difficulty with healing or function after transverse incision of these muscles if this is done in the upper third to avoid injury to the motor nerve supply. The freed margin of the sternocleidomastoid muscle on either side is retracted laterally to avoid its inclusion (FIGURES 20 and 21). Ultrasonic shears may be used to divide the muscle. Alternatively, muscle clamps may be applied over the surgeon's finger as a guide to avoid including any part of the contents of the carotid bundle. The muscle is divided between the clamps, and an incision is made upward and downward from the end of either clamp to facilitate the retraction of the divided muscles (FIGURE 21). If large anterior jugular veins are present, it is advisable first to ligate them with transfixing sutures adjacent to the upper and lower clamps. The muscle clamps can then be lifted out of the wound and will not hinder the subsequent procedure. The muscles on the left side are similarly divided. `CONTINUES`

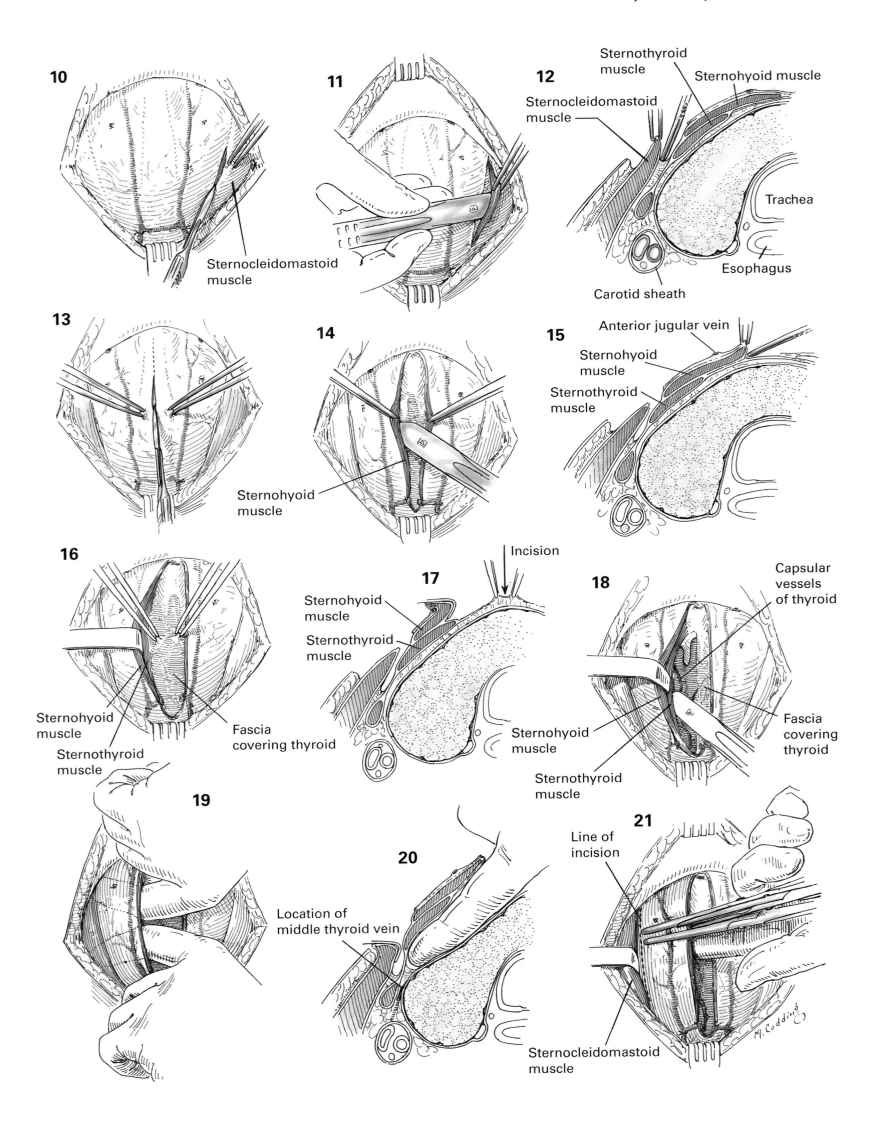

10 Sternocleidomastoid muscle

11

12 Sternothyroid muscle — Sternohyoid muscle — Sternocleidomastoid muscle — Trachea — Esophagus — Carotid sheath

13

14 Sternohyoid muscle

15 Anterior jugular vein — Sternohyoid muscle — Sternothyroid muscle

16 Sternohyoid muscle — Sternothyroid muscle — Fascia covering thyroid

17 Incision — Sternohyoid muscle — Sternothyroid muscle — Sternohyoid muscle

18 Capsular vessels of thyroid — Sternohyoid muscle — Sternothyroid muscle — Fascia covering thyroid

19

20 Location of middle thyroid vein

21 Line of incision — Sternocleidomastoid muscle

M. Codding

DETAILS OF PROCEDURE ◂**CONTINUED** Occasionally, as the upper muscle is retracted upward and outward, a branch of the superior thyroid artery may be encountered, extending from the muscle to the surface of the thyroid gland in the region of the upper pole. This vessel should be carefully clamped and tied (FIGURE 22).

It is customary to begin a subtotal thyroidectomy at the right upper pole or on the larger side. Some surgeons prefer to divide the middle thyroid vein first (FIGURE 26), so as to improve mobility and exposure of the upper pole vessels. A narrow retractor is placed in the wound at the superior pole. Blunt dissection, which allows the thyroid capsule to be pushed away from the larynx, is best accomplished by opening a small, curved fine Crile clamp in the membranous tissue at this point (FIGURE 23). At the uppermost portion of the gland there is a thin fascia that almost encircles the trachea. This area must be clamped carefully, since it contains small blood vessels that, if allowed to retract, are very dangerous to secure because of its proximity to the superior laryngeal nerve. Traction should be maintained on the thyroid gland by means of two babcocks, a curved hemostat, sutures in the thyroid gland itself, or an umbilical tape snugged around the gland in the region of the upper pole. By sharp and blunt dissection the superior thyroid vessels are exposed well above their point of entry into the gland (FIGURE 23). The surgeon now decides whether to leave any thyroid tissue at the upper pole region and places the next clamp either at the upper limits of the gland or in the substance of the gland, perhaps 1 cm below the top of the pole. Hemostasis is effected more easily if the superior thyroid arteries are ligated extracapsularly. Moreover, if much glandular tissue is to be retained, it should be on the posterior surface at the level of the inferior thyroid arteries, as there is more likely to be a recurrence at the superior pole. Three small straight or curved hemostats are applied to the superior thyroid vessels. The vessels are divided, leaving one clamp on the thyroid side and two clamps on the vessels (FIGURE 24). The application of two clamps to the upper pole vessels permits a double ligation and lessens the possibility of active troublesome bleeding. Some surgeons prefer to make the second ligation a transfixing suture of fine silk (FIGURE 25). The superior pole vessels can also be ligated with clips and an ultrasonic shear.

If the middle thyroid vein has not already been identified and ligated, an effort should be made to locate this vessel. Often it is stretched to a thin strand as a result of traction applied to the gland in order to displace it (FIGURE 23). After the superior vessels and middle thyroid vein have been ligated, the narrow retractor is moved to the right lower pole, where the lower pole vessels enter the gland. These vessels are carefully freed from the adjacent structures, either with a small curved clamp or by finger dis-

section (FIGURE 27). Care must be taken not to injure the trachea at the time these vessels are divided and doubly tied (FIGURE 28). Occasionally, a venous plexus (or thyroidea ima) is found over the trachea entering the inferior surface of the gland in the region of the isthmus. This is carefully separated from the trachea with a blunt-nosed hemostat and ligated in the usual fashion.

As an alternative method, the surgeon may decide to start at the lower pole and luxate the gland before the upper pole is ligated. The thyroid tissue over the trachea is divided, and the right lobe is reflected outward (FIGURE 29). The lower pole vessels then are clamped and ligated. The middle thyroid vein is brought into view by medial retraction and can be tied easily. The upper pole is now freed by pushing the index finger behind the superior thyroid vessels. As the superior pole is pushed forward with the finger, a curved clamp may be inserted between the trachea and the medial surface of the superior pole, and the vessels can be doubly clamped (FIGURE 30).

After the middle and inferior veins have been ligated and the superior pole freed by either method, the next step is to expose the inferior thyroid artery. Traction is maintained anteriorly and medially as the artery is exposed on the lateral inferior surface of the gland (FIGURE 31). A narrow retractor is inserted laterally, and by gauze dissection the lateral aspect of the gland in the region of the inferior thyroid artery is visualized clearly. It should be remembered, especially in the presence of a large gland that has been displaced outward, that the recurrent laryngeal nerve may be much higher in the wound than ordinarily is anticipated. If a total lobectomy or extensive removal of thyroid tissue is indicated, it is necessary, by careful dissection, to identify this nerve, which may run between the bifurcation of the inferior thyroid artery as it enters the gland. The fossa posterior of the gland should also be inspected to determine, if possible, the location of the parathyroid glands, which are usually a pinkish chocolate color. Before commencing this dissection, it is wise to place hemostats on the vessels at the margins of the gland where the major branches of the inferior thyroid artery lie. The application of paired clamps to the major blood vessels at a safe distance from the region of the recurrent laryngeal nerve (FIGURE 32) defines the amount of thyroid tissue that will remain and lessens the chance of accidental injury to the nerve. With the trachea in view and the gland lifted into the wound, another row of small, curved hemostats is placed well into the parenchyma so that the desired amount of thyroid tissue is retained along with the posterior capsule (FIGURE 33). The amount of thyroid tissue allowed to remain in relation to recurrent laryngeal nerve is illustrated in FIGURE 3 page 441 and later in this Chapter as FIGURE 41 on page 447. **CONTINUES**▸

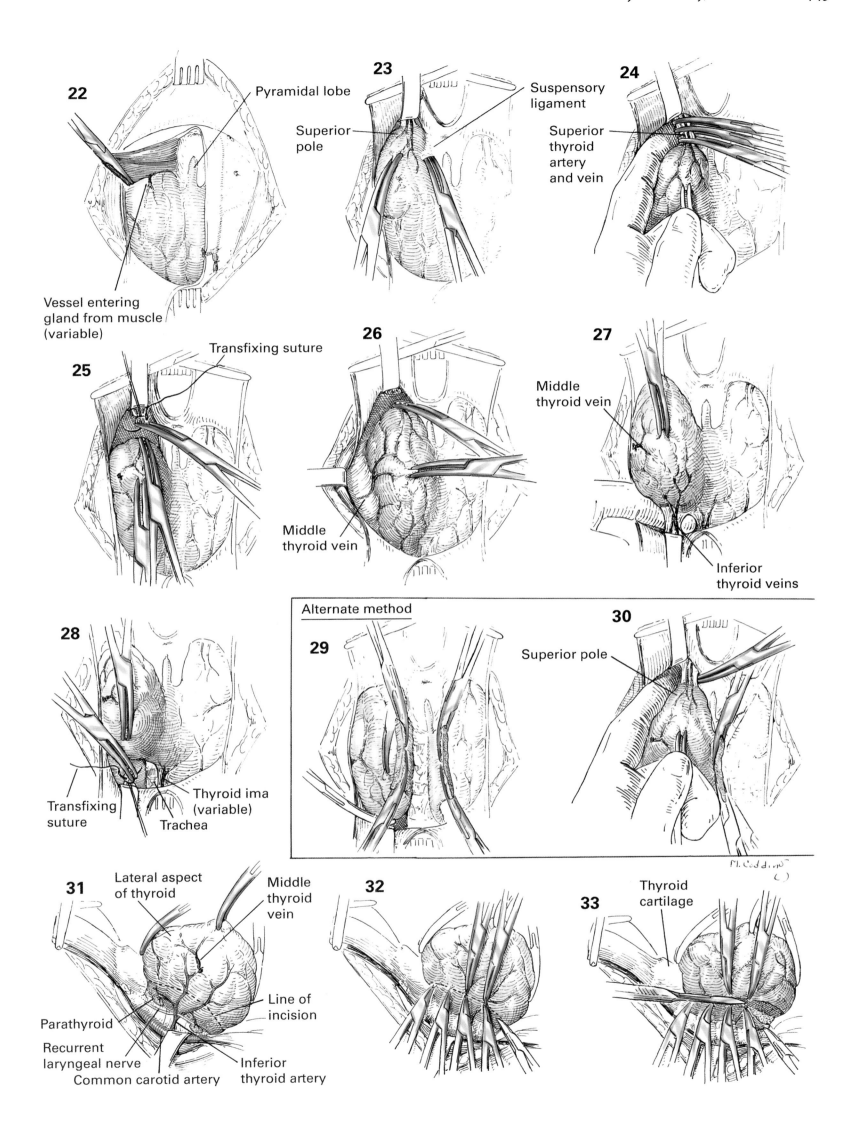

22

Pyramidal lobe

Vessel entering gland from muscle (variable)

23

Suspensory ligament

Superior pole

24

Superior thyroid artery and vein

25

Transfixing suture

26

Middle thyroid vein

27

Middle thyroid vein

Inferior thyroid veins

28

Transfixing suture

Thyroid ima (variable)

Trachea

Alternate method

29

30

Superior pole

31

Lateral aspect of thyroid

Middle thyroid vein

Line of incision

Parathyroid

Recurrent laryngeal nerve

Common carotid artery

Inferior thyroid artery

32

33

Thyroid cartilage

DETAILS OF PROCEDURE **CONTINUED** With the lateral hemostats in place, the right lobe is pushed laterally, and the isthmus is exposed. If this has not already been done, the isthmus is divided. The inferior border immediately over the trachea is grasped with mouse-toothed forceps and pulled upward as a curved clamp is inserted between the trachea and the posterior portion of the gland (FIGURE 34). A similar clamp is inserted from the upper side. After the cleavage plane between the thyroid gland and the anterior surface of the trachea has been developed, the entire isthmus is divided between curved clamps. If the clamps enter the tracheal fascia, there will be added discomfort in the postoperative period. The isthmus is divided close to the right side of the clamps (FIGURE 35). The clamps remain on the left portion of the thyroid as the right lobe margin is retracted laterally (FIGURE 36). Curved clamps are inserted across the trachea into the parenchyma of the gland and pointed toward the lateral row of clamps (on the preceding page 445, FIGURE 32). If the clamps are placed horizontally across the trachea, the points will not injure the recurrent laryngeal nerve (FIGURE 37). The portion to be removed is now lifted and dissected free (FIGURE 38). The bleeding points in the center of the remnant are clamped. Only small amounts of tissue are included. Actively bleeding points that retract, especially along the tracheal margin of the remnant, are controlled by lateral compression with the index finger. Blind clamping of thyroid tissue, particularly at the superior edge, may result in injury to the recurrent laryngeal nerve (FIGURE 39, point x). All bleeding points are carefully ligated. Blind, deep placement of transfixing sutures is avoided because of the risk of injury to the underlying structures. The surgeon must tie beneath these clamps with great care, preferably using a surgeon's knot on the first throw of the tie, so that the subsequent knots can be tied without keeping the ligature under tension. As a rule, the tissues have been clamped under tension, and the vessels tend to retract unless securely held by the first throw of the tie. If transfixion is required, it should be done with a small curved needle, and great care should be exercised to prevent penetration of the posterior capsule and possible injury to the recurrent laryngeal nerve.

When no bleeding points remain, the cavity may be irrigated with saline. The pyramidal lobe, which may be variable in size, is entirely removed. There is usually a bleeding point at the top of this lobe; hemostats are applied and the vessel is ligated (FIGURE 40). In freeing the isthmus, great care is taken to avoid injury to the thin tracheal fascia. If this fascia is torn, postoperative tracheitis and undue soreness may be encountered.

The left side is freed similarly. The additional space left by the removal of a large right lobe somewhat simplifies the removal of the left lobe. The surgeon moves to the left side and takes every precaution to protect the recurrent laryngeal nerve and effect complete hemostasis. The field is inspected for evidence of bleeding (FIGURE 41).

CLOSURE The folded sheet is removed from beneath the neck, and the tension on the chin is relaxed. The wound is repeatedly irrigated with large amounts of saline, and the field is again inspected for any bleeding.

The wound is carefully protected while the anesthesiologist introduces the laryngoscope to inspect the position of the vocal cords. If the position of the vocal cords suggests injury to either nerve, the surgeon should visualize the nerve on the involved side throughout its course and release any sutures that may have included or damaged the nerve. While the anesthesiologist is inspecting the vocal cords, the surgeon should inspect the specimen very carefully for adherent parathyroid glands. Questionable tissue must be closely inspected; any parathyroid substance found should be transplanted, preferably into the sternocleidomastoid muscle.

The operator must be familiar with the appearance of the parathyroid gland, which is a pinkish-brown flattened node about 3 to 4 mm in diameter. The superior glands are usually found on the posterior surface of the thyroid at about the level of the lower portion of the thyroid cartilage. The inferior glands are seen at the lower portion of the thyroid, usually underneath the inferior pole or lying in the fat a little below and deeper than the thyroid substance. Usually, the inferior parathyroids are seen and can be left behind when the small inferior thyroid veins and thyroidea ima vessels are first divided. Regardless of the fact that the surgeon may be certain that the parathyroid glands remain in the wound, any suspected tissue attached to the specimen is transplanted into the neck or forearm muscles.

The prethyroid muscles are then approximated. If the anterior jugular veins have not previously been ligated, they should be tied with a transfixing suture adjacent to the muscle clamps. The anterior margins of the sternocleidomastoid muscles are retracted laterally as the sutures are placed beneath the muscle clamps (FIGURE 42). After closure of the transverse incision, the prethyroid muscles are approximated in the midline with interrupted sutures (FIGURE 43). Drainage is unnecessary in a dry field; however, if a large cavity has resulted following the removal of a large nodular gland, a small closed-suction Silastic drain may be brought out through the center of the incision or through a small stab wound beneath the incision.

The hemostats are removed from the subcutaneous tissue, and all active bleeding points are ligated with fine 0000 silk ligatures or cauterized. The skin flaps are approximated, and the platysma and subcutaneous tissue are repaired in separate layers in order to mound up the tissues and obviate the necessity for tension on the skin sutures (FIGURE 44). The skin may be approximated with an absorbable fine subcuticular suture or with a nonabsorbable subcuticular running pull-out suture that is removed the next day. Skin tapes and a loose dry sterile dressing are applied.

POSTOPERATIVE CARE The patient is immediately placed in a semisitting position. Adequate precautions should be taken to prevent hyperextension of the neck. Oxygen therapy is administered, 4 to 5 L per minute, until the patient has reacted. A sterile tracheotomy set should always be available in the event of acute collapse of the trachea. Parenteral fluids are given until the patient can take adequate fluids by mouth. The addition of sodium iodide and calcium gluconate depends on the patient's general condition. Liquids by mouth are permitted as tolerated. Opiates or sedatives are used as necessary.

Early complications include hemorrhage into the wound, hoarseness and temporary aphonia, vocal cord paralysis, and postoperative thyroid "storm."

The most important postoperative complication is hemorrhage in the wound. If wound hemorrhage is suspected, the dressing is removed, several skin sutures are taken out, the blood is evacuated under aseptic conditions, and major bleeding points are ligated.

Bilateral injury of the recurrent laryngeal nerve may result in paralysis of both vocal cords and may require tracheotomy.

The salient symptoms of postoperative crisis are high fever, severe tachycardia, extreme restlessness, excessive sweating, sleeplessness, vomiting, diarrhea, and delirium. Ice caps or cooling blankets, sedation, and parenteral high-calorie fluids, to which 1 g of sodium iodide and 100 mg of corticoids have been added, are indicated. The continued administration of approximately 15 mg of a satisfactory corticoid preparation per hour in an intravenous drip is recommended. Oxygen, antipyretics, and multivitamin preparations are also administered. Propranolol may be given for the tachycardia.

Postoperative hypoparathyroidism requires calcium gluconate 10% intravenously. Vitamin D_2 is administered at a dosage sufficient to maintain a normal serum calcium level. No added oral calcium other than a glass of milk with each meal is required. Thyroid replacement with levothyroxine is given daily to prevent the recurrence of nontoxic nodular goiter.

Any drains are removed on the first postoperative day. The patient is allowed to go home as soon as he or she is self-sufficient. ■

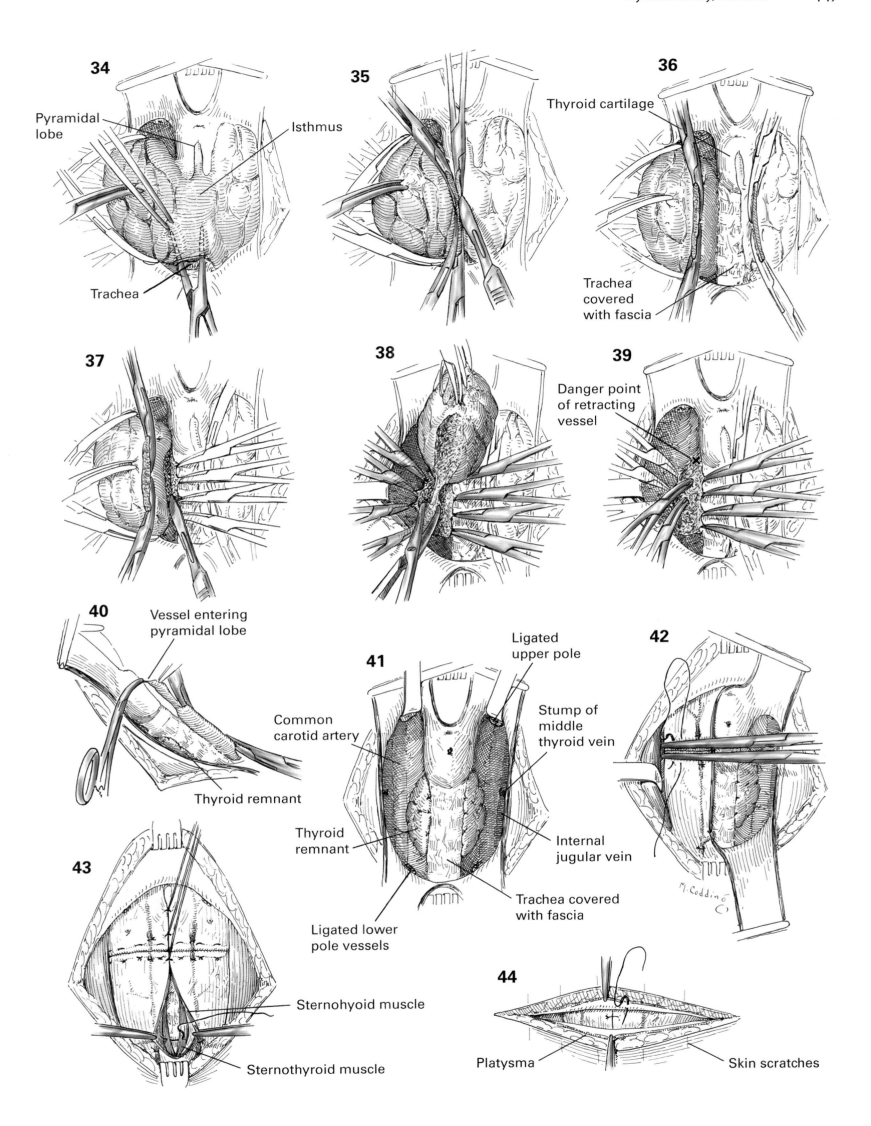

34 Pyramidal lobe — Isthmus — Trachea

35

36 Thyroid cartilage — Trachea covered with fascia

37

38

39 Danger point of retracting vessel

40 Vessel entering pyramidal lobe — Common carotid artery — Thyroid remnant

41 Ligated upper pole — Stump of middle thyroid vein — Thyroid remnant — Internal jugular vein — Ligated lower pole vessels — Trachea covered with fascia

42

43 Sternohyoid muscle — Sternothyroid muscle

44 Platysma — Skin scratches

M. Coddino

Parathyroidectomy

INDICATIONS Hyperparathyroidism is a common endocrine disorder usually cured by subtotal parathyroidectomy. Parathyroid overactivity documented by appropriate laboratory studies may be associated with general hyperplasia of the parathyroid glands or with an adenoma involving one of the four or more parathyroid glands. Kidney stones, gastrinoma, recurrent pancreatitis, or other conditions are some of the clinical disorders that imply a disorder of the parathyroid glands. Hypercalcemia is discovered as a result of more frequent calcium determinations performed as part of a general screening survey. Hyperparathyroidism is associated with gastrinoma in approximately one-third of patients with the familial multiple endocrine syndrome I (MEN I). A mitogenic cause for the relatively high incidence of recurrent hyperparathyroidism in the familial MEN I syndrome suggests the need for a radical approach, which may consist of total parathyroidectomy with autotransplantation of parathyroid slices into the muscle in the nondominant forearm or removal of 3½ parathyroid glands.

Evidence of hyperparathyroidism associated with hypercalcemia of 12 mg/dL after renal transplantation may be an indication to consider a radical parathyroidectomy. Hypercalcemia and extremely high parathyroid hormone (PTH) values may occur after renal transplantation. This condition often resolves spontaneously, usually within a year of the transplantation. In general, a conservative observational approach should be taken within the first 2 years after renal transplantation, with operative intervention on the parathyroids only in patients who demonstrate progressive bone disease and who are clearly symptomatic.

Parathyroidectomy should precede surgical procedures for gastrinoma in patients with the MEN I syndrome. There is an apparent increase in supernumerary parathyroid glands in those with the familial MEN I syndrome, which suggests the need to remove the thymus, where an accessory parathyroid gland may be located when the cervical exploration is negative. More rarely, thyroidectomy may also be considered in a valiant search for a parathyroid gland buried within the thyroid gland if a parathyroid is not visible under the thyroid capsule.

The presence of one endocrine tumor suggests the desirability of a general search for other endocrine tumors, such as gastrinoma, pheochromocytoma, prolactinoma, and others, before parathyroidectomy is performed.

Recurrence of hyperparathyroidism after a parathyroidectomy requires a review of previous surgical procedures and a review of the pathologist's report on the parathyroids. Were the usual four glands found, and where were they? Were any glands verified in the thyroid, thymus, anterior or posterior mediastinum, or above the thyroid? Which glands were removed or verified by frozen section examination? Every effort should be made to localize the parathyroids prior to any reoperation. Computed tomography, magnetic resonance imaging, radionuclide (sestamibi), and ultrasound scans may be useful for identifying large tumors. However, selective venous sampling with hormonal assays may be the last and best diagnostic option.

PREOPERATIVE PREPARATION The surgeon should be familiar with the usual locations of the parathyroid glands as well as their common areas of migration (FIGURE 1). Attempts at localization of the glands are worthwhile, especially if previous surgery has been unsuccessful. Rarely, an adenoma of the parathyroid is large enough to be palpable. A variety of procedures may be used to localize the adenoma, including ultrasound at 10 MHz. Radionuclide imaging with Sestamibi is the preferred test for the localization of parathyroid adenomas. Cross-sectional imaging with CT and MRI may be helpful in evaluating retrotracheal and mediastinal locations but are usually reserved for patients with recurrent hyperparathyroidism. Selective venous

samplings for determination of PTH can be useful in situations of recurrent hyperparathyroidism as well. Because of associated risks and poor accuracy, angiography is rarely used. The superior glands migrate upward or downward into the posterior mediastinum. The lower glands migrate into the thymus or anterior mediastinum (FIGURE 1). In symptomatic patients CT imaging with a stone protocol or intravenous pyelograms are made in a search of renal calculi. The kidney function is carefully reviewed. The vocal cords are inspected. The surgeon should review the variable location of the parathyroid glands, as well as their blood supply and the close relationship with the recurrent laryngeal nerves. A gastrin determination may be advisable if gastric symptoms are present.

ANESTHESIA General anesthesia with orotracheal intubation is desirable. No specific or general anesthetic drugs are specifically indicated. However, the potential exacerbation of renal dysfunction by some anesthetic agents should be considered in patients who have had a renal transplant. If there is a possibility of laryngeal nerve damage, spontaneous respiration should be prolonged with the intratracheal tube in place. There should be sufficient sedation to permit direct laryngoscopy immediately following extubation of the trachea.

POSITION The patient is placed in a semierect position with a folded sheet under the shoulders and the head sharply angulated backward.

OPERATIVE PREPARATION The patient's hair is completely covered to avoid contamination of the field. The skin is routinely prepared. This should include not only the cervical region but also the upper thorax, since an upper sternal incision may be performed in a search for a mediastinal parathyroid adenoma. If available, the laboratory should be notified of the need for determination of parathyroid levels through the operation with rapid PTH assay.

INCISION AND EXPOSURE A low collar incision is made similar to that used in thyroidectomy and all bleeding is carefully controlled. The technical approach is similar to that in subtotal thyroidectomy (Chapter 115, pages 440-447), including division of the strap muscles on both sides. Self-retaining retractors may be inserted to maintain retraction of the skin flaps. A sample for baseline determination of PTH is taken.

DETAILS OF PROCEDURE A four-gland exploration is described. Image guided selective neck exploration is being more frequently employed. This procedure is not described or illustrated. The right lobe is freed by blunt index finger dissection (Chapter 115, FIGURES 19 and 20, page 443) in preparation for identification of the course of the recurrent laryngeal nerve and the tan/yellow-colored parathyroid glands at the upper and lower poles of the thyroid gland. After the two glands on the right side have been identified, a similar search is made on the left side. The parathyroid glands may appear normal or only slightly enlarged when hyperplasia is involved, especially in the MEN I syndrome. A solitary adenoma, when found, may be the size of a small marble or several centimeters in diameter.

Further mobilization of the right lobe results when the middle thyroid vein is ligated and tied (FIGURE 2). A small hemostat is used to grasp the thyroid and retract it upward and medially. The surgeon may retract the thyroid with the left thumb over a piece of gauze on the upper pole of the thyroid. The relationship of the recurrent laryngeal nerve to the middle thyroid artery and the arterial blood supply to the upper pole of the thyroid should be clearly verified (FIGURE 3). The loose tissue is gently pushed aside with forceps and gauze until the color identifiable as parathyroid is visualized. **CONTINUES ▶**

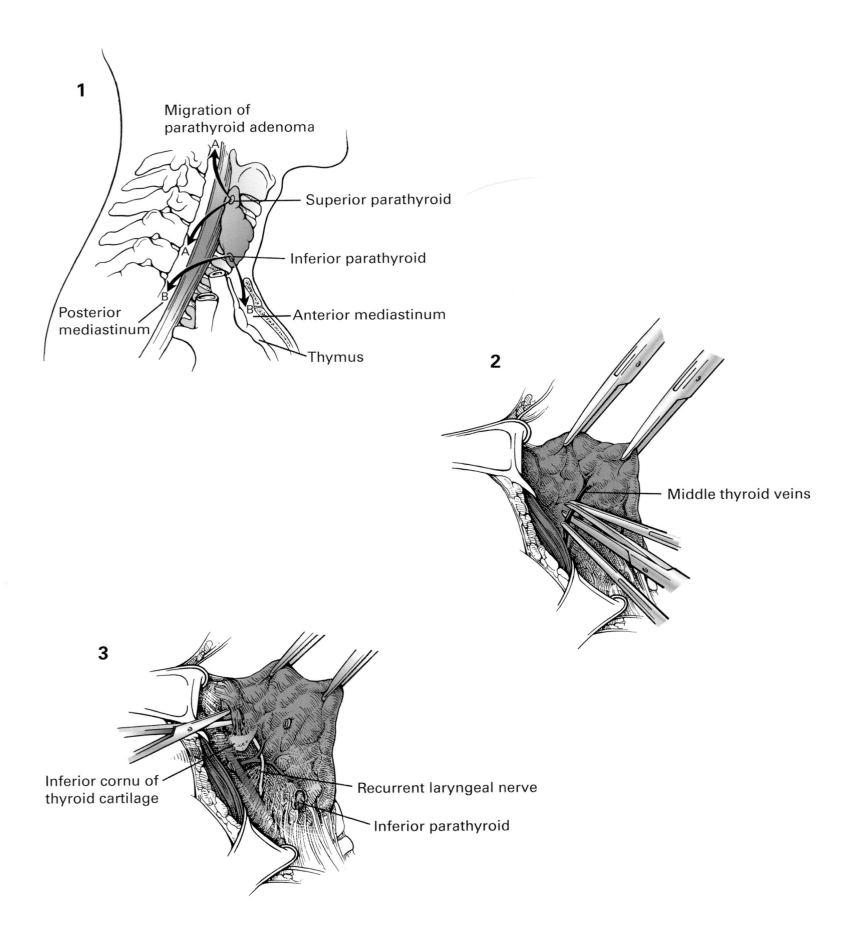

1 Migration of parathyroid adenoma

Superior parathyroid

Inferior parathyroid

Anterior mediastinum

Thymus

Posterior mediastinum

2 Middle thyroid veins

3 Inferior cornu of thyroid cartilage

Recurrent laryngeal nerve

Inferior parathyroid

DETAILS OF PROCEDURE ◀CONTINUED Many times it is difficult to be certain whether discolored tissue is the parathyroid or a hematoma in fatty tissue. Using fine-tooth forceps, the adenoma, if identifiable, is very carefully dissected from the adjacent tissue, constantly keeping in mind the location of the recurrent laryngeal nerve (FIGURE 3). Time is required to develop the rather frail vascular pedicle going to the superior parathyroid, which is double-clamped and ligated (FIGURE 4).

A portion of a gland may be excised for immediate frozen-section examination to determine that it is parathyroid tissue. In some instances, a small biopsy may be taken from several areas believed to be parathyroid glands. A numbered diagram should be made of all biopsy sites along with the individual frozen-section reports of the specimens removed.

The extent of the operation should not be limited to the excision of one obviously enlarged gland that makes a gross diagnosis of adenoma quite likely. If a single enlarged gland is found and removed, repeat determination of a rapid PTH level should show a fall of at least 50% within 10 minutes or 85% by 15 minutes if this was the only abnormal gland. In a four-gland exploration, the other three glands should be identified and their locations recorded. Some prefer a biopsy verification of each one (FIGURE 5), while others attach a fine, deep blue nonabsorbable suture to the gland remnant and bring a long end out into the subcutaneous tissue. The blue suture line serves as a visible guide to the site of the parathyroid biopsy should reoperation become necessary.

In patients with the familial MEN I syndrome, three normal-appearing glands may be excised as well as one-half of the fourth remaining gland. It is advisable to control any oozing with a small silver clip (FIGURE 6) in order to ensure certain identification of the location of any remaining parathyroid tissue should hyperparathyroidism recur.

In rare patients with the familial MEN I syndrome, there is a disturbing rate of recurrent hyperparathyroidism because of the mutagenic potential of the MEN I syndrome. As a result, a radical parathyroidectomy leaving only one-half of one gland should be considered. Resection of the thymus should probably be considered, especially if one of the lower parathyroid glands is missing.

In general, in a patient with recurrent hyperparathyroidism after parathyroidectomy, the surgeon should assume that one or more glands in the cervical region have been overlooked or are aberrantly located or that the patient has the familial multiple neoplasia syndrome. Mediastinal involvement varies but may be present in as little as 2.5% of patients. Upper mediastinal tumors are usually intrathymic, near the innominate vein.

In patients with recurrent hyperparathyroidism, preoperative imaging is helpful if it presents good evidence that a tumor is present in the upper mediastinum. At operation, an effort is made to bring the thymus up into view above the suprasternal notch in the hope of finding a readily recognizable parathyroid gland within it. A transsternal approach to the thymus is rarely required.

POSTOPERATIVE CARE There are two primary complications of great concern. One is injury to the recurrent laryngeal nerve with persistent paralysis of a vocal cord. A second complication is hypocalcemia, even though one-half of one gland has been preserved with meticulous technique. Chvostek's sign, consisting of fascial muscle twitching when the fascial nerve is "thumbed" with the finger, indicates hypocalcemia. Careful monitoring of the serum calcium is carried out with appropriate administration of calcium gluconate daily as well as dehydrotachysterol. Calcium and PTH determinations every 6 months over a long term are worthwhile. ∎

4

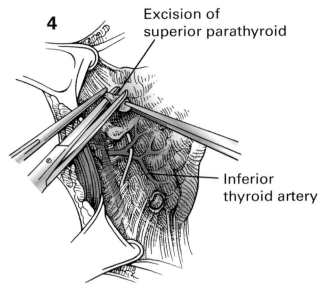

Excision of
superior parathyroid

Inferior
thyroid artery

5

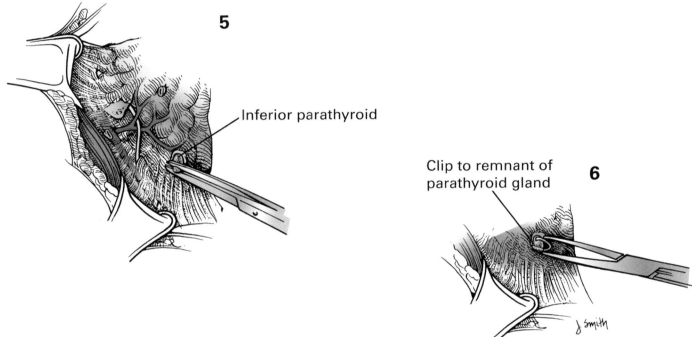

Inferior parathyroid

Clip to remnant of
parathyroid gland

6

J Smith

INDICATIONS The presence of cortical or medullary tumors of either a malignant or benign adenomatous nature is a well-established indication for unilateral adrenalectomy. In recent years, however, the number of indications for bilateral adrenalectomy has gradually increased. It is occasionally performed to control complex endocrine states after partial or unilateral adrenalectomy has failed to alleviate hyperaldosteronism or hypercortisolism, as in Cushing's syndrome.

PREOPERATIVE PREPARATION The most important preoperative procedure is to establish a firm diagnosis. Clinical findings often indicate the altered pathophysiology, but extensive endocrine studies are usually necessary, not only to establish the disorder within the adrenals but also to rule out associated disorders in other endocrine glands. Accordingly, the reader should refer to current texts on diagnostic endocrinology to confirm the diagnosis. Computed tomography scan is usually the preferred imaging modality, but MRI can also be very useful. When adrenalectomy is decided upon, the surgeon should investigate and, if possible, correct many of the secondary systemic and metabolic effects that are the direct result of the altered functional activity of the adrenal. The management of hypertension and its cardiovascular sequelae is a major problem with pheochromocytomas. Problems associated with hypercortisolism include hypokalemia with alkalosis, hypertension, polycythemia, musculoskeletal depletion with osteoporosis and hypercalcemia, abnormal glucose tolerance, multiple areas of skin furunculosis, and, finally, poor wound healing. Thus, the surgeon must be aware that many organ systems and their responses to surgery are profoundly affected by adrenal malfunction.

ANESTHESIA Preoperative consultation and communication among endocrinologist, surgeon, and anesthesiologist are necessary. The anesthesiologist must be prepared for adequate blood and endocrine replacement and occasionally for a prolonged procedure that may be extended into the chest. Electrolytes should be in optimum condition. Parenteral steroids need to be available at the time of surgery for hypercortisolism or bilateral adrenalectomy. Adequate blood must be available, as hypertension plus increased vascularity and fragile veins around the adrenals all tend to increase blood losses.

General anesthesia with endotracheal intubation is preferred. Patients with pheochromocytomas should have adequate preoperative preparation with a long-acting adrenergic (alpha receptor) blocking agent, such as phenoxybenzamine hydrochloride (Dibenzyline) or doxazosin (Cardura) for an extended period of time, if possible. Administering IV fluids the day and evening prior to surgery helps alleviate the dehydration associated with pheochromocytomas. To minimize wide fluctuations of blood pressure, an intra-arterial line should be placed and hypertension controlled with an intravenous infusion of sodium nitroprusside (Nipride). After assuring that adequate fluid and blood replacement has been accomplished, an infusion of norepinephrine (Levophed) may be necessary to treat hypotension. A beta-blocker and lidocaine hydrochloride (Xylocaine) may be needed to control tachycardia and cardiac arrhythmias. Once the tumor is out, norepinephrine may be needed for several days with gradual tapering as tolerated.

POSITION The patient is placed supine with the foot of the table slightly down, so that moderate hyperextension can be obtained if necessary. A posterior approach to the adrenals can be used, and may be useful for normal-sized adrenal glands but is not described here.

OPERATIVE PREPARATION The patient's hair should be completely removed with minimal trauma to the skin. In the anterior approach, the skin of the lower chest and abdomen well into the flanks should be included in the preparation, since, in making a transverse incision, it may be necessary to go far into the flanks in obese patients.

INCISION AND EXPOSURE The surgeon stands on the patient's right side and outlines an incision about two to three fingerbreadths below the costal margin with its apex about two fingers below the tip of the xiphoid process (FIGURE 1). A thoracoabdominal approach through the ninth interspace may be used for large adrenal tumors occurring on the right side. When the posterior approach is used, the incision extends from the level between the 11th and 12th ribs 5 cm from the midline and curved downward to the midportion of the ileum. Increased vascularity in the subcutaneous tissue is common in these cases, particularly in Cushing's syndrome. Meticulous ligation of all bleeding points or control with electrocoagulation should be carried out before the peritoneal cavity is opened. Both rectus muscles are divided, and then the transversus muscle and peritoneum are incised through a liberal incision. This is necessary since many of these patients tend to be obese. Additional exposure may be obtained by dividing the internal oblique muscles in the direction of their fibers out into the flanks. The falciform ligament to the liver is divided between curved hemostats and then ligated. In some patients it may be prudent to mobilize the right lobe of the liver by dividing the falciform and right triangular ligaments (Chapter 81, FIGURES 1 and 2).

DETAILS OF PROCEDURE The surgeon must first be aware of the anatomic differences of the two adrenal glands (FIGURE 2). The right adrenal is close to the superior pole of the kidney, the vena cava medially, and the right lobe of the liver superiorly. Its main arterial supply comes directly to its medial edge from the aorta (FIGURES 2, Label 11), and the main right adrenal vein (5) comes directly from the inferior vena cava in a parallel manner. In contrast, the left adrenal is in proximity to the aorta medially, the renal vein inferiorly, and the superior pole of the left kidney. Its main arterial supply comes directly from the aorta (12), but the main left adrenal vein (6) usually comes from the left renal vein (8). Both adrenal glands, however, have many arterial twigs from both the inferior phrenic arteries (9 and 10) and both renal arteries.

The operative exposure of the right adrenal is shown first (FIGURE 3); it is begun with a classic Kocher maneuver, after the transverse colon and omentum have been carefully packed away and the right lobe of the liver has been retracted gently. The right lobe of the liver should be fully mobilized to gain a better exposure of the right adrenal. After the peritoneum lateral to the duodenum has been incised, it is mobilized in the usual manner by blunt dissection with the surgeon's index finger under the head of the pancreas. The inferior vena cava is exposed in its position directly posterior to the second portion of the duodenum (FIGURE 4) and then cleared to show the right renal vein. The superior pole of the right kidney is located and exposed with further blunt finger dissection. The adrenal is identified by its characteristic yellowish color, lobulated appearance, and clearly definable blunt lateral edge. This generally avascular area is then incised (FIGURE 5), and additional exposure and mobility of the adrenal gland may be obtained by gentle blunt finger dissection directly posterior to the gland. The surgeon should bear in mind that the vascular attachments are usually on or near the medial and superior edges of the gland rather than on its anterior and posterior broad surfaces. If preoperative studies show a large adrenal tumor, especially on the right side, a thoracoabdominal incision should be considered in order to provide exposure for mobilizing the right lobe of the liver. It may be necessary to remove the kidney along with the invading adrenal neoplasm. **CONTINUES**

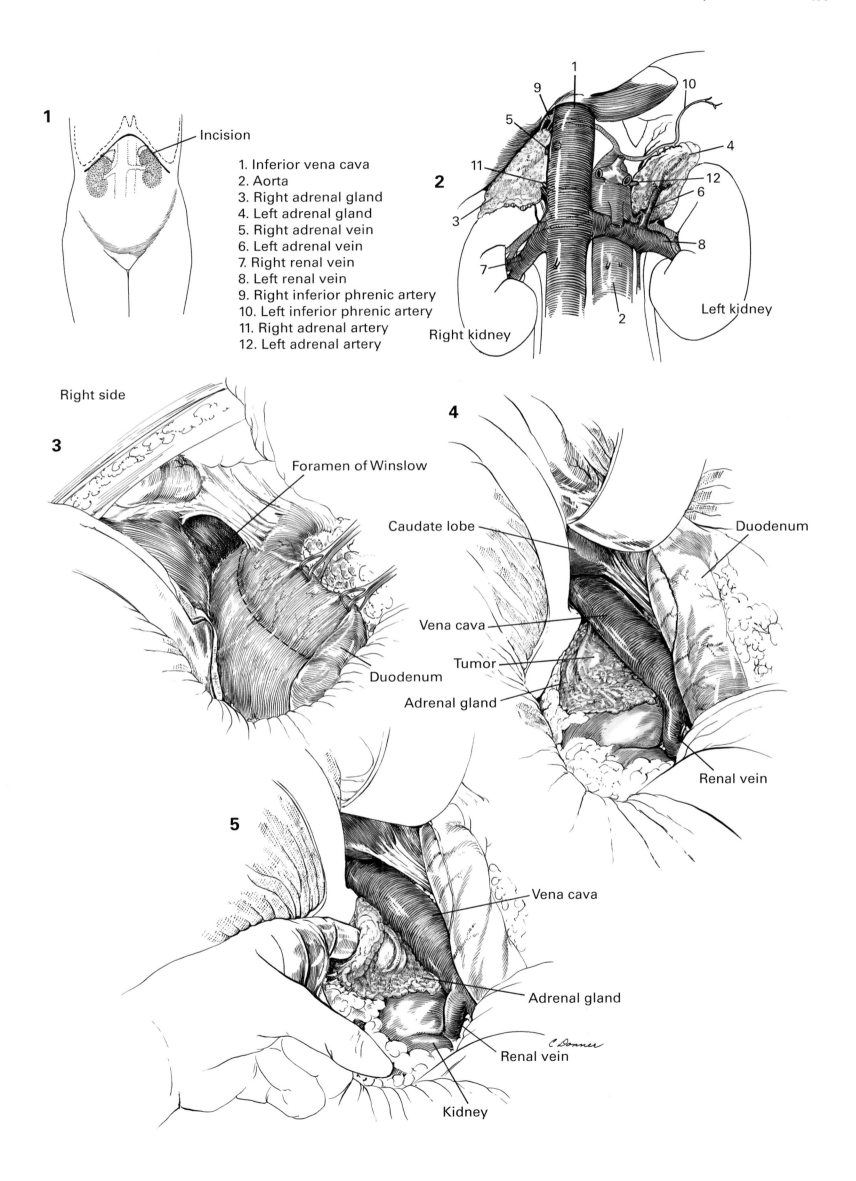

1

Incision

1. Inferior vena cava
2. Aorta
3. Right adrenal gland
4. Left adrenal gland
5. Right adrenal vein
6. Left adrenal vein
7. Right renal vein
8. Left renal vein
9. Right inferior phrenic artery
10. Left inferior phrenic artery
11. Right adrenal artery
12. Left adrenal artery

2

Right kidney

Left kidney

3

Right side

Foramen of Winslow

Duodenum

4

Caudate lobe

Duodenum

Vena cava

Tumor

Adrenal gland

Renal vein

5

Vena cava

Adrenal gland

Renal vein

Kidney

DETAILS OF PROCEDURE ◀CONTINUED▶ Usually, the principal adrenal vein is first identified and then doubly ligated with 00 silk (FIGURE 6). The surgeon then cautiously works about the medial and inferior edges of the gland and ligates the principal artery or accessory arteries in a similar manner. The many minor vessels encountered must also be either carefully ligated or secured with clips.

The approach to the left adrenal via the transabdominal route may take either of two courses, as demonstrated in FIGURES 7 to 10. The usual approach is shown in cross section in FIGURES 7 and 8. The abdominal contents are carefully packed toward the surgeon and then, carefully grasping the spleen, the surgeon divides the avascular splenorenal ligament so that the spleen is mobilized somewhat toward himself or herself. With blunt dissection, it is then possible to dissect above Gerota's fascia but beneath the pancreas and primary splenic artery and vein. This dissection may be carried medially as far as the superior mesenteric vein, which will give a degree of mobilization as shown in FIGURE 11. The surgeon then incises Gerota's fascia over the left kidney (FIGURE 8) and, with blunt dissection, clears the superior pole of the left kidney and comes upon the adrenal, which is shown here in a somewhat medial and inferior location. The left lobe of the liver is also identified, but it is usually not necessary to mobilize or retract it. The same general principles of exposure apply to the left adrenal gland except that the prominent adrenal vein (FIGURE 11) is shown being secured first. The surgeon then works about the periphery of the gland, ligating all prominent vessels. This is often slow, meticulous work, but—if in doubt—it is safer to ligate or clip each suspicious vascular area.

Many surgeons have found it useful to approach the left adrenal through the transverse mesocolon, after mobilizing the inferior border of the body and tail of the pancreas (FIGURE 9). This is accomplished by first removing most of the greater omentum from its attachment along the transverse mesocolon and carefully securing any bleeding points in this generally avascular area. Care must be taken to preserve the middle colic vessels, since the omentum is sometimes closely blended with the mesocolon, and these vessels therefore are susceptible to damage during the procedure. An incision is then made along the distal or inferior margin of the pancreas from the tip of its tail, back along the body to the region of the inferior mesenteric vein (danger point [central arrow], FIGURE 9). This allows the surgeon to mobilize the distal pancreas with blunt finger dissection so that it may be elevated in a cephalad manner and to expose Gerota's fascia directly over the left kidney, whose midportion is usually directly encountered by this approach. This fascia is then incised and the dissection carried about the superior pole of the kidney, where the adrenal can be identified (FIGURE 12). Its lateral edge is then approached and its removal performed as in the procedure described above.

CLOSURE The incision is closed in the routine manner. However, retention sutures are recommended in hypercortisolism, as poor wound healing is a known complication.

POSTOPERATIVE CARE Blood losses must be replaced carefully, and patient observation and blood pressure monitoring must be unfailingly frequent, preferably by an intra-arterial line. Should blood pressure continue to fall in the recovery area or during closure despite adequate endocrine replacement, retroperitoneal hemorrhage from an unsecured vessel must be strongly suspected. In patients who have had a pheochromocytoma removed and for whom adequate fluid and blood replacement has been accomplished, a postoperative vasopressor in the form of norepinephrine may be necessary for 24 to 36 hours, after which time it is gradually tapered as tolerated. Propranolol hydrochloride (Inderal) and lidocaine hydrochloride (Xylocaine) may be needed to control tachycardia and cardiac arrhythmias.

Patients will experience a drop in the level of circulating corticosteroids after removal of a hyperfunctioning tumor or after subtotal or total adrenalectomy. Therefore they must have cortisone support before, during, and after surgery. Hydrocortisone (Cortef) in the dose of 100 mg is given intravenously during the surgery. This is gradually tapered down over the next 7 to 10 days to 30 to 50 mg per day, which may be given orally in divided doses (frequently 20 mg in the morning and 10 mg in the afternoon). It is felt that 30 to 50 mg per day of hydrocortisone represents reasonable maintenance therapy. However, it may be necessary to add an active mineralocorticoid, such as fludrocortisone (Florinef) at 0.1 mg per day to this if maintaining sodium and potassium balance is difficult. In the immediate postoperative period, however, the major problem is to ensure adequate cortisone replacement, as it is easy to undertreat but almost impossible to overtreat with cortisone.

The postoperative ileus and return to alimentation should be handled the same as for any laparotomy. Wound healing, however, will be impaired in patients with hypercortisolism, and infection is a possibility, as many of these patients also have extensive furunculosis. Finally, it is important that the patient's long-term medical management and endocrine replacement be clearly defined. ■

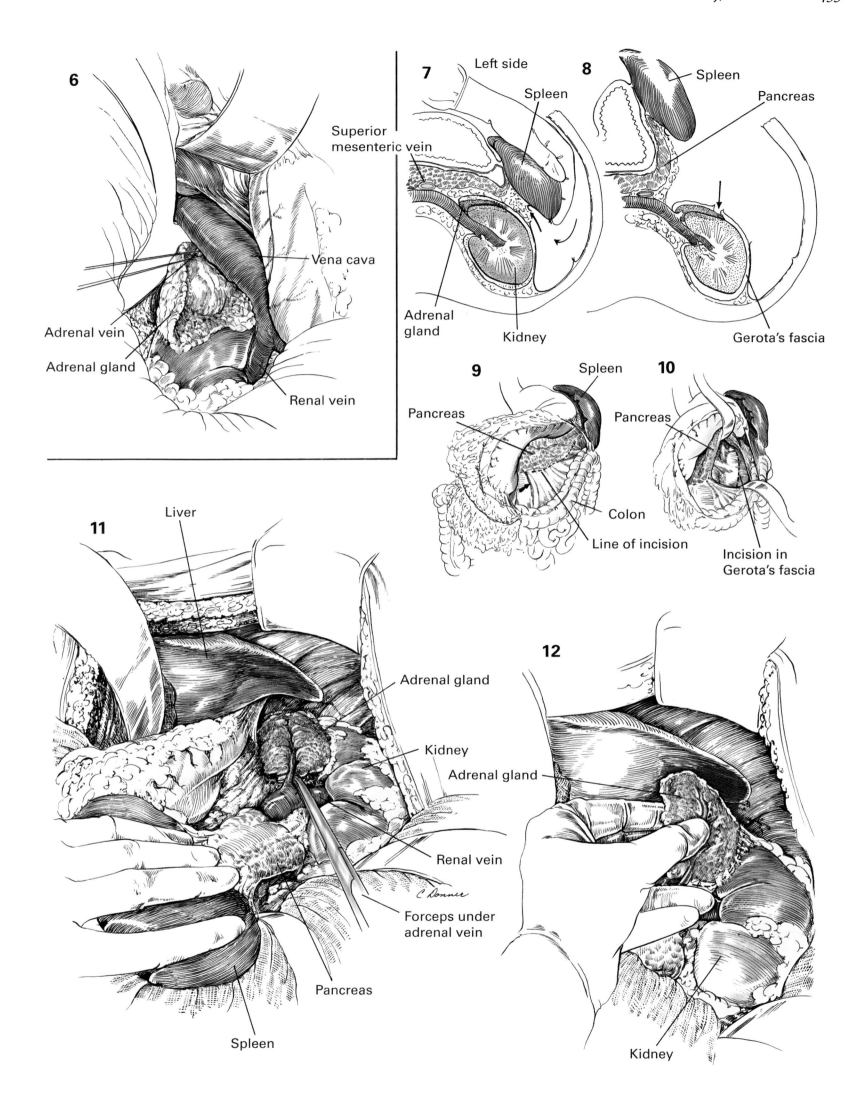

6

Adrenal vein

Adrenal gland

Vena cava

Renal vein

7 Left side

Spleen

Superior mesenteric vein

Adrenal gland

Kidney

8 Spleen

Pancreas

Gerota's fascia

9 Spleen

Pancreas

Colon

Line of incision

10 Spleen

Pancreas

Incision in Gerota's fascia

11 Liver

Adrenal gland

Kidney

Renal vein

Forceps under adrenal vein

Pancreas

Spleen

12 Adrenal gland

Kidney

C. Donner

ADRENALECTOMY, LEFT LAPAROSCOPIC

INDICATIONS The presence of cortical or medullary tumors of a benign nature is a well-established indication for unilateral laparoscopic adrenalectomy. These tumors may be functional and produce cortisol, aldosterone, catecholamines, and rarely testosterone and other sex hormones. In many cases the tumors are nonfunctional and are removed because of the concern for cancer. In these situations the adrenal mass is frequently found during abdominal imaging done for unrelated indications. These so-named adrenal "incidentalomas" should generally be removed if they have a cross-sectional diameter 4 cm or greater or if they are proven to be functional. Patients with nonfunctional adrenal masses less than 4 cm should be followed with periodic imaging to monitor changes in the size of the mass. A benign adenoma on CT is typically a homogeneous mass with a low attenuation value (less than 10 HU on a noncontrast image or a greater than 50% washout on an adrenal protocol CT). It is recommended that patients with an incidentaloma should have a 1-mg dexamethasone suppression test and a measurement of plasma-free metanephrines. In addition, patients with hypertension should have determinations of serum potassium and plasma aldosterone concentrations to plasma renin activity for an activity ratio. Surgery is considered in all patients with functional adrenal cortical tumors. All patients with biochemical evidence of pheochromocytoma should undergo surgery except in rare instances. Although size is not an absolute contraindication to laparoscopic adrenalectomy, the procedure may be difficult on lesions greater than 10 cm. Open adrenalectomy with en bloc excision is the mainstay for primary and recurrent adrenocortical carcinoma due to the lack of effective adjuvant therapy and the difficulty of maintaining oncologic principles with laparoscopy.

PREOPERATIVE PREPARATION The most important preoperative procedure is to establish a firm diagnosis. Accordingly, the reader should refer to current texts on diagnostic endocrinology for the required procedures. When adrenalectomy is decided upon, the surgeon should investigate and, if possible, correct many of the secondary systemic and metabolic effects that are the direct result of the altered functional activity of the adrenal. The management of the hypertension and its cardiovascular sequelae is the major problem with pheochromocytomas. Preoperative treatment with an alpha-receptor antagonist such as phenoxybenzamine hydrochloride or doxazosin (Cardura) and volume expansion is necessary in patients with pheochromocytoma in order to control the associated hypertension. This may take 2 weeks or more. Beta-blockers are reserved for patients with tachycardia or cardiac arrhythmias. Problems associated with hypercortisolism have been reviewed in the section on bilateral adrenalectomy.

ANESTHESIA Preoperative consultation and communication among endocrinologist, surgeon, and anesthesiologist are necessary. A type and screen is acceptable for small tumors. Autologous donation or type and cross to ensure the availability of blood products is recommended for tumors greater than 6 cm and for a right-sided tumor due to its proximity to the inferior vena cava. General anesthesia with endotracheal intubation is preferred in all cases. A catheter should be placed in the urinary bladder for monitoring urine output. The stomach should be decompressed with an orogastric or nasogastric tube. For patients with nonfunctional tumors, there are no special considerations for anesthesia. Patients with hyperaldosteronism should have the blood pressure controlled preoperatively, but rarely have life-threatening intraoperative hypertension. Patients with hypercortisolism should have correction of the metabolic abnormalities and be given a stress dose of steroids.

Patients with pheochromocytoma should have an arterial line and central line placed. In some patients with associated hypertensive cardiomyopathy, a pulmonary artery catheter may be helpful. During the procedure the anesthesiologist should be prepared to control hypertension with an intravenous infusion of sodium nitroprusside (Nipride). After the pheochromocytoma is removed and ensuring that adequate fluid and blood replacement has been accomplished, an infusion of norepinephrine (Levophed) may be necessary to treat hypotension. Propranolol hydrochloride (Inderal) and lidocaine hydrochloride (Xylocaine) may be needed to control tachycardia and cardiac arrhythmias.

ANATOMY The surgeon must first be aware of the anatomic differences of the two adrenal glands (see preceding Chapter 117, FIGURE 2 Labels 1-12). The left adrenal is in proximity to the aorta medially, the renal vein inferiorly, and the superior pole of the left kidney. It may be located near the renal hilum. Its main arterial supply comes directly from the aorta (Label 12), but the main left adrenal vein (Label 6) usually comes from the left renal vein (Label 8). In contrast, the right adrenal is close to the superior pole of the kidney, the vena cava medially, and the right lobe of the liver superiorly. Its main arterial supply comes directly to its medial edge from the aorta (Label 11), and the main right adrenal vein (Label 5) comes directly from the inferior vena cava in a parallel manner. Both adrenal glands, however, have many arterial twigs from both the inferior phrenic arteries (Labels 9 and 10) and both renal arteries. Both adrenal glands are within Gerota's fascia.

POSITION An adjustable vacuum beanbag should be placed on the operating table prior to bringing the patient into the room. The patient is positioned with

the bag being at the level of their flank below the ribs and above the iliac crest over the break position of the table so as to allow a "jack knife" extension that may be useful in obese patients.

For a left adrenalectomy the patient is placed in a lateral position with the left arm crossing the chest and supported on a padded arm board (FIGURE 1). The right arm is placed on a separate arm board and an axillary roll is used. Liberal padding is used between and around both arms. The abdomen and flank area should be exposed and the left knee flexed, with a padding of blankets or pillows between the legs.

OPERATIVE PREPARATION The patient's hair should be removed with electric hair clippers with minimal trauma to the skin.

INCISION AND EXPOSURE For a left adrenalectomy the surgeon stands on the patient's right side (FIGURE 1A). The camera operator stands to the left or right of the surgeon and the assistant on the left side of the patient. A 10-mm 30-degree laparoscope is placed either above the umbilicus or in the left lateral midsubcostal position in the mid-clavicular line just above the level of the umbilicus using the open technique of Hasson as described in Chapter 11, page 40. The abdominal space is inflated to 15 cm of pressure, the laparoscope is introduced, and all four quadrants of the abdomen are examined for abnormalities, safety of other planned port sites, and evidence of any metastatic disease. A 5-mm port is placed in the far left lateral subcostal position and a 5-mm port is placed just to the left of the midline through the upper rectus muscle sheath just to the left of the round ligament. This reduces the chance of lacerating the epigastric artery, which might require suture ligation. These ports are in a line about two fingerbreadths or so below the edge of the costal margin. A third 5-mm port is placed in the anterior axillary line midway between the costal margin and the iliac crest (FIGURE 1B).

DETAILS OF PROCEDURE The operative exposure of the left adrenal is shown first. The splenic flexure of the colon is mobilized using an ultrasonic device so as to expose the kidney. The dissection is continued cephalad and the lesser sac is entered by separating the greater omentum from the splenic flexure and transverse colon (FIGURE 2). It is not necessary to mobilize the spleen. The lesser sac is entered and the pancreas identified (FIGURE 2). The retroperitoneum is exposed to show the kidney and posterior surface of the pancreas (FIGURES 2 and 3). Gerota's fascia is incised and opened to expose the upper pole of the kidney (FIGURES 2 and 3). Dissection is continued under Gerota's fascia while the assistant lifts the tail of the pancreas anteriorly (FIGURE 3). This dissection should be continued as far cephalad as possible. The inferior pole of the adrenal gland will be seen as a bright yellow organ and the adrenal tumor exposed (FIGURE 3). It may be difficult to identify in obese patients with excessive retroperitoneal fat. If one cannot identify the left adrenal, it is usually because the operative field is too caudad and more superior dissection is needed. In these cases, identifying the left renal vein will allow the identification of the left adrenal vein that may be traced to the adrenal gland (FIGURE 3). It is usually necessary to place a retractor device under Gerota's fascia and the tail of the pancreas in order to expose the operative field (FIGURE 3).

Once the gland is identified, dissection is begun with the ultrasonic device along the inferior pole working medially. The adrenal vein is dissected with a Maryland dissector so as to visualize its entire circumference. It is doubly clipped on the patient side using a 5-mm clip applier (FIGURE 4). The vein is cut sharply leaving a longer stump on the renal vein side. The ultrasonic device is used to dissect around the adrenal gland beginning medially. Clips may be used to secure prominent blood vessels (FIGURES 5 and 6). The ultrasonic dissector effectively seals small arterial vessels that enter the adrenal gland like the spokes of a wheel. In some patients it is necessary to dissect the entire lateral border of the adrenal gland in order to mobilize it and retract the gland superiorly, thus permitting identification of the adrenal vein. The inferior attachments are divided. Finally, the avascular lateral and superior attachments are dissected (FIGURE 7). The gland is now free for extraction in a laparoscopic retrieval bag (FIGURE 8). The technique for extraction is described under laparoscopic right adrenalectomy (see Chapter 119, page 458).

The tumor bed is then inspected for any evidence of bleeding and any additional hemostasis obtained. The retraction on the pancreas is released and it is returned to its normal position.

POSTOPERATIVE CARE If the patient does not have a pheochromocytoma, the orogastric tube and Foley catheter are removed in the postoperative recovery area. Intravenous fluids are administered and a clear liquid diet is ordered. Vital signs are monitored every 4 hours. The hemoglobin is checked on postoperative day 1 and the diet advanced. The patient is discharged on postoperative days 1 to 3. If the patient has a pheochromocytoma, the patient may need to be in the ICU. Monitoring of urinary output with a urinary Foley catheter is required. In addition, blood pressure is monitored with an arterial line. The patient is transferred from the ICU when stable and the diet advanced. For patients with a functional tumor, discussion with the endocrinologist about resumption of preoperative medications is helpful. ∎

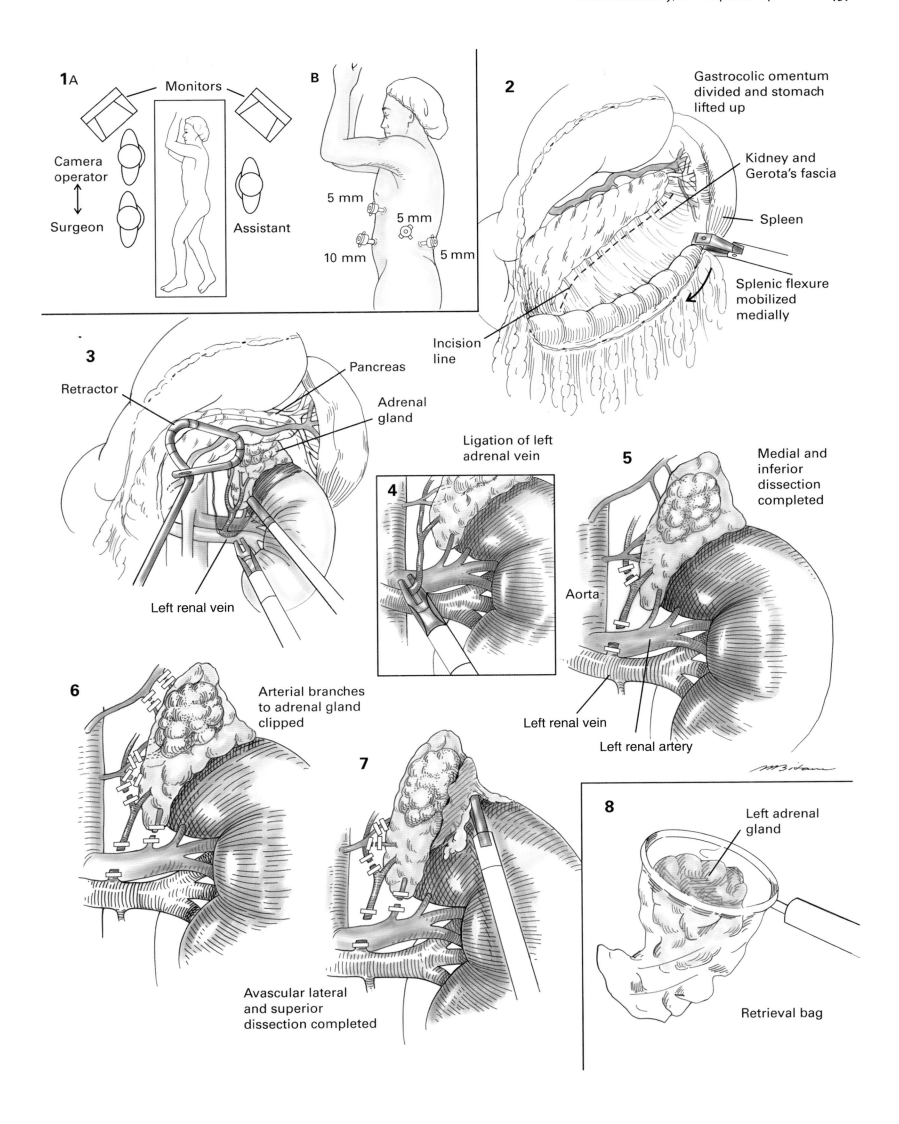

1A Monitors

Camera operator

Surgeon

Assistant

B

5 mm

5 mm

10 mm

5 mm

2 Gastrocolic omentum divided and stomach lifted up

Kidney and Gerota's fascia

Spleen

Splenic flexure mobilized medially

Incision line

3

Retractor

Pancreas

Adrenal gland

Left renal vein

Ligation of left adrenal vein

4

5 Medial and inferior dissection completed

Aorta

Left renal vein

Left renal artery

6 Arterial branches to adrenal gland clipped

7

Avascular lateral and superior dissection completed

8 Left adrenal gland

Retrieval bag

ADRENALECTOMY, RIGHT LAPAROSCOPIC

INDICATIONS The indications are as previously described for laparoscopic left adrenalectomy.

PREOPERATIVE PREPARATION The same steps in preparation are taken as described for the laparoscopic left adrenalectomy.

ANESTHESIA The anesthetic considerations as described for the left adrenalectomy are followed.

ANATOMY See Chapter 117, FIGURE 2.

POSITION A vacuum-assisted beanbag should be placed on the operating table prior to bringing the patient into the room. The patient is positioned with the bag being at the level of their flank below the ribs and above the iliac crest over the break position of the table so as to allow a "jack knife" extension that may be useful in obese patients.

For a right adrenalectomy the patient is placed in the right lateral position with the right arm crossing the chest and supported on an arm board (FIGURE 1A). The left arm is placed on an arm board and an axillary roll used. In general the left and right positions are mirror images of each other. After the patient is positioned, the air is suctioned from the beanbag in order to secure the position. In addition, the patient is secured across the chest and hips to the table with wide adhesive tape, as the operating room table will be tilted. Some surgeons may prefer to improve tape adhesion with a skin preparation.

INCISION AND EXPOSURE For a right adrenalectomy the surgeon stands on the patient's left side (FIGURE 1A). The camera operator stands to the surgeon's left or right and the assistant on the patient's right. A 10-mm 30-degree laparoscope is inserted using the aforementioned technique either in a supraumbilical position or the right lateral subcostal position in the midclavicular line just above the level of the umbilicus. A 5-mm port is placed in the right lateral subcostal area in the anterior axillary line and another 5-mm port is placed just to the right of the midline and the right of the round ligament. A third 5-mm port is placed on the right side in the anterior axillary line midway between the costal margin and the iliac crest (FIGURE 1B). Additional ports or larger ports may be placed depending on the preference of the surgeon, the size of the tumor, and the shape and size of the patient. The patient is then placed in a reverse Trendelenburg (head-up) position.

DETAILS OF THE PROCEDURE On the right side, the hepatic flexure of the colon is mobilized from the lateral gutter using the ultrasonic device. Any adhesions about the lateral liver or even the gallbladder may need to be incised with sharp dissection (FIGURE 2). A Kocher maneuver is done to expose the inferior vena cava in its position directly posterior to the second portion of the duodenum and possibly the right renal vein as it is essential to know the location of these structures before entering Gerota's fascia (FIGURE 3). The right lobe of the liver should be mobilized by dividing posterior and lateral attachments until the diaphragm is exposed so as to gain a better exposure of the right adrenal (FIGURES 2 and 3). A retractor is placed to hold the liver superomedially (FIGURES 2 and 3). This may require an additional port—either a 5-mm or a 10-mm one depending upon which retractor device is used. The peritoneum lateral to the duodenum is

then incised, and it is mobilized in the usual Kocher maneuver manner by using a blunt tip dissector or the ultrasonic device (FIGURE 3). This area is then incised, and the duodenum is mobilized to show the right renal vein. Gerota's fascia is incised and the superior pole of the right kidney is located (FIGURE 3). The adrenal is identified by its characteristic yellowish color, lobulated appearance, and its clearly definable blunt lateral edge.

The surgeon should bear in mind that the vascular attachments are usually on or near the medial and superior edges of the gland rather than on its broad surfaces (as shown in Chapter 117, page 453). After initial lateral and inferior mobilization, the adrenal gland may be retracted laterally. It is essential to identify the inferior vena cava (FIGURE 4) and then the right adrenal vein. The right adrenal vein is identified and doubly clipped proximally and distally using a 5-mm clip applier and divided (FIGURES 4 and 5). The superior attachments of the adrenal gland are then divided and the superior arterial supply clipped or coagulated freeing the gland. Next the inferior portion of the gland is further dissected exposing the adrenal artery arising from the right renal artery. This is doubly clipped (FIGURE 6). The generally avascular lateral area is then incised and additional exposure and mobility of the adrenal gland may be obtained by gentle blunt dissection directly posterior and lateral to the gland (FIGURE 7). The suction tip is an excellent tool for this blunt dissection. The gland should be free at this point for extraction (FIGURE 8). The tumor bed is inspected for bleeding and any additional hemostasis obtained.

EXTRACTION OF THE ADRENAL GLAND The same technique is used to remove either the right or the left gland from the peritoneal cavity. The 10-mm laparoscope is removed, and the video camera is mounted on a 5-mm laparoscope. This is inserted through the most inferior 5-mm trocar. A clear plastic specimen retrieval bag device is inserted into the peritoneal cavity through the 10-mm Hasson port. The bag is opened and the adrenal gland is grasped by some periadrenal fat or connective tissue. The gland is delivered into the bag (FIGURE 8). The bag is closed and separated from its insertion device. Using gentle traction, the bag with the adrenal gland is pulled from the abdominal cavity through the Hasson insertion site. The incision may need to be enlarged for larger tumors. It is not necessary to fragment the adrenal gland into pieces as it is soft and pliable, permitting it to be removed through a relatively small opening. The camera is then placed back on the 10-mm laparoscope and the bed of the adrenal gland is irrigated and inspected for bleeding, which may be controlled by electrocautery, the harmonic scalpel, or clips.

CLOSURE The Hasson trocar site is closed with interrupted absorbable sutures. In the patient with hypercortisolism, nonabsorbable sutures may be necessary. For Hasson incisions in the lateral abdomen or flank, the use of a Thompson closure device may be helpful. The skin is closed with subcuticular absorbable sutures or staples.

POSTOPERATIVE CARE The general principles are the same as those for open adrenalectomy and those specific to laparoscopic adrenalectomy are described in the section on laparoscopic left adrenalectomy (see Chapter 118). ■

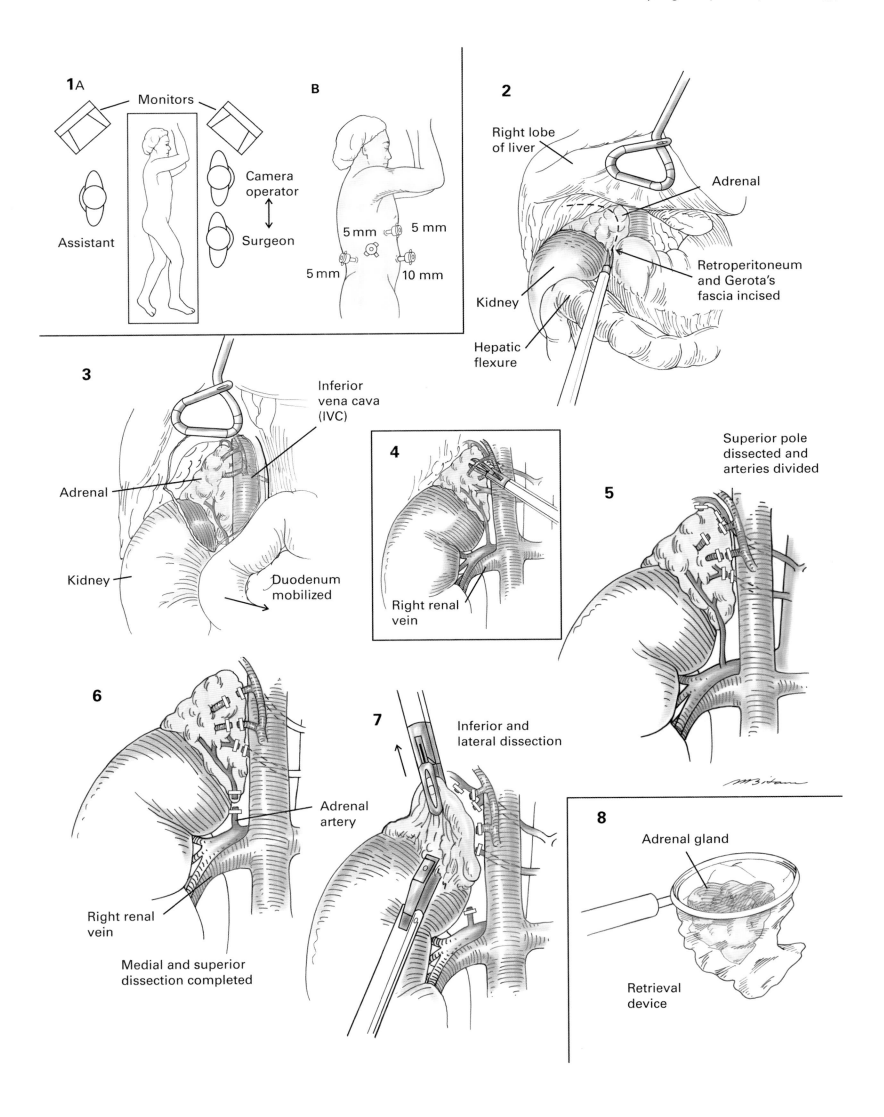

1A

Monitors

Assistant

Camera operator

Surgeon

B

5 mm   5 mm

5 mm   10 mm

2

Right lobe of liver

Adrenal

Retroperitoneum and Gerota's fascia incised

Kidney

Hepatic flexure

3

Inferior vena cava (IVC)

Adrenal

Kidney

Duodenum mobilized

4

Right renal vein

5

Superior pole dissected and arteries divided

6

Adrenal artery

Right renal vein

Medial and superior dissection completed

7

Inferior and lateral dissection

8

Adrenal gland

Retrieval device

HEAD AND NECK

INDICATIONS Tracheotomy is performed for two groups of patients. The first group comprises those with an obstruction of the airway at or above the level of the larynx. Such obstruction may result acutely from laryngeal tumors, edema, fracture, foreign bodies, burns about the oropharynx, or severe throat and neck infections.

The second group consists of patients with chronic or long-term respiratory problems. Inability to cough out tracheobronchial secretions in paralyzed or weakened patients may be an indication for tracheotomy, which allows frequent and easy endotracheal suctioning. This group of patients includes those with prolonged unconsciousness after drug intoxication, head injury, or brain surgery and those with bulbar or thoracic paralysis, as in poliomyelitis. To this group are added patients with general debility, especially in the presence of pulmonary infection or abdominal distention, where a temporary course of respiratory support with an endotracheal tube and mechanical ventilator for 10 to 14 days must be converted into a longer course of pulmonary assistance. In these patients inability to maintain an adequate gas exchange or oxygen or carbon dioxide may dictate conversion of the endotracheal tube to a tracheotomy tube. Frequently, checks of arterial blood gases will reveal hypoxemia or hypercarbia, while simple measurements of vital capacity and negative inspiratory force will detect insufficient respiratory muscular effort. These tests are important in the decision to continue tracheal intubation with ventilator assistance. Other candidates for tracheotomy may include patients undergoing major operative or radical resections of the mouth, jaw, or larynx, where this procedure often is done as a precautionary measure. Antibiotics may be indicated.

PREOPERATIVE PREPARATION Because the patient is usually in respiratory difficulty, preoperative preparation is generally not possible.

ANESTHESIA In cooperative patients, in both elective and emergency situations, local infiltration anesthesia is preferred. In patients who are comatose or are choking, no anesthesia may be necessary or possible. Because it helps to ensure a good airway during tracheotomy, endotracheal intubation is especially useful in patients whose laryngeal airway is very poor and who may obstruct at any moment. It is also an aid in palpating the small, soft trachea of infants.

POSITION A sandbag or folded sheet under the shoulders helps extend the neck (FIGURE 1), as does lowering the head rest of the operating table. The chin is positioned carefully in the midline.

OPERATIVE PREPARATION In emergency tracheotomy, sterile preparation is either greatly abbreviated or omitted entirely. In routine tracheotomy, a sterile field is prepared in the usual manner.

A. EMERGENCY TRACHEOTOMY

INCISION AND EXPOSURE Emergency tracheotomy is done when there is no time to prepare for a routine tracheotomy. There may be no sterile surgical instruments available and no assistants.

An emergency airway is made by a transverse cut or stab through the cricothyroid membrane. Here the airway is immediately subcutaneous, yet the level is still under the vocal cords (FIGURE 2). The wound is held open by twisting the handle of the knife blade in the wound. Later, with the airway ensured, the patient is removed to the operating room and a routine tracheotomy is done.

B. ELECTIVE TRACHEOTOMY

INCISION AND EXPOSURE A transverse incision is most commonly used. It is made at roughly the midpoint between the notch and the thyroid cartilage. The procedure is demonstrated with a vertical incision which is made in the midline of the neck from the middle of the thyroid cartilage to just above the suprasternal notch (FIGURE 3). The skin, subcutaneous tissues, and strap muscles are retracted laterally to expose the thyroid isthmus (FIGURES 4 and 5). The isthmus may be either divided and ligated or retracted upward after the pretracheal fascia is cut. Usually, upward retraction is the better method.

After the cricoid cartilage is identified (FIGURE 6), the trachea is opened vertically through its third and fourth rings (FIGURES 7 and 8). In order to facilitate insertion of the tracheotomy tube, either a cruciate incision is made or a very narrow segment of one ring may be removed (FIGURE 9). The transverse incision, preferred by some surgeons for cosmetic reasons, is more time-consuming. The difference in the final cosmetic result is negligible, since it is the tube and not the incision that causes scarring.

DETAILS OF PROCEDURE A tracheal hook is used to pull up the trachea and steady it for incision (FIGURE 9). Great care must be taken not to cut through the trachea too deeply, since the posterior wall of the trachea is also the anterior wall of the esophagus.

After the trachea has been incised, a previously selected tracheotomy tube is inserted. A No. 6 tube is ordinarily suitable for an adult male and a No. 5 or 6 tube for an adult female. Correspondingly smaller tubes are used in children and infants. The trachea of a newborn will accept only a No. 00 or 0 tube. The assistant must be careful to keep the tube in the trachea by holding one finger on the flange; otherwise the patient may cough it out. Plastic endotracheal tubes with an inflatable cuff usually of the size similar to oral intubation are used.

CLOSURE Closure should be loose to prevent subcutaneous emphysema. Only skin sutures are used. Ties hold the tube in place (FIGURE 10). A dressing is made by cutting a surgical gauze and pulling the gauze under the flange of the tube.

POSTOPERATIVE CARE Special and frequent attention is very desirable in the first few postoperative days. The inner tube must be cleaned every hour or two; otherwise it may block off with accumulated secretions. After a tract has formed, usually in 2 or 3 days, the outer tube may be removed, cleaned, and replaced. Even then, however, the tube should be replaced rapidly, since the stoma constricts sufficiently in only 15 or 20 minutes to make replacement difficult. An obturator is provided with each tracheotomy tube to make insertion of the outer tube easier. There must always be a duplicate tracheal tube at the patient's bedside.

Suctioning of the trachea is done as needed. In the alert patient who can cough, suctioning may not be needed at all; but in the comatose patient suctioning may be required every 15 minutes. It is essential that moisture be added to the air, since the nasal chambers are bypassed and the usual means by which the body moistens the air are lost. This can be accomplished by the use of aerosol bubblers or ultrasonic nebulizers.

Blood gases and blood pH should be monitored frequently until stable and satisfactory levels have been attained. ∎

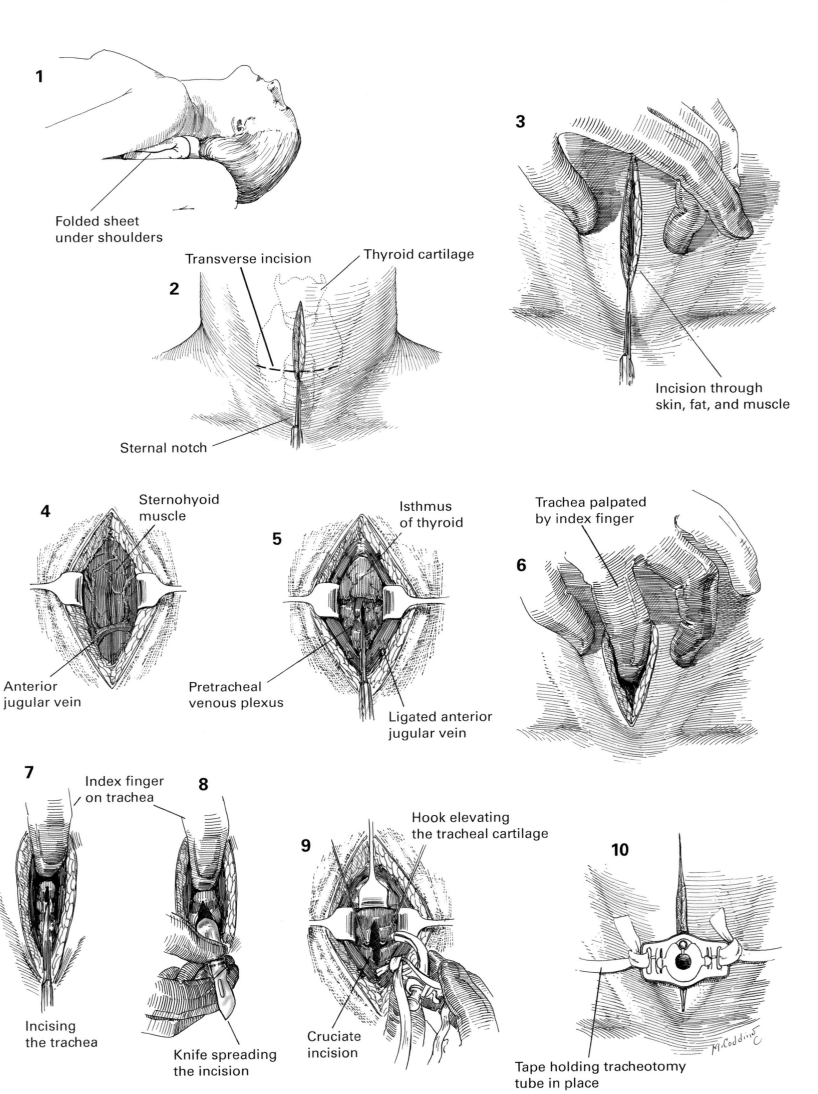

1 Folded sheet under shoulders

2 Transverse incision   Thyroid cartilage   Sternal notch

3 Incision through skin, fat, and muscle

4 Sternohyoid muscle   Anterior jugular vein

5 Isthmus of thyroid   Pretracheal venous plexus   Ligated anterior jugular vein

6 Trachea palpated by index finger

7 Index finger on trachea   Incising the trachea

8 Knife spreading the incision

9 Hook elevating the tracheal cartilage   Cruciate incision

10 Tape holding tracheotomy tube in place

M. Coddins

INDICATIONS Indications for percutaneous dilational tracheotomy (PDT) are similar to those for open tracheotomy (OT) and include providing a portal for pulmonary toilet in debilitated patients or patients with neuromuscular disease, and providing a means for prolonged ventilatory support. Similar to OT, PDT should be considered in patients requiring mechanical ventilation 7 to 10 days following initial intubation. If prolonged intubation is expected based on patient circumstances (high spinal cord or traumatic brain injury), earlier tracheotomy may be considered.

Advantages of PDT over a prolonged translaryngeal intubation include a reduced risk of direct endolaryngeal injury, decreased risk of ventilator-associated pneumonia (VAP), more effective pulmonary toilet, increased airway security and ease in weaning from mechanical ventilation, improved patient comfort with decreased requirements for sedation, and earlier discharge from the intensive care unit (ICU). In suitable patients, the major advantage of PDT to OT is that it is performed as a bedside procedure, obviating the need for operating room time and patient transport, as well as being significantly more cost effective.

When evaluating a patient for PDT, a thorough history and physical examination will identify anatomic contraindications, including previous difficult tracheal intubation, morbid obesity, obscure cervical anatomy, goiter, short thick neck, previous neck surgery (especially tracheotomy), cervical infection, facial or cervical trauma/fractures, halo traction, or known presence of subglottic stenosis. Physiologic contraindications to PDT include hemodynamic instability, requirement of FiO_2 >0.60, a positive end-expiratory pressure (PEEP) >10 cm H_2O, or uncontrolled coagulopathy. Cervical deformity, previous radiation therapy, edema, or tumor can also make tracheal cannulation difficult and increase the risk of morbidity. The need for emergency control of the airway is an absolute contraindication to PDT.

Complications of PDT include injury to posterior tracheal wall resulting in a tracheoesophageal fistula, injury to cupula of lung with pneumothorax, tracheal ring rupture, recurrent laryngeal nerve injury, paratracheal insertion, tube dislodgement with loss of airway, stomal hemorrhage, peristomal cellulitis, subglottic or tracheal stenosis, or a tracheoinnominate fistula. A guidewire placed too deep in the trachea during the procedure can potentially cause bronchoconstriction or lung injury.

PREOPERATIVE PREPARATION Several components are required for PDT placement, and these include bronchoscope, medications, tracheotomy insertion kit, and tracheotomy tube. Kits are available for either the single or the serial dilator technique, and either a standard or a percutaneous tracheotomy tube may be used. The tube cuff must be checked for leaks and then be well lubricated prior to placement. We recommend that the operator develop a materials checklist to facilitate gathering of the critical components prior to the procedure.

ANESTHESIA A three-drug regimen including sedative, analgesic, and nondepolarizing muscle relaxant agents facilitates placement. It is important to maintain immobility during insertion of the introducer needle, guidewire, dilators, and tracheotomy tube to prevent inadvertent puncture of the posterior tracheal wall. Direct manipulation of the trachea (particularly during dilation) is cough provoking, thus the recommendation for paralytics.

POSITION Positioning is aided with a shoulder roll to allow maximal extension of the neck during the procedure. Neck extension elevates the trachea out of the mediastinum and displaces the chin to allow greater access to the anterior neck. The palpable anatomic landmarks are shown in FIGURE 1. The exposed neck can then be prepped with a standard surgical scrub and sterile drapes applied.

OPERATIVE PREPARATION The procedure requires two operators: one performing the tracheotomy and the second providing tracheal visualization with flexible fiberoptic bronchoscopy. Identification and transillumination of the area between the second to fourth tracheal rings with visual confirmation of proper tracheotomy tube positioning improves success in patients with poorly palpable surface anatomy. A respiratory therapist maintains the endotracheal tube (ETT) position and ventilation with 100% oxygen. After all equipment is gathered, the correct level of placement of the ETT being used for control of ventilation is verified by passing a fiberoptic bronchoscope into the trachea by way of a special anesthesia adapter (FIGURE 2). The skin is prepped with an antiseptic, and a sterile draping is done.

INCISION AND EXPOSURE The tracheotomy is performed between the second and fourth tracheal rings. Placing the tracheotomy tube above this level may result in injury to the first ring or cricoid cartilage, which increases the risk of subglottic stenosis or bleeding from the thyroid isthmus. Placing it too low can predispose to tracheoinnominate fistula. A point midway between the cricoid cartilage and the sternal notch is palpated and marked. Local anesthesia is infiltrated in the skin and subcutaneous tissues, as well as into the trachea (FIGURE 3). A vertical skin incision is made in the midline from the level of the cricoid cartilage and extending 1.0 to 1.5 cm downward.

The second or third tracheal interspace is visualized in preparation for the tracheotomy.

DETAILS OF PROCEDURE The ETT should be withdrawn to 1 cm above the anticipated needle insertion site under bronchoscopic or transillumination guidance. In average-sized adults, the tube can be withdrawn to about the 17-cm mark at the teeth. The bronchoscope can show indentation of the trachea with palpation, locating the tracheotomy site. A 17-gauge sheathed introducer needle is then advanced in the midline, angling posterior and caudad (FIGURE 4). Aspiration with an attached syringe containing a small amount of water will indicate when the tracheal wall has been punctured. Puncture of the trachea is confirmed bronchoscopically to ensure midline needle placement (FIGURE 4). The stylet or needle is removed leaving the outer cannula in the trachea. The "J"-tip guidewire is advanced through the cannula into the trachea toward the carina (FIGURE 5). After cannula removal, a short 14-French mini-dilator is advanced over the guidewire using a slight twisting motion and then removed (FIGURE 6). **CONTINUES ▶**

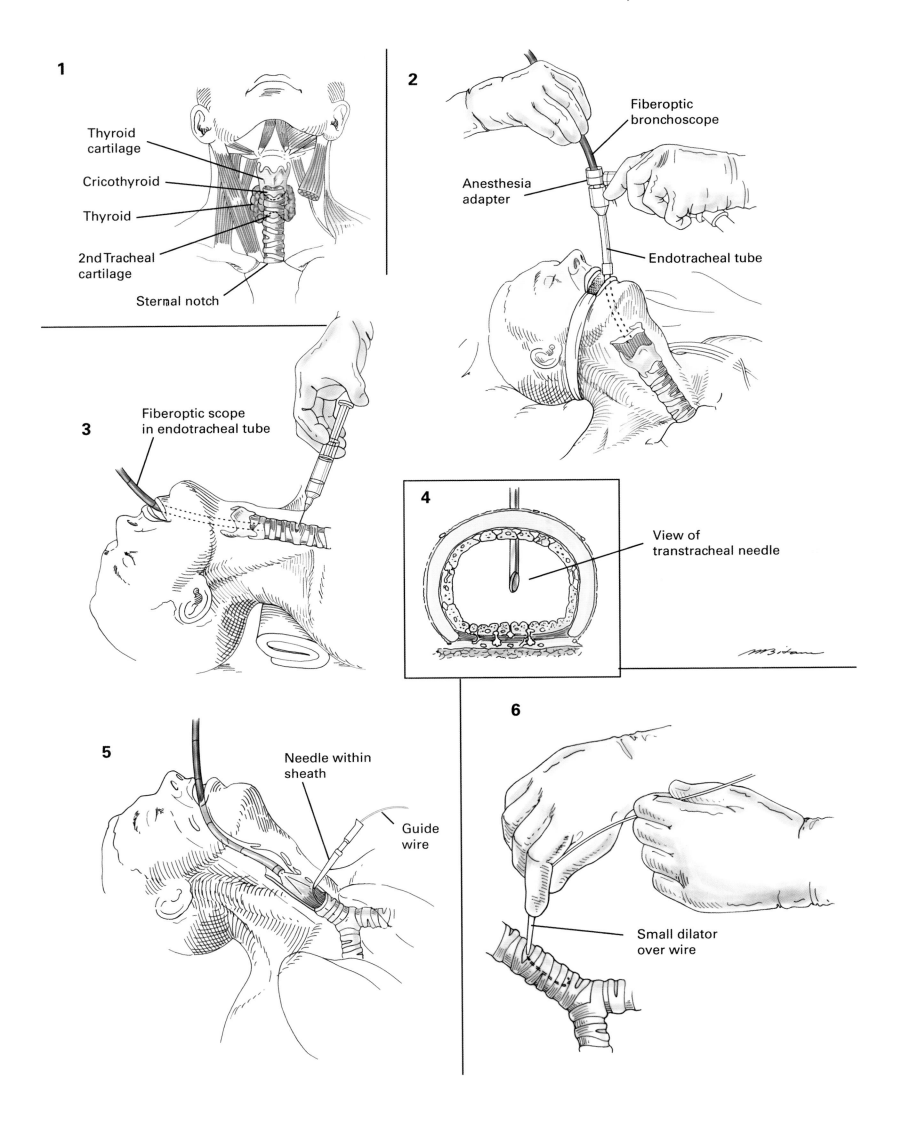

1

Thyroid cartilage

Cricothyroid

Thyroid

2nd Tracheal cartilage

Sternal notch

2

Fiberoptic bronchoscope

Anesthesia adapter

Endotracheal tube

3

Fiberoptic scope in endotracheal tube

4

View of transtracheal needle

5

Needle within sheath

Guide wire

6

Small dilator over wire

DETAILS OF PROCEDURE **◄CONTINUED►** For the single dilator systems, activate the coating by immersing the distal end of the dilator in sterile water or saline. Slide the dilator up to the safety ridge on the guiding catheter, then with concurrent bronchoscopic visualization, advance the dilator assembly using the Seldinger technique over the guidewire into the trachea. After passage to the appropriate depth (marked on the dilator), it is withdrawn and advanced several times to dilate the tract (FIGURE 8). For multiple dilator systems, serial dilation is performed with incrementally larger dilators (FIGURES 7 and 8).

The lubricated tracheotomy tube (loaded on a dilator/guiding catheter unit) is then advanced over the guidewire into the trachea (FIGURE 9). The guidewire and dilator are then removed, leaving the tracheotomy tube in place. The cuff of the tracheotomy tube is inflated and the inner cannula inserted. The ventilator tubing or an Ambu bag device is disconnected from the ETT and attached to the PDT tube (FIGURE 10). The translaryngeal ETT is not removed until correct intratracheal placement of the tracheotomy tube has been confirmed visually by bronchoscopy (FIGURE 10).

CLOSURE The incision is typically just large enough to accommodate the tracheotomy tube and does not require closure. Nonabsorbable suture is used to secure the tracheotomy cuff to the skin and securing tapes are placed to hold the PDT tube in place usually over a dry sterile gauze dressing (FIGURE 11).

POSTOPERATIVE CARE A chest x-ray is ordered to confirm tracheotomy tube position and evaluate for pneumothorax or pneumomediastinum. Elevate the head of the patient's bed 30 to 40 degrees immediately following the procedure and suction any bloody secretions. The tracheal tapes and cuff sutures should not be removed until the first tracheotomy tube change. Ideally, the first tube change should not be attempted until the tract has matured, which requires at least 7 to 10 days. If accidental decannulation occurs within the first 7 days of PDT, an oral ETT should be placed instead of attempting reinsertion of the tracheotomy tube through the stoma. Dislodgement of a tracheotomy tube that has been in place 2 weeks or longer can often be managed simply by replacing the tube through the mature tract. Humidification and frequent tracheal suctioning is recommended to prevent inspissation of secretions, which can result in mucous plugging and tracheotomy tube obstruction. ∎

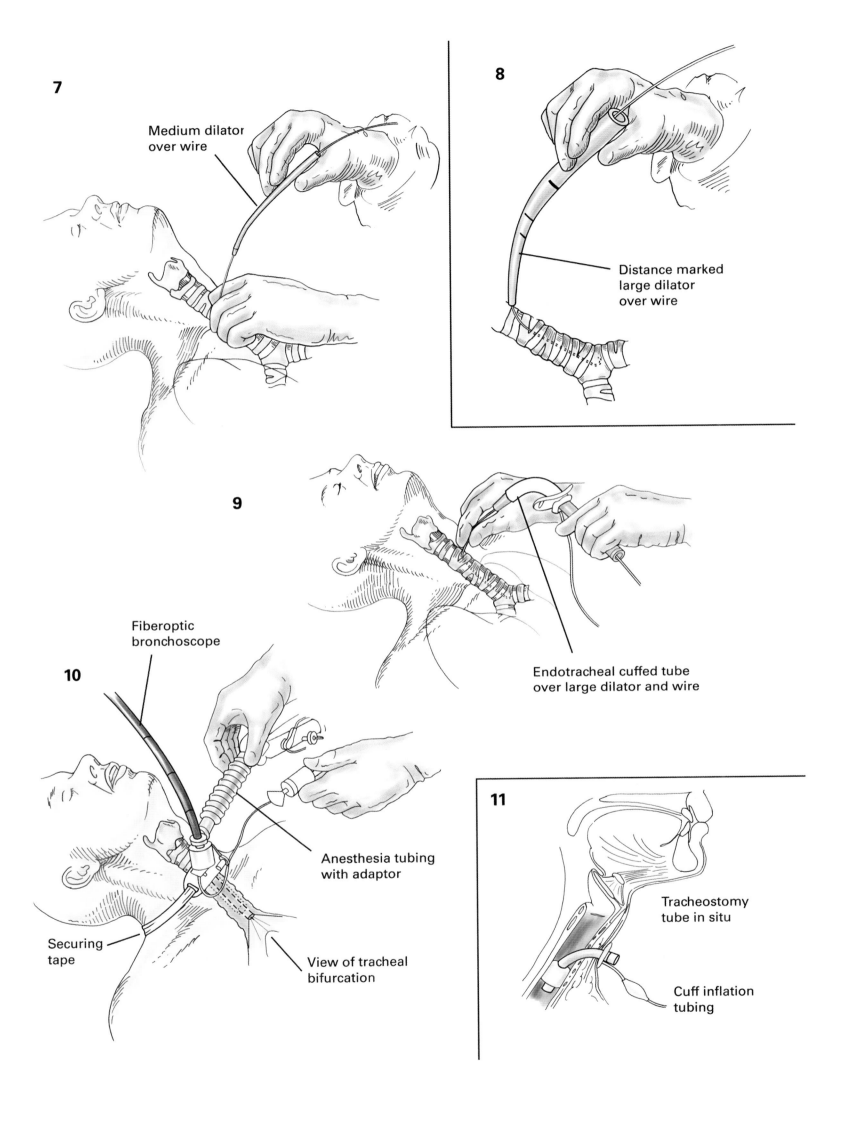

7

Medium dilator over wire

8

Distance marked large dilator over wire

9

Endotracheal cuffed tube over large dilator and wire

10

Fiberoptic bronchoscope

Anesthesia tubing with adaptor

Securing tape

View of tracheal bifurcation

11

Tracheostomy tube in situ

Cuff inflation tubing

RADICAL NECK DISSECTION

INDICATIONS There are two major indications for radical neck dissection. The first is for the removal of palpable metastatic cervical lymph nodes, and the second is for the removal of presumed occult metastatic disease in the neck. The latter indication has been termed "prophylactic neck dissection." "Elective neck dissection" better describes this operation, since it is not intended to prevent metastasis but to remove occult metastatic lymph nodes.

Before radical neck dissection is performed, the surgeon must have assurance that the primary lesion can be controlled either by simultaneous en bloc removal with the radical neck dissection or by radiation therapy. However, curative radiation for cervical metastases must be confined to a single node or small group of nodes, because patients cannot tolerate radical surgery plus radiation therapy to the entire neck. Node fixation, invasion of adjacent tissues, bilateral or contralateral, and distant metastases are relative contraindications to this procedure. In general, radical dissection of the cervical lymph nodes in a patient who is a reasonable surgical risk remains the preferred treatment for metastatic disease of the neck.

The usual patient with metastatic cancer in the neck from an unknown primary source should be treated as if the primary tumor were controlled. If surgical treatment of the cervical metastasis is deferred until the primary neoplasm becomes obvious, the opportunity to control the neck disease is sometimes lost.

PREOPERATIVE PREPARATION The patient's general medical status should be assessed and corrective measures instituted for any treatable abnormalities. Intraoral ulcerations represent a potential source of pathogenic material. The liberal preoperative use of nonirritating solutions (e.g., diluted hydrogen peroxide) can significantly reduce the danger of postoperative infection.

Only rarely will primary cancers of the hypopharynx, cervical esophagus, larynx, and so forth produce respiratory obstruction or interference with alimentation significantly enough to require preoperative tracheostomy or insertion of a feeding tube.

ANESTHESIA The major consideration is a free airway. The equipment should allow free movement of the head and easy access to the endotracheal tube.

The choice of anesthetic agents varies. Consideration must be given to the individual needs of the patient and to the need for cautery. General endotracheal anesthesia is preferred.

Complications at surgery are the carotid sinus syndrome, pneumothorax, and air embolus. The carotid sinus syndrome, consisting of hypotension, bradycardia, and cardiac irregularity, can usually be corrected by infiltrating the carotid sinus with a local anesthetic agent. Intravenous atropine sulfate will usually control the syndrome if the local anesthetic fails. Pneumothorax may result from injury of the apical pleura. It is treated with a closed-tube thoracostomy through the second intercostal space anteriorly.

POSITION The patient is placed in a dorsal recumbent position. The head of the table is somewhat elevated to lessen the blood pressure, particularly the venous pressure, in the head and neck and thus reduce blood loss. The bend of the neck should be placed on the hinge of the headpiece so that the head may be either flexed or extended as needed. A small sandbag should be placed under the shoulders so that the head and neck are extended while the chin remains on a plane horizontal with the shoulders.

OPERATIVE PREPARATION The patient's hair should be completely covered by a snug gauze cap to avoid contamination of the operative field. Once the patient has been correctly positioned on the table, the skin is prepared routinely. The preparation should include a large portion of the face on the side of the dissection, the neck from the midline posteriorly to the sternocleidomastoid muscle of the opposite side of the neck, and the anterior chest wall down to the nipple. The entire field of dissection is outlined with sterile towels secured by either skin staples or sutures. A large sheet about the head and neck area completes the draping.

INCISION AND EXPOSURE Radical neck dissection is described and illustrated. Radical neck dissection refers to the removal of all ipsilateral cervical lymph node groups extending from the inferior border of the mandible superiorly to the clavicle inferiorly and from the lateral border of the sternohyoid muscle, hyoid bone, and contralateral anterior belly of the digastric muscle anteriorly to the anterior border of the trapezius muscle posteriorly. Today most surgeons employ a modified radical neck dissection or functional neck dissection.

Modified radical neck dissection is defined as the excision of all lymph nodes routinely removed in a radical neck dissection with preservation of one or more nonlymphatic structures (spinal accessory nerve, internal jugular vein, and sternocleidomastoid muscle).

The surgeon stands on the side of the proposed dissection. Many types of incision have been used. The incision illustrated allows maximum anatomic visualization, whereas many surgeons prefer two nearly parallel, oblique incisions with an intervening skin bridge that is broadly based at both ends. The most useful incision is a modification of the double trifurcate incision (FIGURE 1), in which the angles of the skin flaps are obtuse and connected by a short vertical incision. Some prefer to make only the upper transverse incision with a single vertical extension that proceeds to the sternocleidomastoid muscle edge and then takes a lazy-S posterior course to the clavicle, as shown by the dashed line in FIGURE 1. The upper arm of the double Y extends from the mastoid process to just below the midline of the mandible. The lower arm extends from the trapezius in a gentle curve to the midline of the neck. This incision allows the greatest exposure of the neck area while producing a good cosmetic result. Creation of the skin flaps includes the platysma muscle (FIGURE 2). In most instances, if the skin flaps are developed without inclusion of the platysma muscle, poor wound healing and uncomfortable scarring with fixation of the skin to the deep neck structures will result. The two lateral skin flaps are turned back, the posterior flap is extended as far as the anterior edge of the trapezius muscle, and the anterolateral flap is extended to expose the strap muscles covering the thyroid gland. In developing the superior skin flap, care must be taken to preserve the mandibular marginal branch of the facial nerve (FIGURE 2). This branch of the facial nerve innervates the lower lip. In the majority of cases the nerve can be identified as it crosses over the external maxillary artery and the anterior facial vein beneath the platysma muscle. Usually, it lies parallel to the lower border of the mandible. Occasionally, the nerve will lie much higher, and it may not be visualized during the neck dissection. As suggested by others, a useful maneuver to preserve this nerve is to identify the external maxillary artery and the anterior facial vein at least 1 cm below the lower border of the mandible (FIGURE 2). After identification, the nerve is retracted and covered by securing the upper end of the vascular stump to the platysma muscle. If obvious or strongly suspected tumor is present in this area, the branches of this nerve are sacrificed voluntarily. The inferior skin flap should be reflected down to expose the superior aspect of the clavicle.

DETAILS OF PROCEDURE Once the four skin flaps have been created, the inferior limits are outlined. The sternocleidomastoid muscle is severed just above its insertion into the clavicle and the sternum (FIGURE 3). The dissection is then shifted to the posterior cervical triangle. Using both sharp and blunt dissection, the surgeon exposes the anterior border of the trapezius muscle (FIGURE 4). **CONTINUES▶**

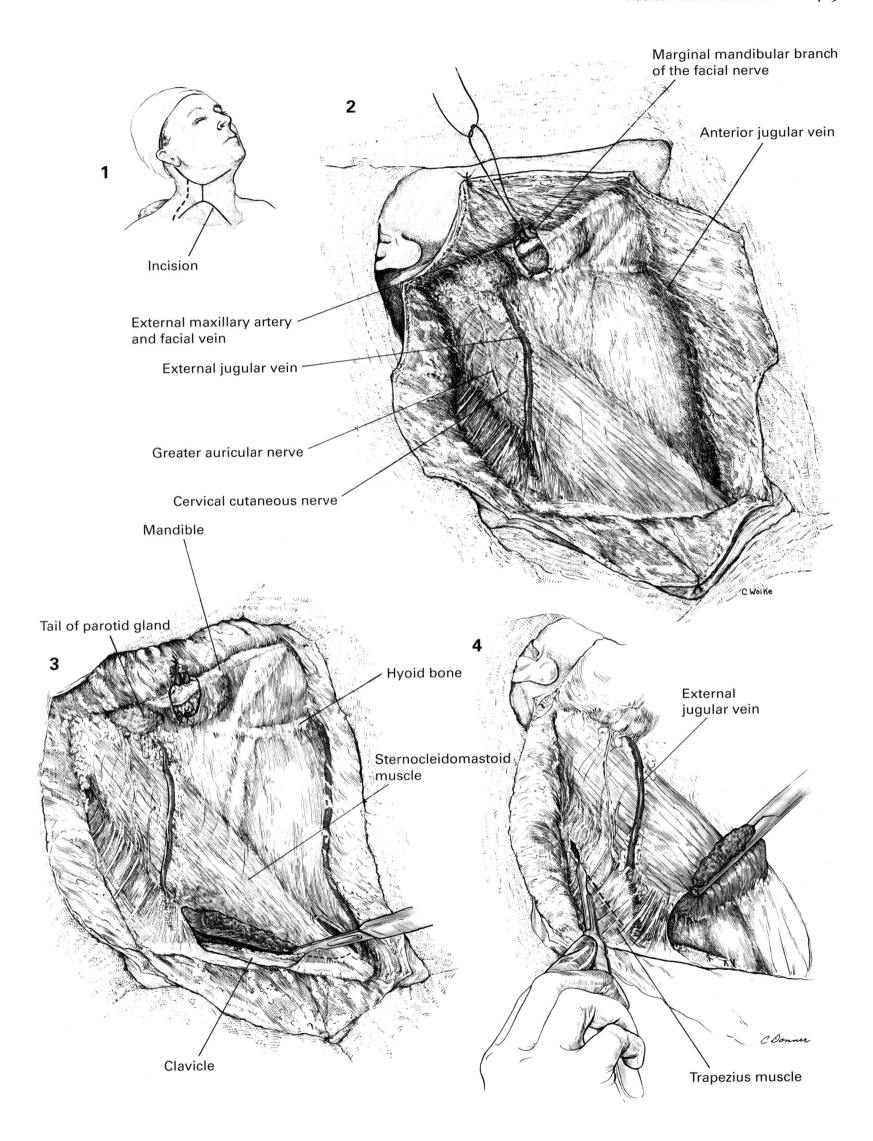

1 Incision

2 Marginal mandibular branch of the facial nerve

Anterior jugular vein

External maxillary artery and facial vein

External jugular vein

Greater auricular nerve

Cervical cutaneous nerve

Mandible

Tail of parotid gland

3

Hyoid bone

Sternocleidomastoid muscle

Clavicle

4

External jugular vein

Trapezius muscle

C. Woike

C. Donner

DETAILS OF PROCEDURE `CONTINUED` As one approaches the most posteroinferior angle of the neck dissection, the first important structure to be seen is the external jugular vein. It is ligated and divided at the posteroinferior corner (FIGURE 5). Then the posterior cervical triangle can be completely cleaned of its areolar and lymphatic tissues. The spinal accessory nerve should be preserved as long as it is not involved with tumor or enlarged lymph nodes. The spinal accessory nerve must be divided (FIGURE 6) if clean dissection of this area is impossible. Dissection is carried forward along the superior aspects of the clavicle. The posterior belly of the omohyoid muscle and the transverse cervical artery and vein are visualized (FIGURE 6). The posterior belly of the omohyoid muscle is severed (FIGURE 7) in order to allow greater exposure of the deep muscles and the brachial plexus. The phrenic nerve is found lying upon the anterior scalene muscle between the brachial plexus and the internal jugular vein (FIGURE 8A). To avoid paralysis of the corresponding leaf of the diaphragm, this nerve should be preserved unless it has been invaded by the cancer. The phrenic nerve lies upon the scalenus anticus muscle. Its exposure has been facilitated by the previous transection of the lower end of the sternocleidomastoid muscle. Just medial to the phrenic nerve, the internal jugular vein is seen (FIGURE 8A). This vessel, which lies within the carotid sheath (FIGURE 8B), is dissected free (FIGURE 9), doubly ligated by a stick tie on the inferior ligation, and then divided (FIGURE 10). By division of the internal jugular vein, avoiding the thoracic duct on the left side, the dissection has been carried down to the prevertebral fascia overlying the deep muscle structures of the neck. The inferior compartment of the neck is then outlined medially by division of the pretracheal fascia just lateral to the strap muscles of the thyroid (FIGURE 11). This facilitates exposure of the common carotid artery, which permits the dissection to be carried superiorly. With the lateral limits of the dissection defined and the common carotid artery exposed, dissection is started inferiorly and extended superiorly, following the floor of the neck or the prevertebral fascia. `CONTINUES`

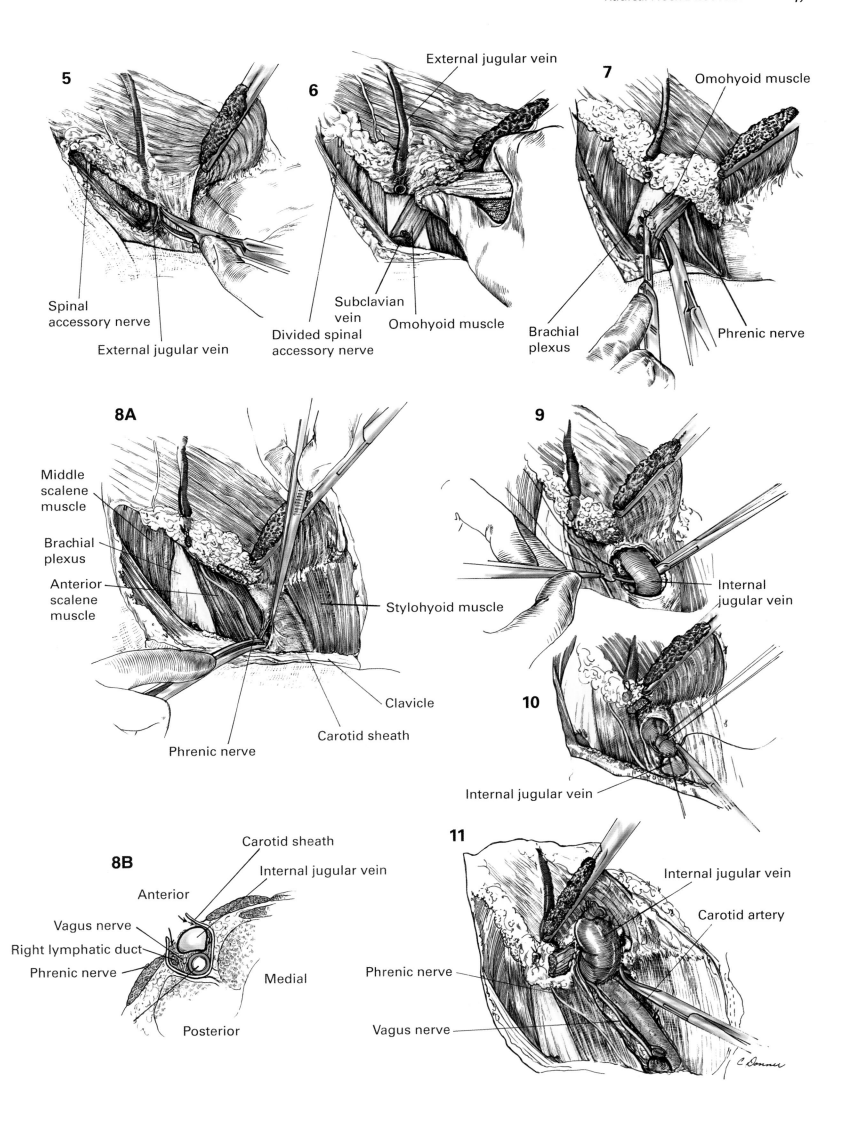

5

Spinal
accessory nerve

External jugular vein

6

External jugular vein

Subclavian
vein

Divided spinal
accessory nerve

Omohyoid muscle

7

Omohyoid muscle

Brachial
plexus

Phrenic nerve

8A

Middle
scalene
muscle

Brachial
plexus

Anterior
scalene
muscle

Phrenic nerve

Stylohyoid muscle

Clavicle

Carotid sheath

9

Internal
jugular vein

10

Internal jugular vein

8B

Carotid sheath

Internal jugular vein

Anterior

Vagus nerve

Right lymphatic duct

Phrenic nerve

Medial

Posterior

11

Internal jugular vein

Carotid artery

Phrenic nerve

Vagus nerve

C. Donner

DETAILS OF PROCEDURE ◄CONTINUED This dissection consists of turning up the areolar and lymphoid tissues of the neck lying along the course of the internal jugular vein, which is reflected upward with these structures (FIGURE 12). All loose areolar tissue about the carotid artery is completely removed. This dissection may be carried out without danger to any of the vital structures, since both the vagus nerve and the common carotid artery are in full view and the other important nerve structures—namely, the phrenic nerve and the brachial plexus—are covered by the prevertebral fascia (FIGURE 12). As the dissection proceeds superiorly, branches of the cervical plexus are seen penetrating the fascia; they should be divided as they emerge through the fascia.

In the anterior part of this phase of the dissection, tributaries of the superior thyroid, superior laryngeal, and pharyngeal veins are seen as they cross the operative field to enter the jugular vein. These may be ligated as the dissection proceeds. The carotid bifurcation can usually be identified by the appearance of the superior thyroid artery (FIGURE 12). With reasonable care this vessel can be preserved. After exposure of the bifurcation, dissection proceeds superiorly with some caution to expose the hypoglossal nerve as it crosses both the internal and external carotid arteries 1 cm or so above the carotid bifurcation (FIGURE 12). The surgeon should watch for this nerve as it emerges deep to the posterior belly of the digastric muscle.

The hypoglossal nerve continues forward into the submaxillary triangle, where it lies inferior to the main submaxillary salivary duct.

After identification of the hypoglossal nerve, attention should be directed to the submental area of the neck. The fascia from the midline of the neck is divided (FIGURE 13). This facilitates exposure of the anterior belly of the digastric muscle and the underlying mylohyoid muscle. Complete exposure of the digastric muscle in the submental compartment is necessary to remove the paired submental nodes (FIGURES 13 and 14). By following the anterior digastric muscle from anterior to posterior, the submaxillary gland is exposed. The submaxillary gland is dissected from its bed by approaching the gland anteriorly (FIGURE 15). By mobilizing the gland from its bed from anterior to posterior, the lingual nerve, which lies in the most superior aspect of the submaxillary space, the submaxillary duct, which lies in the midportion of the compartment, and the hypoglossal nerve, which lies in the most inferior aspect of the area, are identified (FIGURE 16). This exposure may be eased by traction on the submaxillary gland with a tenaculum. This allows the surgeon to visualize the posterior edge of the mylohyoid muscle and to retract this muscle anteriorly (FIGURE 16), thereby exposing the three important structures: the lingual nerve, the salivary duct, and the hypoglossal nerve. To facilitate removal of the submaxillary gland, the major salivary duct is divided and ligated. CONTINUES►

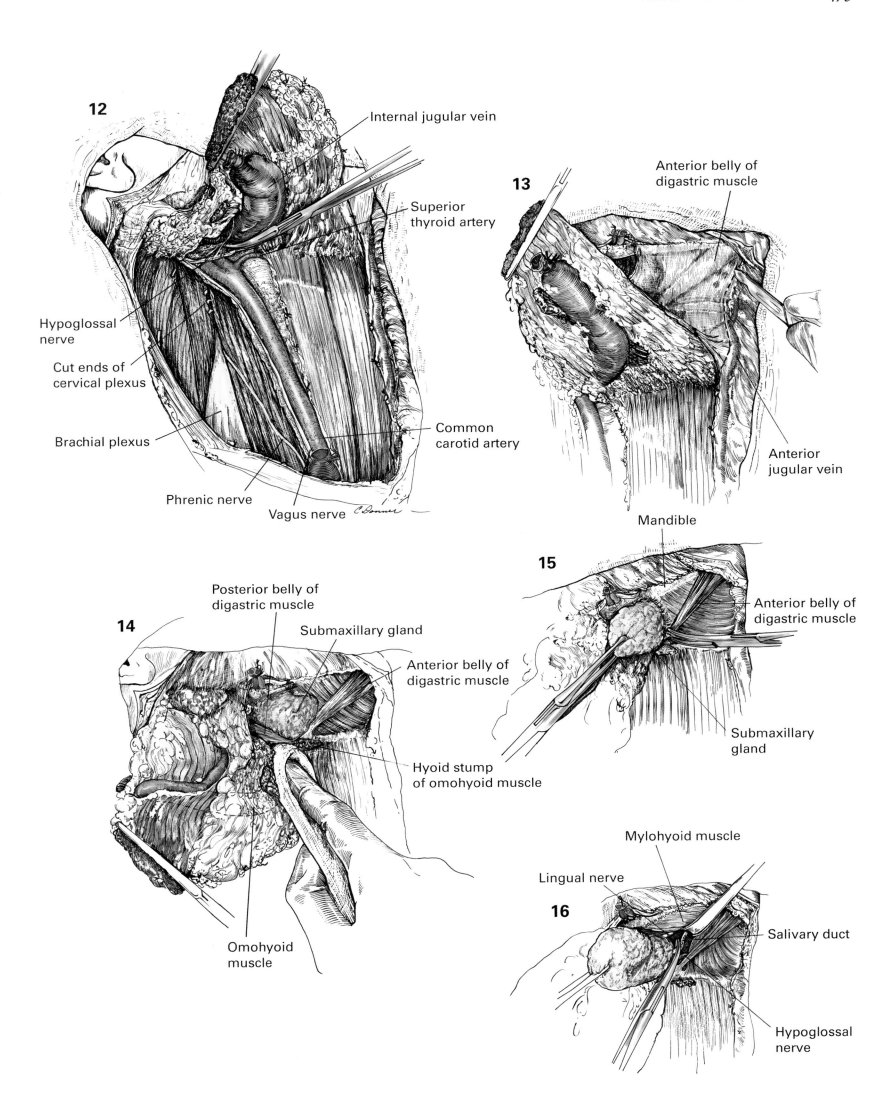

12

Internal jugular vein

Superior thyroid artery

Hypoglossal nerve

Cut ends of cervical plexus

Brachial plexus

Common carotid artery

Phrenic nerve

Vagus nerve

13

Anterior belly of digastric muscle

Anterior jugular vein

Mandible

Posterior belly of digastric muscle

Submaxillary gland

14

Anterior belly of digastric muscle

Hyoid stump of omohyoid muscle

Omohyoid muscle

15

Anterior belly of digastric muscle

Submaxillary gland

Mylohyoid muscle

Lingual nerve

Salivary duct

16

Hypoglossal nerve

DETAILS OF PROCEDURE CONTINUED The anterior belly of the omohyoid muscle is divided from the sling of the digastric muscles; the dissection can then be completed after the posterior belly of the digastric muscle is exposed (FIGURE 17). Retraction of the posterior belly of the digastric superiorly exposes the internal jugular vein for clamping and division (FIGURE 18). Retraction of the posterior belly of the digastric muscle also allows complete exposure of the hypoglossal nerve (FIGURE 18). The internal jugular vein must be clamped high, since the upper limit of the internal jugular chain of lymphatics is one of the most common areas for metastatic cancer in the neck. To ensure that it has been divided high, the tail of the parotid (FIGURE 19) is sacrificed as the complete surgical specimen is excised. If extensive node involvement is present in the upper jugular chain of lymphatics, additional exposure can be obtained by total division of the posterior belly and its subsequent total removal. The dissection is completed with the division of the sternocleidomastoid muscle at the mastoid process.

CLOSURE Hemostasis is secured in all areas of the neck. The platysma is closed using interrupted 0000 sutures. The skin is approximated with interrupted 0000 subcutaneous nonabsorbable sutures. Before closure of the platysma and the skin, closed-suction Silastic catheters are placed beneath both the anterior and posterior skin flaps and connected to suction (FIGURE 20). The placement of the catheters is important to ensure complete removal of fluid from beneath the flaps and to eliminate dead space in the area of dissection. A vacuum-type suction source can be attached to the patient, thus permitting early ambulation. Such catheters have eliminated bulky and uncomfortable pressure dressings.

POSTOPERATIVE CARE The patient is placed immediately in a semi-sitting position to reduce venous pressure within the neck. Oxygen therapy is administered at 4 to 5 L/min until the patient has reacted. The most immediate danger is airway obstruction, especially when the neck dissection has been combined with an intraoral resection. Elective tracheostomy is done when either radical neck dissection is combined with removal of a portion of the mandible or the patient has had significant intraoral excision. If tracheostomy has not been performed, it is advisable to have a sterile tracheostomy set at the bedside.

Another early complication is hemorrhage. The wound should be inspected frequently for such a difficulty. Only moderate analgesia is necessary to control the patient's pain, since the operative site has been almost completely denervated by division of the cervical cutaneous nerves. Excessive sedation is unwise owing to the danger of asphyxia by airway obstruction.

The suction catheters can usually be removed by the fourth or fifth postoperative day.

Tube feedings are necessary only in those patients who have had a combined neck dissection with intraoral dissection. ■

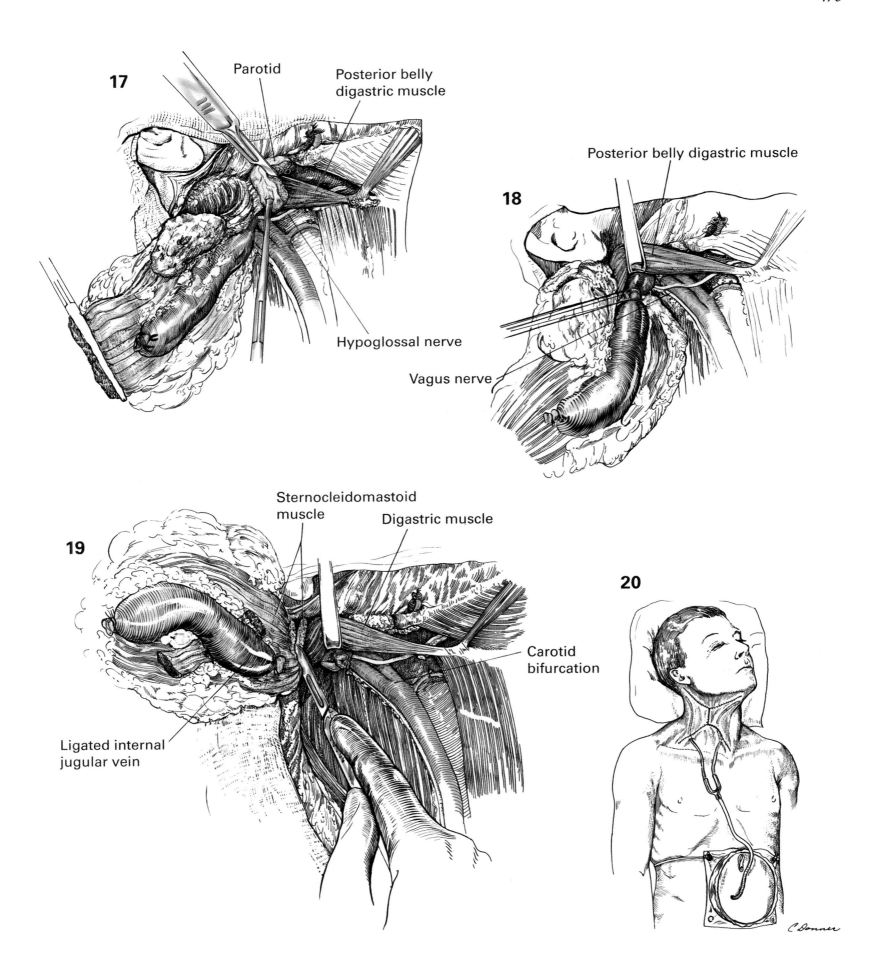

17 Parotid
Posterior belly digastric muscle
Hypoglossal nerve

18 Posterior belly digastric muscle
Vagus nerve

19 Sternocleidomastoid muscle
Digastric muscle
Carotid bifurcation
Ligated internal jugular vein

20

C Donner

ZENKER'S DIVERTICULECTOMY

INDICATIONS The indications for repairing Zenker's diverticulum are partial obstruction, dysphagia, a choking sensation, pain on swallowing, or coughing spells associated with aspirations of fluid from the diverticulum. The diagnosis is confirmed by a barium swallow. The pouch appears suspended by a narrow neck from the esophagus. Zenker's diverticulum is a hernia of mucosa through a weak point located in the midline of the posterior wall of the esophagus where the inferior constrictors of the pharynx meet the cricopharyngeal muscle (FIGURE 1). The neck of the diverticulum arises just above the cricopharyngeal muscle, lies behind the esophagus, and usually projects left of midline. Swallowed barium collects and remains in the herniated mucosa of the esophagus. The procedure described is an open technique and should be applied when a peroral stapling technique is not feasible. The open approach has the advantage of complete removal of the pouch with a low chance of recurrence. Furthermore, it provides a histological specimen to exclude carcinoma within the pouch. It may be useful in treating small pouches, with cricopharyngeal myotomy alone, which cannot be treated endoscopically. Disadvantages of the open procedure consist of a longer hospital stay and significant complications including recurrent laryngeal nerve injury and pharyngeal leak with mediastinitis.

PREOPERATIVE PREPARATION The patient should be on a clear liquid diet for several days before operation. He or she should gargle with an antiseptic mouthwash. Antibiotic therapy may be initiated.

ANESTHESIA Endotracheal anesthesia is preferred through a cuffed endotracheal tube that is inflated to prevent any aspiration of material from the diverticulum. If general anesthesia is contraindicated, the operation can be performed under local or regional infiltration.

POSITION The patient is placed in a semi-erect position with a folded sheet under the shoulders. The head is angulated backward (FIGURE 2). The chin may be turned toward the right side if the surgeon wishes.

OPERATIVE PREPARATION The patient's hair is covered with a snug gauze or mesh cap to avoid contamination of the field. The skin is prepared routinely, and the line of incision is marked along the anterior border of the sternocleidomastoid muscle, centered at the level of the thyroid cartilage (FIGURE 2). Skin towels may be eliminated by using a sterile adherent transparent plastic drape. A large sterile sheet with an oval opening completes the draping.

INCISION AND EXPOSURE The surgeon stands on the patient's left side. He or she should be thoroughly familiar with the anatomy of the neck and aware that a sensory branch of the cervical plexus, the cervical cutaneous nerve, crosses the incision 2 or 3 cm below the angle of the jaw (FIGURE 3). The surgeon applies firm pressure over the sternocleidomastoid muscle with a gauze sponge. The first assistant applies similar pressure on the opposite side. The incision is made through the skin and platysma muscle along the anterior border of the sternocleidomastoid muscle. Bleeding in the subcutaneous tissues is controlled by hemostats and ligation with fine 0000 sutures.

DETAILS OF PROCEDURE As the surgeon approaches the upper extent of the wound, he or she must avoid dividing the cervical cutaneous nerve, which lies in the superficial investing fascia (FIGURE 3). The sternocleidomastoid muscle is then retracted laterally and its fascial attachments along the anterior border are divided. The omohyoid muscle crosses the lower portion of the incision and is divided between clamps (FIGURE 4). Hemostasis is obtained by a 00 ligature. The inferior end of the omohyoid muscle is retracted posteriorly, while the superior end is retracted medially (FIGURE 5). As the middle cervical fascia investing the omohyoid and strap muscles is divided in the upper portion of the wound, the superior thyroid artery is exposed, divided between clamps, and ligated (FIGURES 4 and 5). The cervical visceral fascia containing the thyroid gland, trachea, and esophagus is entered medial to the carotid sheath. The posterior surfaces of the pharynx and esophagus are exposed by blunt dissection. The diverticulum is then usually easy to recognize unless inflammation is present, causes adhesions to the surrounding structures (FIGURES 6 and 7). If difficulty is encountered in outlining the diverticulum, the anesthesiologist can pass a rubber or plastic catheter down into it. Air is injected into this catheter to distend the diverticulum. The lower end of the diverticulum is freed from its surrounding structures by blunt and sharp dissection, its neck is identified, and its origin from the esophagus located (FIGURES 6 and 7). Special attention is given to the removal of all connective tissue surrounding the diverticulum at its origin. This area must be cleaned until there remains only the mucosal herniation through the defect in the muscular wall between the inferior constrictors of the pharynx and the cricopharyngeal muscle below. The cricopharyngeal muscle is divided (FIGURE 8). This is a critical portion of the operation. Care must be taken not to divide the two recurrent laryngeal nerves, which may lie on either side of the neck of the diverticulum or in the tracheoesophageal groove, more anteriorly (FIGURE 7). The NG tube is palpated in the esophagus and the diverticulum is pulled away from the cervial esophagus (FIGURE 8). A linear stapling device is applied to the neck of the esophagus and closed with care taken not to narrow the esophageal lumen (FIGURE 9). The neck of the diverticulum is divided with the stapling device and the diverticulum removed (FIGURE 10). A row of horizontal sutures closes the muscular defect between the inferior constrictors of the pharynx and the cricopharyngeal muscle below. These muscles are brought together by interrupted 0000 sutures (FIGURE 10).

CLOSURE After thorough irrigation, careful hemostasis is obtained. A small closed-suction Silastic drain may be placed, and the omohyoid is rejoined with several interrupted sutures. The platysma is reapproximated with fine absorbable sutures, and 0000 nonabsorbable sutures are used to close the skin in a subcutaneous manner. Adhesive skin strips and a lightweight sterile gauze dressing are applied. These must not be circumferential about the neck.

POSTOPERATIVE CARE The patient is kept in a semi-sitting position and not allowed to swallow anything by mouth. Water and tube feedings are provided through the nasogastric tube to maintain fluid and electrolyte balance for the first 3 days. The drain is removed on the second postoperative day unless contraindicated by excessive serosanguineous drainage or by saliva draining from the wound. The nasogastric tube is removed on the second or third postoperative day, and the patient is started on clear fluids. The diet is advanced as tolerated. The patient is permitted out of bed on the first postoperative day and may ambulate with the nasogastric tube in place but clamped off. Antibiotic coverage is optional, depending upon the amount of contamination. ■

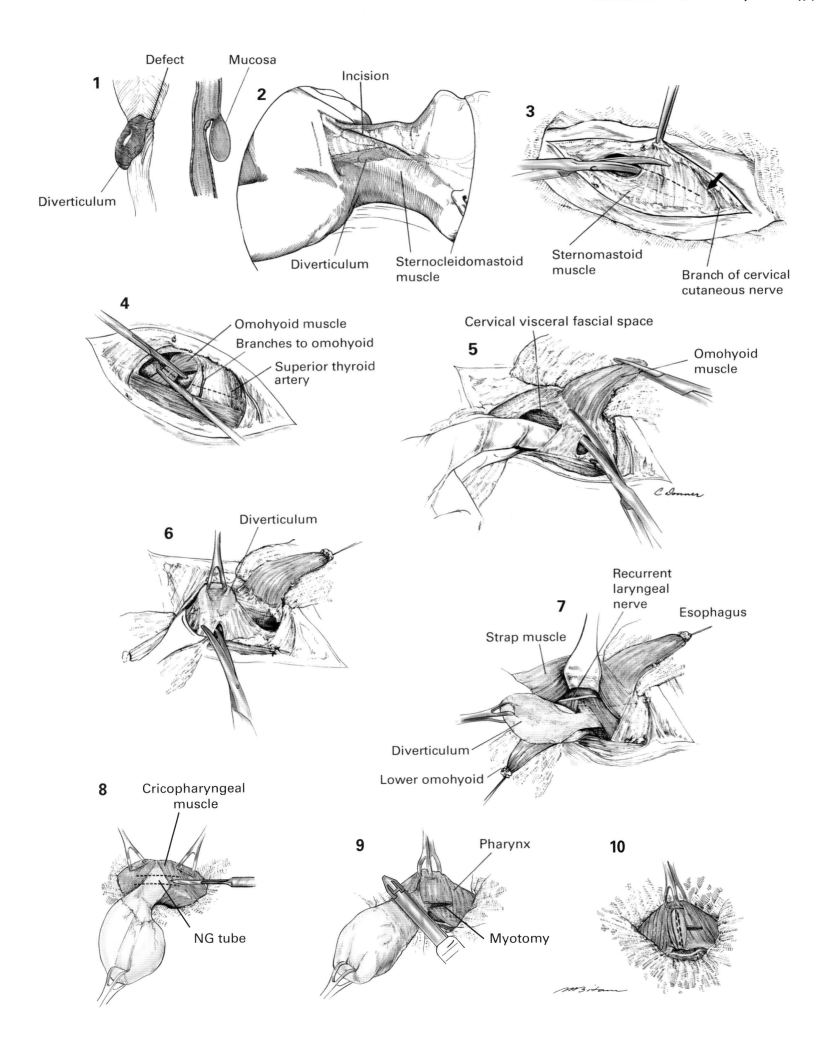

1 Defect Mucosa Diverticulum

2 Incision Diverticulum Sternocleidomastoid muscle

3 Sternomastoid muscle Branch of cervical cutaneous nerve

4 Omohyoid muscle Branches to omohyoid Superior thyroid artery

5 Cervical visceral fascial space Omohyoid muscle

6 Diverticulum

7 Strap muscle Recurrent laryngeal nerve Esophagus Diverticulum Lower omohyoid

8 Cricopharyngeal muscle NG tube

9 Pharynx Myotomy

10

PAROTIDECTOMY, LATERAL LOBECTOMY

INDICATIONS Tumors are the most common indication for surgical exploration of the parotid gland. Most are benign mixed tumors that arise in the lateral lobe and are treated with wide excision, including a margin of normal tissue to prevent local recurrence. Exploration of the parotid area must include careful identification of the facial nerve and its branches, thus avoiding the major complication of facial nerve palsy. Malignant tumors are also seen and require a wide excision, which may include all or a portion of the facial nerve if it is involved. Lesions of the medial lobe may necessitate a total parotidectomy; a superficial parotidectomy is carried out first to identify and preserve the facial nerve before the medial lobe is explored.

PREOPERATIVE PREPARATION It is essential that all patients undergoing parotid surgery be made aware of the possible loss of facial nerve function, with its resultant functional and cosmetic consequences. Men should shave themselves early on the morning of surgery; the hair about the ear may be cleared by the surgeon before draping.

ANESTHESIA Oral endotracheal anesthesia with a flexible coupling is utilized so that the anesthesiologist may be located at the patient's side, thus giving the surgeon adequate room. A short-acting muscle relaxant should be used for the endotracheal intubation. This allows the surgeon to identify motor nerves by direct stimulation (gentle pinch) during the dissection.

POSITION The patient is positioned on his or her back, and the face is turned to the side opposite the lesion. The head and neck are placed in slight extension, and the head of the table is elevated to reduce venous pressure in the head and neck.

OPERATIVE PREPARATION After appropriate skin preparation with detergents and antiseptic solutions, sterile towel drapes are positioned to allow visualization of the entire ipsilateral side of the face.

INCISION AND EXPOSURE The incision is carried in the crease immediately in front of the ear, around the lobule and up in the postauricular fold (FIGURE 1). It then curves posteriorly over the mastoid process and swings smoothly down into the superior cervical crease. The superior cervical crease is located approximately 2 cm below the angle of the mandible. It should be remembered that with the patient's neck extended and head turned to the side, the facial skin is pulled down onto the neck, and the incision should be made low enough that when the patient's head is returned to normal position, the incision does not lie along the body of the mandible. No incisions are made on the cheek itself. The cervical-facial skin flap is then elevated with sharp dissection to expose adequately the area of the tumor. This elevation takes place to the anterior border of the masseter muscle. A traction suture may be placed through the earlobe to hold this out of the operator's visual field (FIGURE 2). The masseteric parotid fascia has then been exposed, and the parotid gland can be seen within its capsule, bounded superiorly by the cartilages of the ear, posteriorly by the sternocleidomastoid muscle, and medially by the digastric and stylohyoid muscles.

DETAILS OF PROCEDURE The surgeon must understand clearly the surgical anatomy of the facial nerve. The main trunk of the facial nerve emerges from the stylomastoid foramen. It courses anteriorly and slightly inferiorly between the mastoid process and the membranous portion of the external auditory canal. The main trunk of the nerve usually bifurcates into the temporofacial and cervicofacial divisions after it enters the gland, but occasionally this occurs before entrance. The parotid gland is commonly described as being divided into superficial and deep lobes, the nerve passing between the two. These lobes are not anatomically distinct, because the separation is defined by the location of the nerve, which actually passes directly through the glandular parenchyma. The cervicofacial division bifurcates into the small platysmal or cervical branch and the marginal mandibular branch at the inferior margin of the gland. The latter courses within the platysma muscle just inferior to the horizontal ramus of the mandible, where it innervates the lower lip. Whereas most other branches of the facial nerve have numerous cross-anastomoses, the marginal mandibular branch has none; therefore division of this branch will always result in paralysis of half of the lower lip. Identification of the marginal mandibular branch before the main nerve trunk is defined is facilitated by the fact that 97% of the time it lies superficial to the posterior facial vein.

The buccal zygomatic division emerges from the anterior margin of the gland with numerous filamentous branches that innervate the muscles of facial expression, including the periorbital muscles and circumoral muscles of the upper lip. The temporal branch runs superiorly and innervates the frontal muscles. This branch has poor regenerative potential and no cross-anastomosis; injury to it will lead to permanent paralysis of the frontalis muscle.

The safest way of identifying the facial nerve is to locate and expose the main trunk. The anterior border of the sternocleidomastoid muscle is identified, as are the posterior facial vein and the greater auricular nerve, in the inferior portion of the incision (FIGURES 2 and 3). The capsule of the parotid gland then is mobilized from the anterior border of the sternocleidomastoid muscle, and dissection is carried down in an area inferior and posterior to the cartilaginous external auditory canal.

Several landmarks are utilized here in the search for the main trunk of the facial nerve. The sternocleidomastoid muscle is retracted posteriorly and the parotid gland anteriorly. The posterior belly of the digastric can be visualized as it pushes up into its groove (FIGURE 4), and the nerve lies anterior to this. The membranous portion of the canal is the superior landmark, and the nerve lies approximately 5 mm from the tip of this cartilage. By using these landmarks as well as a Faradic stimulator or gentle mechanical stimulation with forceps, the surgeon safely can locate the main trunk of the nerve (FIGURE 5). If mechanical stimulation is used, the instruments must not be clamped firmly on the tissue as a form of testing, but rather the tissue should be pinched gently as the muscles of the face are observed for motion. If an electrical nerve stimulator is used, it must be tested regularly to be certain that it is functioning in each test situation. A final landmark is a branch of the postauricular artery just lateral to the main trunk of the facial nerve. If the position or bulk of the tumor makes exposure of the main trunk of the facial nerve difficult, it may be identified distally. As indicated previously, the marginal mandibular branch lies superficial to the posterior facial vein in most circumstances. The buccal branch lies immediately superior to Stensen's duct, and identification of this duct will lead the operator to the buccal branch of the nerve. Dissection from distal to proximal must be carried out carefully, because the junction of other branches of the nerve may not be seen as easily as divisions of the nerve when the dissection is carried out in the opposite direction.

Numerous methods have been described for freeing the gland from the nerve. The safest dissection technique is the hemostat-scissors dissection. By dissecting bluntly with a fine hemostat and then cutting only the tissue exposed in the open jaws, the surgeon can protect the nerve (FIGURE 6). The gland may be elevated by clamping the tissue or by the use of holding sutures, and the two major divisions of the facial nerve are identified. Dissection may proceed anteriorly along any or all of the major divisions, depending upon the tumor's position. Since the majority of tumors occur in the lower portion of the lateral lobe, the upper segment of the gland is usually mobilized first (FIGURE 7). A moderate amount of bleeding may be expected, but this will be controllable with finger pressure, electrocoagulation, or fine ligatures. Once the tumor has been freed from the facial nerve, Stensen's duct will appear in the midanterior portion of the gland (FIGURE 8). Only the lateral lobe tributary is ligated, because medial lobe atrophy will occur if the main duct is tied. After removal of the lateral lobe, the isthmus and the medial lobe remain deep to the facial nerve; they will appear as small islands of parotid tissue and should represent only 20% of the total parotid gland. The lobe may be transected when the tumor and a surrounding portion of normal tissue have been completely separated from the facial nerve.

CLOSURE The wound is thoroughly irrigated and meticulous hemostasis obtained. A small perforated closed-suction Silastic catheter may be brought up through a stab wound and attached to a suction apparatus. The subcutaneous tissue is approximated with fine absorbable sutures followed by adhesive skin strips.

POSTOPERATIVE CARE Temporary paresis from traction on the facial nerve may occur and usually clears in a few days to a week. If the greater auricular nerve has been divided in the course of the procedure, anesthesia in its distribution will be permanent. ■

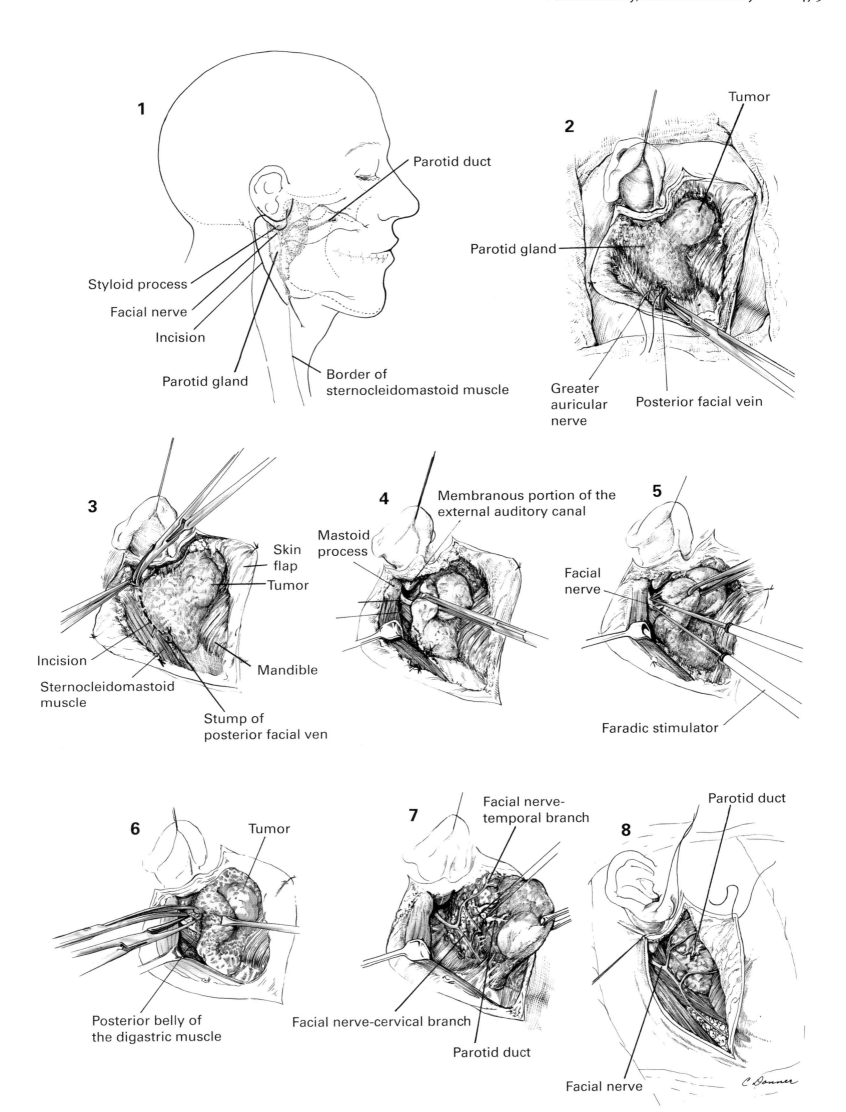

1

Parotid duct

Styloid process

Facial nerve

Incision

Parotid gland

Border of
sternocleidomastoid muscle

2

Tumor

Parotid gland

Greater
auricular
nerve

Posterior facial vein

3

Skin
flap

Tumor

Incision

Sternocleidomastoid
muscle

Mandible

Stump of
posterior facial ven

4

Membranous portion of the
external auditory canal

Mastoid
process

5

Facial
nerve

Faradic stimulator

6

Tumor

Posterior belly of
the digastric muscle

7

Facial nerve-
temporal branch

Facial nerve-cervical branch

Parotid duct

8

Parotid duct

Facial nerve

C Donner

SECTION XII
SKIN, SOFT TISSUE, AND BREAST

INDICATIONS Sentinel lymph node dissection (SLND) is an important procedure in the staging of patients with cutaneous melanoma. Skin melanomas have a straightforward lymphatic flow that can be mapped. The metastases rarely skip to higher lymph nodes; therefore, an SLND can provide the first evidence of metastatic spread of the melanoma. This operation is indicated in patients who do not have palpable regional lymph nodes. The original melanoma on histologic studies following wide excision should be of intermediate or greater thickness (>1 mm). If thinner, the melanoma should have associated high risk factors such as ulceration or mitotic count/mm² ≥1. Additional risk factors to be considered are age, site, Clark's level of invasion, and gender. An SLND that uses both radionuclide and blue dye is highly accurate in finding positive lymph nodes. It allows a focused pathologic examination by the pathologist with both routine hematoxylin and eosin (H&E), plus immunohistochemical staining on the lymph nodes that are most likely to contain metastases. Finally, an SLND should be considered prior to a wide excision of the primary melanoma site. This is especially important if a rotational skin flap is planned for closure, as the resultant scar will alter the dermal lymphatic flow.

PREOPERATIVE PREPARATION In the example shown (FIGURE 1), the cutaneous melanoma was excised from the midportion of the patient's back. This is considered a watershed area—that is to say, the lymphatic drainage may go to either axilla or groin. Accordingly, a preoperative scintigram is required to demonstrate which lymphatic basin receives the lymphatic drainage from the tumor site. The most common areas are the axillary and inguinal regions for extremity or truncal lesions and cervical or supraclavicular regions for head and neck primaries. Other sites include deep iliac, hypogastric, and obturator regions and the popliteal or epitrochlear regions for legs and arms, respectively. Finally, ectopic sites are also possible.

The skin must be cleared of any active infections, as must the excision site for the melanoma. Preparation, inspection, and monitoring of the radionuclide solution must be coordinated with the nuclear medicine staff.

A few hours before operation, the patient is injected with a radionuclide solution intradermally about the perimeter of the surgical site, using sterile technique. This may be done by the radiologist or the surgeon. The commercially available human serum albumin or sulfur colloid solution tagged with technetium 99m is filtered and sterilized. Four syringes of approximately 100 µC Tc 99m filtered sulfur colloid and 0.1 mL of normal saline each are prepared, for a total dose of about 400 µC. The area for injection is prepared with an antiseptic solution. Disposable paper drapes are widely placed and the physician is gloved. Extensive shielding for radioactivity is not required, but the site and supplies are monitored with a radiation survey meter. The gloved physician injects the radionuclide in an intradermal pattern about the incision (FIGURE 2). The area is washed and all the disposable items are surveyed and disposed of in a radiologically safe manner.

The lymphatic drainage area or basin is noted on a large or whole-body scintigram; a hand-held gamma detector is used to identify the hottest area. This spot is marked with indelible ink as a temporary tattoo and the patient is transported to the operating room.

ANESTHESIA Deep sedation plus local or a general anesthesia may be used.

POSITION The patient is placed in a comfortable supine position. If an axillary SLND is planned, that arm should be out at a 90-degree angle on a padded arm board. Alternative positions, such as the lateral decubitus position, can be utilized if wide excision of a lesion on the back is planned in conjunction with the sentinel node procedure. The arm can be sterilely draped with a stockinet if desired to allow manipulation of the extremity to facilitate identification of the sentinel node. If the dissection is planned in the neck, the head of the table may be elevated and the patient's head turned to the opposite side.

OPERATIVE PREPARATION The hair is shaved about the tattoo and a routine skin preparation and draping is performed. The surgeon performs another intradermal injection about the perimeter of the melanoma excision site using 1 to 3 mL of isosulfan blue vital dye (FIGURE 3). The area is massaged for a few minutes, and a faint blue streaking of the dye may be seen in the dermal lymphatics heading toward the SLND site. In this illustration, the sentinel node is within the left axilla. Using a hand-held gamma probe in a sterile cover (FIGURE 4), the surgeon verifies that the tattoo marks the hottest spot. A small 5-cm transverse incision is made over the tattoo and dissection is carried into the subcutaneous fat (FIGURE 5). The fat is retracted laterally and the probe explores the open incision to find the area of maximum radioactivity (FIGURE 6). **CONTINUES**

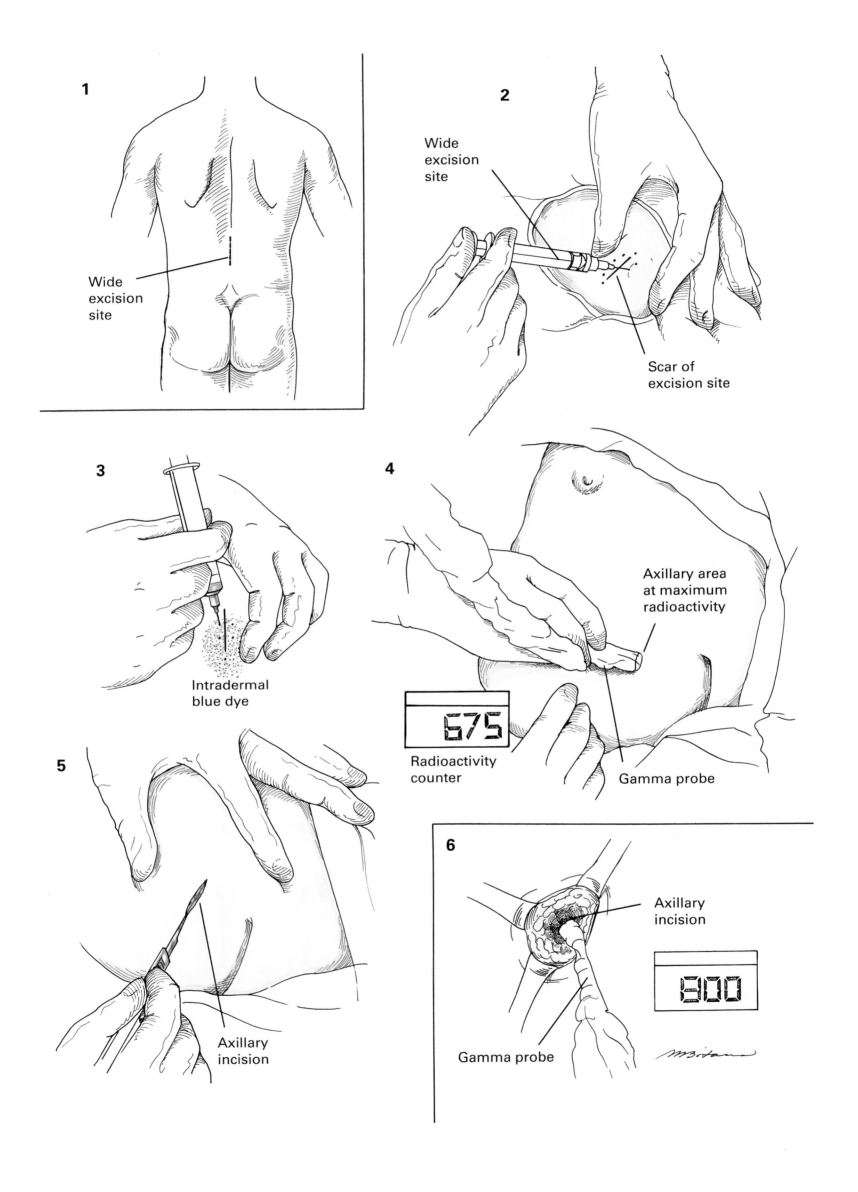

1

Wide
excision
site

2

Wide
excision
site

Scar of
excision site

3

Intradermal
blue dye

4

Axillary area
at maximum
radioactivity

675

Radioactivity
counter

Gamma probe

5

Axillary
incision

6

Axillary
incision

Gamma probe

900

OPERATIVE PREPARATION `CONTINUED` The blue dye may be seen in lymphatic channels flowing into a now palpable lymph node (FIGURE 7). This node should be blue and hot. The node is dissected free, as are any neighboring lymph nodes that are faintly blue, have significant radioactivity counts, or are clinically suspicious (FIGURE 8). Significant radioactivity is identified as a level ≥10% of the counts of the hottest sentinel node or a level greater than two or three times the background activity of the axillary tissue. A small cluster, usually two or three lymph nodes, is excised (FIGURE 9), as often there is more than one sentinel node. The nodal basin is scanned with the probe to verify that no other hot areas or potential sentinel lymph nodes exist. The probe demonstrates a basal background level (FIGURE 9). The nodal cluster removed is examined and the lymph nodes are separated. One node, the principal sentinel lymph node, should be blue and quite hot (FIGURE 10A). In this illustration, lymph nodes B and C are considered sentinel lymph nodes, as they have significant radioactivity counts. Any other regional nodes that have any blue coloration are also considered sentinel nodes, even if they do not have elevated radioactivity counts. A final visual and gamma probe survey is performed about the operative site and careful hemostasis is obtained.

CLOSURE Subcutaneous tissue and Scarpa's fascia are closed with interrupted 000 absorbable sutures. The skin is approximated with fine subcuticular sutures. Adhesive skin strips and a dry sterile dressing are applied. Skin adhesive may be used as an alternative or adjunct to subcuticular closure, and if used, no dressing is applied.

POSTOPERATIVE CARE In most cases, this procedure can be performed in an ambulatory surgery setting. The patient returns home when discharge criteria for this surgery are met. The patient is given written instructions concerning activities and signs of bleeding or infection. Simple oral pain medication should suffice. At the follow-up visit, the surgeon reviews the pathology findings with the patient, who may require a formal lymphadenectomy if any sentinel lymph nodes show metastases. ∎

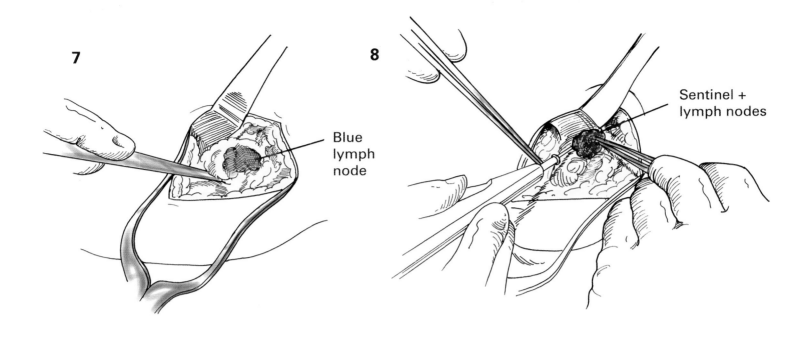

7

8

Blue
lymph
node

Sentinel +
lymph nodes

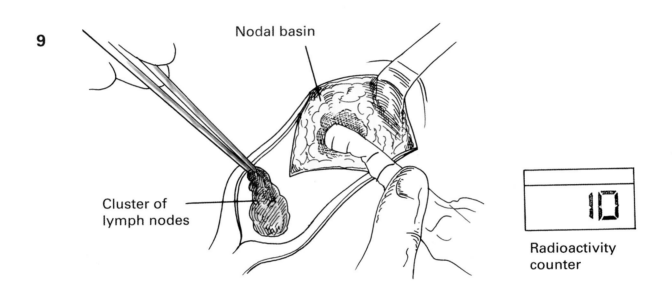

9

Nodal basin

Cluster of
lymph nodes

10

Radioactivity
counter

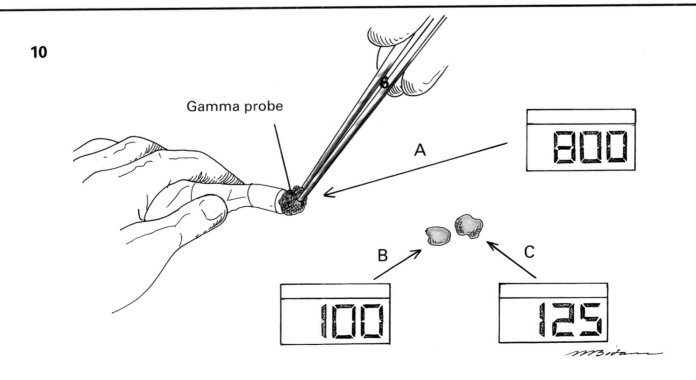

10

Gamma probe

A

B

C

BREAST ANATOMY AND INCISIONS

A. ANATOMY

The regional anatomy of the breast is illustrated in FIGURES 1 and 2. The principal blood supply to the breast comes from the medial perforating branches of the internal mammary artery and vein after they transverse the pectoralis major muscle and its anterior investing fascia. The medial aspect of the breast has lymphatic drainage into the internal mammary chain of lymph nodes within the chest; however, this is quite variable. The majority of the lymphatics from the breast drain to the axillary lymph node basin. The most proximal node or nodes may be located in atypical locations such as within the breast in the axillary tail of the upper/outer quadrant or very low on the lateral chest wall. The identification of these nodes using radionuclide tags and blue dye localization techniques is one of the additional benefits of a sentinel lymph node dissection. Axillary lymph nodes have been grouped into three levels defined by their anatomic relationship to the pectoralis minor muscle (FIGURE 2). Level I nodes are defined as those lateral to the edge of the pectoralis minor muscle. This area includes the external mammary, subscapular, and lateral axillary nodes. Level II nodes are behind or posterior to the muscle and are commonly defined as the central axillary lymph nodes. Level III nodes are located medial or superior to the pectoralis minor muscle. This group includes the subclavicular or apical lymph nodes. They reside in the apex of the axillary space behind the clavicle and deep to the axillary vein. In general, level I and II nodes are removed in axillary lymph node dissections (ALNDs). The overall boundaries of this standard ALND are the chest wall (serratus anterior muscle) medially, axillary vein superiorly, subscapularis muscle plus thoracodorsal and long thoracic nerves posteriorly, and latissimus dorsi laterally.

The axillary vein is the major structure defining the superior border of the surgical dissection. The axillary artery (posterior and pulsatile) plus the brachial plexus (superior and solid) are palpable but not exposed. Common regional findings are dual axillary veins or a very large, long thoracic vein running longitudinally along the lateral chest. After the axillary vein is exposed by the surgeon, a key landmark aids in finding the thoracodorsal nerve, which is deep upon the subscapularis muscle. A pair of subscapular veins are identified (FIGURE 1). The more superficial one is divided, revealing the deep subscapular vein and the adjacent subscapular artery, which may be mistaken for the thoracodorsal nerve. This nerve, however, is posterior to the axillary vein and medial to the deep subscapular vein. It tends to angle toward the deep subscapular vein, whereas the subscapular artery is more parallel. A gentle mechanical stimulation of this nerve will result in muscle contraction.

Also running parallel to the axillary vein and rising perpendicularly from between the ribs on the chest wall are the sensory intercostal brachial skin nerves. One or more of these nerves may pass directly through the axillary fat and lymph nodes that will be removed in the dissection. Division results in hypesthesia in the posterior axillary web and in the upper/inner arm. Conversely, the long thoracic nerve runs longitudinally over the serratus anterior at the depth of an axillary dissection. If the surgeon dissects the axillary fat and specimen cleanly off of the serratus anterior muscle, the long thoracic nerve will be found not on the muscle but rather out in the axillary fat about 7 or 8 cm deep to the lateral edge of the pectoralis minor muscle. Gentle mechanical stimulation will elicit contraction of the serratus anterior muscle. It is also important to note that the long thoracic nerve tends to arch anteriorly as it proceeds caudally.

B. BREAST INCISIONS FOR EXCISIONAL BIOPSY

The principal indication for biopsy is the presence of clinically suspicious findings on physical examination or diagnostic studies. Palpable masses may be sampled with fine needle aspiration (FNA) for cytologic evaluation. A better diagnosis is obtained with a core needle biopsy and histologic study. Asymmetric nodularity, architectural distortion, or suspicious patterns of microcalcifications may require excisional biopsy guided by wire localization when percutaneous biopsy cannot be performed or is not concordant. In general, a wide excisional biopsy with a clear margin of several millimeters of surrounding normal glandular tissue is planned. The placement of the incision is determined by the location of the lesion (FIGURE 3). If possible, incisions in the upper/inner quadrants should be avoided, as they are most visible. Circumareolar or inframammary incisions tend to give the best cosmetic result. Curvilinear incisions along Langer's lines may be used in most areas; however, some surgeons prefer radial incisions, especially in the medial breast. The incision should be kept small and placed over the lesion. The incision for a wire localization need not be placed about the entrance site of the wire, because most wires are flexible enough to be drawn through the skin and subcutaneous fat into an open biopsy site.

C. SIMPLE OR TOTAL MASTECTOMY

INDICATIONS A simple or total mastectomy is indicated in patients who are not candidates for breast-conserving (lumpectomy) operations or who prefer this approach. The principal indications are for large cancers that persist after neoadjuvant therapy, especially in a smaller breast, in multicentric disease, and in elderly poor-risk patients with localized lesions. This procedure may also be utilized for breast cancer risk reduction in high-risk populations.

PREOPERATIVE PREPARATION (See Chapter 127, page 488).

ANESTHESIA General anesthesia is given via an endotracheal tube. Short-acting muscle depolarizing agents are used for the intubation.

POSITION The patient is placed in a comfortable supine position with the arm on the involved side abducted approximately 90 degrees, in order to give maximum exposure of the region.

OPERATIVE PREPARATION A routine skin prep is performed and the area is draped in a sterile manner.

INCISION AND EXPOSURE A horizontal elliptical incision is inked so as to include the entire areolar complex (FIGURE 4). The two skin edges should be of equivalent length, as measured with a free suture between hemostats at each end. The two incisions should come together without tension. Incisions may vary if immediate reconstruction is planned. Skin- or nipple-sparing techniques may be appropriate depending on the indication for surgery.

DETAILS OF PROCEDURE The skin incision is made sharply with the scalpel and carried through the dermis. Any significant vessels should be secured with fine ligatures or controlled with electrocautery. The skin flaps are elevated with large skin hooks that are lifted vertically so as to provide countertraction as the surgeon elevates the skin flaps using a scalpel or electrocautery. The dissection proceeds superiorly almost to the clavicle, medially to the sternal edge, and inferiorly to the costal margin near the insertion of the rectus sheath. This should include virtually all of the glandular tissue of the breast. The lateral flap dissection is carried to the edge of the pectoralis major muscle. This leaves the axillary fat and lymph nodes for a separate dissection.

A subfascial dissection is performed, lifting the breast off of the pectoralis major muscle. It is easier to begin superiorly. As the dissection continues medially, the perforating internal branches of the mammary vessel are controlled with electrocautery or ligature, using fine silk. Finally, the axillary flap is developed such that the breast is removed from the lateral chest wall. The specimen is oriented for the pathologist. The wound is irrigated and careful hemostasis is obtained. The perimeter may be infiltrated with a long-acting local anesthetic. This allows the anesthesiologist to awaken the patient sooner and lessens the amount of pain medication required after surgery. One or two closed suction drains are placed via separate stab incisions and secured in position with nylon suture. The dermis is approximated with interrupted 000 absorbable sutures. These sutures are often placed so as to serially bisect the incision, thus giving the best approximation if the two skin incisions are not of equal length. Finally, a 0000 absorbable suture is placed for subcuticular approximation of the skin. Adhesive skin strips and a dry sterile dressing complete the procedure. Some prefer skin adhesive to the subcuticular suture, and if this is utilized, adhesive skin strips are not utilized and a dressing is not required.

POSTOPERATIVE CARE The patient may use the arm immediately for normal activities. Vigorous use should be curtailed for about a week, when it is determined that the skin flaps are well sealed to the pectoralis major muscle without accumulation of serum or hematoma. The drain is generally removed when the output is <30 mL per day.

D. MODIFIED RADICAL MASTECTOMY

An elliptical incision is placed more obliquely, being angled toward the axilla. The entire areolar complex as well as the lesion or its biopsy scar should be included within the ellipse. If no reconstruction is planned, the wider ellipse illustrated in FIGURE 5 is used. After the patient is prepped and draped, the incision is marked with ink. The incisions are created to be of equal length. There should be no redundant or excess skin at either end of the incision upon closure. In overweight patients or those with very large breasts, a more lateral incision with a wider angle is required. Conversely, very creative or comma-shaped incisions that encircle only the areolar area and then proceed laterally as a single curvilinear extension to the base of the axilla may be used in coordination with the plastic surgeon, who will be performing a concurrent reconstruction (see also Chapter 127, page 488, Modified Radical Mastectomy). This incision may be combined with a separate elliptical incision about a preceding biopsy site.

The full radical mastectomy is no longer included in this atlas, as most surgeons do not remove the entire pectoralis major muscle. Instead, a modified radical mastectomy is performed with a wedging out of a full-thickness section of the underlying pectoralis major muscle where the cancer is attached. ■

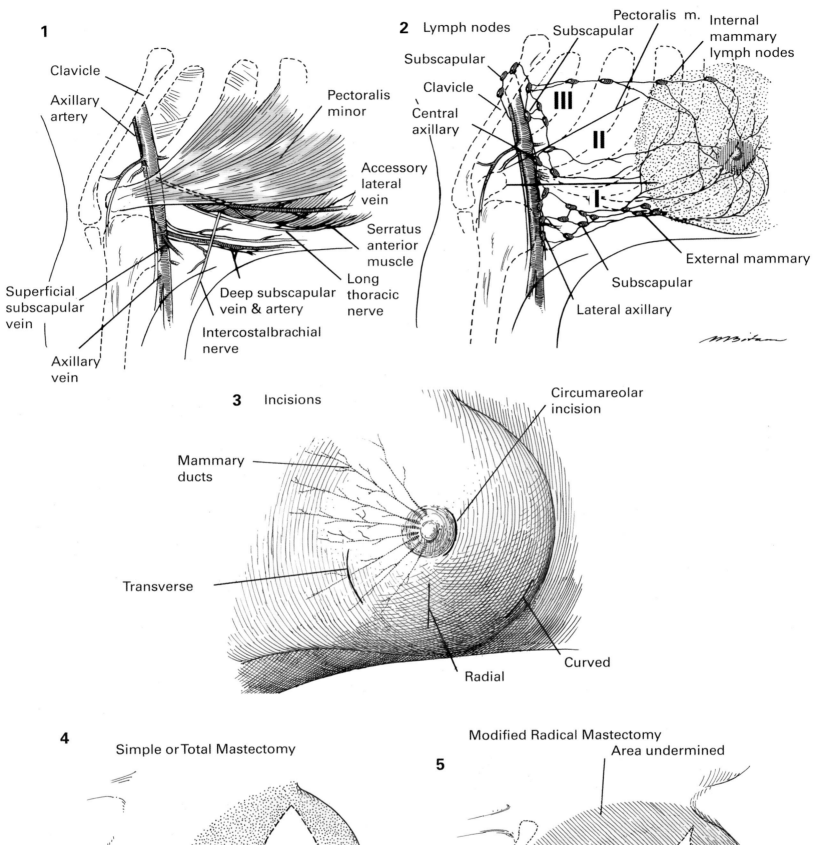

1

Clavicle

Axillary artery

Pectoralis minor

Accessory lateral vein

Serratus anterior muscle

Long thoracic nerve

Deep subscapular vein & artery

Superficial subscapular vein

Intercostalbrachial nerve

Axillary vein

2 Lymph nodes

Pectoralis m.

Internal mammary lymph nodes

Subscapular

Subscapular

Clavicle

Central axillary

III

II

I

External mammary

Subscapular

Lateral axillary

3 Incisions

Circumareolar incision

Mammary ducts

Transverse

Radial

Curved

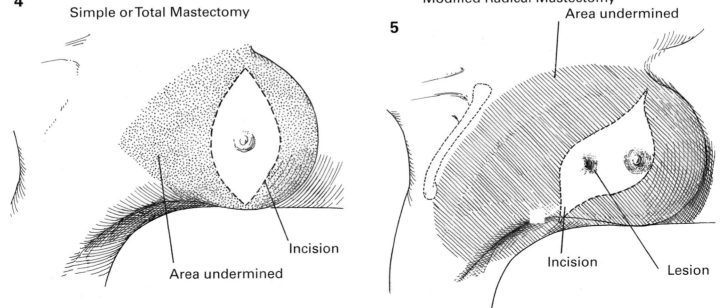

4 Simple or Total Mastectomy

Incision

Area undermined

Modified Radical Mastectomy

5 Area undermined

Incision

Lesion

MODIFIED RADICAL MASTECTOMY

INDICATIONS Over the past 20 years, multiple international clinical studies have shown equivalent survival between patients treated with modified radical mastectomy and appropriately selected patients treated with breast-conserving surgery and adjuvant radiation, hormonal therapy, and/or chemotherapy. Accordingly, breast-conserving surgery has become the dominant mode of treatment, with modified radical mastectomy becoming the alternate choice in certain circumstances. A residual large cancer after neoadjuvant therapy (especially in a small breast), multicentric cancers, and patient preference or concerns about the complications of radiation therapy are the principal indications for the operation. Prior to surgery, the opposite breast should be evaluated by physical examination and mammography. The role of MRI to screen the contralateral breast is still an area of controversy. Appropriate blood tests and imaging scans and mammographic studies are made in a search for potential metastases to the lung, liver, or bone. The standard preadmission physical examination and laboratory evaluations are done in an ambulatory setting, as most patients are admitted to the hospital on the day of operation.

PREOPERATIVE PREPARATION The skin over the involved area should be inspected for signs of infection. The skin is shaved and electrical hair clippers may be used over the axillae. Some surgeons give a single perioperative dose of parenteral antibiotics, particularly if a regional breast biopsy has recently been performed.

ANESTHESIA General anesthesia is given via an endotracheal tube. Short-acting muscle depolarizing agents should be requested for the intubation, such that the motor nerves will be responsive during the axillary node dissection.

POSITION The patient is placed nearest the edge of the operating table on the side of the surgeon. The arm is abducted and held by an assistant or placed upon a support at right angles to the patient to facilitate the preparation of the skin. Some prefer to wrap the arm, including the hand, in sterile drapes so that the arm can be moved upward as well as medially to facilitate the subsequent dissection of the axilla.

OPERATIVE PREPARATION The skin is widely prepared with topical antiseptics. This includes not only the involved breast but also the area over the sternum; the supraclavicular region, shoulder, axilla, and collateral chest wall; as well as the upper abdomen on the involved side. A slight Fowler position with a tilt away from the surgeon improves the exposure. The surgical drape should be secured to the skin at appropriate points around the margin of the proposed field of operation. The arm should be free to be moved by an assistant as required for exposure in the axilla.

INCISION AND EXPOSURE The diagnosis of malignancy is usually established by core needle biopsy under ultrasound guidance or stereotactic biopsy prior to mastectomy. If the diagnosis of malignancy has not been documented by previous biopsy, the diagnosis is first confirmed by a biopsy of excised tumor using frozen-section examination by the pathologist. The specimen is also sent for hormone binding and other immunoassays. The underlying pectoralis muscle should not be involved in any way by the biopsy; otherwise that section of the muscle should be excised en bloc with the specimen. After the biopsy wound is closed and sealed, all instruments and gloves used in the procedure are discarded. Some prefer to have a second sterile table available, which results in a repeated complete skin preparation and sterile draping. An oblique elliptical incision is made that may include a short

extension laterally up toward the axilla to ensure a better exposure for the axillary dissection and a more cosmetically acceptable closure (FIGURE 1). The transverse segment of the elliptical incision includes the nipple and areola and an appropriate distance beyond the limits of the tumor whenever possible. If reconstructive surgery is planned, a more limited incision (FIGURE 1, dashed line) that preserves skin can be made in consultation with the plastic surgeon. The entire nipple plus an adequate margin about the biopsy site must be taken, while a lateral, comma-like extension provides the exposure for the axillary dissection.

The initial incisions through the skin should be only through dermis, as it is advisable to include most of the subcutaneous tissue, especially in the region of the axilla, with the final specimen (FIGURE 2). The skin flaps require careful elevation, with control of all bleeding points as the dissection progresses. With good retraction, a plane between the breast tissue and subdermal fat can be visualized and the dissection carried out in this plane to assure removal of all possible breast tissue while maintaining viability of the skin. The flaps are elevated to the level of the clavicle superiorly, to the edge of the sternum medially, to the rectus sheath and costal margin inferiorly (some prefer elevation to the level of the inframammary fold when reconstruction is planned), and then laterally to the edge of the latissimus dorsi muscle. Particular attention is required to remove as much subcutaneous fat as possible in the axillary region, because the lymph nodes and breast tissue are very close to the skin in this region.

The fascia over the pectoralis major muscle as well as the breast is resected as a subfascial dissection starting near the clavicle and extending downward over the midportion of the sternum (FIGURE 3). The fascia is meticulously dissected off the pectoralis muscle without including any of the latter within the gross specimen. If the cancer has penetrated this fascia and invaded the pectoralis major muscle, that section of the muscle can be excised en bloc with the specimen. It is usually not necessary to perform a full radical mastectomy with removal of the entire pectoralis major muscle. The perforating intercostal arteries and veins near the sternal margins must be carefully clamped and ligated.

The axillary flap is retracted upward, and the fascia over the edge of the pectoralis major is incised (FIGURE 4), exposing the pectoralis minor muscle beneath and the junction of the coracobrachialis and pectoralis minor origins superiorly at the coracoid process. Electrodiathermy is often used in this operation, but it should be avoided about the axillary vessels and nerves and for control of bleeding from intercostal perforating vessels lateral to the sternum. The loose tissue over the axillary vein is incised and the vein wall gently exposed for a short distance beyond the subscapular vessels (FIGURE 5).

Level I and II lymph nodes are removed in the axillary node dissection that begins by incising the clavipectoral fascia along the lateral edge of the pectoralis minor muscle. Precautions are taken to avoid the medial and lateral nerves to the pectoralis major muscle. The medial nerve is so named because it arises from the medial cord of the brachial plexus and then passes through the pectoralis minor muscles in about 60% of patients or passes laterally around the pectoralis minor in 40% en route to innervating the lower region of the pectoralis major muscle (FIGURE 6). The dominant lateral nerve to the pectoralis major muscle arises from the lateral cord. It passes medial to the pectoralis minor muscle near its insertion and is closely associated with the acromial thoracic artery. **CONTINUES ▶**

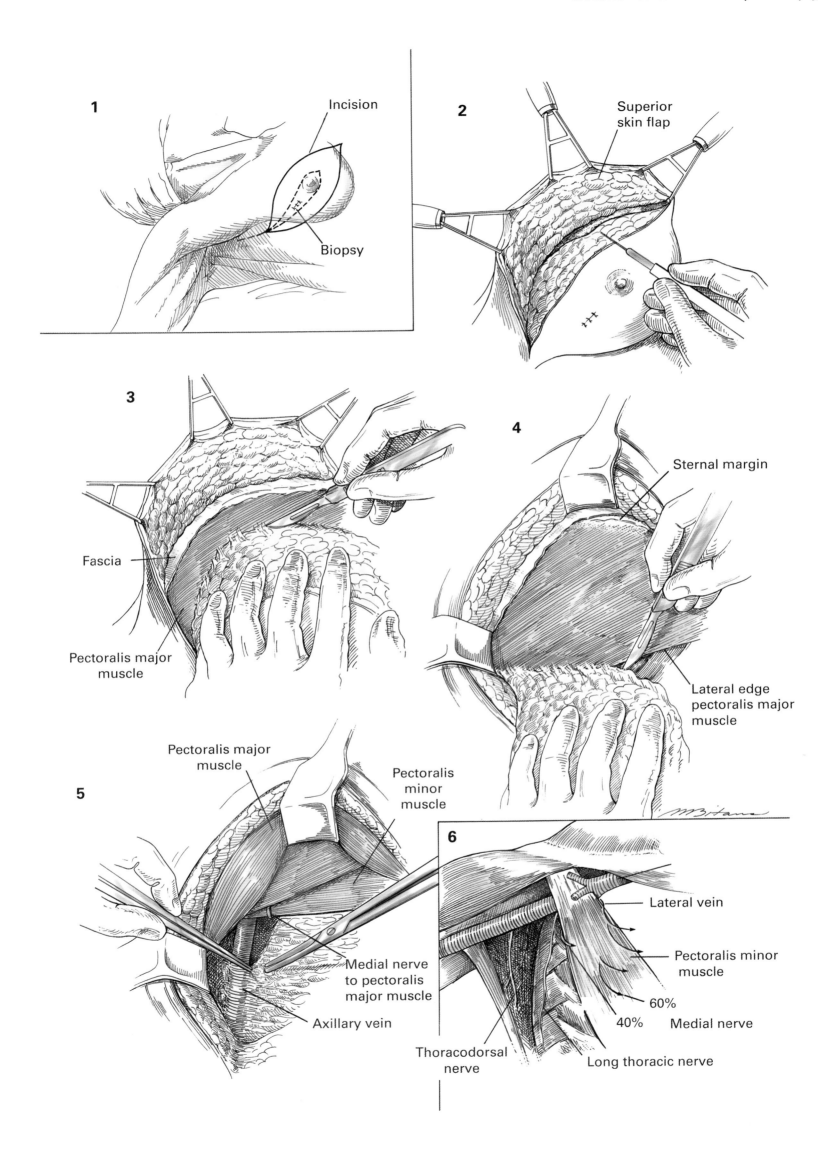

1 Incision

Biopsy

2 Superior skin flap

+++

3 Fascia

Pectoralis major muscle

4 Sternal margin

Lateral edge pectoralis major muscle

5 Pectoralis major muscle

Pectoralis minor muscle

Medial nerve to pectoralis major muscle

Axillary vein

6 Lateral vein

Pectoralis minor muscle

60%

40% Medial nerve

Thoracodorsal nerve

Long thoracic nerve

DETAILS OF PROCEDURE ◀CONTINUED▶ The lateral edge of the pectoralis minor is cleared of fascia to near its insertion on the corticoid process and several veins are ligated as they drain into the axillary vein (FIGURE 7). A careful search is made for the medial nerve to the pectoralis major, which is preserved. Ligation rather than electrocoagulation is preferred for all vessels about the axilla and for those adjacent to the sternum.

The pectoralis major and minor are retracted upward and medially, exposing the uppermost tissues to be divided over the axillary vein. Some prefer to divide the pectoralis minor muscle from its insertion on the coracoid process as to gain better exposure of the medial area of the axillary vein and its lymph nodes.

The fascia over the serratus anterior muscle is dissected free, and the axillary fat and lymph nodes are mobilized off the chest wall and axillary vein (FIGURE 8). The arm, wrapped in sterile drapes, is lifted up or manipulated to enhance the exposure as the dissection progresses in the axilla. The long thoracic nerve should be identified deep to the axillary vein. As it lies within the loose fascia over the serratus anterior muscle, it is possible to lift this nerve away from the muscle; hence, it must be carefully sought and dissected out from the axillary contents to be contained within the resected specimen. This nerve should be retained intact, because a "winged" scapula will result if it is divided. A sensory nerve that is often sacrificed is the more transverse intercostobrachial that appears beneath the second rib and provides sensory innervation to the upper inner aspect of the arm (see Chapter 129, page 497, FIGURE 5).

As the breast is retracted laterally (FIGURE 9), the long thoracic nerve as well as the thoracodorsal nerve should be free of redundant tissue. The thoracodorsal nerve is characteristically located adjacent to the deep subscapular vein and artery. Division of the thoracodorsal nerve is avoided unless there is tumor involvement, since its sacrifice has only a partial effect upon the latissimus dorsi muscle.

The specimen is freed from the latissimus dorsi muscle (FIGURE 10) and finally from the suspensory ligaments in the axilla, where large veins and lymphatics should be carefully ligated. The operative area is repeatedly inspected for any bleeding points, which are ligated. The two major nerves are checked to be certain that their course is free of ligature, and their integrity is verified by a brisk but gentle pinch that results in an appropriate muscle twitch. The wound is irrigated with saline, and a final inspection is made for hemostasis prior to closure. Two closed system perforated suction catheters are inserted for drainage. They are usually introduced through separate stab wounds made in the lower flap posteriorly. One catheter is directed up to the axilla. The other catheter is secured anterior to the pectoralis major muscle for drainage from under the skin flaps. The catheters are secured to the skin with nonabsorbable sutures and attached to a closed system of suction (FIGURE 11).

It is very important that the surgeon spends the necessary time and effort to compress the skin flaps into place in the axilla and elsewhere as the skin is finally closed. If the skin flaps are so thin that there is minimal subcutaneous tissue, interrupted sutures are used in the skin. Alternatively, some surgeons use a few interrupted absorbable sutures in the subcutaneous fat in medium-thickness skin flaps. Some surgeons will run a subcuticular suture with fine absorbable material. Others will close the wound with topical skin adhesive.

The skin is cleaned, dried, and may be prepared with tincture of benzoin, and approximated with steri-strips. Others apply a simple gauze dressing and a surgical bra, whereas some prefer bulky fluffed dressings followed by gauze or elastic bandage wrappings.

POSTOPERATIVE CARE Skin sutures, if present, are removed in 3 to 5 days, with the incision being reinforced with "butterfly" adhesive strips. The suction catheters are removed when the drainage is less than 30 mL per day. The duration the drain tubes are in place is variable, extending from as short as several days to a week to as long as 1 month. Any collections of fluid may be aspirated in the surgeon's office using strict adherence to aseptic precautions. Normal use of the arm is encouraged for the first week; thereafter, active shoulder exercises are performed to ensure return of full range of motion within the ensuing 2 weeks. Physical therapy may be necessary if progress is not apparent in this interval. The patient is cautioned to minimize cuts and possible infection in this arm and to report immediately any injury that results in infection, since a rapidly spreading lymphangitis is possible. Finally, a systematic regimen for lifelong follow-up is instituted even if the final pathologist's report does not indicate the need for additional therapy at the time. ■

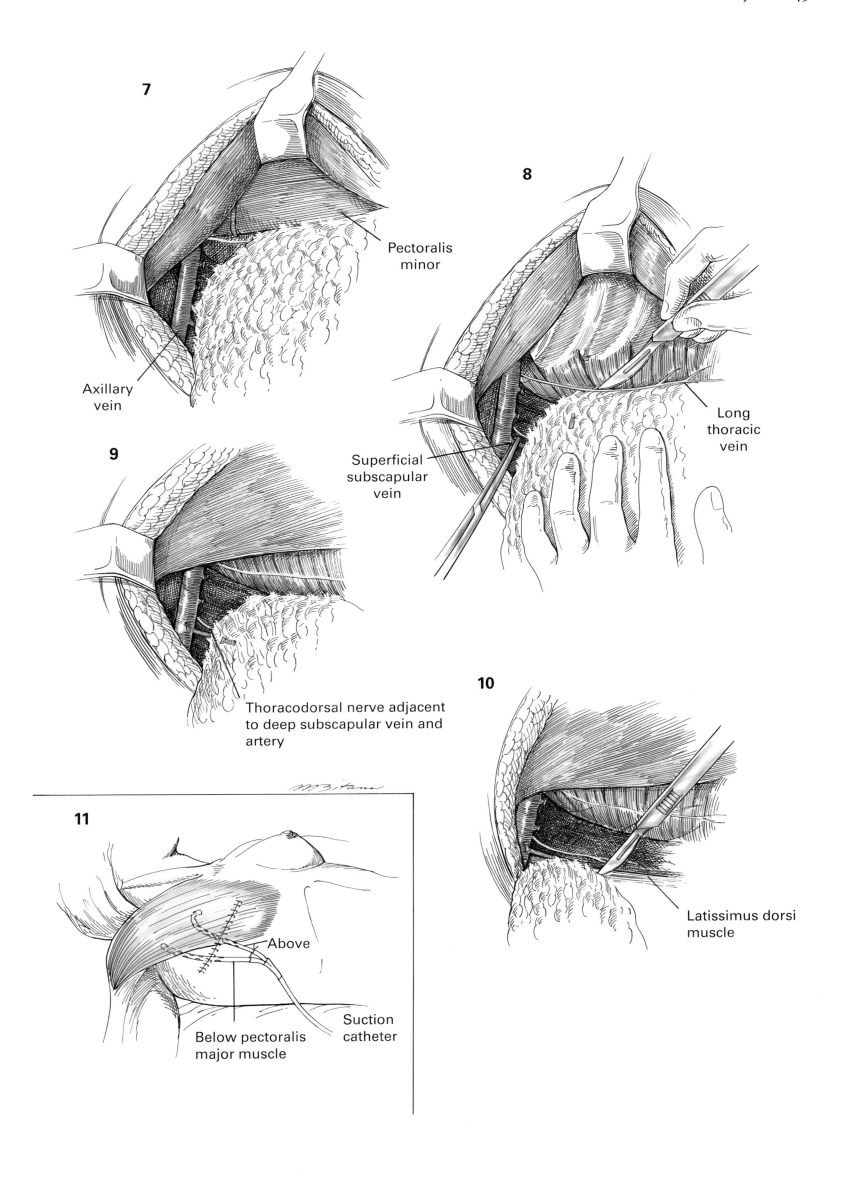

7

Pectoralis minor

Axillary vein

8

Long thoracic vein

Superficial subscapular vein

9

Thoracodorsal nerve adjacent to deep subscapular vein and artery

10

Latissimus dorsi muscle

11

Above

Below pectoralis major muscle

Suction catheter

INDICATIONS Breast cancer patients undergoing a mastectomy or breast-conserving procedure are candidates for axillary sentinel lymph node dissection (SLND) if there is no palpable or clinical evidence of axillary lymph node involvement. The finding of breast cancer metastases in axillary lymph nodes changes the staging of the disease, predicts the rate of recurrence and survival, and results in adjuvant treatment with chemotherapy, hormone therapy, or radiation therapy. The standard axillary lymph node dissection (ALND) of level I and II nodes has significant morbidity, of which lifelong lymphedema is the most feared by patients. Using a combination of radionuclide and dye injections, the correlation of SLND and standard ALND in finding positive lymph nodes is quite high (95%) in the hands of an experienced surgeon. Although at least one sentinel lymph node can be identified in the majority of cases, in a small percentage, identification may not be possible, necessitating complete axillary node dissection. In addition, a false-negative finding occurs in 3% to 10% of the patients having SLND—that is to say, the sentinel nodes are negative, but higher nodes are found to be positive. The advantages of SLND are the fewer complications versus ALND and the ability to identify sentinel lymph nodes that are not in the traditional level I or II areas. The identification of sentinel lymph nodes focuses the histopathologic examination, which may include immunohistochemical staining as well as the traditional hematoxylin and eosin (H&E). The importance of micrometastases (<2 mm) is under study; however, the total number of nodes involved with metastases may influence the adjuvant therapy that is offered. Contraindications to SLND include suspicious, palpable axillary lymphadenopathy; and regional breast operations (e.g., breast reduction) that alter normal lymphatic flow. Sentinel lymph node biopsy may be considered after prior axillary surgery, but lymphatic mapping may be necessary to identify alterations in drainage patterns and the identification rate of sentinel nodes may be lower.

PREOPERATIVE PREPARATION The skin should be free of infection, as should the preceding breast biopsy site. The preparation, delivery, and monitoring of the radionuclide solution for injection must be coordinated with the nuclear medicine staff.

ANESTHESIA General anesthesia with endotracheal intubation is preferred, as some patients will also have ALND and may be having a concurrent operation upon the breast. Most surgeons prefer that the anesthesiologist uses a short-acting muscle paralyzing agent for placement of the endotracheal tube such that the motor nerves can still be identified with mechanical stimulation during the ALND.

POSITION The patient is placed in a comfortable supine position with the arm out at 90 degrees on a padded arm board (FIGURE 1). This position allows easy access of the breast and axilla. Some prefer to wrap the arm, including the hand, in sterile drapes so that the arm can be moved upward as well as medially to facilitate the subsequent dissection.

OPERATIVE PREPARATION Approximately 90 minutes before the start of the operation, the surgeon injects the radionuclide solution into the breast, using sterile technique. A commercially available sulfur colloid solution using a technetium-99m tag is sterilized after passage through a 0.22-µm filter. Many techniques are used for injection of the radionuclide and blue dye. The injections may be placed (1) deeply about the tumor or biopsy cavity (FIGURE 2), (2) superficially in the subdermal or intradermal site over the tumor or about the biopsy site scar, and (3) superficially about the perimeter of the nipple in a subareolar manner. The total dose of radionuclide is generally about 400 µC. Shielding is not required, but the site is monitored with a radiation survey meter. The breast is prepared with an antiseptic solution and sterile paper drapes are applied. The pattern shown (FIGURE 2A) allows infiltration above, below, and at either end of the incision from a preceding biopsy. A long 1½-in 25-gauge needle is used for this injection about the biopsy site or breast cancer. Care must be taken not to inject into a biopsy cavity. The breast is washed and the disposal items are surveyed and disposed of in a radiologically safe manner. The patient proceeds to the operating room. After induction of anesthesia, the breast, chest, and upper arm are prepared and draped in the usual manner.

INCISION AND EXPOSURE The same three techniques are available for injection of about 3 to 5 mL of 1% isosulfan blue vital dye (FIGURE 3). After injection, the area is massaged for a few minutes. The dermal lymphatics may then manifest a faint blue blush streaming toward the axilla. Using a hand-held gamma detector with a sterile cover, the surgeon scans toward the axilla (FIGURE 4) looking for the area with the highest count rate. This may be difficult to find if the breast tumor or biopsy site is high in the upper/outer quadrant, as a regional "shine through" of the injection site radioactivity may create a very high background level. The angled head of the gamma counter can be used to advantage, as it allows more medial placement of the detector with an angled view that is away from the injection site but still points into the axilla. If the hottest spot is near the base of the hair-bearing axilla, a transverse incision is made directly over it (FIGURE 5) in such a manner that the incision can be extended later in a medial manner for a standard ALND. Sharp dissection with a scalpel or electrocautery is made through the first 1 to 2 cm of fat. The probe explores the open incision to find the hottest area (FIGURE 6). **CONTINUES ▶**

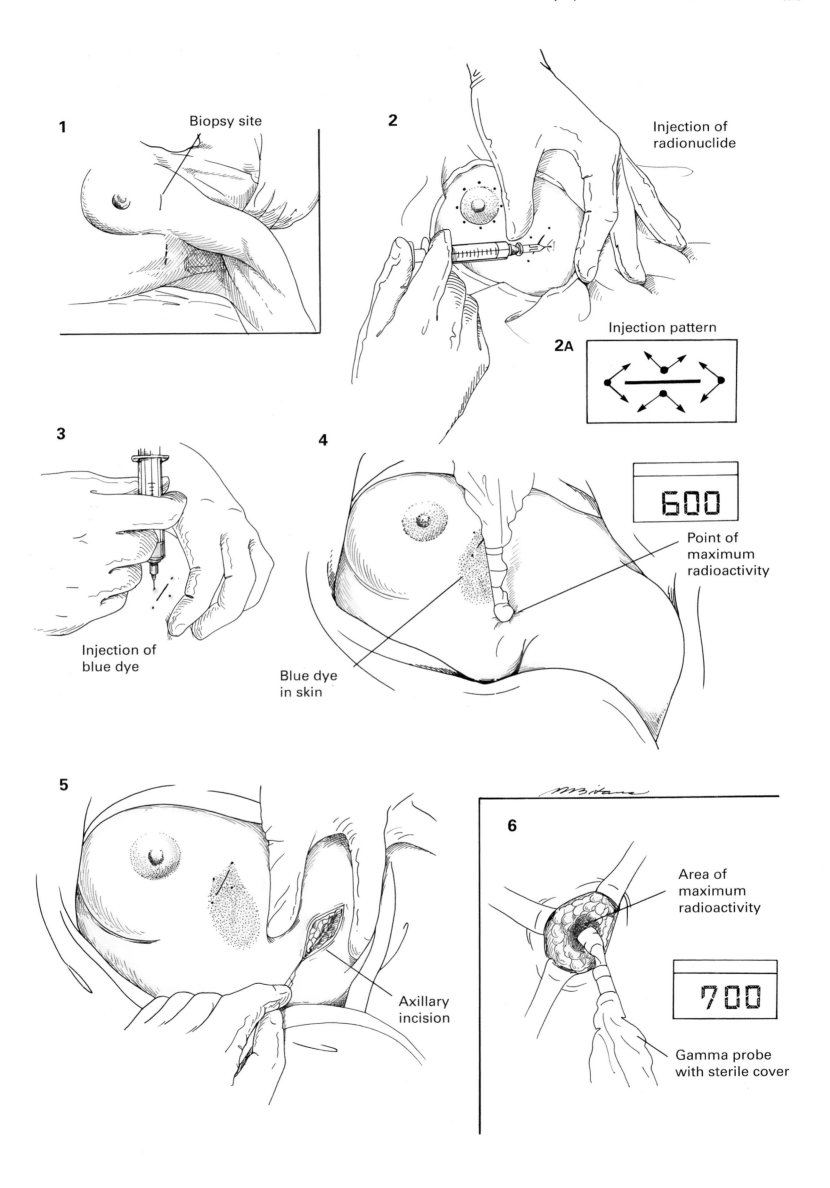

1   Biopsy site

2   Injection of radionuclide

2A   Injection pattern

3   Injection of blue dye

4   600   Point of maximum radioactivity

Blue dye in skin

5   Axillary incision

6   Area of maximum radioactivity

700

Gamma probe with sterile cover

DETAILS OF PROCEDURE <u>CONTINUED</u> Deeper dissection may reveal some blue lymphatic channels (FIGURE 7) flowing toward the hot region where a lymph node may be palpable. The lymph node is dissected free along with any neighboring lymph nodes that are blue or significantly hot (FIGURE 8). The definition of "significant" is any lymph node that has a radioactivity level greater than 10% of the hottest sentinel node (or a level greater than two or three times the background level of the axillary tissue). Following removal of the sentinel nodal tissue, the incision is explored with the gamma probe for any other lymph nodes with significant radioactivity. A basal background level (FIGURE 9) should be present except when the detector is pointed toward the tumor or biopsy injection site. In addition, the axilla should be palpated and any firm or abnormal lymph nodes should be removed.

The nodal tissue removed is examined and the individual lymph nodes are separated (FIGURE 10). In the example shown, lymph node A is labeled as the principal sentinel lymph node. Lymph node B is labeled as a sentinel node. Node C is not a sentinel node, as its counts are less than 10% of the principle sentinel node and it is not blue.

CLOSURE If the sentinel lymph node is in the typical low axillary region, careful hemostasis is obtained. A decision must be made as to whether to proceed with a standard ALND through a new incision or through extension of the existing incision. If a new incision is required, then closure is performed. Scarpa's fascia and the subcuticular fat are closed with interrupted oo absorbable sutures. The skin is approximated with oooo absorbable sutures.

POSTOPERATIVE CARE Most patients who have both SLND and ALND are observed overnight until the effects of the general anesthesia have cleared. Oral intake is resumed as tolerated and oral pain medications are given. The serous output of the closed-suction Silastic drain is monitored. Often it is removed before the patient is discharged or whenever the output falls to less than 30 mL per 24 hours.

Patients with only an SLND are usually operated in an ambulatory setting. They can be discharged home within a few hours when they are alert and have stable vital signs according to the discharge protocol of the surgical unit. ■

7

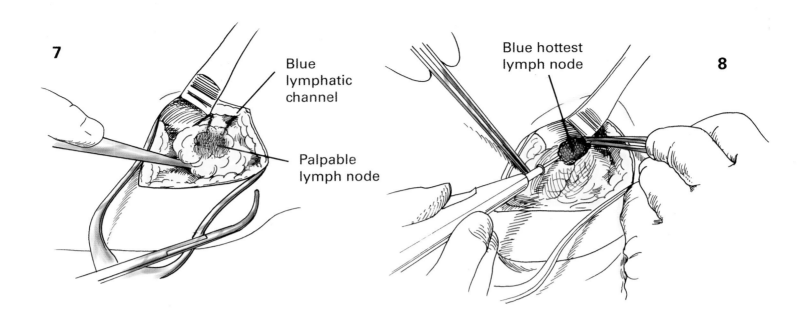

Blue lymphatic channel

Palpable lymph node

Blue hottest lymph node

8

9

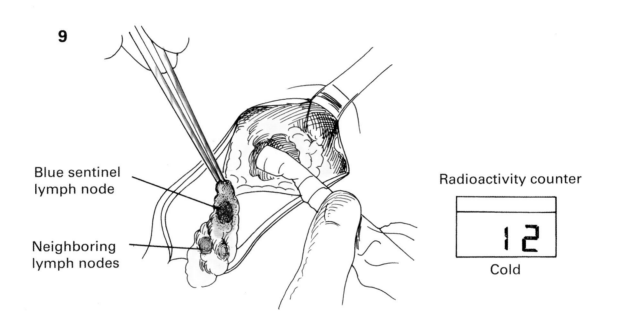

Blue sentinel lymph node

Neighboring lymph nodes

Radioactivity counter

| 1 2 |

Cold

10

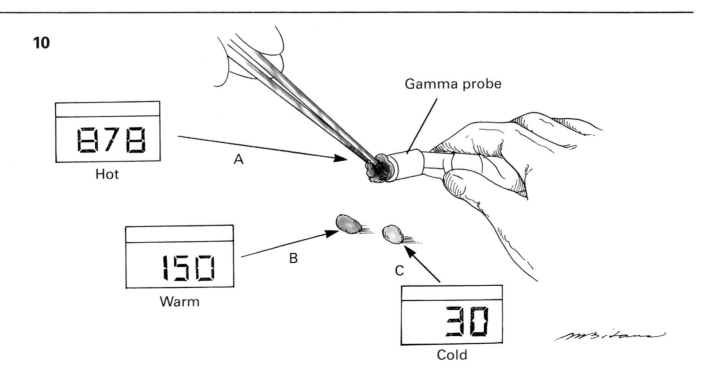

Gamma probe

8 7 8

Hot

A

1 5 0

Warm

B

3 0

Cold

C

AXILLARY DISSECTION, BREAST

INDICATIONS Axillary lymph node dissection is indicated for the management of clinically positive nodes secondary to breast cancer or melanoma. It is also the current standard of care after a positive axillary sentinel node for melanoma and selected cases of breast cancer. Axillary node dissection is also considered for breast cancers when the sentinel lymph node cannot be identified.

PREOPERATIVE PREPARATION The skin of the axilla should be inspected for signs of infection. The skin is shaved, preferably with electric clippers. Most surgeons administer a perioperative dose of parenteral antibiotics.

ANESTHESIA General anesthesia is administered via endotracheal tube. If muscle depolarizing agents are used for induction, they should be short acting to allow recovery of the motor nerves for evaluation during the procedure.

POSITION The patient is placed with the operative side close to the edge of the table. The arm is abducted and placed upon a support at a right angle to the body. Some surgeons wrap the arm in sterile drapes so that the arm is freely mobile to facilitate exposure (FIGURE 1).

INCISION AND EXPOSURE Incisions may vary slightly depending on the disease process being addressed. For melanoma, transverse incisions are preferred to allow easier access to the level III axillary nodes (FIGURE 1). For breast cancer, curvilinear incisions in a skin fold inferior to the hair-bearing area are generally preferred. If a previous sentinel node biopsy incision exists, this should be excised.

DETAILS OF PROCEDURE The incision is extended through the subcutaneous tissues and clavipectoral fascia to expose the pectoralis major muscle medially and the latissimus dorsi muscle laterally. The medial border of the pectoralis major muscle is cleared to allow medial retraction of the muscle (FIGURE 2). The interpectoral, or Rotter's nodes, are swept laterally and included with the specimen. The pectoralis minor muscle is then exposed and the lateral edge cleared to facilitate medial retraction and exposure of the deeper nodes. The medial pectoral bundle is identified and traced back to identify the axillary vein. The inferior border of the vein is cleared between the chest wall and latissimus dorsi muscle (FIGURE 3). The axillary vein is the superior extent of dissection for breast cancer, but for melanoma, some authors suggest continuing the dissection superior to identify the coracobrachialis muscle and carefully dissecting the fibrofatty tissue overlying the brachial plexus down to be included with the specimen, taking care to maintain the fascial covering overlying the brachial plexus.

As the dissection of the vein proceeds, the thoracodorsal bundle is identified (FIGURE 4). Usually, there is a vein superficial to the thoracodorsal vein that will require division and ligation. The thoracodorsal bundle, including the vein artery and nerve, is generally preserved, but can be sacrificed with minimal consequence if necessary due to bulky adenopathy.

Once the thoracodorsal bundle has been identified, its course can be gently dissected using a Kitner. Attention is then directed to the chest wall, where at approximately the same depth, the long thoracic nerve can

be identified (FIGURE 4). The course of this nerve is determined and is protected during the dissection. Damage to the nerve results in a winged scapula.

Once the nerves have been identified, the pectoralis major and minor muscles are retracted medially and the fibrofatty tissue containing lymph nodes is retracted laterally. The fascia over the serratus anterior muscle is dissected free and the axillary fat and lymph nodes are mobilized off the chest wall. Level I (lateral to the pectoralis minor) and II (deep to the pectoralis minor) nodes are routinely removed. Level III nodes (medial to the pectoralis minor) are removed if clinically suspicious. Some melanoma surgeons routinely remove level III nodes as well. If exposure cannot be adequately attained with retraction, the pectoralis minor can be removed by dividing the muscle at the coracoid process and at the chest wall. The arm, if prepped into the field, can be lifted or manipulated at this point to facilitate exposure.

Care is taken to preserve the motor nerves. As the dissection proceeds, one or more intercostobrachial nerves will be identified running through the specimen (FIGURE 5). Depending on surgeon preference, these nerves, which are sensory, can either be preserved or divided. If sacrificed, numbness in the axillary region and the upper inner arm will result. This will often be permanent, although the area of numbness may decrease in size. If preserved, traction on the sensory nerves may result in a burning paresthesia, which usually resolves over time.

The specimen is removed from the floor of the axilla, the subscapularis muscle. The dissection proceeds laterally to the latissimus dorsi muscle. Once removed, the specimen is passed off the field. The two major motor nerves are checked to verify their integrity. This can be accomplished by a gentle pinch, demonstrating the appropriate muscle contraction. The cavity is irrigated and inspected for hemostasis.

A closed system perforated suction catheter is placed into the wound via a separate stab incision. The drain is secured in position with nonabsorbable suture and attached to a closed system of suction (FIGURE 6).

The wound is then closed in layers. Some surgeons attempt to reapproximate the clavipectoral fascia with absorbable sutures. The deep dermis is reapproximated with 3-0 absorbable sutures. Depending on surgeon preference, the skin may be closed using fine absorbable subcuticular sutures or the skin can be reapproximated with skin adhesive.

POSTOPERATIVE CARE The closed suction drains are generally removed when the drainage is <30 mL per day. Any collections of fluid that occur after drain removal can be aspirated in the office. Normal use of the arm is encouraged once the drain is out.

Physical therapy may be helpful to improve shoulder range of motion. The patient is instructed to minimize cuts and possible infections of the affected extremity and to report immediately any injury to the arm, since lymphangitis and lymphedema are possible consequences. A systematic regimen for lifelong follow-up should be instituted to identify and manage potential lymphedema at an early stage. ■

1

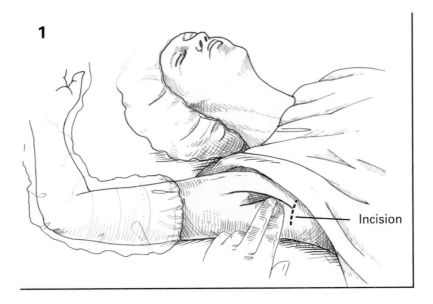

Incision

2

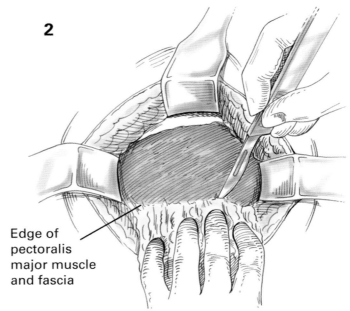

Edge of pectoralis major muscle and fascia

3

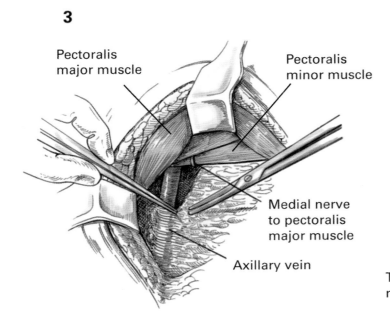

Pectoralis major muscle

Pectoralis minor muscle

Medial nerve to pectoralis major muscle

Axillary vein

4

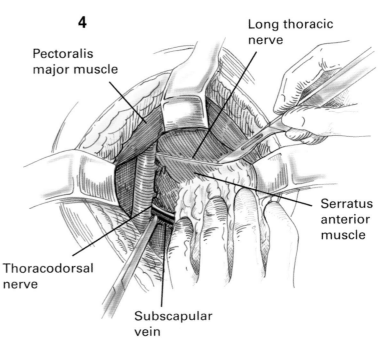

Pectoralis major muscle

Long thoracic nerve

Serratus anterior muscle

Thoracodorsal nerve

Subscapular vein

6

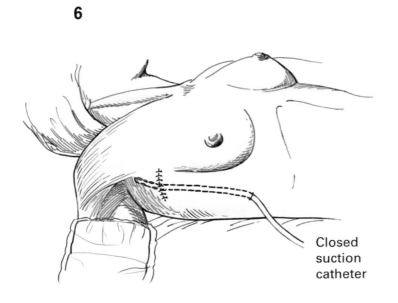

Closed suction catheter

5

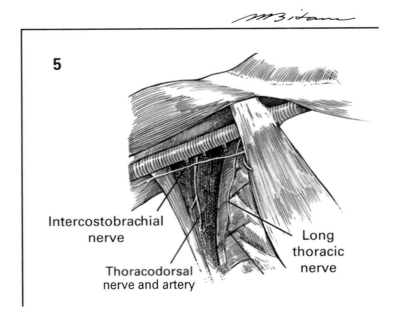

Intercostobrachial nerve

Thoracodorsal nerve and artery

Long thoracic nerve

SKIN GRAFT

INDICATIONS Full-thickness skin loss can occur from burn, trauma, infection, or surgical excision. A skin graft should be considered when the defect cannot be closed primarily or with local tissue flaps and the wound base can adequately support a skin graft. Exposed bone, joint, tendon, blood vessels, and other significant structures are not good candidates for skin grafting and need other methods of reconstruction (pedicled or free flaps). Active infection and poor blood supply to the recipient sites are contraindications. Weight bearing is a relative contraindication for skin grafting, although glabrous skin grafts can sometimes provide an adequate reconstruction.

Skin grafts can be categorized as split thickness or full thickness (FIGURE 1). Full-thickness skin grafts (FTSGs) remove all layers of the skin and create a secondary defect at the donor site, which must be closed primarily or left open to heal secondarily. For this reason, FTSGs are not frequently used for large defects. Split-thickness skin grafts (STSGs) can be of variable thickness, with the amount of dermis taken with the graft the determinant of graft thickness. In general, the thinner the skin graft, the more likely the graft will survive or "take" and quicker the donor site will re-epithelialize. Donor sites heal by epithelial cells in the sweat gland and hair follicles dividing and migrating superficially and then across the donor site until contact inhibition occurs. Thicker skin grafts tend to have better cosmesis because they display less secondary contracture and deformity. In cosmetic areas, including the face and hands, full-thickness grafting is more common because of its better cosmesis.

Because of the large amount of dermis present, the buttock and lateral hip can supply large quantities of STSG when needed (FIGURE 2). The thinner the graft taken, the higher the number of skin grafts that can be harvested from that donor site. The surgeon should be reluctant to use a donor site that will be exposed with normal dress patterns. In the face, color match is important for cosmesis. For this reason, the supraclavicular area, neck, and scalp are better color matches for defects on the face, if available.

PREOPERATIVE PREPARATION In the case of the burn patient, early excision of the burned tissue and skin grafting (within 2 weeks) will limit the amount of hypertrophic scarring and contracture. For all cases of skin grafting, the wound bed must be clean and clear of any evidence of infection. Frequent debridements and dressing changes may be required prior to skin grafting. Negative pressure dressings may help stimulate granulation tissue and prepare the wound bed. Medical issues (including nutritional status) should be optimized.

ANESTHESIA Generally, local anesthesia can be used for small excisions and skin grafts. Where extensive skin grafting must be carried out, general anesthesia is usually indicated.

POSITION The patient's position is determined by the field of operation. Frequent position changes are required sometimes because of the multisite nature of the surgery. Care must be taken to cover the patient at all times except for the area being operating on, as hypothermia can become a serious problem. If possible, the donor and recipient sites should be ipsilateral to allow the patient to have one part of his body without any surgical site, allowing for improved comfort.

DETAILS OF PROCEDURE A variety of instruments are available for use in obtaining STSGs. The choice will depend on the individual case and the surgeon's experience. The most common method of harvesting STSGs is using a powered dermatome (FIGURE 3), although free-hand harvesting with a scalpel or skin knife can be performed for small grafts. For irregular donor site areas, infiltration of a tumescent solution under the skin can provide increased tissue turgor that may make harvesting the graft easier.

ELECTRICAL AND AIR-POWERED DERMATOMES

The donor site must be a flat, firm surface, the back and thighs being commonly used. The blade is checked carefully, inserted into the dermatome, and secured. When the desired width and thickness calibrations are determined (FIGURE 3) and settings made using a graft sizer (FIGURE 3A), a thin layer of mineral oil is spread over the donor site and carefully on the dermatome. A surgical assistant helps to keep tension on the donor site. As the graft is lifted the assistant gently picks up the end to the graft to apply tension (FIGURE 4). The dermatome should be started prior to making contact with the skin and approached at approximately a 45-degree angle. Once the dermatome has engaged the skin and a couple of centimeters of advancement occurred, the dermatome should be lowered to approximately a 30-degree angle. The dermatome is advanced until the desired length of skin is obtained. The amount of pressure exerted becomes important, as too great a pressure may produce a thicker graft of skin than is desired. If large areas need grafting, as in extensive burns, the skin graft can be placed through a mesher (FIGURES 5 and 6) to increase the surface area grafted with each graft. In most applications, meshing beyond a ratio of 3:1 makes handling the mesh difficult with mixed results. Most meshing occurs with a ratio of 1.5:1.0 (FIGURE 6A). In general, meshing should not take place for grafting of the face or hands. Hemostasis must be complete in the recipient area before application of the graft. The recipient site is then sprayed with a thin layer of fibrin glue and the graft is carefully placed into the defect. Grafts are very sensitive to crush injury and should be handled with extreme care. Excessive skin is trimmed from the edges so that no graft overlies normal skin, and the graft is carefully sutured to the adjacent skin with interrupted absorbable sutures (FIGURE 7). Before application of the dressing, the wound is checked for the presence of any blood clots under the graft. The external dressing is then applied with nonadherent gauze adjacent to the graft, supported by a firm compression dressing that is carefully applied and immobilized. If a bolster dressing is required a negative pressure dressing placed on low, continuous suction can be placed over the graft with a nonadherent, oil immersion gauze providing a barrier layer between the graft and dressing sponge (FIGURE 8). Immobilization of joints in proximity to the newly applied graft is important to prevent movement of the graft, thus improving graft take. At the same time, however, patients should be encouraged to be out of bed and ambulate as their condition will allow. Strict bedrest is not mandatory for most patients receiving skin grafts.

MANAGEMENT OF THE DONOR AREA

There are several options for dressing the donor area. Any of the silver-containing barrier dressings can be used to cover the donor site. Conversely, nonadherent gauze can be applied as a single layer over the donor area and supported by a bulky nonocclusive gauze dressing. On the following day, the outer dressing is removed from the donor site, leaving the inner gauze adjacent to the wound and allowed to dry, preferably with assistance of a heat lamp. This dressing can be left in place until it falls off as the donor site re-epithelializes.

POSTOPERATIVE CARE The frequency with which the dressing is changed will vary with the case. When a bolster or negative pressure dressing is used, it may be left in place for 3 to 5 days. When the dressing is changed, the presence of a fluid collection beneath the graft does not necessarily indicate a loss of the graft. The graft should be incised over the fluid collection and evacuated, and a firm dressing reapplied for 24 to 48 hours. After the graft has healed fully, the daily application of a moisturizing cream will help keep it from scaling and make it pliable. The donor area should be healed in 8 to 14 days and be ready for harvesting of a new graft if necessary. ■

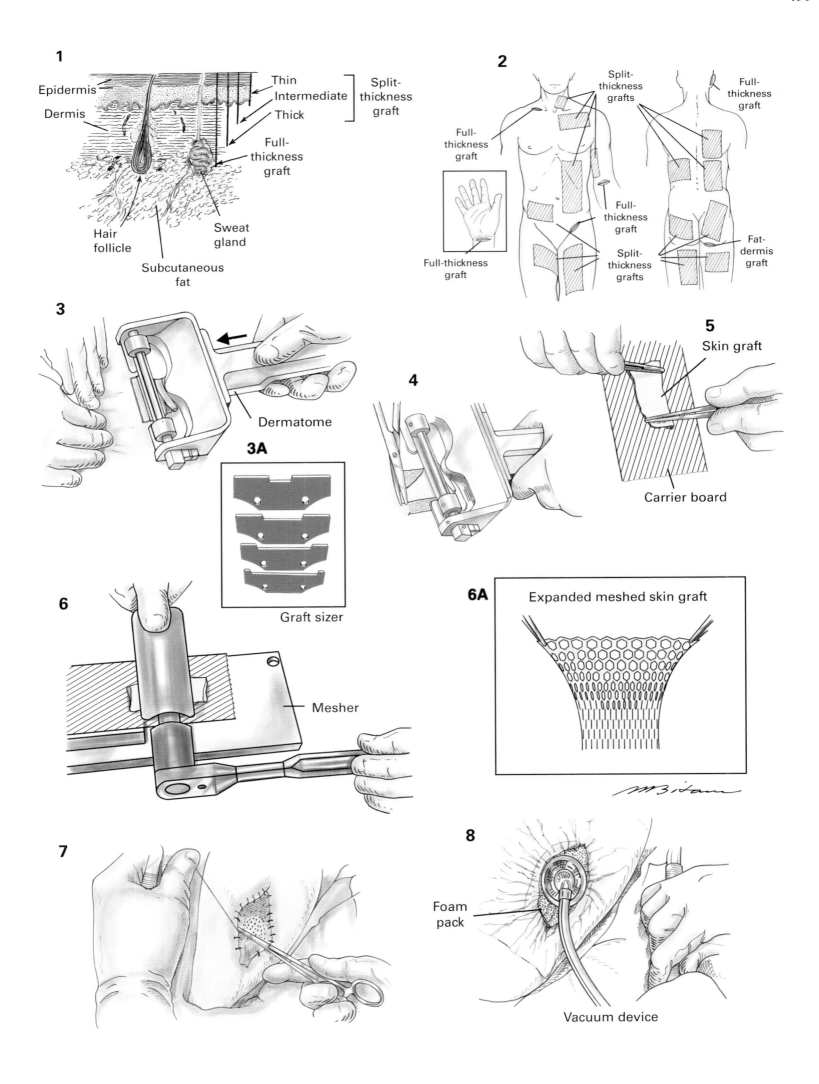

1

Epidermis

Dermis

Hair
follicle

Subcutaneous
fat

Sweat
gland

Thin
Intermediate
Thick

Split-
thickness
graft

Full-
thickness
graft

2

Split-
thickness
grafts

Full-
thickness
graft

Full-
thickness
graft

Full-
thickness
graft

Full-
thickness
graft

Split-
thickness
grafts

Full-
thickness
graft

Fat-
dermis
graft

3

Dermatome

3A

Graft sizer

4

5

Skin graft

Carrier board

6

Mesher

6A   Expanded meshed skin graft

7

8

Foam
pack

Vacuum device

Section XIII
VASCULAR

CAROTID ENDARTERECTOMY

INDICATIONS The role of carotid endarterectomy is the prevention of strokes in patients with systemic disease of the vascular system. The indications for the procedure are varied, but the chief indication is transient ischemia. When the symptoms of cerebral ischemia are transient, intermittent, and self-resolving, the results of surgical correction of the area of carotid stenosis are excellent. The operation may be considered in some patients who have recovered from old strokes who develop new symptoms. Mild intracranial disease with severe proximal disease is another indication for carotid endarterectomy. The two principal indications are asymptomatic high-grade stenosis and transient ischemia.

Duplex ultrasound blood-flow imaging studies with or without magnetic resonance angiography (MRA) or contrast angiography are used to visualize the arch, carotids, and vertebral vessels. This allows accurate documentation of any areas of stenosis as well as the extent of the collateral blood supply. Surgical improvement is minimal in patients with complete occlusion of the internal carotid artery, and operation is not recommended for patients with established long-standing occlusion. The risks of increasing cerebral damage or of the patient suffering hemiplegia are ever present, and the patient and family should be thoroughly informed of the risks.

A thorough medical evaluation of the cardiovascular system with special attention to the coronary arteries is indicated. Other medical problems, including diabetes, must be under complete control. The incidence of stroke is greater in patients with contralateral carotid occlusion, and one-stage bilateral carotid endarterectomy is inadvisable because of the increased incidence of complications. At least a week or more should separate two procedures. The operation may be delayed in patients with acute strokes, allowing them to stabilize for 4 to 6 weeks, but there is increasing evidence that earlier intervention may be indicated in specific cases. At that time, imaging studies and operation can be considered.

POSITION The patient is placed in a supine position with the head slightly extended and turned toward the contralateral side.

OPERATIVE PREPARATION After routine skin preparation, the operative field is draped to expose the mastoid process superiorly, the angle of the mandible anteriorly, the manubrium and clavicle inferiorly, to the trapezius posteriorly.

INCISION AND EXPOSURE The incision is made along the anterior border of the sternocleidomastoid muscle from the mastoid process to a point two-thirds of the distance to the sternoclavicular joint (FIGURE 1). The incision is carried through the platysma muscle exposing the anterior border of the sternocleidomastoid muscle, which is then retracted laterally to expose the carotid sheath. Care must be taken to avoid making the upper end of the incision too far anteriorly, where the marginal mandibular branch of the facial nerve may be injured in its course just inferior to the horizontal ramus of the mandible. Such an injury results in paralysis of the lower lip. In the cephalad portion of the incision, the greater auricular nerve and sensory branches of the cervical plexus often can be identified and preserved if exposure is not compromised. Injury to these nerves will result in a sensory deficit involving the earlobe or the angle of the mandible. Gentle self-retaining retractors may be positioned at this time to provide maximal exposure. The omohyoid muscle may be retracted inferiorly or divided to permit exposure of the common carotid artery, depending upon the required extent of the procedure.

DETAILS OF PROCEDURE The anatomy of the neck must be understood clearly so that inadvertent injury to nearby cranial nerves can be avoided (FIGURE 2). The vagus nerve lies within the carotid sheath generally in a posterolateral position; injury will result in vocal cord paralysis. The hypoglossal nerve passes superficial to the carotid arteries 1 to 2 cm cephalad to the carotid bifurcation; injury will result in deviation of the tongue and dysphagia. The ansa hypoglossi branches from the hypoglossal nerve as it crosses the internal carotid artery and passes inferiorly to innervate the strap muscles. This may be sacrificed without significant consequence to facilitate exposure of the more distal internal carotid artery, allowing the hypoglossal nerve to be gently retracted superiorly. The carotid body is in the crotch of the carotid bifurcation. Dissection in this area may result in hypotension and bradycardia, cardiovascular effects that can be blocked effectively by injecting the carotid body with 1% lidocaine. The facial nerve is at the most cephalad extent of the incision and should be well out of the field anteriorly (FIGURE 2).

After the described exposure has been obtained, the facial vein is divided, exposing the carotid bifurcation (FIGURE 3). The carotid sheath is entered and opened superiorly and inferiorly. A vessel loop is passed about the common carotid artery proximally. A vessel loop is passed around the external carotid artery to facilitate later placement of a vascular clamp. A vessel loop or a 00 silk ligature then is passed doubly around the superior thyroid artery as a Potts tie to provide vascular control. The internal carotid artery is then dissected circumferentially at a point 1 cm distal to palpable disease and encircled with a vessel loop. Great gentleness is required and care is taken during this dissection to prevent plaque embolization.

If selective shunting is to be used, appropriate monitoring equipment (a transducer, extension tubing, and a 22-gauge needle) must be readied and carefully flushed with saline to free it of bubbles or particulate debris. Clamps are placed across the external carotid artery and common carotid artery, after which the needle is placed within the carotid artery to measure the carotid stump pressure (FIGURE 4). Stump pressures greater than 40 to 50 mm Hg document significant collateral blood flow and are associated with a lower incidence of cerebrovascular accident. Care must be taken in the presence of extensive or ulcerated plaques to avoid plaque embolization with this maneuver. Some rely upon continuous electroencephalographic monitoring to gauge the adequacy of collateral blood flow and the requirement for intraluminal shunting; others choose to shunt all patients routinely; and still others may choose not to shunt patients at all but attain acceptable results.

Heparin is now given intravenously by the anesthesiologist at the surgeon's discretion. Bulldog clamps are placed across the internal carotid artery, external carotid artery, and common carotid artery in sequence. An incision then is made on the anterolateral surface of the common carotid artery just inferior to the bifurcation. Potts scissors then are used to elongate the incision proximally and distally across the area selected for endarterectomy (FIGURE 5). Care must be taken to extend the arteriotomy distally to a point beyond the end of the atheromatous plaque so that the endarterectomy can be performed entirely under direct vision. The incision is carried through the thickened intima into the lumen. The line of cleavage is within the media, leaving the adventitia and media externa for closure as indicated by the arrows (FIGURE 6). **CONTINUES▶**

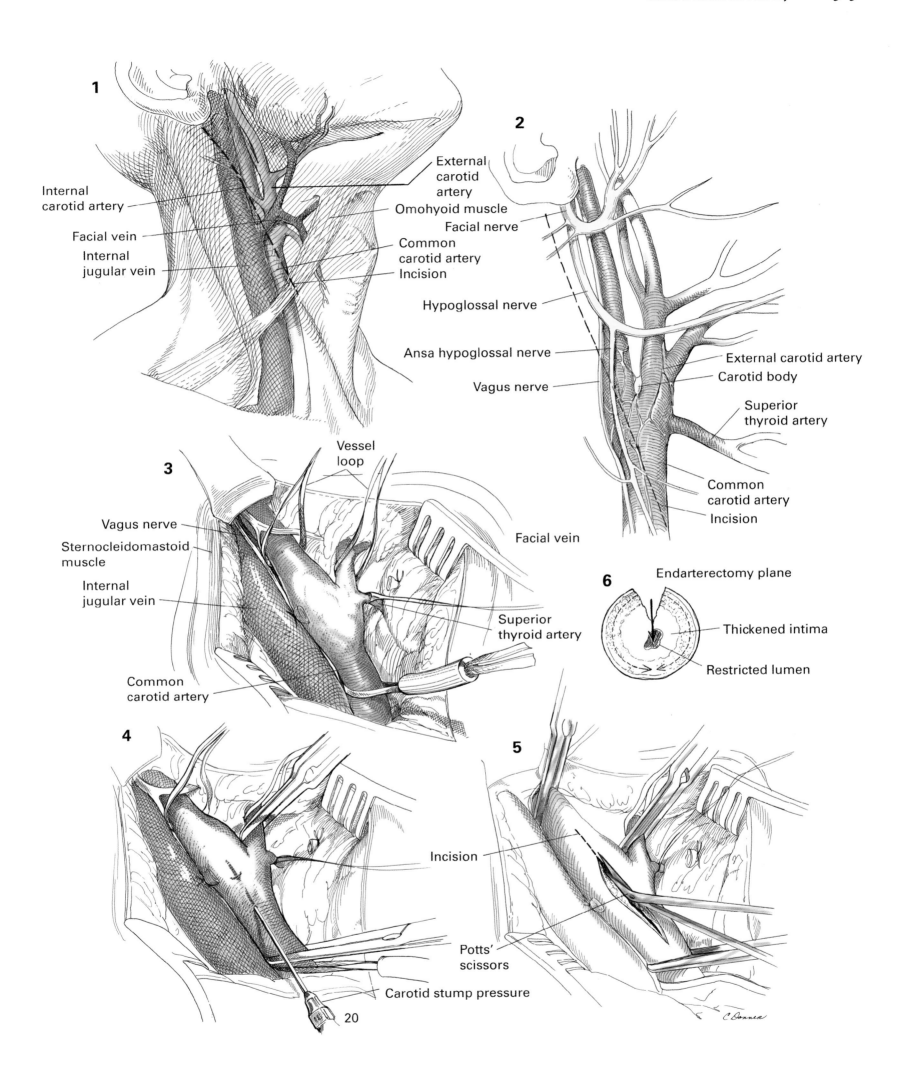

1

Internal carotid artery

Facial vein

Internal jugular vein

External carotid artery

Omohyoid muscle

Facial nerve

Common carotid artery

Incision

2

Hypoglossal nerve

Ansa hypoglossal nerve

Vagus nerve

External carotid artery

Carotid body

Superior thyroid artery

Common carotid artery

Incision

3

Vessel loop

Vagus nerve

Sternocleidomastoid muscle

Internal jugular vein

Common carotid artery

Facial vein

Superior thyroid artery

6

Endarterectomy plane

Thickened intima

Restricted lumen

4

Incision

Carotid stump pressure

20

5

Incision

Potts' scissors

DETAILS OF PROCEDURE ◂CONTINUED▸ If intraluminal shunting is elected with a Pruitt-Inahara shunt it needs to be flushed and prepped ahead of time. Heparinized saline is flushed through the irrigating port and hemostats are placed on the proximal and distal limbs of the shunt directly adjacent to the irrigating port. The distal end is inserted first and the balloon is gently inflated to seal off back bleeding around the shunt (FIGURE 7). The distal hemostat is opened and the distal limb aspirated back through the irrigating limb to remove all air. The hemostat is reapplied. The proximal end of the shunt is then inserted into the common carotid artery and the balloon gently inflated to prevent any antegrade flow around the shunt (FIGURES 8 and 9). Overinflation is to be avoided to prevent tearing of the intima or prolapsing of the balloon over the end of the shunt and occluding flow. The proximal hemostat is removed and the limb aspirated through the irrigating port to remove any air or debris. The aspirating process should be repeated one more time and the hemostats removed to establish flow through the shunt. The shunt is checked with the Doppler probe to check for flow and the endarterectomy is then commenced. With experience and planning, placement of such a shunt should consume no more than 60 to 90 seconds.

Endarterectomy is begun in the distal common carotid artery, using a Freer elevator, blunt spatula, or a mosquito hemostat. The appropriate endarterectomy plane usually is identified easily in the mid to outer media, leaving a smooth, glistening reddish-brown arterial wall behind (FIGURE 10).

This dissection is continued quite carefully in an attempt to elevate the plaque circumferentially. A blunt-tipped right-angle clamp is often valuable (FIGURE 11). The plaque then is divided proximally with the Potts scissors to facilitate exposure. The endarterectomy proceeds distally in a meticulous fashion, care being taken to maintain a single endarterectomy plane. The most important aspect of the procedure is the delicate feathering of the endarterectomy at the distal boundary of the atheromatous plaque. No flap or shelf can be tolerated, since a technical fault will result in dissection after restoration of prograde flow with subsequent thrombosis and probable neurologic catastrophe. Plaque is removed similarly from the external carotid orifice by eversion endarterectomy allowing removal of the specimen (FIGURE 12). All residual debris is removed carefully with forceps in a circumferential direction. A Kittner sponge also may be helpful in clearing the field of debris. Heparinized saline is used to irrigate the field, allowing free removal of clot. Forceful irrigation distally may reveal elevation of a distal flap that may require attention or tacking sutures (FIGURE 13). CONTINUES▸

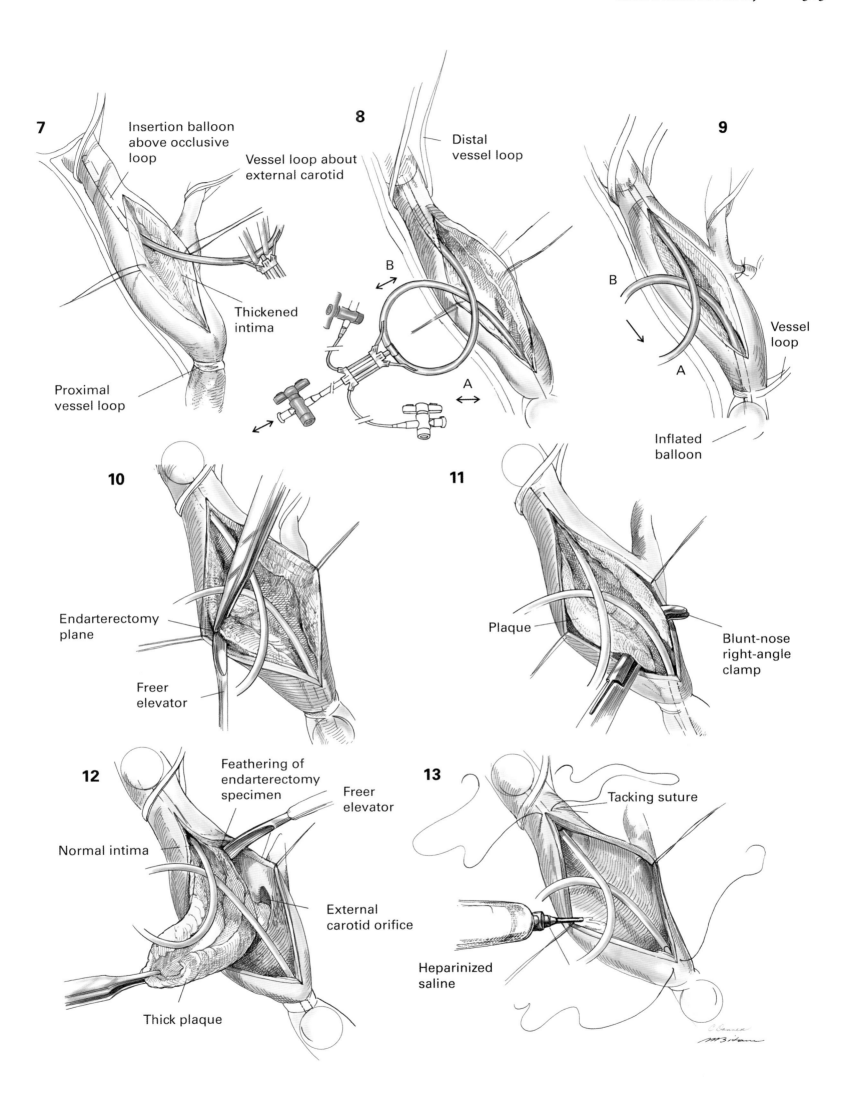

7

Insertion balloon above occlusive loop

Vessel loop about external carotid

Thickened intima

Proximal vessel loop

8

Distal vessel loop

B

A

9

B

A

Vessel loop

Inflated balloon

10

Endarterectomy plane

Freer elevator

11

Plaque

Blunt-nose right-angle clamp

12

Feathering of endarterectomy specimen

Freer elevator

Normal intima

External carotid orifice

Thick plaque

13

Tacking suture

Heparinized saline

DETAILS OF PROCEDURE CONTINUED Often, tacking sutures will be required to prevent subintimal dissection (FIGURE 14). These horizontal mattress sutures of 7/0 polypropylene are placed at intervals circumferentially, using double-ended sutures passed from inside out and tied externally (FIGURE 14).

Occasionally a very large artery with a short length of arteriotomy can be closed primarily, however, patch angioplasty with prosthetic material (dacron, PTFE, or bovine pericardium) or autologous vein is the preferred technique for closure. Mattress sutures of double-ended 6/0 polypropylene are placed at either end (FIGURE 15). Both needles of each end suture pass through the patch from outside to in and then pass from lumen to the outside of the carotid artery where the knots are tied (FIGURE 16). This provides a broad-based loop that anchors the graft. The inferior or proximal suture B' is run superiorly in a continuous manner on the medial side of the graft and tied to A' (FIGURE 16). Sutures A and B are then run toward the midpoint on the lateral side of the arteriotomy (FIGURE 17). When approximately 1 cm of arteriotomy remains to be closed in the midportion of the incision, the balloons are deflated and the shunt is cross clamped with a straight mosquito hemostat. A brisk inflow and backflow are allowed so as to flush the area as the two ends of the shunt are removed, first distally, then proximally (FIGURE 18). The bulldog clamps are reapplied or the vessel loops cinched down so as to secure active bleeding. The remainder of the arteriotomy then is closed rapidly, with great care being taken to flush the region of particulate debris and air (FIGURE 18). Following completion of closure, the clamps are removed in a specific order: external carotid artery, common carotid artery, and finally internal carotid artery. This sequence minimizes the possibility of cerebral embolization, permitting potential emboli to be flushed into the external carotid system preferentially. The completed endarterectomy must have thorough hemostasis and no residual stenosis (FIGURE 19).

Upon completion, a Doppler or duplex ultrasound study is performed to verify an unobstructed blood flow. Any suspicion of recurrent thrombosis is an urgent indication to reopen the arteriotomy and remove the thrombus. Finally, many surgeons keep the patient in the operating room until they awaken without a neurologic deficit. If any neurologic changes are present, the operative site is re-explored immediately.

CLOSURE Meticulous hemostasis must be obtained to prevent cervical hematoma and possible respiratory embarrassment from tracheal compression. If heparinization has been used, protamine sulfate may be given to reverse anticoagulation. The wound is closed in layers, approximating the sternocleidomastoid muscle and cervical fascia, the platysma, and the skin. A small closed-suction Silastic drain may be brought out the inferior margin of the incision at the surgeon's discretion.

POSTOPERATIVE CARE Bleeding into the wound may occur from excessive anticoagulation, improper hemostasis, seeping from the suture line, or postoperative hypertension. Tracheal obstruction may occur and requires endotracheal intubation. Re-exploration of the wound may be indicated for hematoma evacuation.

The effects of injury to sensory as well as motor nerves can range from minor losses in skin sensation to drooping of the corner of the mouth resulting from injury to the marginal branch of the facial nerve.

The patient should remain on underphysiologic monitoring and neurologic assessment for the postoperative period. Postoperative hypotension must be avoided by adequate blood and fluid replacement. Overmedication and cardiovascular complications must be considered. Likewise, hypertension is to be avoided because of the danger of an acute stroke or disruption of the arterial closure. The patient must be assessed for unimpaired swallowing prior to self-feeding and discharge. ■

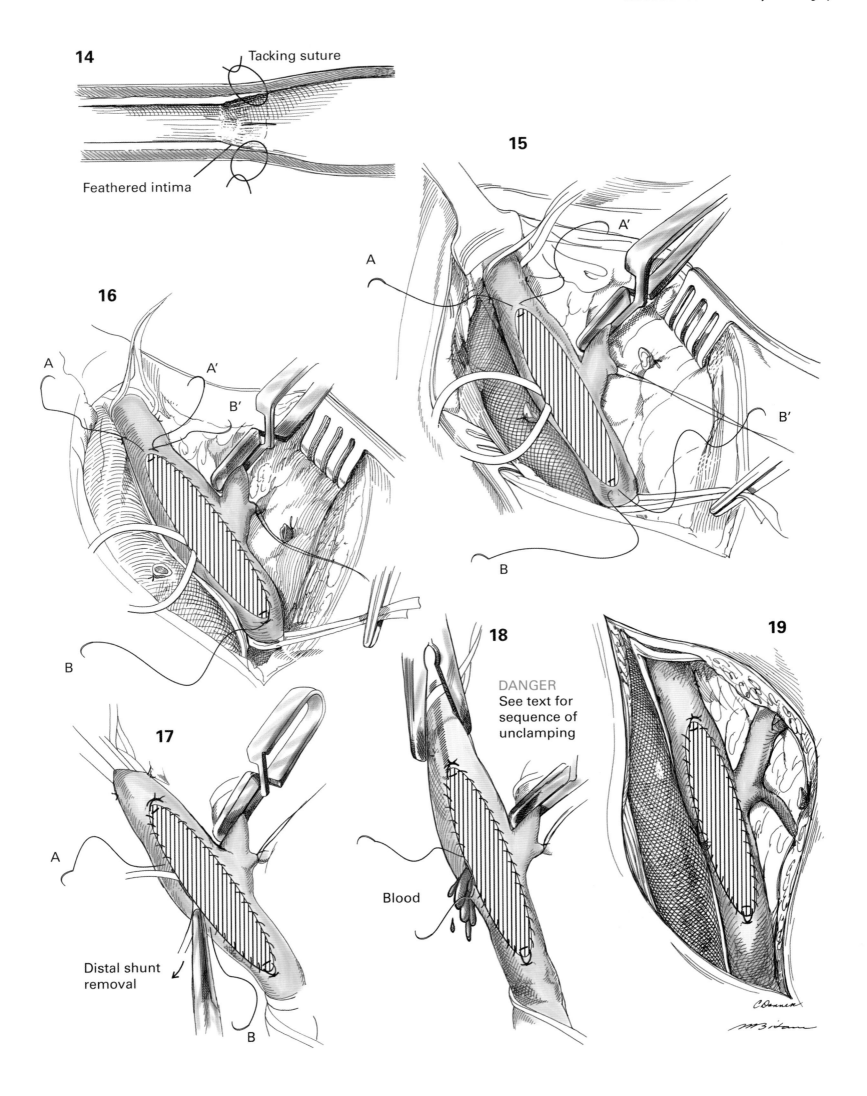

14
Tacking suture

Feathered intima

15

A

A′

B′

B

16

A

A′

B′

B

17

A

Distal shunt removal

B

18

DANGER
See text for sequence of unclamping

Blood

19

VASCULAR ACCESS, ARTERIOVENOUS FISTULA

INDICATIONS The most common indication for creation of an arteriovenous (AV) fistula is renal failure requiring chronic hemodialysis. It is preferable to create a native fistula, although prosthetic material may be needed if a suitable vein is not available.

PREOPERATIVE PREPARATION The goal is to place an AV fistula prior to the patient starting dialysis. The day of surgery, electrolytes should be checked to verify the absence of hyperkalemia. Many of the patients are diabetic and close monitoring of blood glucose levels during the procedure is warranted. Antibiotic prophylaxis is administered within 1 hour of the incision. A single dose is usually sufficient. In patients with a poorly defined superficial venous system, venous mapping may be done preoperatively to define the anatomy.

ANESTHESIA The patients requiring chronic hemodialysis are poor risks for general anesthesia. An axillary block on the side that is to be used provides excellent regional anesthesia. If regional anesthesia cannot be done, local anesthesia is a valid option.

POSITION The patient is placed in the supine position. The arm to be used for the fistula is placed on an arm board (FIGURE 1). The opposite arm may be tucked with a sheet or placed on an arm board.

OPERATIVE PREPARATION Hair is removed with clippers. The arm is prepped circumferentially from the fingers to the axilla. After draping, a sterile knit stocking is placed over the arm. This covers the fingers and arm to the axilla (FIGURE 2).

DETAILS OF PROCEDURE The surgeon palpates the radial pulse. The location of the incision is planned (FIGURE 3). A vertical incision is made in the forearm close to the wrist and lateral to the radial pulse (FIGURE 4). Once the incision is carried to the deep subcutaneous tissue, self-retaining retractors are placed. Sharp and blunt dissection is used to identify the cephalic vein. The vein is skeletonized for a distance of 2 to 3 cm. It is encircled with vessel loops proximally and distally. Side branches of the vein are ligated with 4-o silk (FIGURE 5). The radial artery is then dissected for a distance of 2 to 3 cm. There is a vein on either side of the radial artery that may be ligated or freed from the artery. The artery is encircled with vessel loops proximally and distally. Side branches are ligated as necessary with 4-o silk. Both vessels must be freely mobilized to enable a tension-free anastomosis. The artery and vein are then encircled with a single vessel loop both proximally and distally to allow alignment of the structures (FIGURE 6).

A longitudinal venotomy is made in the cephalic vein with a number 11 blade and extended for 1 cm with iris scissors. The vein is dilated to size 3.5 mm and a Silastic catheter is passed cephalad to ensure patency of the vein. The vein is irrigated with heparinized saline (FIGURE 7).

The patient is administered intravenous heparin. Fine curved or straight bulldog clamps are placed proximally and distally on the radial artery. A longitudinal arteriotomy of 1 cm is made. In some cases the arterial wall may be much calcified and it will be necessary to probe the artery proximally to ensure patency. Once patency is established, the proximal bulldog clamp is reapplied. The artery and vein are aligned. A side-to-side anastomosis is then created between the cephalic vein and radial artery using running 6-o nonabsorbable monofilament sutures. The needle on the arterial side must be passed from the endothelial surface outward, ensuring the endothelium is tacked down (FIGURES 8 and 9). Needle B' (FIGURE 8) is passed back into the lumen and then run continuously on the back wall—always beginning into the arterial intima. At the end, it is tied externally to suture A (FIGURE 10). Needle A' is passed back into the lumen and then run continuously on the front wall. Once the anastomosis is nearly complete, the proximal bulldog clamp is released transiently to ensure inflow and to flush out any clot. The distal bulldog is likewise released to ensure back bleeding and clear any clot and debris (FIGURE 11). The suture is then tied. The vessel loops are released on the vein and the distal and proximal bulldog clamps are removed from the radial artery. The vein proximal to the anastomosis is then palpated for a thrill to determine patency. Absence of a thrill may indicate a technical problem and the anastomosis should be re-explored. This is done by making a small venotomy in the cephalic vein distal to the anastomosis and a dilator is used to explore the anastomosis as well as the artery and vein. It is important to ligate the cephalic vein distal to the anastomosis, usually with double 2-o silk (FIGURE 12). After ligation, the vessel is transacted, as this releases any tension on the anastomosis and reduces the incidence of venous hypertension of the hand. The presence of a thrill is reverified. Hemostasis is achieved and the subcutaneous layers are closed with interrupted 4-o absorbable suture. The skin is closed with a running subcuticular 4-o absorbable suture. A sterile dressing is then placed.

POSTOPERATIVE CONSIDERATIONS The patient is discharged the day of the procedure. If needed, dialysis is continued by the temporary access achieved prior to the operation. Occasionally, a venous side branch creating diversion of flow may need ligation. It usually takes 6 weeks for the AV fistula to mature and be ready to be used for hemodialysis. ■

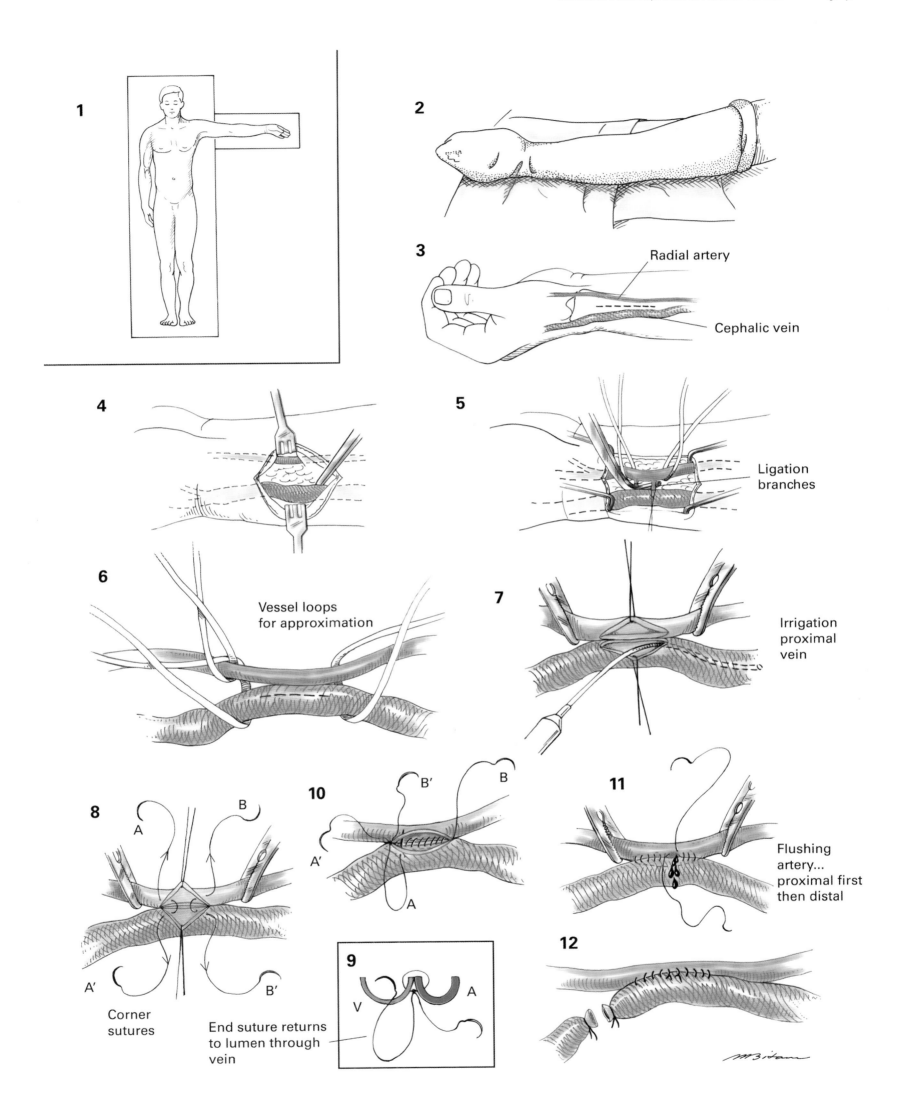

3
Radial artery

Cephalic vein

5
Ligation branches

6
Vessel loops for approximation

7
Irrigation proximal vein

8
A   B

A'   B'

Corner sutures

9
V   A

End suture returns to lumen through vein

10
B'   B

A'

A

11
Flushing artery... proximal first then distal

12

CHAPTER 133

VENOUS ACCESS, PORT PLACEMENT, INTERNAL JUGULAR VEIN

INDICATIONS The most common indication is for the administration of chemotherapy or long-term parenteral nutritional support. For these purposes, a port is usually used. For short-term therapies, alternatives include a tunneled central venous catheter or a peripherally inserted central catheter (PICC).

PREOPERATIVE PREPARATION The procedure is usually performed as an outpatient. Electrolytes and clotting studies should be checked prior to the procedure. If the patient has had previous central catheters, a careful history should be obtained, as this will help with site selection. Transcutaneous ultrasound can assist with vein localization. A single dose of preoperative antibiotics provides for prophylaxis.

ANESTHESIA Moderate sedation and local anesthesia is preferred.

POSITION The patient is placed in the supine position. Fluoroscopy should be available. The arms are tucked at each side.

OPERATIVE PREPARATION The hair is removed with clippers. The chosen side of the neck/upper thorax is prepped and draped using the maximum sterile barrier technique.

DETAILS OF PROCEDURE

INTERNAL JUGULAR VEIN ACCESS The internal jugular vein may be safer than subclavian venous access. The internal jugular vein is located posterior to the sternocleidomastoid muscle (FIGURE 1). It is usually accessed by a percutaneous route. This chapter demonstrates a right internal jugular cannulation.

Preliminary ultrasound of the right side of the neck is done in order to document the patency of the internal jugular vein. With real-time ultrasound guidance and employing a modified Seldinger technique, a small incision is made in the skin of the neck with a 15 blade and the internal jugular vein is cannulated with a small-diameter needle (FIGURE 2A). After removing the syringe, the surgeon places a flexible guidewire (FIGURE 2B). The needle is removed, and over this wire, a 5-French dilator is placed to create a track (FIGURE 3). A 3- to 4-cm transverse incision is made on the upper right thorax two fingerbreadths below the clavicle and a hemostat is passed to create a tunnel between the two incisions (FIGURE 4). Blunt dissection is done to create a subcutaneous pocket on top of the pectoralis muscle fascia for the reservoir (FIGURE 4). The Silastic catheter is advanced through the

subcutaneous tissues from the upper thoracic subcutaneous pocket to the neck incision (FIGURE 4). The 5-French dilator is exchanged over a wire for an introducer with a peel-away sheath (FIGURE 5). The dilator and wire are removed from the introducer. The Silastic catheter is advanced through the peel-away sheath (FIGURE 6) and is positioned under fluoroscopy with its tip in the right atrium (FIGURE 7). Keeping the catheter in place with a forceps (FIGURE 6), the sheath is "peeled away" by pulling it apart laterally until it is completely split and out. The catheter is cut to length at the pocket and the slide-on boot is placed over the catheter. The catheter is pushed onto the chamber hubs (FIGURE 8A), and the boot is slid down over the catheter in order to secure its attachment to the hub (FIGURE 8B). Immediately following placement, each of the ports is aspirated and flushed to verify patency. If any resistance is encountered, then obstruction of the catheter in the vein insertion site, the tunnel, or at the junction of the catheter with the reservoir should be suspected. These sites should be inspected. The position of the catheter with its tip in the right atrium should be verified by fluoroscopy. The reservoir is then secured with nonabsorbable monofilament suture to the pectoralis fascia. The subcutaneous tissues of the reservoir pocket are closed using interrupted 3-0 absorbable suture. The port must be easily palpable, and in very obese patients, the subcutaneous fat may need to thinned directly above the port. The skin edges are approximated using a continuous subcuticular 4-0 absorbable suture. The neck incision is closed using a single subcuticular 4-0 absorbable suture and the port is checked for flow in both infusion and aspiration after which it is loaded with a dilute heparin solution. The final configuration is shown in FIGURE 9 and all personnel who access the port must remember to use the special needles that do not cut or core out a segment of the Silastic access dome as they are inserted into the port.

ALTERNATIVELY The central venous system may be accessed via the subclavian vein as shown in the following Chapter 134, page 512. In this operation the subclavian skin entrance site is opened a few millimeters and a tunnel is created with a small hemostat to the port-site pocket. The subcutaneous fat at the entrance may require some spreading so as to allow the Silastic catheter to round this corner without an obstructing angulation. The remainder of the procedure is the same except for the need to close this skin incision with a few absorbable subcuticular sutures followed by adhesive skin strips. The port is then aspirated, checked for free flow in both directions, and finally loaded with a dilute heparin solution. ■

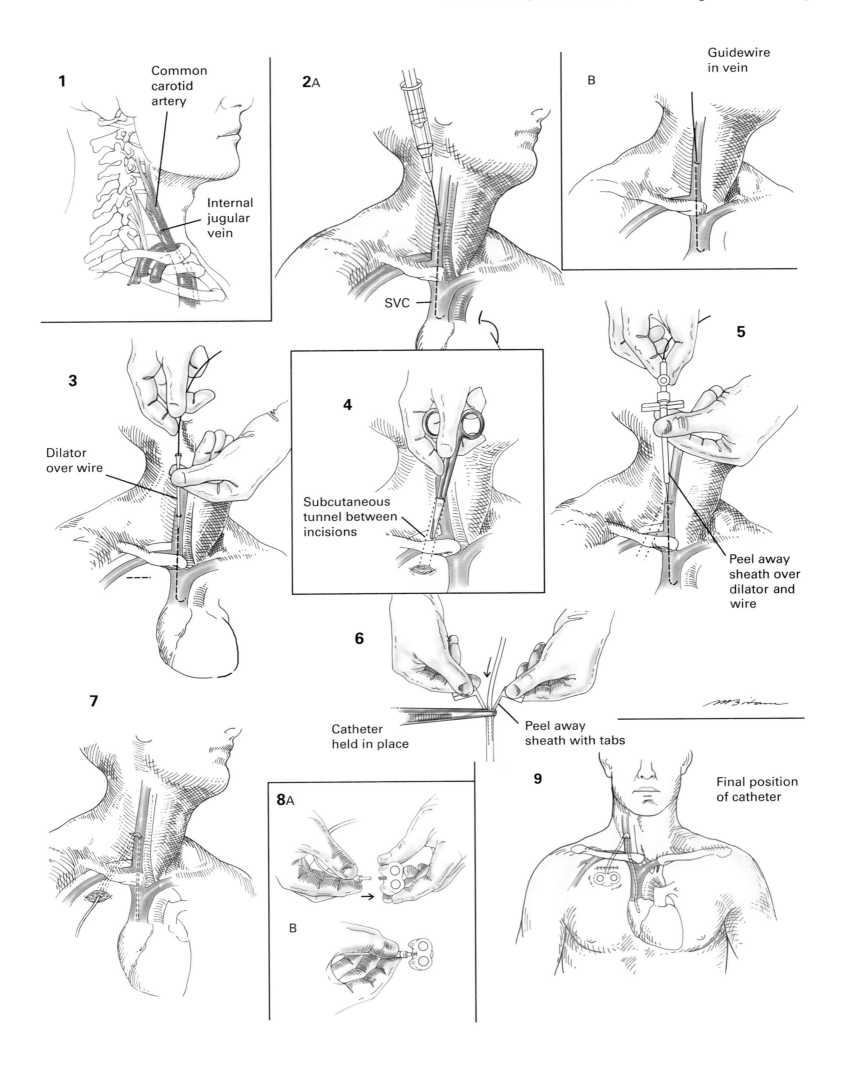

1 Common carotid artery

Internal jugular vein

2A

SVC

B   Guidewire in vein

3 Dilator over wire

4 Subcutaneous tunnel between incisions

5 Peel away sheath over dilator and wire

6 Catheter held in place   Peel away sheath with tabs

7

8A

B

9 Final position of catheter

CHAPTER 134

VENOUS ACCESS, CENTRAL VENOUS CATHETER, SUBCLAVIAN VEIN

INDICATIONS The most common indication is for the short-term (7–10 days) administration of fluids, electrolytes, antibiotics, or other concentrated parenteral medications that are not well tolerated in peripheral veins. Absence of suitable peripheral veins and patient comfort are alternative indications, as is the inability to place a peripherally inserted central catheter (PICC).

PREOPERATIVE PREPARATION The procedure may be performed at the bedside, in the operating room, or in an outpatient ambulatory setting. Electrolytes and clotting studies should be checked prior to the procedure. If the patient has had previous central catheters, a careful history should be obtained, as this will help with site selection. Transcutaneous ultrasound can assist with vein localization.

ANESTHESIA Moderate sedation and local anesthesia is preferred.

POSITION The patient is placed in the supine position, and the arms are tucked at each side. Fluoroscopy should be available.

OPERATIVE PREPARATION The hair is removed with clippers. The chosen side of the neck and upper thorax are prepped and draped using the maximum sterile barrier technique.

DETAILS OF PROCEDURE FIGURES 1 and 2 show the relevant anatomy of the subclavian vein. It may be cannulated on the right or the left side. The chapter shows cannulation on the right side. On the right, the subclavian vein courses behind the medial third of the clavicle and joins the internal jugular vein to drain into the superior vena cava. It lies anterior and inferior to the subclavian artery. The dome of the right lung lies behind the vessels. Ultrasound is used to confirm the patency of the vein and location. The same modified Seldinger technique is used as described in the preceding Chapter 133. The patient is placed in a supine position. A rolled towel or sheet is placed in the interscapular area to allow the shoulder to drop to the side away from the infraclavicular site (FIGURES 1 and 3). The patient is placed in a 20-degree Trendelenburg position (head down) in order to minimize the risk of air embolism and increase the size of the vein. The head is turned slightly to the opposite side. After installation of local anesthetic to include the periosteum of the clavicle, the subclavian vein is cannulated with a small caliber needle (FIGURE 3). Ultrasound guidance may be used to provide assistance. A key landmark is the point one fingerbreadth lateral to the junction of the middle and medial thirds of the clavicle. The needle is inserted at this point and passed along a straight line toward the sternoclavicular joint on a plane parallel to the chest wall. A flexible guidewire is inserted into the needle (FIGURE 4), and if any arrhythmia is noted, the wire is withdrawn until the electrocardiogram returns to its usual pattern. The position of the wire is fluoroscopically verified. The triple-lumen catheter is thread over the guidewire (FIGURE 5). Topical antiseptic and a dry sterile dressing are placed over the entrance site. The catheter hub and wings are secured to the chest skin with fine nonabsorbable sutures (FIGURE 6). A chest x-ray is obtained to verify the position of the catheter and exclude complications such as a pneumothorax. ■

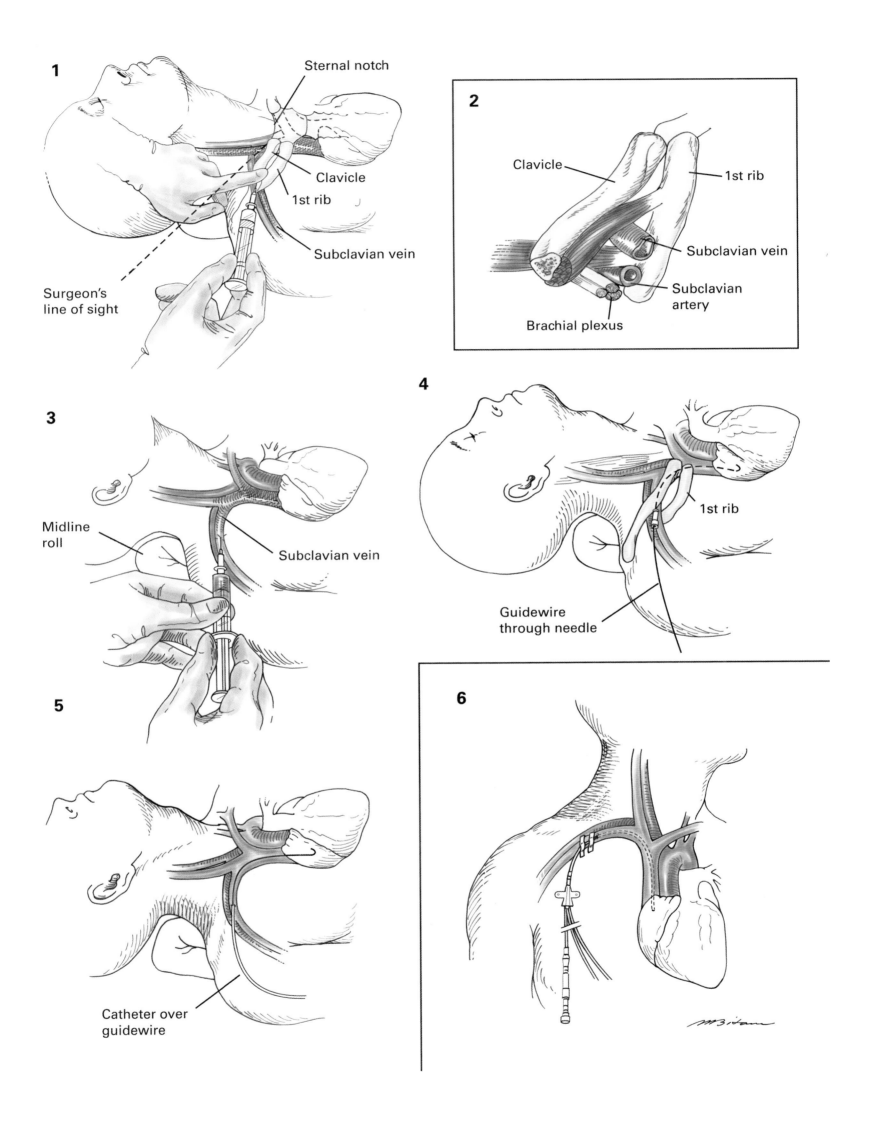

1

Sternal notch

Clavicle

1st rib

Subclavian vein

Surgeon's line of sight

2

Clavicle

1st rib

Subclavian vein

Subclavian artery

Brachial plexus

3

Midline roll

Subclavian vein

4

1st rib

Guidewire through needle

5

Catheter over guidewire

6

RESECTION OF ABDOMINAL AORTIC ANEURYSM

INDICATIONS Aneurysms of the abdominal aorta occurring distal to the renal arteries should, in general, be replaced. This is particularly true if they are enlarging, 5.5 cm or greater in males and 5.3 cm or greater in females, producing pain or if there is evidence of impending or actual rupture. In poor-risk patients with small aneurysms less than 5 cm in diameter, observation may be the better course. Many aneurysms are corrected by endovascular techniques, but an open operative approach is acceptable and a sometime necessary alternative. Although the operation is of considerable magnitude, anticipated mortality associated with spontaneous rupture and exsanguination from an aneurysm is such as to warrant the risk of surgery in the great majority of patients. Emergency operations may offer the only chance of a patient's survival if there is evidence of leakage or rupture of the aneurysm. A past history of coronary artery disease is not a contraindication to surgery.

PREOPERATIVE PREPARATION CT scan best defines the size and contour of these aneurysms. Transabdominal ultrasound is a good screening tool, but CT best defines size and proximal and distal extent. Aortography is carried out if there is a question about the extent of the aneurysm, if distal occlusive disease is present, and when renal vascular disease or mesenteric insufficiency is suspected. A thorough cardiac evaluation with an electrocardiogram, echocardiogram, and imaging stress test is performed.

In elective resection of an aneurysm, the preoperative preparation consists of emptying the large intestine by administering a mild cathartic. A fluid load of "crystalloid" is given at approximately 100 to 150 mL per hour beginning the evening before operation if the patient is hospitalized. Intravenous antibiotic coverage is started 1 hour before the anticipated incision. A nasogastric tube is inserted, and constant bladder drainage is initiated to follow accurately the hourly output of urine, especially during the immediate postoperative period. Catheters are placed for central venous and arterial monitoring, while a Swan–Ganz catheter may be useful in complex cardiac cases.

ANESTHESIA General anesthesia with endotracheal intubation is routine. The arterial line permits instantaneous evaluation of blood pressure changes, and blood gas sampling can be done when required. Several large-bore (16-gauge) catheters should be placed intravenously for adequate control of fluid and blood replacement, including a central venous line.

POSITION The patient is placed in a slight head-down position to aid in natural retraction of the small intestine from the region of the lower abdomen. Intravenous catheters are secured in place in both arms and adequately protected from dislodgement. The urethral catheter is connected to a constant bladder drainage bottle. Since the presence of pedal pulsations must be verified before and after the prosthesis has been inserted, some type of low support should be provided over the feet and lower third of the legs to assist in evaluating the presence of arterial pulsations.

INCISION AND EXPOSURE A long midline incision is made from xiphoid to pubis (FIGURE 1). Many surgeons use a large open ring retractor for exposure. This retractor is secured to the side rail of the operating table and allows for the placement of multiple individual curved or angled adjustable retractors.

DETAILS OF PROCEDURE After rapid palpation and visualization of the aorta and confirmation of the diagnosis of aneurysm, steps are taken to empty the abdominal cavity of small intestine. Unless the abdominal wall is quite thick, the greater portion of the small intestine can be retracted upward and to the right and inserted into a plastic bag, the mouth of which can be partly constricted by a tape (FIGURE 2). Saline is added to the plastic bag to keep the intestine moist. A sterile gauze pad is inserted into the neck of the plastic bag to avoid undue constriction and prevent the escape of the small intestine from the bag. It may be advisable (if the aneurysm is sizable and involves the right common iliac) to mobilize the appendix, terminal ileum, and cecum and to retract the right colon upward. The small and large bowels are retracted laterally and superiorly using multiple adjustable retractors. Additional exposure can be gained by dividing the peritoneum about the ligament of Treitz to permit further retraction of the small intestine upward and to the right (FIGURE 2). In thinner individuals, the small intestine may be tucked within the right side of the abdomen to minimize heat loss. What at first may appear to be an inoperable aneurysm eventually may prove to be rather easily resectable, since the aneurysm tends to bulge anteriorly and seems to extend up so high as to suggest involvement of the renal vessels (FIGURE 3). The bulk of the aneurysm tends to come forward from under the left renal vein. The incised peritoneum over the anterior surface of the aneurysm is reflected by blunt and sharp dissection until the left renal vein is visualized. Blunt and sharp dissection frees the left renal vein from the underlying aorta (FIGURE 4). The left renal vein is retracted upward with a vein retractor (FIGURE 5) to gain additional space for the application of the occluding clamp to the aorta above the aneurysm. The left renal vein can be divided, if necessary, to gain the final exposure. It does not need to be reanastomosed if the adrenal and gonadal vessel veins are intact. **CONTINUES** ➤

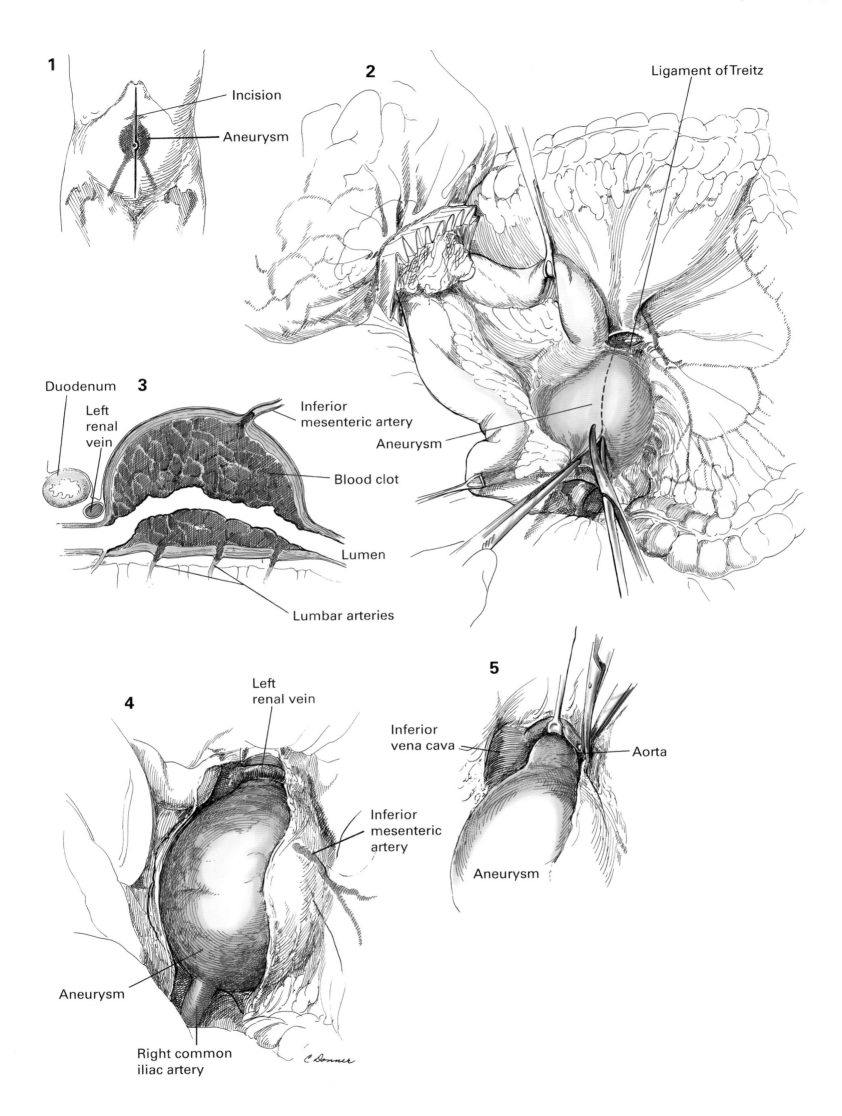

1

Incision

Aneurysm

2

Ligament of Treitz

Aneurysm

3

Duodenum

Left renal vein

Inferior mesenteric artery

Blood clot

Lumen

Lumbar arteries

4

Left renal vein

Inferior mesenteric artery

Aneurysm

Right common iliac artery

5

Inferior vena cava

Aorta

Aneurysm

C. Donner

DETAILS OF PROCEDURE <CONTINUED> The inferior mesenteric artery is clamped (FIGURE 6). The aortic side may be divided and ligated from without or, more commonly, oversewn from within after the aneurysm is opened. Usually, this vessel is small and sclerotic, in which case its sacrifice is of little consequence. In some instances, it is large and serves as a major contributor to the left colon blood supply, especially if internal iliac and mesenteric occlusive disease is present. In such cases the vessel will be patent but will not exhibit back bleeding. Reimplantation of this vessel into the aortic graft may be required to protect the colon.

The common iliac arteries then are exposed on their anterior, lateral, and medial surfaces in preparation for clamp placement. It is not necessary to encircle these vessels completely, and dissection posteriorly can result in troublesome hemorrhage from the underlying iliac veins. During the iliac artery exposure the ureters are identified and protected from injury throughout the procedure (FIGURE 6).

In the past, certain grafts required preclotting; however, this is not necessary with woven grafts, knitted grafts sealed with collagen or gelatin, or expanded polytetrafluoroethylene grafts.

Heparin is then injected systemically to provide protective anticoagulation for the extremities during aortic clamping.

Angled vascular clamps are applied to the distal common iliac arteries. An aortic clamp is used to occlude the aorta proximal to the aneurysm and distal to the renal arteries. A careful identification of the position of the renal arteries is mandatory before clamp application. The aneurysm is then opened through a linear arteriotomy (FIGURE 7). The mural thrombus is extracted (FIGURE 8). Bleeding from the paired lumbar arteries is controlled with full-thickness mattress or figure-of-eight nonabsorbable suture ligatures (FIGURE 9). The aortic cuff is next prepared by dividing all but the posterior wall. Leaving this portion attached prevents troublesome bleeding from lumbar veins often found in this area (FIGURE 10). The iliac arteries are prepared in similar fashion; the posterior wall is undisturbed to protect the iliac veins (FIGURE 10). Alternatively, some surgeons prefer to completely transect the proximal aorta and the distal iliac arteries so as to provide free circumferential cuffs for graft anastomoses. <CONTINUES>

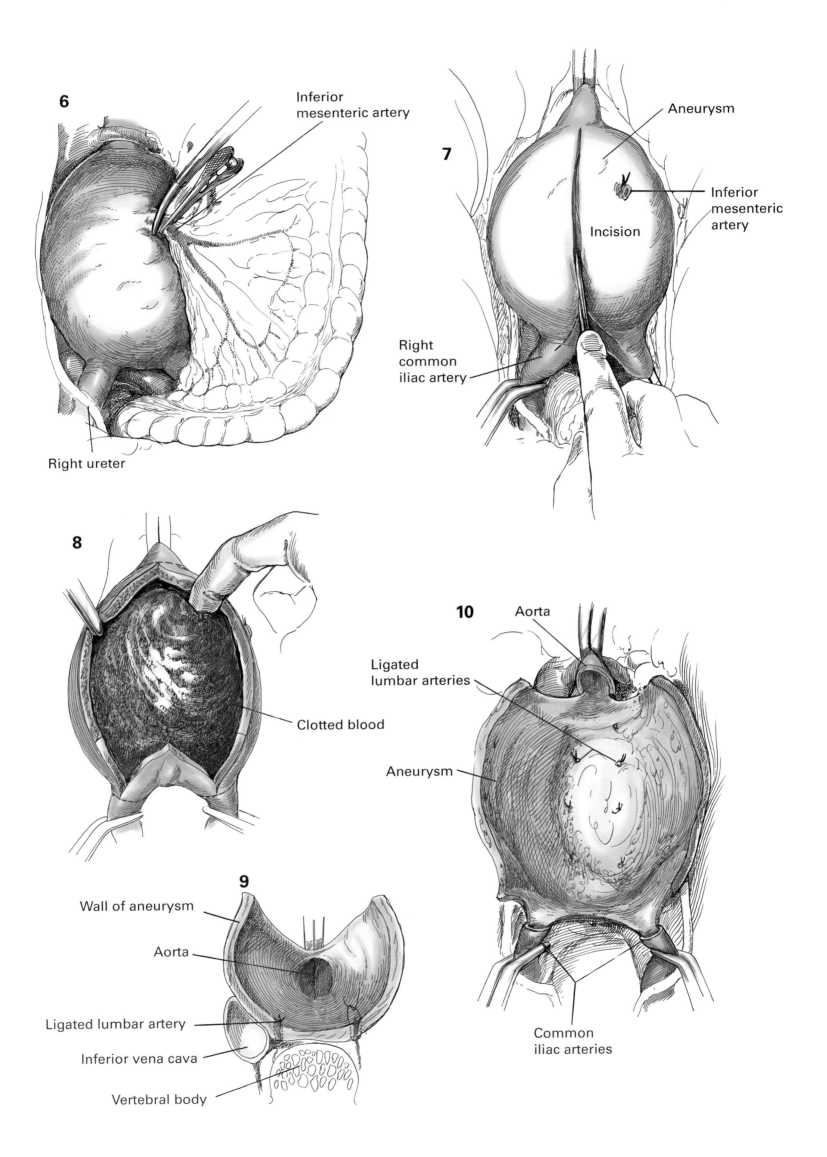

6

Inferior mesenteric artery

Right ureter

7

Aneurysm

Incision

Inferior mesenteric artery

Right common iliac artery

8

Clotted blood

9

Wall of aneurysm

Aorta

Ligated lumbar artery

Inferior vena cava

Vertebral body

10

Aorta

Ligated lumbar arteries

Aneurysm

Common iliac arteries

DETAILS OF PROCEDURE ◄**CONTINUED**► A graft of appropriate size is then stretched and tailored to fit the aortic defect (FIGURE 11). Suturing of the graft begins in the midline posteriorly with a double-arm swedged 00 or 000 nonabsorbable suture usually made of monofilament nylon or polypropylene. The initial stitch begins by passing both needles from outside inward on the graft and from inside outward on the aorta. This suture is then tied (FIGURE 12). Over-and-over suturing is then carried from the midline position, proceeding from outside inward on the graft to inside outward on the aorta. At the midline anteriorly, this suture is again tied (FIGURE 13).

Vascular clamps are temporarily applied to the iliac limbs of the graft, and the aortic clamp is momentarily released to check the proximal suture line for hemostasis and the preclotting of the graft. Should leaks be noted in the anastomosis, they can be controlled by individual mattress sutures.

The iliac anastomoses are done in the same manner as that of the aorta (FIGURE 14). Just before completion of the anastomosis, the aortic clamp is opened momentarily to flush any clots that may have accumulated in the aorta or graft (FIGURE 15). This flushing out greatly lessens the incidence of subsequent thrombosis in either extremity and justifies a modest loss of blood. **CONTINUES►**

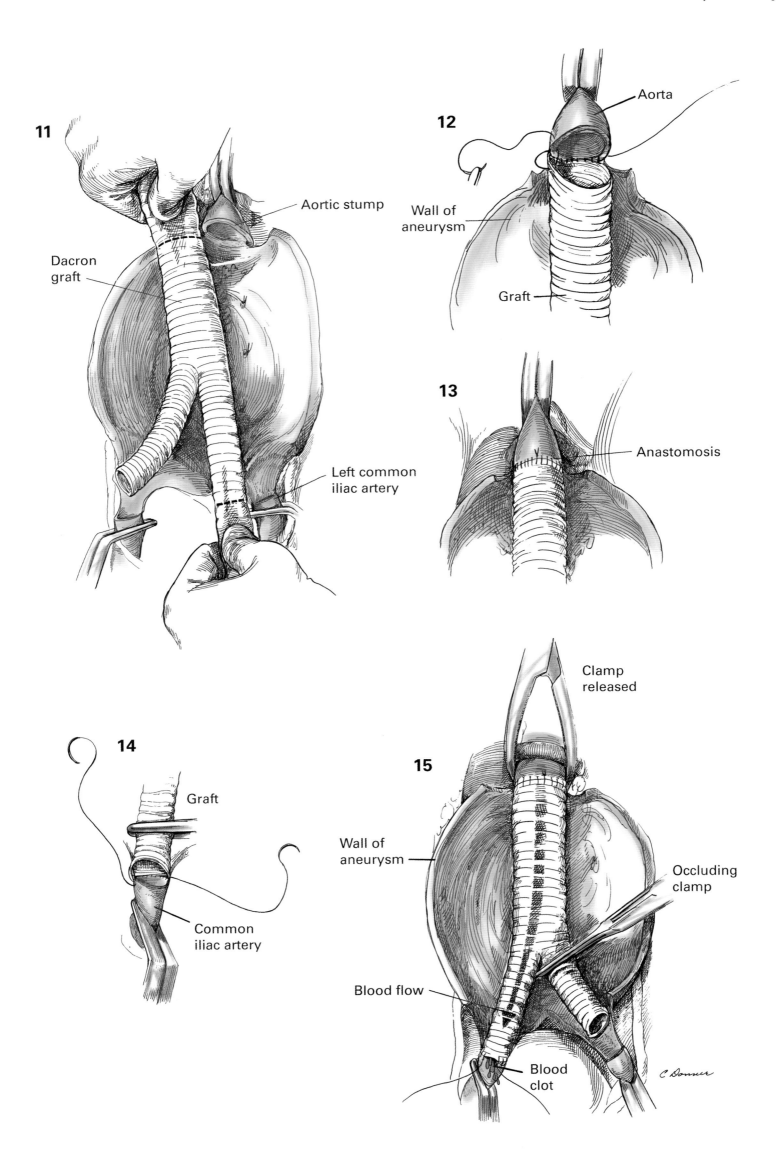

11

Aortic stump

Dacron graft

Left common iliac artery

12

Aorta

Wall of aneurysm

Graft

13

Anastomosis

14

Graft

Common iliac artery

15

Clamp released

Wall of aneurysm

Occluding clamp

Blood flow

Blood clot

DETAILS OF PROCEDURE ◀CONTINUED The clamp is closed and the suture line completed and tied. The completed limb is occluded by finger control, and the aortic clamp is removed slowly. Blood flow is gradually reestablished to the limb to prevent hypotension (FIGURE 16). Flow should be established first to the hypogastric artery to minimize the risk of distal embolization. Close coordination between the surgeon and anesthesiologist is required at this point so that the rate of opening the graft is compensated by fluids and blood administration with maintenance of stable blood pressure.

The other iliac anastomosis is carried out in similar fashion (FIGURE 17). The aneurysm sac, if adequate, is closed over the graft with a running suture (FIGURE 18). If at all possible, closure of the proximal aneurysmal sac should cover the aortic anastomosis so as to provide tissue between it and the duodenum. Alternatively, some surgeons tuck a segment of omentum in this region. The posterior peritoneum is reapproximated, with care taken not to injure the ureters.

In the presence of occlusive disease of the common iliac in addition to the aneurysm, the common iliac may be divided and oversewn with a continuous suture (FIGURE 19) on both sides following removal of the aneurysm. The graft is tailored to permit anastomosis of the aorta above the aneurysm with end-to-side anastomosis to the external iliacs beyond the points of stenosis (FIGURE 20). This bypass procedure makes extensive endarterectomy unnecessary and prevents sacrifice of the hypogastric arteries, which are important in maintaining colonic viability.

CLOSURE The small intestine is returned to the peritoneal cavity from the plastic bag, and the peritoneal cavity is cleared of blood clots and sponges. Before closure, particular attention is given to the adequacy of the blood supply to the sigmoid. Ordinarily, the blood supply is adequate after ligation of the inferior mesenteric artery, but occasionally reimplantation into the graft or bypass of the inferior mesenteric artery with saphenous vein may be necessary to preserve the viability of the left colon and rectum. Evidence of bleeding from the prosthesis or at the site of anastomosis is thoroughly searched for before the closure is finally completed. The femoral vessels should be palpated from time to time to ensure that thrombosis has not occurred and that a good flow of blood is going through to the lower extremities. In case of doubt it may be necessary to reexplore one or both sides and remove any blood clots that are found. Routine abdominal closure is done.

POSTOPERATIVE CARE Postoperative care usually is provided in an intensive care unit for the first 24 to 48 hours. In the postoperative period it is particularly important to ensure that there is a good blood supply to the lower extremities and a good hourly output of urine. Blood should be given until all major blood loss has been replaced, and the blood pressure is satisfactory. The use of a cell saver system during surgery should lessen this need for blood replacement. Intravenous fluids are administered slowly during the first 24 hours to ensure a steady output of urine from the indwelling catheter. The presence or absence of pulsation in the dorsalis pedis arteries should be recorded. Confirmation may be difficult at first, but the pulsations usually become more apparent later in the postoperative period. If pulsations are absent and there is a cold extremity, thrombosis may have occurred, and reexploration and removal of the blood clot should be considered.

Cardiac monitoring and daily laboratory studies to evaluate the blood volume and kidney function are performed until the convalescence becomes uneventful. A tendency to paralytic ileus should be combatted by gastric suction until there is evidence that peristalsis has returned. Renal failure should be suspected if there has been preoperative evidence of impaired renal function or if there has been a prolonged period of hypotension.

If adequate hourly output of urine is not maintained despite an adequate intake, anuria should be suspected and appropriate therapy instituted. ∎

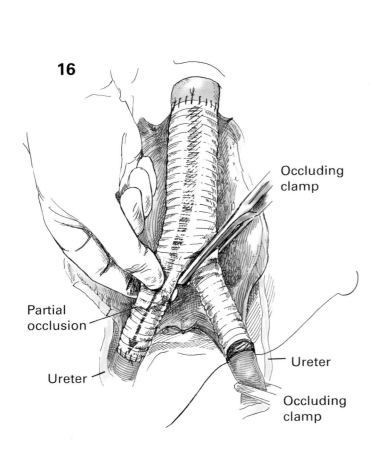

16

Occluding clamp

Partial occlusion

Ureter

Ureter

Occluding clamp

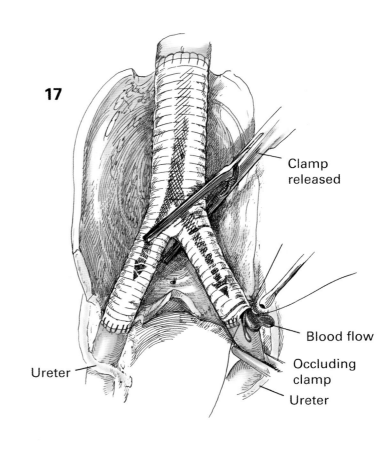

17

Clamp released

Blood flow

Occluding clamp

Ureter

Ureter

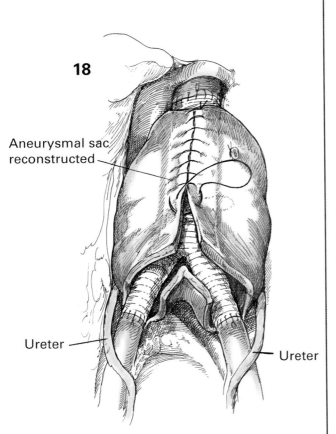

18

Aneurysmal sac reconstructed

Ureter

Ureter

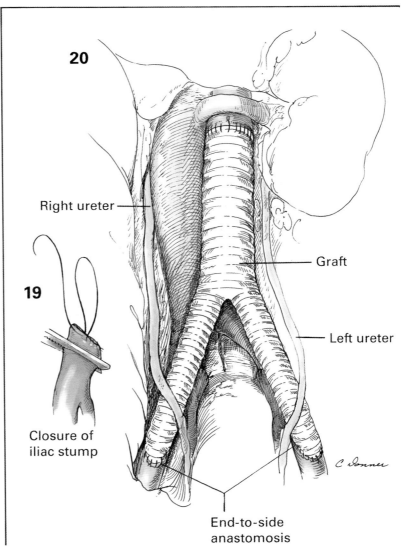

20

19

Right ureter

Graft

Left ureter

Closure of iliac stump

End-to-side anastomosis

C. Donner

CHAPTER 136 AORTOFEMORAL BYPASS

INDICATIONS Only patients with severe and debilitating occlusive disease of the aortoiliac segment should be considered for surgery. Initial management of aortoiliac occlusive disease is often via endovascular methods. In general, these patients will have claudication that is progressing or disabling. Patients with rest pain, ulceration, or gangrene may require surgery to preserve limb function. These patients are generally elderly and have associated generalized atherosclerosis with a high incidence of coronary artery disease and hypertension. In addition, the majority are long-time smokers, and it is not unusual for them to have impaired pulmonary function. The risks associated with these comorbidities must be carefully weighed against the benefits expected from a successful surgical procedure. The careful selection of patients is of the utmost importance.

PREOPERATIVE PREPARATION See preceding Chapter 135, Resection of Abdominal Aortic Aneurysm.

ANESTHESIA See preceding Chapter 135.

POSITION See preceding Chapter 135.

OPERATIVE PREPARATION See preceding Chapter 135.

INCISION AND EXPOSURE A midline incision is made from the xiphoid to the pubis to afford maximum exposure (FIGURE 1). The abdomen is explored for the presence of other pathology, and the intraabdominal arterial tree is carefully assessed. FIGURE 2 demonstrates typical aortoiliac occlusive disease. The aorta is exposed by entering the retroperitoneal space. The posterior peritoneum is divided, and the fourth portion of the duodenum is mobilized until the renal vein is identified. Sharp and blunt dissection is used to clear the aorta on its anterior, lateral, and medial surfaces (FIGURE 3). It is usually not necessary to encircle the aorta or to free it completely; this often leads to troublesome bleeding from lumbar arteries and veins. In addition, if the left renal vein is not visualized, it may lie behind the aorta and be injured by such a dissection.

DETAILS OF PROCEDURE An aortic clamp is used to clamp the aorta proximally just below the renal arteries (FIGURE 4). A second aortic clamp is placed tangentially to occlude the iliac vessels and the lumbar arteries, as depicted in FIGURES 4 and 5. It is important to have the distal aorta freed sufficiently so that this clamp can be placed far posteriorly to avoid interference with the arteriotomy and the anastomosis. A small vascular clamp should be applied to the inferior mesenteric artery, close to its origin, so as not to impair collateral circulation to the left colon. A linear arteriotomy is made in the aorta to a point just above the inferior mesentery artery takeoff (FIGURE 5). An attempt is made to preserve that vessel if at all possible. The graft is beveled (FIGURE 6A), and an end-to-side anastomosis is then created (FIGURES 6B, 7 to 9) with a running 3-0 monofilament vascular suture much as described in Chapter 135. The running suture then is carried around each side of the arteriotomy, and finally the anastomosis is completed in the middle of the arteriotomy.

ALTERNATIVE TECHNIQUE Many vascular surgeons prefer a direct end-of-aorta to end-of-graft ("end-to-end") proximal anastomosis. In this technique, the aorta is dissected free circumferentially at the same level below the renal arteries and proximal to the lumbar vessels. A pair of vascular clamps are applied, one distal to the renal arteries and one on the distal aorta, and the aorta is transected below the proximal clamp, leaving an adequate cuff for anastomosis proximally while oversewing the distal cuff with a 3-0 monofilament vascular suture. **CONTINUES** ▶

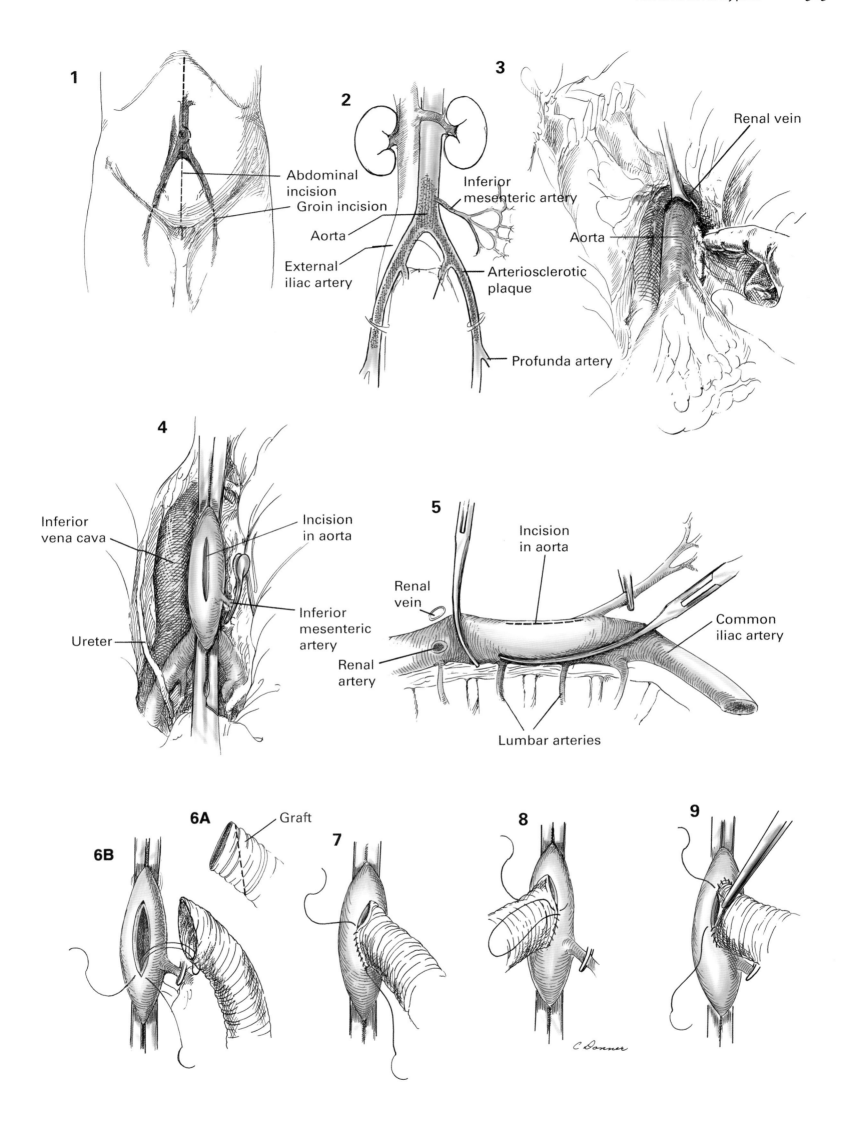

1

Abdominal incision
Groin incision
Aorta
External iliac artery

2

Inferior mesenteric artery
Arteriosclerotic plaque
Profunda artery

3

Renal vein
Aorta

4

Inferior vena cava
Ureter
Incision in aorta
Inferior mesenteric artery

5

Incision in aorta
Renal vein
Renal artery
Common iliac artery
Lumbar arteries

6A   Graft

6B

7

8

9

C Donner

DETAILS OF PROCEDURE ◀CONTINUED A linear incision is made in each groin over the femoral artery (FIGURE 10), and the common femoral, the profunda femoris, and the superficial femoral artery are carefully isolated. It is important to dissect at least several centimeters of the profunda femoris to evaluate the presence of disease in this vessel, especially if indicated on preoperative imaging. If it is significantly involved, profunda endarterectomy or a profundoplasty should be considered, because this procedure appears to increase the longevity of graft function, especially if it is the main runoff vessel. A retroperitoneal tunnel is then made overlying the iliac artery and extending into the femoral incision (FIGURE 10) by blunt finger dissection from above as well as from below, under the inguinal ligament. It is important to make this tunnel directly on top of the artery so that the ureter does not become entrapped or injured. Care should be given to anterior displacement of the ureter so that after the procedure it will overlie the prosthetic graft. Finally, it is important to remember that all of the dissections, aortic and femoral, and tunneling should be completed *before* the patient is systemically heparinized.

The graft is pulled into the groin incision through the previously created tunnel, taking care not to twist the limbs (FIGURE 11). Vascular clamps have been gently placed on the common femoral, the profunda femoris, and the superficial femoral arteries (FIGURE 12), and the linear arteriotomy is made. Stay sutures may be placed to retract the edges of the artery if necessary. It is not necessary to excise a button of artery wall. The slack is removed from the graft and the end is beveled to match the arteriotomy (FIGURE 13).

The anastomosis is carried out in the same manner as the upper end-to-side anastomosis of the graft to the aorta, typically with 5-0 or 6-0 monofilament vascular suture (FIGURES 14 and 15). Just before completion of the femoral anastomosis, a clamp is placed on the origin of the opposite iliac limb of the graft. The aortic clamp is opened momentarily to allow any thrombus and debris to be flushed out from the graft (FIGURE 16). The clamp is replaced and the femoral anastomosis is completed. Then the aortic clamp is removed, with digital compression of the graft in order to ensure gradual increased flow to the limb (FIGURE 17). The limb is allowed to slowly reperfuse so that hypotension does not occur, much as was outlined in the aortic aneurysm procedure. A similar procedure is followed in completing the anastomosis of the graft to the contralateral common femoral artery.

CLOSURE The incisions are closed in the routine manner. The retroperitoneum is closed over the entire graft with absorbable suture to protect the graft from the intra-abdominal organs, and especially the duodenum. If the retroperitoneum is inadequate for closure, omentum should be mobilized and brought through the transverse mesocolon. It is then tacked to the retroperitoneum over the graft. A running (0 or #1) monofilament suture with large wide bites is used for the midline incision, whereas the groin incisions are closed in layers with absorbable sutures.

POSTOPERATIVE CARE See preceding Chapter 135, page 520. ∎

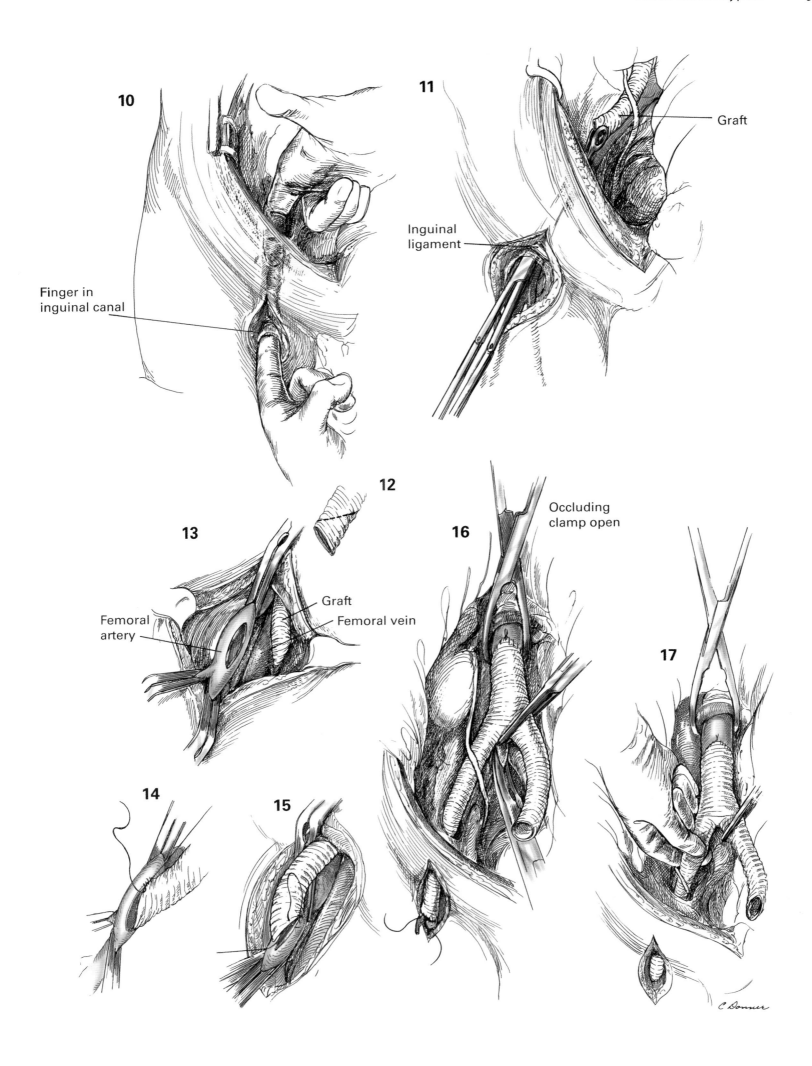

10

Finger in inguinal canal

11

Graft

Inguinal ligament

12

13

Femoral artery

Graft

Femoral vein

16

Occluding clamp open

17

14

15

C. Bonner

THROMBOEMBOLECTOMY, SUPERIOR MESENTERIC ARTERY

INDICATIONS Acute mesenteric fischemia may develop on top on chronic mesenteric ischemia due to an underlying atherosclerotic lesion, but may also occur de novo due to an embolic event. Typically this is a result of cardiac dysfunction, including acute MI, cardiac aneurysm, and dysrhythmia. The usual presentation is "pain out of proportion to physical findings," where the patient complains of the worst abdominal pain they have ever had, but physical examination elicits a soft abdomen with no discrete tender areas. Acute mesenteric ischemia is a surgical emergency where time is of the essence to avoid full-thickness bowel necrosis and even death.

PREOPERATIVE PREPARATION Diagnosis is often made on computed tomographic angiography (CTA) where lack of contrast is noted in one or more of the mesenteric vessels. The superior mesenteric artery is the most commonly affected, and often the thrombus lodges at the site of the first branch. The arteries should be surveyed for any signs of atherosclerosis and the bowel examined for any thickening, implying early ischemia or evidence of full-thickness necrosis. As soon as a diagnosis is made, intravenous heparin bolus should be administered and arrangements are made for transfer to the operative suite made. Meanwhile, the patient should be hydrated, given prophylactic antibiotics, and hemodynamically monitored.

ANESTHESIA General anesthesia is employed with meticulous attention to hemodynamic monitoring.

POSITION The patient is positioned supine on the operating table and the entire abdomen and anteromedial thighs should be prepared and draped, in case saphenous vein be needed for mesenteric bypass. Some prefer to "frog leg" the patient so that the medial thigh is more accessible. A nasogastric tube is inserted and left in place at the completion of the procedure.

PROCEDURAL DETAILS A vertical midline abdominal incision is made. The abdomen is explored and note made of any area of ischemia of the bowel or other organs. The small bowel is eviscerated to the right and the root of the mesentery palpated for the presence of a pulse (FIGURE 1A). In FIGURE 1B the relevant anatomy is illustrated. The superior mesenteric artery is exposed by dissecting parallel to it within the base of the mesentery. A self-retaining retractor is used for exposure purposes. Mesenteric venous branches and lymphatics are carefully ligated and divided. Silastic vessel loops are placed around the artery proximally, near the takeoff from the aorta, and distally, as well as on any side branches which should all be preserved (FIGURE 2). Depending on the status of anticoagulation, additional IV heparin may be given.

If the source of acute mesenteric ischemia is felt to be a more proximal, embolic source, then the artery may be opened transversely, so that closure is accomplished more rapidly and patch angioplasty closure avoided (FIGURE 3A). If the etiology is thought to be thrombosis due to underlying atherosclerotic plaque, then a longitudinal incision is preferred (FIGURE 3B), in order to perform endarterectomy or a bypass if necessary. Once the transverse arteriotomy is made, an appropriately sized Fogarty catheter (usually a 3 mm, but 2 mm or 4 mm may be used as well, depending on the size of the native vessel) is passed proximally and distally until thrombus removal is complete (FIGURE 4). There should be pulsatile inflow and adequate back bleeding. The Silastic vessel loops are briefly loosened, first distally and then proximally to verify blood flow. The artery is flushed antegrade and retrograde with heparinized saline solution (FIGURE 5). The transverse arteriotomy is closed using interrupted 6-0 polypropylene sutures and the clamps/Silastic loops are removed in order to restore distal flow (FIGURE 6). The bowel is reinspected throughout its entirety and any portions that are nonviable are resected; typically plans are made for a second look laparotomy the next day to reassess the remaining intestine. ■

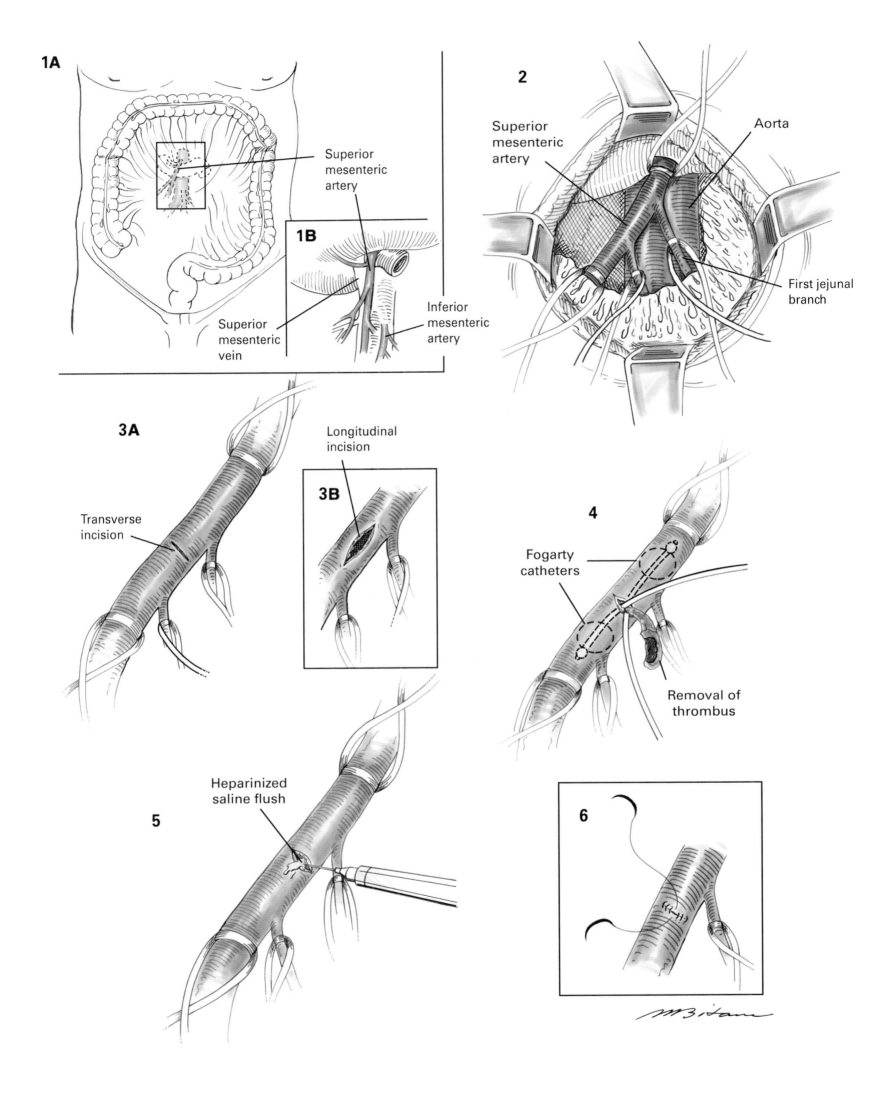

1A

Superior mesenteric artery

1B

Superior mesenteric artery

Superior mesenteric vein

Inferior mesenteric artery

2

Superior mesenteric artery

Aorta

First jejunal branch

3A

Transverse incision

Longitudinal incision

3B

4

Fogarty catheters

Removal of thrombus

5

Heparinized saline flush

6

FEMOROFEMORAL BYPASS

INDICATIONS Only patients with severe and debilitating occlusive disease of a unilateral aortoiliac segment should be considered for femorofemoral bypass. Today, endovascular angioplasty and stenting have reduced the indications for both aortofemoral bypass and femorofemoral bypasses, but there remains the occasional patient in whom bypass is the preferred treatment. Not all patients with a long-standing unilateral aortoiliac occlusion can be recannulated by endovascular techniques. In those patients where recannulation cannot be accomplished, femorofemoral bypass may be the preferred operative option. The contralateral, or donor aortoiliac segment should be free of occlusive disease. In the case where there is occlusive disease on the donor side, balloon angioplasty and stenting may need to be performed first to assure adequate inflow. Unilateral claudication is the leading indication for femorofemoral bypass, but occasionally rest pain, ulceration and gangrene may be the indication especially in the presence of significant comorbidities in the elderly. In younger patients with unilateral claudication, femorofemoral bypass may be preferred over the more durable aortofemoral bypass to eliminate the risk of retrograde ejaculation in those patients desiring children. While the younger patients are generally healthier and the operation is less invasive than aortofemoral bypass, the long-term patency is reduced and these factors need to be considered in the decision making. Elderly patients may still have generalized arteriosclerosis, including coronary artery disease and hypertension, and careful selection remains important.

PREOPERATIVE PREPARATION The anatomy is best defined by contrast angiography, CTA or MRA (FIGURE 1) and the final reconstruction is shown in FIGURE 2. Medical clearance is obtained as indicated. Intravenous antibiotic coverage is started on call to the operating room.

ANESTHESIA Regional epidural anesthesia is most commonly used, but general anesthesia may be preferred by the patient or anesthesiologist.

POSITION Patient is placed in the supine position.

DETAILS OF PROCEDURE A linear incision is made in each groin over the femoral artery and the common femoral, the profunda femoris, and the superficial femoral artery are carefully isolated and encircled with Silastic vessel loops for control. It is important to dissect at least several centimeters of the profunda femoris to evaluate the presence of disease in this vessel, especially if indicated on preoperative imaging. If it is significantly involved, profunda endarterectomy or a profundoplasty should be considered, because

this procedure appears to increase the longevity of graft function, especially if it is the main runoff vessel. Prior to giving heparin, a suprapubic subcutaneous tunnel is started with gentle subcutaneous finger dissection (FIGURE 3) in both groins. A tunneling device then joins the 2 groin incisions and a Penrose drain is pulled through to secure the passageway. From the suprapubic position the tunnel must form a gentle curve to each groin to avoid kinking of the graft when it is pulled into place by too acute of an angle. Generally the graft is sutured to the common femoral artery and extended toward the profunda femoris as needed. However, in some cases the common femoral artery does not extend far enough below the inguinal ligament to allowing suturing, and the arteriotomy is made on the profunda femoris or superficial femoral artery to avoid kinking as well.

Generally an 8-mm ringed Dacron or PTFE graft is used as the conduit and brought onto the field. Following adequate heparinization, tension is placed on the vessel loops in the donor groin to stop flow and the arteriotomy made with an 11 or 15 blade and extended with Potts scissors. The graft is beveled as shown in Chapter 136, FIGURE 12 and is sutured into place with 5-0 or 6-0 polypropylene as shown in the succeeding FIGURES 13 to 15. Separate sutures are started in the heel and toe of the anastomosis, flushed to evacuate air and debris and completed. A noncrushing vascular clamp is applied to the graft just proximal to the suture line and flow is restored to the leg and hemostasis obtained. The end of the Penrose drain in the contralateral groin is grasp with the graft passer and the graft passer is pulled into the opposite groin. The end of the newly attached graft is grasp and pulled into the contralateral groin (FIGURE 4). Again acute angulation is avoided. The vessels in this groin are then occluded by gentle traction on the vessel loops, the site for arteriotomy chosen. Generally the common femoral artery is the preferred site with extension to the profunda femoris artery. Gentle traction is applied to the graft to remove redundancy and the graft is cut to appropriate length and beveled (FIGURE 4). The graft is anastomosed in a similar fashion as done in the opposite groin with 5-0 or 6-0 polypropylene (FIGURES 5 and 6). All vessels are back bled and the graft flushed prior to completion of the suture line (FIGURES 7 and 8). The suture line is completed and flow restored to the leg. Once hemostasis is complete, the groins are closed with absorbable suture in layers with a subcuticular skin closure.

POSTOPERATIVE CARE Postoperative care is generally provided on the general vascular surgery floor and intensive care is not required. The patient is discharged on the first or the second postoperative day. ■

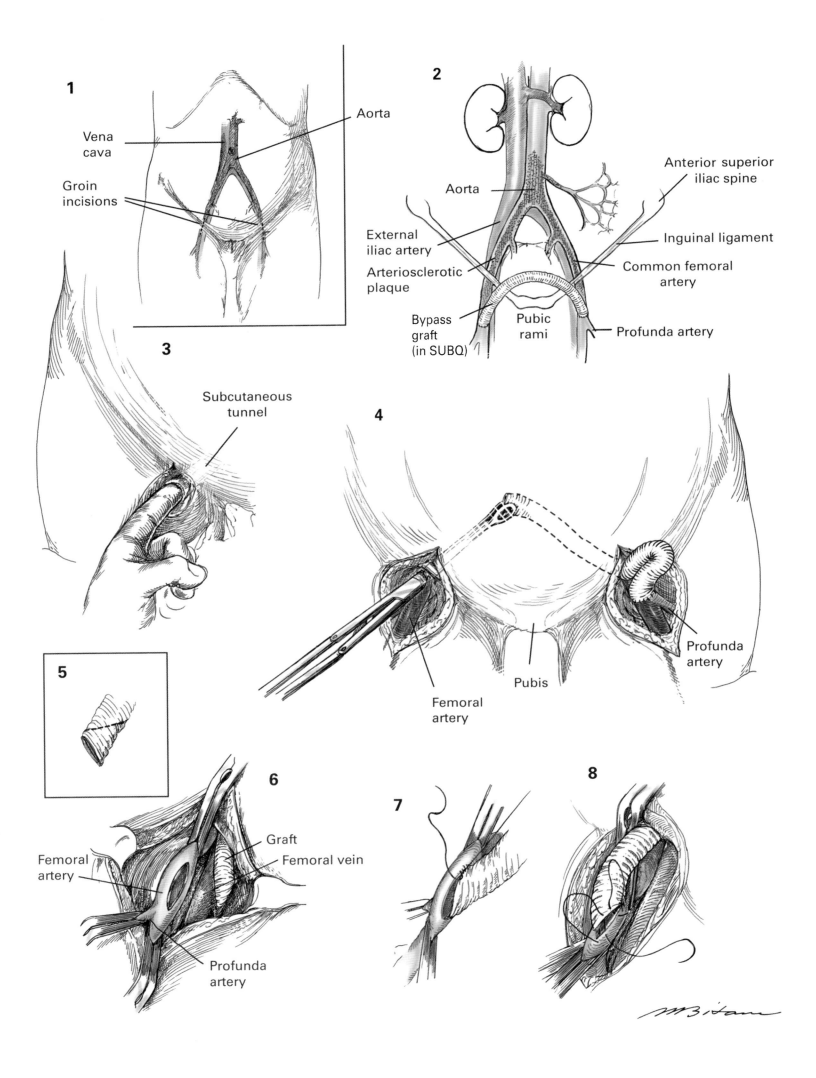

1

Vena cava

Groin incisions

Aorta

2

Aorta

External iliac artery

Arteriosclerotic plaque

Bypass graft (in SUBQ)

Pubic rami

Anterior superior iliac spine

Inguinal ligament

Common femoral artery

Profunda artery

3

Subcutaneous tunnel

4

Femoral artery

Pubis

Profunda artery

5

6

Femoral artery

Profunda artery

Graft

Femoral vein

7

8

FEMOROPOPLITEAL RECONSTRUCTION

INDICATIONS Surgical bypass of the femoropopliteal segment is reserved for patients with severe claudication or impending limb loss manifested by ischemic rest pain or tissue necrosis. Often the first-line treatment is via endovascular techniques. Typically, such patients have generalized atherosclerosis and a high incidence of significant coronary artery or extracranial carotid artery occlusive disease. Multiple risk factors—including cigarette smoking, hypertension, diabetes mellitus, and hyperlipidemia—can be identified in the majority. Careful selection of candidates for operation is of utmost importance, weighing the expected benefit against the potential risk.

PREOPERATIVE PREPARATION Catheter-based aortography or computed tomographic angiography with full evaluation of the distal runoff is mandatory to identify and exclude more proximal occlusive disease and to ensure adequate distal runoff. Noninvasive vascular laboratory studies—including duplex ultrasound scanning, segmental limb pressures and segmental limb plethysmography—aid accurate physiologic assessment and serve as a baseline for estimation of the response to therapy. Preoperative saphenous vein mapping with duplex ultrasound is the preferred method for assessment of the vein. It demonstrates the patency and anatomy of the saphenous vein, as it is prone to variation, double systems, or unexpectedly large perforating connectors.

Careful assessment of cardiopulmonary function is most important. An electrocardiogram and chest x-ray are obtained and further investigations may be prompted by the history or physical examination. Cardiac evaluation with an echocardiogram or a radionuclide imaging stress test may be prudent in order to risk stratify patients, as may be pulmonary function studies. Further investigation may be prompted by history, physical examination, or these initial studies. Immediately preceding operation, catheters are placed for monitoring the central venous pressure, arterial pressure, and urinary output. Prophylactic antibiotic therapy is begun before operation and continued for 24 hours. The groin and lower extremity hair is clipped in the preoperative prep area.

ANESTHESIA General or regional anesthesia is employed with careful attention given to maintaining satisfactory hemodynamic parameters.

POSITION The patient is placed supine on the operating table.

OPERATIVE PREPARATION The lower abdomen and appropriate limb are prepared in the usual manner to allow full mobility and exposure of the extremity. The foot is placed in a clear plastic Lahey bag (FIGURE 1) after which a clear occlusive drape may be applied to the skin with special care anteromedially over the areas of planned incision. If the contralateral greater saphenous vein is to be used as the graft, the opposite extremity must be prepared in a similar fashion. Any question concerning the adequacy of inflow from the aortoiliac segment should have already been addressed with concomitant or previous inflow procedure.

INCISION AND EXPOSURE The initial incision, which follows the course of the greater saphenous vein (FIGURE 1), is made vertically across the inguinal crease, and early identification is made of the greater saphenous vein at the fossa ovalis. Dissection is continued distally in a progressive fashion to expose the entire length of vein required for the bypass. Alternatively, multiple incisions with intervening skin bridges may be elected. The creation of large skin flaps must be avoided to prevent skin necrosis and serious wound problems. After exposure of a suitable length of saphenous vein (FIGURE 2), the venous tributaries are ligated and divided between 4-0 silk ties and clips (FIGURE 3). Flow is maintained with both ends intact as tributaries are ligated. Precautions are taken not to gather venous adventitia by ligating these tributaries excessively close to the vein wall, which will result in stenosis of the bypass graft (FIGURE 4). The vein should be kept in situ with flow maintained until just before the bypass graft is to be performed. After the saphenous vein is removed, a ball-tipped needle is inserted into the distal lumen (FIGURE 5) to permit flushing and distention during graft preparation (FIGURE 6). The proximal vein is then clamped gently with a bulldog clamp, and the vein is distended gently with heparinized saline. This maneuver may reveal leaks resulting from division of unidentified tributaries and stenotic areas that may require attention. Overdistention by forceful irrigation is avoided, as this may irreversibly damage the vein graft. At the completion of vein distention, an ink line is drawn down the graft to help avoid twisting the segment as it is brought through the tunnel later in the procedure (FIGURE 7). The graft is temporarily placed in dilute Papaverine solution to maintain vasodilation and to keep the graft moist. The femoral arterial exposure is performed as for aortofemoral bypass grafting with vessel loops passed around the common femoral artery proximally, and the profunda femoris and the superficial femoral arteries distally (FIGURE 8). Care is taken to ligate the overlying lymphatic tissue to prevent formation of a lymphocele or lymph fistula. **CONTINUES**

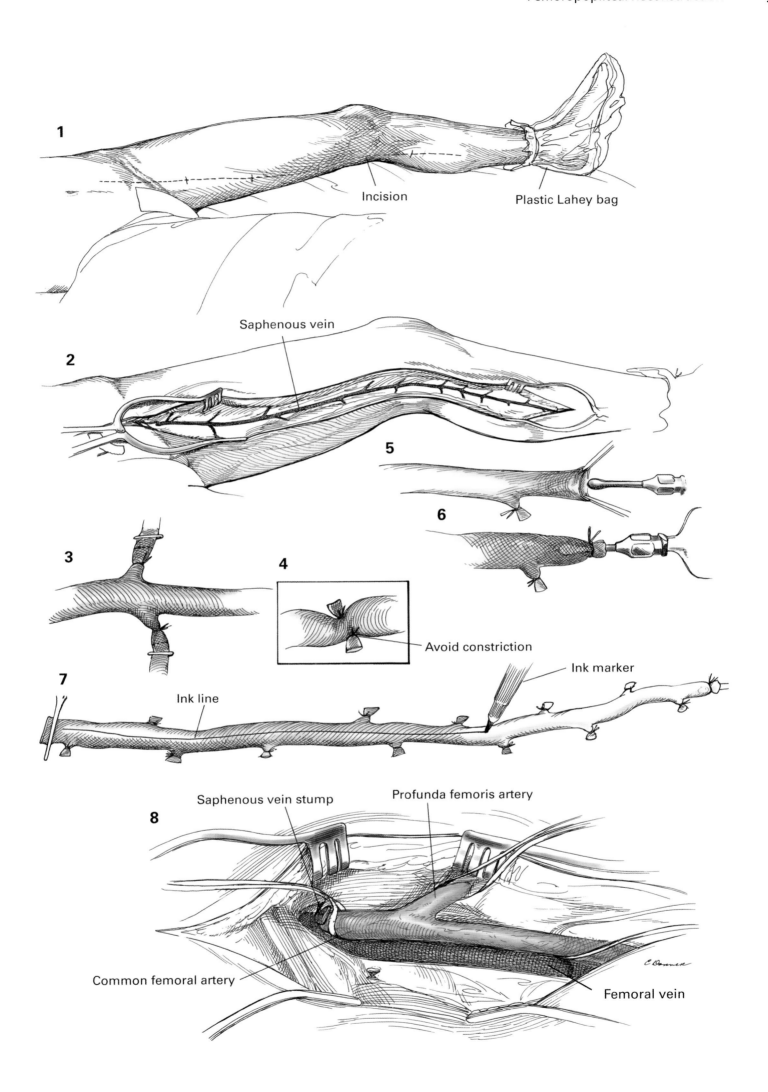

1

Incision

Plastic Lahey bag

2

Saphenous vein

3

4

Avoid constriction

5

6

7

Ink line

Ink marker

8

Saphenous vein stump

Profunda femoris artery

Common femoral artery

Femoral vein

INCISION AND EXPOSURE `CONTINUED` The distal popliteal artery is exposed immediately above the medial knee or below the knee, posterior to the tibia (depending on the distal target vessel). This is done below the knee by opening the fascial compartment and retracting the gastrocnemius and soleus muscles posteriorly and entering the popliteal space. Insertion of a self-retaining retractor greatly facilitates the exposure (FIGURE 9). The popliteal artery is identified medial to the posterior tibial nerve and the popliteal vein. Often, the popliteal vein, which may be duplicated, must be mobilized in order to get to the more lateral artery. It is carefully dissected free over a distance of 4 to 5 cm (FIGURE 10), controlling any small branches with double loops of silk ties, vessels loops, or temporarily applied clips. Vessel loops are then passed around the vessel proximally and distally to elevate the vessel and improve exposure (FIGURE 11). To tunnel to the below knee incision, the proximal popliteal space then is entered above the knee by incising the fascia anterior to the sartorius muscle. The graft tunnel is developed by blunt finger dissection (FIGURE 12) or a tunneling instrument behind the knee in the anatomic plane. A Penrose drain is placed to temporarily mark the tract. `CONTINUES`

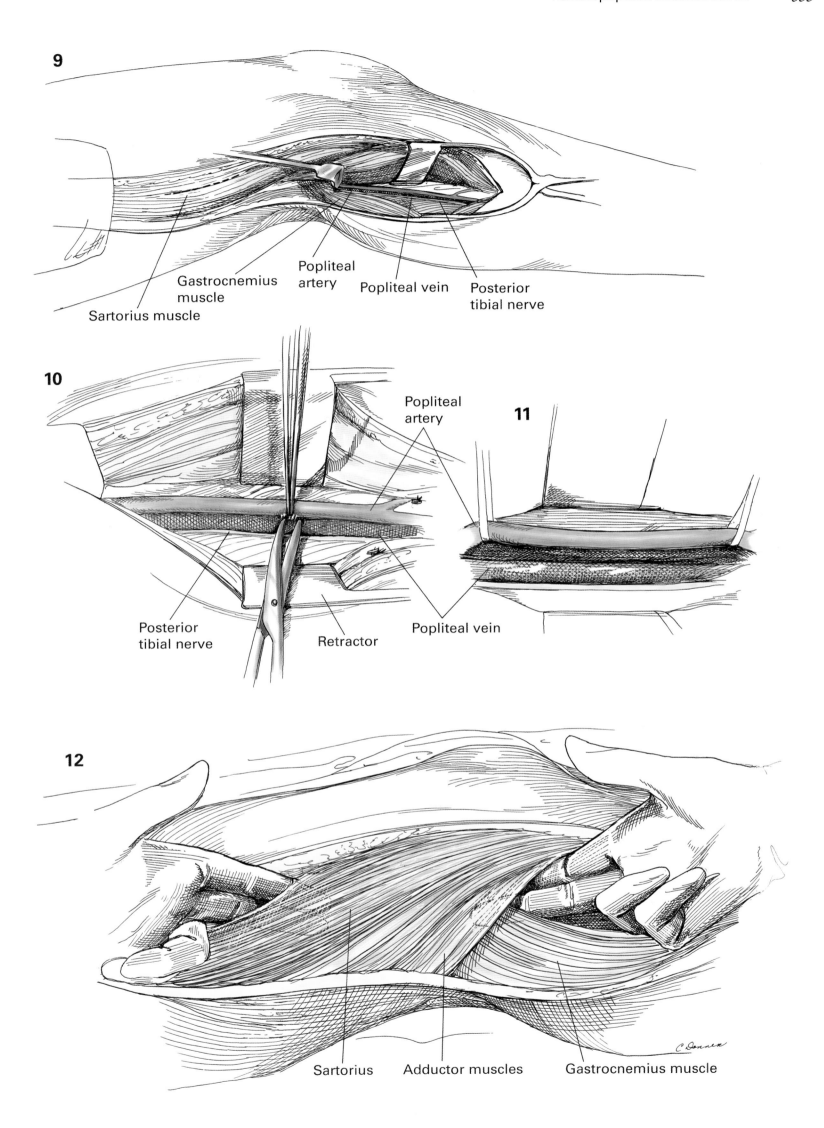

9

Sartorius muscle

Gastrocnemius muscle

Popliteal artery

Popliteal vein

Posterior tibial nerve

10

Popliteal artery

11

Posterior tibial nerve

Retractor

Popliteal vein

12

Sartorius   Adductor muscles   Gastrocnemius muscle

INCISION AND EXPOSURE **◄CONTINUED** A tunnel is fashioned from the femoral incision through to the proximal popliteal space by similar blunt dissection in the subsartorial muscle plane. These tunnels are temporarily marked with Penrose drains (FIGURE 13).

The patient is systemically anticoagulated with heparin. The femoral artery at the site chosen for anastomosis is occluded proximally and distally. The arteriotomy site is carefully chosen to avoid significant disease or a decision is made to perform an endarterectomy with possible patch angioplasty. The artery is incised with a small-bladed knife and the arteriotomy completed with Potts scissors (FIGURE 14). The vein is reversed and the distal end of the saphenous vein graft is then tailored to match the femoral arteriotomy. The vein is incised longitudinally (FIGURE 15), and the edges of the tips are removed to create a "cobra-head" tip (FIGURE 16). The anastomosis is started with a double ended 6-0 polypropylene suture at the heel of the graft (FIGURE 17). The anastomosis is then created by running one end of the suture toward the sidepoint of the anastomosis, using a running continuous technique proceeding from outside-in on the vein and inside-out on the artery to avoid elevating an intimal flap (FIGURES 18 and 19). **CONTINUES►**

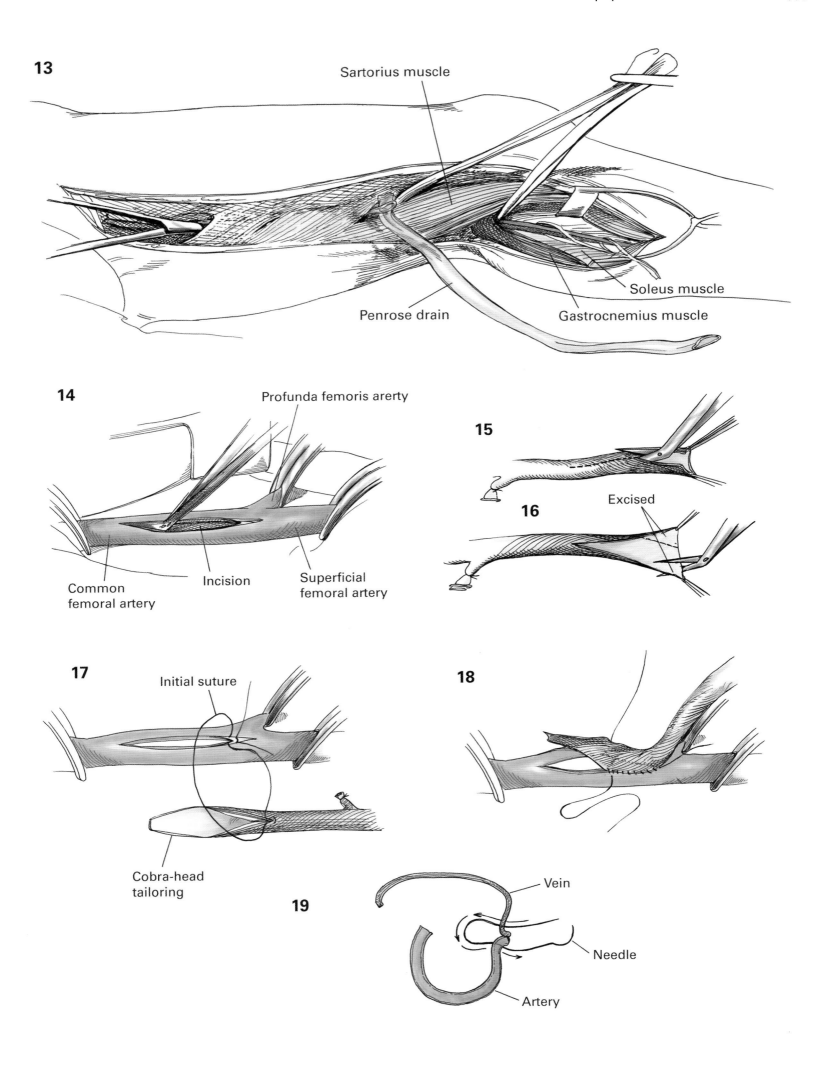

13

Sartorius muscle

Soleus muscle

Gastrocnemius muscle

Penrose drain

14

Profunda femoris arerty

Common
femoral artery

Incision

Superficial
femoral artery

15

16

Excised

17

Initial suture

Cobra-head
tailoring

18

19

Vein

Needle

Artery

INCISION AND EXPOSURE <small>◄CONTINUED</small> The other suture end is then run around the opposite direction. (FIGURE 20). One method is to suture down the toe of the graft with a horizontal mattress suture (FIGURE 21). The anastomosis is completed by carefully running one suture all the way around to meet the other end at its midpoint position (FIGURE 22). The two suture ends are tied together (FIGURE 23).

When the anastomosis is completed, the graft is tested by releasing the proximal femoral control and flushing the graft first. Any significant suture line bleeding can be repaired at this time. Blood flow can be restored to the profunda femoris and superficial femoral artery as well. Next any bleeding from venous side branches can be repaired at this time with 7-0 polypropylene suture (FIGURE 24). <small>CONTINUES►</small>

20

21

22

23

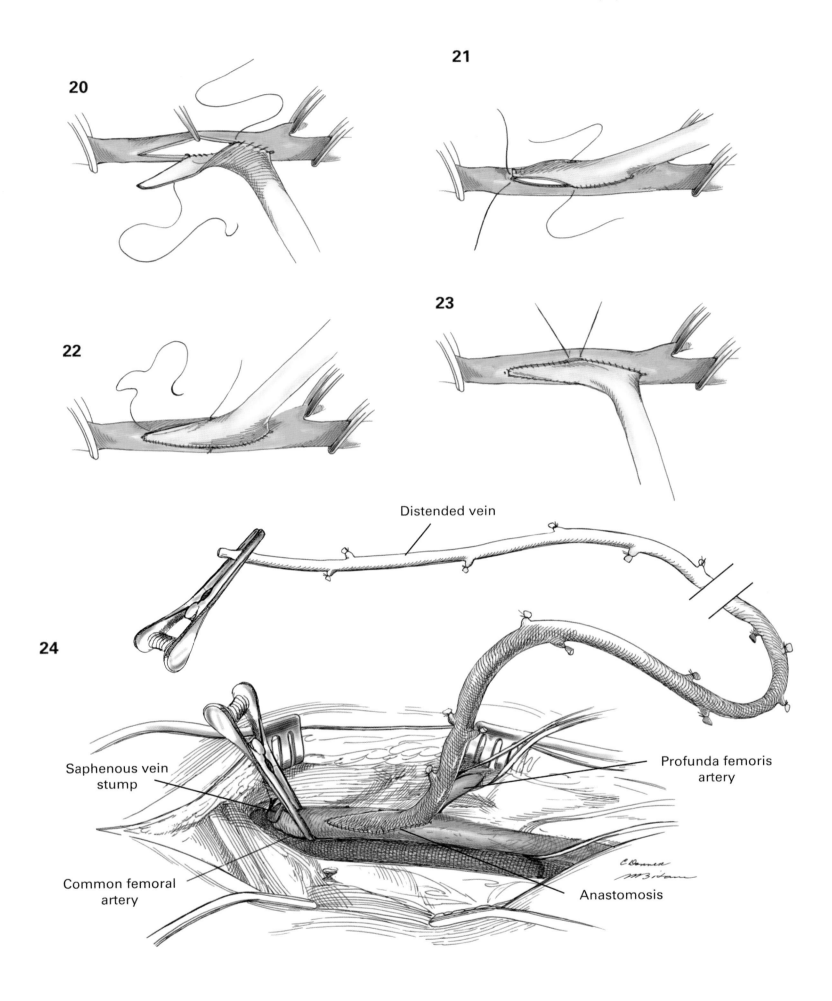

Distended vein

24

Saphenous vein stump

Profunda femoris artery

Common femoral artery

Anastomosis

INCISION AND EXPOSURE `CONTINUED` The graft is brought through the previously made subsartorial tunnel, with great care being taken to avoid kinking or twisting of the graft. If the distal target vessel is below the knee, the graft is further tunneled through the popliteal space in the previously created tunnel. The leg must be straightened to ensure that the length of the graft is adequate and the tension appropriate when crossing the knee joint (FIGURE 25). The popliteal artery is now cross-clamped, and an arteriotomy is performed in the usual manner (FIGURE 26. The anastomosis is then performed in a similar fashion as to the proximal (FIGURES 27 and 28) (Prior to completion, an appropriately sized dilator is carefully passed through the toe of the graft into the native artery to ensure patency. If there is any technical problem, the anastomosis is taken down and redone). Flushing maneuvers are performed immediately before completion, including back bleeding of the distal arterial tree (FIGURE 29). The completed femoropopliteal reconstruction should lie comfortably within its tunnel with no tension, twisting, or kinking (FIGURE 30).

Careful palpation for pulsation of the vein graft distally and the artery distal to the popliteal anastomosis is performed to confirm patency. Completion arteriography should be performed via a butterfly needle introduced into the saphenous vein graft with injection of 15 to 25 mL of contrast over 5 seconds. Routine arteriography confirms a technically perfect reconstruction and provides accurate assessment of the graft runoff. Any defects must be corrected if a successful outcome is to be expected. Pedal pulses should be documented by Doppler or palpable for postoperative comparison.

CLOSURE Meticulous hemostasis must be attained. Anticoagulation may be reversed with protamine sulfate if required by continued oozing. The incisions are then closed in layers in the usual fashion. Skin staples are typically utilized. Dry sterile dressings are employed.

POSTOPERATIVE CARE The cardiopulmonary status must be observed carefully and often in an intensive care setting. Postoperative cardiac events are the most common medical complication. Distal pulses should be assessed hourly for the first 24 hours and subsequently at regular intervals. Antiplatelet therapy is begun soon in the postop period and continued after discharge. The patients begin ambulation on the day after surgery and many can be discharged home within 2 to 3 days typically. Special attention is given to the care of the feet. All efforts should be directed to controlling risk factors, such as smoking, and careful postoperative follow-up is imperative to enhance long-term benefit.

Noninvasive vascular laboratory testing in the postoperative period is valuable to assess hemodynamic improvement and the success of the bypass procedure. Graft occlusion can be manifested by loss of pulses, pallor, pain, paresthesias, and loss of function. If noninvasive testing is found to be unexpectedly abnormal, duplex imaging or angiography may be helpful to verify occlusion or technical problem in order to revise the surgery in a timely fashion. After discharge, patients are monitored in 3, 6, 9, and 12 months intervals during the first year with duplex imaging of the graft to assess for stenotic areas at the proximal and distal anastomoses, as well as in the body of the graft at sclerotic valves. If identified, these areas may require revision to prolong the patency of the graft. ∎

25

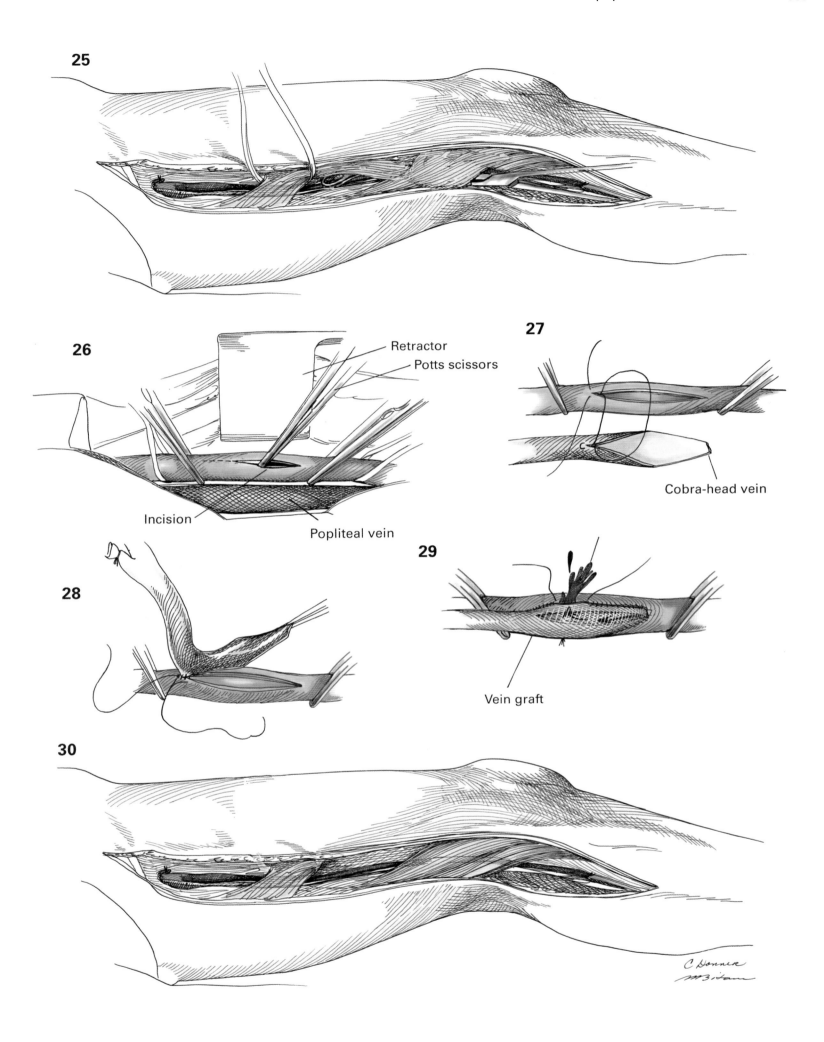

26

Retractor

Potts scissors

Incision

Popliteal vein

27

Cobra-head vein

28

29

Vein graft

30

INDICATIONS Infrainguinal arterial bypass procedures may be indicated in patients with critical limb ischemia, including rest pain, tissue loss such as gangrene of the toes or ulceration of the foot or ankle, or with progressive, severe claudication. Compared to bypass procedures using either a synthetic graft or a reversed autogenous saphenous vein, the use of the in situ saphenous vein technique is preferred by some surgeons. Currently, there are no significant differences in patency rates between the in situ and reversed vein grafts. Hence, the choice is largely a matter of surgeon preference. In addition, this technique may be preferred when the distal anastomosis is to the tibial and peroneal arteries. This is because the vein size tapers in the anatomic direction, in contrast to reversed vein grafts. The taper results in a more well-matched anastomosis as the sizes are more comparable, and potentially in improved hemodynamic flow. It is believed that all these factors contribute to the improved results over prosthetic material for a biologically living bypass graft whose natural lining is not thrombogenic.

PREOPERATIVE PREPARATION Most patients are older and have generalized arteriosclerotic cardiovascular disease. A general medical assessment is necessary, with special attention being given to associated risk factors such as diabetes and smoking. Cardiopulmonary function should be assessed with a chest x-ray, electrocardiography, and additional studies as indicated while the patient's overall condition is optimized.

Segmental Doppler pressures and waveforms are useful in evaluating the extent of the arterial disease and serve as baseline for postoperative studies to document improvement. However, most surgeons believe that the best evaluation is obtained with contrast angiogram, either computed tomography or digital subtraction. Visualization from the aorta to the foot is essential so as to evaluate any possible obstruction of inflow, the levels of occlusion, and the suitability of target arteries in the lower leg, ankle, or foot. Venous mapping with duplex ultrasound is the preferred method for assessment of the saphenous vein. It demonstrates the patency and anatomy of the saphenous vein, as it is prone to variation, duplication, and unexpectedly large perforating connectors.

ANESTHESIA General or regional anesthesia may be used while hemodynamic parameters are monitored carefully.

POSITION The patient is placed supine on the operating table.

OPERATIVE PREPARATION The lower abdomen and entire leg are prepared with the usual antiseptic solutions. The sterile drapes are applied so as to allow access to the entire leg. Gangrenous toes or a foot ulcer should be enclosed in a sterile, impervious plastic wrap or bag.

DETAILS OF PROCEDURE A two-team approach may be used to prepare both groin and ankle incisions simultaneously, but a single-team procedure will be presented. FIGURE 1 shows the femoral incision site for exposure of the proximal termination of the saphenous vein and the femoral artery and its branches. Two ankle incisions are shown for a planned in situ bypass to the posterior tibial artery. A slightly curved incision is made just anterior to

the medial condyle for the vein whereas a secondary posterior one is made for the posterior tibial artery. Additional short incisions will be made later along the vein sites for the division of major side branches of the saphenous vein as determined by venogram and ultrasound after arterial inflation of the in situ graft.

A proximal incision is made to expose the common femoral, superficial femoral, and profunda femoris arteries. The region for proximal arterial takeoff of the graft is chosen, and Silastic loops are placed around each artery (FIGURE 2). The greater saphenous vein is dissected back to the fossa ovalis. The medial circumflex iliac artery lies at the lower margin of the fossa ovalis and consequently is a reliable anatomic reference to the saphenofemoral junction just above it. The proximal saphenous vein is exposed, and 2-0 silk ligatures are tied around each branch (FIGURE 3), including the fairly large and constant superficial epigastric (c), superficial external pudendal (d), medial and lateral superficial circumflex iliacs (a and b), and the medial superficial femoral cutaneous vein (e). The superficial or Scarpa's fascia of the fossa ovalis is incised to allow complete exposure of the saphenofemoral venous junction. This junction is usually just at the level of the profunda artery.

The end of the saphenous vein is exposed in the distal incision as is the chosen area of the posterior tibial artery (FIGURE 4). Next the patient is given systemic heparin. The vein is transected distally with an adequate length to reach the arterial site. A venogram catheter is inserted into the cut end of the saphenous vein (FIGURE 4) and a retrograde on-table venogram is obtained. Side branches are marked on the leg (FIGURE 5). This process can be assisted by the use of a disposable ruler tape on the leg.

The proximal end of the saphenous vein is next evaluated for sufficient length to reach the planned anastomotic site on the femoral artery. Ordinarily, a Satinsky curved vascular clamp is applied to the saphenous side of the junction. A small cuff of saphenous vein is left above the clamp for closure with a running 6-0 monofilament vascular suture such that there will be no constriction of the common femoral vein when the vascular clamp is removed (FIGURE 6). If needed, additional venous length can be obtained by excising a portion of the anterior common femoral vein in continuity with the saphenous bulb. This technique can also be used to create a larger inflow anastomosis. The common femoral vein is then repaired with a monofilament 6-0 vascular continuous suture, taking care not to impinge on the flow lumen of the common femoral vein.

The proximal 5 to 7 cm of the saphenous vein is mobilized as its major tributaries are ligated and divided. Using Potts scissors, the first valve, about 1 cm into the saphenous bulb, is excised in the translucent central portion of each valve under direct vision (FIGURE 7). The second valve is typically 3 to 5 cm farther distal. This second valve and the remainder of the saphenous vein valves are cut with the retrograde valvulotome method shown in FIGURES 11 and 12 on page 543.

The proximal arterial inflow site is controlled and the common femoral artery is opened at about the level of the profunda femoris (FIGURE 8). This allows inspection of the profunda stoma and possible endarterectomy, if necessary. CONTINUES ▶

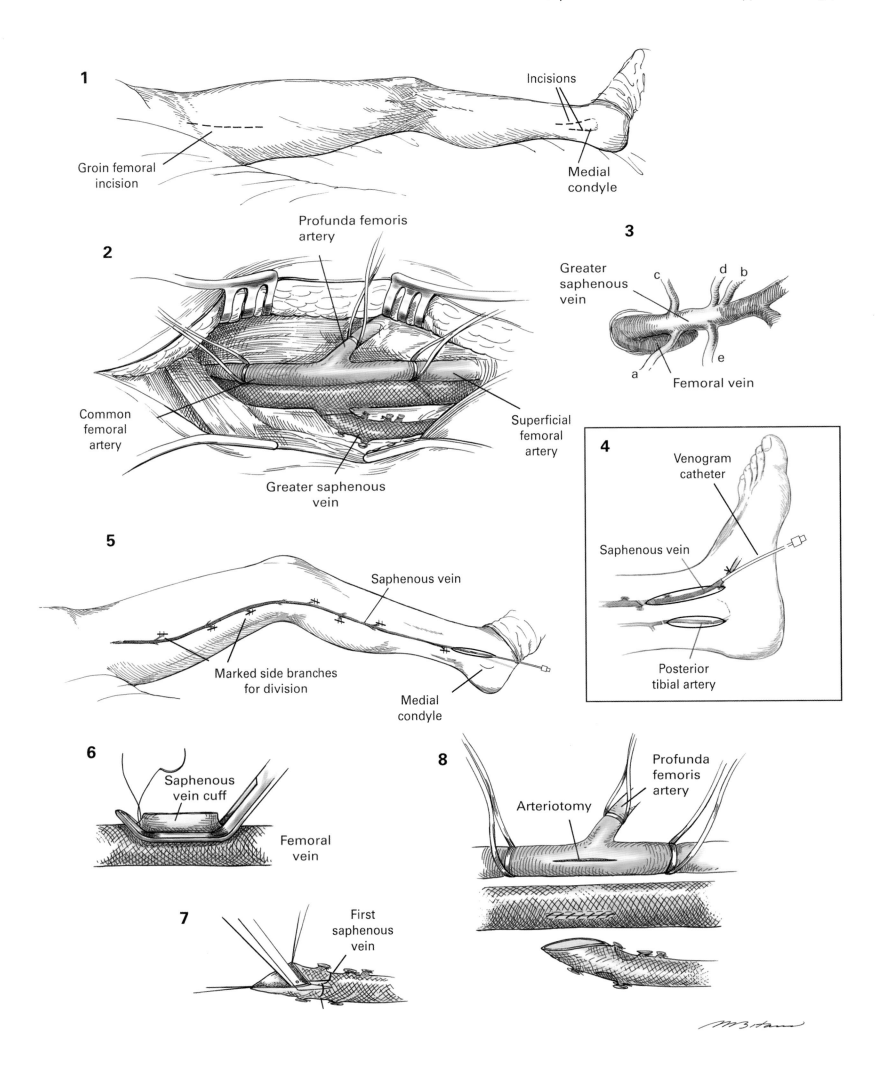

1
Groin femoral incision

Incisions

Medial condyle

2
Profunda femoris artery

Common femoral artery

Greater saphenous vein

Superficial femoral artery

3
Greater saphenous vein

c   d   b

a   e

Femoral vein

4
Venogram catheter

Saphenous vein

Posterior tibial artery

5
Saphenous vein

Marked side branches for division

Medial condyle

6
Saphenous vein cuff

Femoral vein

7
First saphenous vein

8
Arteriotomy

Profunda femoris artery

DETAILS OF PROCEDURE CONTINUED The open proximal end of the saphenous vein is tailored to match the arteriotomy. The edges of the tip may be removed to create a more oval taper and the vein may be opened in a longitudinal direction posteriorly to create a larger opening if needed. The anastomosis is performed with a 6-0 monofilament polypropylene suture that is double ended with a needle at each end. As shown in FIGURE 9A, the course of each stitch in this running suture begins by entering the vein from the outside to lumen and proceeds from lumen to outside on the artery. This avoids raising an intimal flap in the artery. The suture line is begun with a mattress-type suture at the "heel" end of the vein (FIGURE 9). The lateral or far side is run first and brought around the tip or "toe" end to join the medial or near-side suture in the mid-portion (FIGURE 10). The anastomosis is flushed with heparinized saline, and the sutures are tied. The arterial vessel loops are released, and the proximal saphenous vein will dilate with a pulsatile arterial inflow. Flow will stop at the first of any residual venous valves.

EXPANDABLE VALVULOTOME METHOD In order to avoid the long incisions required for total saphenous vein exposure and the use of a hand held valve cutter passed sequentially via side branches, this method employs a disposable, expandable valve cutter. By limiting lower extremity incisions, trauma from vein dissection may be minimized, surgical site infections may be reduced, and post-op pain control may be better.

As the new arterial blood flow enters the vein there will be little flow beyond the first valve. The disposable, expandable valvulotome is tested for function and loaded with heparinized saline as per the manufacturer's instructions for use. The closed unit with the valvulotome in the sheath is inserted through the distal transected vein (FIGURE 11) and carefully passed to just distal to the femoral artery anastomosis. The presence of the bulbous blunt tip is confirmed by palpation (FIGURE 11A) and care is taken not to cross the fresh anastomotic suture line. The valvulotome is deployed according to the manufacturer's instructions for use and carefully withdrawn. There will be a slight pulling sensation when valves are crossed. The valvulotome is self-centering to prevent injury to the vein walls as the vein dilates over the central cage and the leaflets are cut as the vein passes down the tapered cage into its cutting section (FIGURE 12). This maneuver may need to be done several times to render all the valves incompetent as manifest by full dilation of the entire saphenous vein under arterial pressure and possibly pulsatile inflow.

Next, small incisions (1–2 cm) are made at the previously marked side branch sites and the branches are ligated with 3-0 silk ties. Seven typical ligation and branch division sites are illustrated (FIGURE 11). This should improve the flow through the vein so that it is pulsatile. If not, another pass with the valvulotome can be performed.

The choice of site for the distal bypass anastomosis is determined according to the preoperative studies. It is important that the vein have a clear path without angulation. Also, the vein must be of sufficient length for it to reach the anastomotic site without tension when the leg or ankle is straightened. An anastomosis to the posterior tibial artery is shown. The peroneal artery may be approached in a similar manner, whereas the anterior tibial artery is approached by tunneling through the interosseous membrane in its upper two-thirds or by tunneling around the anterior tibia in its lower one third. The appropriate arterial segment has been previously dissected over a 3- to 4-cm zone and isolated with Bulldog vascular clamps (FIGURE 13). An advantage of the in situ vein bypass technique is now apparent as the sizes of the two vessels (distal artery and bypass vein) are nearly the same.

Most surgeons use magnifying loupes for the end-of-vein-to-side-of-artery anastomosis, which is performed in a manner similar to the proximal anastomosis (FIGURES 9A and 10). The vein may be incised longitudinally and tapered to create a larger stoma. All vessels are occluded with the elastic loops or small Bulldog vascular clamps. The artery is opened longitudinally (FIGURE 14). A double-ended 6-0 or 7-0 monofilament vascular suture is placed into the heel of the vein and then out of the artery in a mattress-suture manner at the proximal angle. A continuous, running suture is placed such that it enters through the vein and exits through the artery. This prevents the raising of an intimal flap as the needle point is pressed from the lumen outward on the artery.

The posterior suture line is run first and usually carried around the distal tip to the mid-portion of the anterior line. This allows better visualization in the placement of the completed anterior line suture. The artery and vein are flushed with heparinized solutions and the loops and clamps are transiently released to flush all segments clear of thrombus, debris, and air. The two suture ends are tied.

Pulsations within the in situ vein and artery are palpated or verified with a Doppler instrument. An intraoperative on-the-table completion angiogram should be performed, with attention to the distal anastomosis and to verify that all the side branches are ligated and that there are no residual saphenous valves. The distal anastomosis should also be inspected for any technical errors.

The leg is flexed and straightened to be certain that the vein does not kink. A careful search is made along the entire vein to reveal any arteriovenous fistulas in the venous branches that were not recognized and ligated. These fistulas may be palpated as a hum or thrill, which can also be localized with a Doppler instrument. Simple division between 3-0 silk ligatures is sufficient.

After the distal anastomosis is secured, a completion on-table angiogram of the entire vein graft should be obtained.

CLOSURE The superficial fascia is approximated with interrupted or running absorbable 3-0 sutures, taking care not to constrict or kink the vein, and the skin is closed in the routine manner.

POSTOPERATIVE CARE The hemodynamic status of the patient is monitored carefully in the recovery or intensive care setting. Cardiac parameters should be optimized. A record of distal pulses obtained by palpation or Doppler is made hourly for the first day and at sequentially regular intervals thereafter. The patient is usually not anticoagulated but is kept well hydrated. An ankle-brachial index is typically performed on postoperative day 1 to ensure graft patency. ■

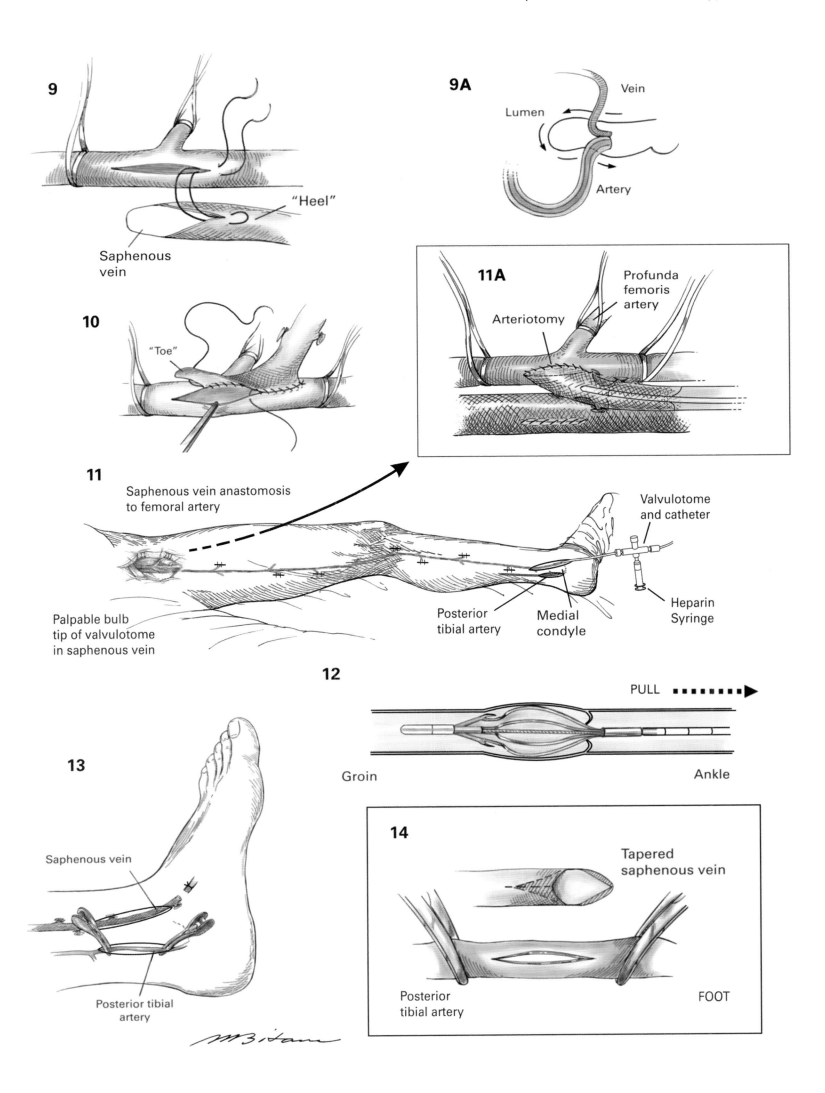

9

"Heel"

Saphenous
vein

9A

Lumen

Vein

Artery

10

"Toe"

11A

Arteriotomy

Profunda
femoris
artery

11

Saphenous vein anastomosis
to femoral artery

Palpable bulb
tip of valvulotome
in saphenous vein

Valvulotome
and catheter

Heparin
Syringe

Posterior
tibial artery

Medial
condyle

12

PULL ▪▪▪▪▪▪▪➤

Groin

Ankle

13

Saphenous vein

Posterior tibial
artery

14

Tapered
saphenous vein

Posterior
tibial
artery

FOOT

THROMBOEMBOLECTOMY, FEMORAL

INDICATIONS Acute lower limb ischemia may be caused by distal embolization from a more proximal source or by thrombosis of an underlying atherosclerotic lesion or previously constructed bypass graft. The clinical presentation is often an emergency situation with varying degrees of limb threatening ischemia. If a patient's ischemia is not as severe and allows more time for treatment, catheter-based thrombolytic therapy may be preferred as first line, since lysis may reveal an underlying lesion that also requires treatment. If ischemia is more profound, then proceeding to emergency surgical intervention is the best, most expeditious approach.

PREOPERATIVE APPROACH Preoperative imaging, such as catheter-based angiography, CT angiography, and duplex ultrasound, can be helpful to localize the extent of the thrombus/embolus, but is not always necessary depending on the urgency of the procedure. Since these are often emergency surgeries, rapid preparation of the patient is essential to increase the chances of limb salvage. As patients with embolic phenomenon often have a cardiac source, including acute myocardial infarction, dysrhythmia, and aneurysm, attention should be given to close hemodynamic monitoring and maximizing cardiac function as much as possible in an emergency situation.

History of prior claudication or previous surgical bypass graft points more toward a diagnosis of thrombotic disease. An understanding of the patient's vascular disease history is critical to determining the underlying etiology. Heparin administration is extremely important as soon as a diagnosis of thromboembolic phenomenon is made. Prophylactic antibiotic therapy is administered just before the operation and continued for 24 hours.

ANESTHESIA General or regional anesthesia is generally employed; however, local with monitored anesthesia care is sometimes preferred in this group of patients who may have other significant comorbidities. The feasibility of local anesthesia depends on the location of incision and extent of surgery. Careful attention should be given to maintaining satisfactory hemodynamic parameters.

OPERATIVE PREPARATION The patient is positioned supine on the operating table. It is usually best to prep and draped the lower abdomen and contralateral groin area in case an adjuvant in flow procedure, such as a femoral-femoral bypass, becomes necessary. The entire affected leg should be circumferentially prepared and draped as well, with the foot preferentially placed in a sterile plastic (Lahey) bag, so that the foot may be inspected at the end of the case (FIGURE 1). Anticoagulation with heparin is usually not interrupted; often with an extra dose given during surgery.

PROCEDURAL DETAILS A vertical groin incision is made and the femoral vessels are dissected free from surrounding structures. Silastic vessel loops are placed around the arteries proximally and distally (FIGURE 2). If additional heparin is warranted, then a dose is given a few minutes prior to occluding the vessels.

If the etiology is felt to be due to an embolic source and the vessel feels soft and free from atherosclerosis, then a transverse arteriotomy is made (FIGURE 3). The advantage is closing the arteriotomy primarily, which is usually fairly quick. If a thrombotic etiology is implicated or if chronic plaque is palpable, then a longitudinal arteriotomy may be the best choice. This longitudinal incision is made in the common femoral artery for plaque in the area so that the vessel may be directly inspected and an endarterectomy with patch angioplasty performed if needed. For the common plaque at the origin of the profundus artery, an oblique longitudinal incision is made as shown in FIGURE 4A,B for the same reason.

A Fogarty® thrombectomy catheter (usually a 3 mm, but 2 mm or 4 mm may be used as well, depending on the size of the native vessel) is passed proximally and distally into all the major branches (FIGURE 5A). Several passes will be required until adequate pulsatile inflow is restored, as well as appropriate back bleeding confirmed. The catheter is then passed proximally (FIGURE 5B) to be certain that all clot has been cleared. The artery is flushed antegrade and retrograde with heparinized saline solution (FIGURE 6). A transverse arteriotomy can be closed primarily with interrupted 6-0 polypropylene sutures, passed inside to outside to prevent lifting any flap inside the artery (FIGURE 7). All air and debris are vented prior to completing the vessel closure and restoring flow to the leg. The foot is now reassessed for perfusion (color, capillary refill, warmth, motor function, Doppler signals) and if adequate, the wound is irrigated and closed in multiple layers with absorbable sutures and skin staples. If the leg remains ischemic, then the level of impairment is reassessed and further thrombectomy performed if needed. Lower-leg fasciotomies are performed at this time if deemed necessary (see Chapter 145, pages 554-555).

POSTOPERATIVE CARE It is critical to maintain close observation of these patients, not only for recurrent leg thrombosis OR ischemia, but also for delayed compartment syndrome if a fasciotomy was not done. The patient is kept on a heparin drip and converted to oral anticoagulation if deemed appropriate. In addition, depending on the patient's clinical status, intensive care and hemodynamic monitoring will most likely be in order. ■

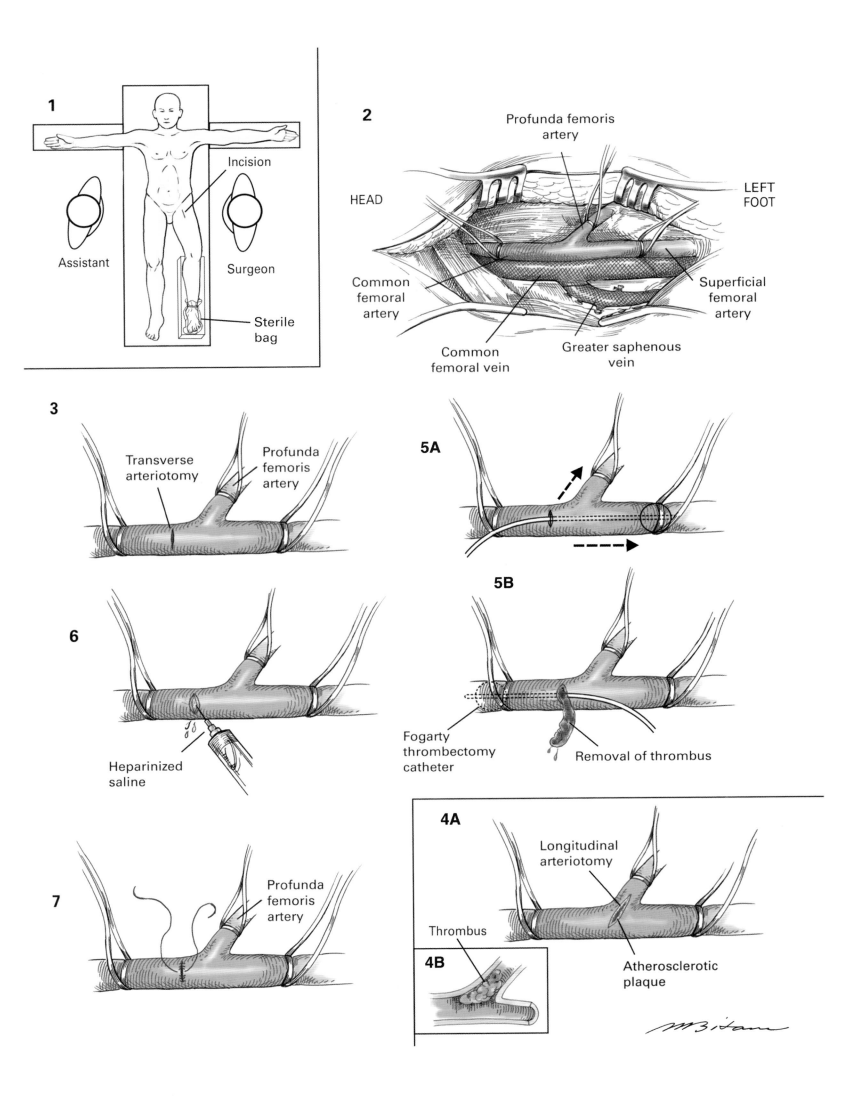

1

Assistant

Surgeon

Incision

Sterile bag

2

HEAD

Profunda femoris artery

LEFT FOOT

Common femoral artery

Common femoral vein

Greater saphenous vein

Superficial femoral artery

3

Transverse arteriotomy

Profunda femoris artery

5A

5B

Fogarty thrombectomy catheter

Removal of thrombus

6

Heparinized saline

7

Profunda femoris artery

4A

Longitudinal arteriotomy

Thrombus

4B

Atherosclerotic plaque

INDICATIONS Life-threatening pulmonary embolism is a frequent complication of many medical illnesses and surgical procedures when antecedent venous thrombosis is associated with low-flow states, venous injuries, obesity, prolonged immobilization, hypercoagulability, and the poorly understood effects of certain malignancies.

Anticoagulation is generally accepted as the primary therapy for thromboembolic disease. Venous interruption, proximal to the site of venous thrombosis, is usually reserved for patients who have recurrent pulmonary emboli despite well-controlled, adequate anticoagulation; those who have a large, life-threatening embolus such that an additional one might be fatal; those who cannot be anticoagulated because of potential bleeding problems or other contraindication for anticoagulation; or those who are developing progressive pulmonary hypertension from repeated emboli.

Superficial femoral ligation has been largely abandoned because of the inability to precisely localize the proximal extent of the process and the likelihood of undetected thrombus in the opposite extremity or deep pelvic veins. Inferior vena caval interruption avoids these uncertainties. Caval filters placed via the femoral or jugular veins are commonly used today for prophylaxis against pulmonary emboli and their use has replaced the application of partially occlusive serrated clips. Temporary and permanent filters are now commercially available, with the advantage of being able to remove the temporary filter when its presence is no longer clinically needed.

PREOPERATIVE PREPARATION Since intravenous contrast is usually used during the procedure, absence of contrast allergy is imperative and if present, may require premedication. Kidney function should be assessed as well as the patient's ability to lie flat for a period of time during and after the procedure. These patients may have impaired cardiac function and abnormal ventilation/perfusion of the lung, requiring vigorous cardiac and pulmonary support, and perhaps monitoring by an anesthesiologist.

ANESTHESIA Local anesthesia is favored. A secure intravenous catheter for medications (especially sedation) is essential. An anesthesiologist to manage the patient may be imperative if there is impaired cardiopulmonary function.

POSITION The patient is supine with the groin or right jugular area exposed and clipped of any hair. Fluoroscopy should be available. This procedure may be done preferably in a dedicated angiography suite.

DETAILS OF PROCEDURE The groin or neck access area is prepped and draped in the usual fashion and local anesthesia is administered. The jugular or femoral (FIGURE 1) vein is accessed with an entry needle under ultrasound guidance if needed below the level of the inguinal ligament (FIGURE 2). Using fluoroscopy a fine (0.018) access wire is guided up into the inferior vena cava in preparation for passage of a pigtail catheter into the inferior vena cava (FIGURE 3). A venacavagram is obtained (FIGURE 4). The position of the renal veins relative to a given vertebral body level is noted. If the infrarenal cava is found to be <28 mm, nonduplicated, and free from thrombus formation, the pigtail is advanced superiorly to above the renal veins before the stiffer insertion wire (0.025) for the deployment sheath is inserted. This maneuver lessens the chance that the new wire may enter a caval branch or the renal veins. The filter deployment sheath is inserted and the position of its tip verified using the previously noted vertebral body as a marker (FIGURE 5). The filter is placed into the deployment sheath and advanced to just the end of the sheath. While the filter is held in place, the sheath is withdrawn inferiorly leaving the filter at the correct level. Do not push or advance the filter out of the sheath, but rather withdraw the sheath from the filter (FIGURE 6). The filter is expanded with the anchoring barbs being well seated into the wall of the cava as per the manufacturer's instructions for use. The superior end of the filter should be just below the level of the renal veins (FIGURE 6). After removal of the insertion device a completion venacavagram is obtained to ensure proper placement and lack of complications. You may use the sheath or reinsert the guidewire and pigtail catheter for this contrast dye injection.

CLOSURE After removal of the sheath, appropriate pressure is held for several minutes to prevent bleeding (FIGURE 7). The patient should be instructed to lay flat for 1 to 2 hours afterward and the site should be monitored for bleeding or hematoma formation.

POSTOPERATIVE CARE Heparin should be continued before, during, and after the procedure unless there is significant access site bleeding or a contraindication. The patient should be monitored and the temporary filter removed when it is no longer necessary for the purpose for which it was placed. ■

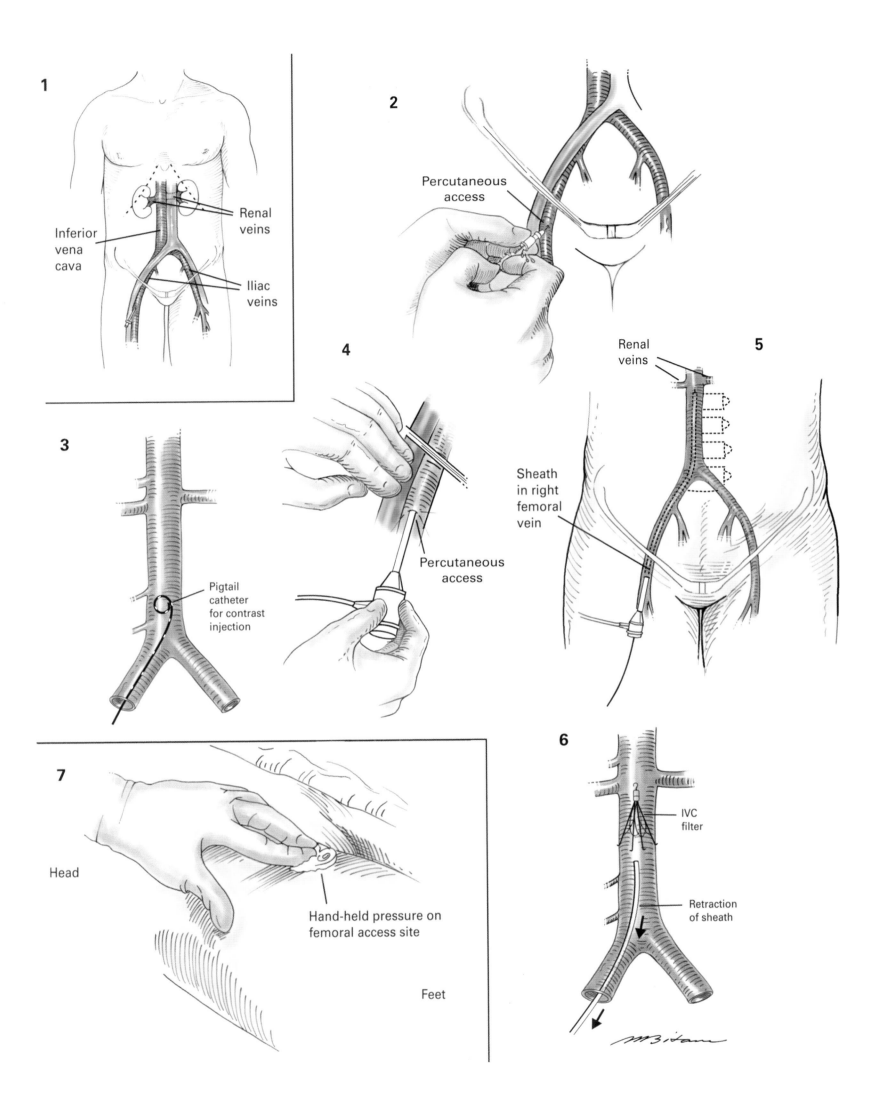

1

Inferior vena cava

Renal veins

Iliac veins

2

Percutaneous access

3

Pigtail catheter for contrast injection

4

Percutaneous access

5

Renal veins

Sheath in right femoral vein

6

IVC filter

Retraction of sheath

7

Head

Feet

Hand-held pressure on femoral access site

ENDOVENOUS LASER ABLATION OF THE GREAT SAPHENOUS VEIN AND STAB PHLEBECTOMY

INDICATIONS Endovenous laser ablation of the great saphenous vein has replaced high ligation and stripping of this vein for many centers in patients exhibiting symptoms related to the valvular incompetence of this vein, usually with varicose veins (FIGURE 1). In some centers radiofrequency ablation is preferred over laser ablation, but the technics are similar. Before considering ablation, these patients must have a complete peripheral vascular examination to determine whether the varicosities are primary or secondary, to evaluate the status both the superficial and deep venous systems, and to ascertain the adequacy of the arterial system. Venous duplex scanning is used to check for patency and the presence of reflux in both venous systems.

CONTRAINDICATIONS Evidence of obstruction in the deep system may contraindicate ablation of the superficial system because of reliance upon it for venous return from the leg. Other contraindications include discontinuity or tortuosity of the greater saphenous vein, pregnancy, and active breastfeeding, allergy to local anesthetics, liver dysfunction, and severe coagulation disorders. Patients are required to wear compression stocking in the postoperative period, and inability to tolerate them is a relative contraindication.

ANESTHESIA Some patient prefer general anesthesia, but more commonly, tumescent anesthesia is preferred, especially in the office setting. Tumescent anesthesia consists of the infusion of a dilute local anesthetic solution (usually 0.1% lidocaine) into the subcutaneous space surrounding the veins to be treated. Epinephrine may be added to the solution for its vasoconstrictive effect, and sodium bicarbonate is included for buffering to minimize discomfort on infusion.

POSITION The patient is supine with moderate Trendelenburg position to reduce venous hypertension and is prepped from the umbilicus through the entire lower extremity and foot. The toes are covered with a sterile plastic bag or glove. If phlebectomy, which is the removal of visible varicose veins through tiny stab incisions, is to be performed as well, the veins are marked with indelible ink in the preoperative holding area with the patient upright to assure adequate filling.

DETAILS OF PROCEDURE Using a 7.5 MHz ultrasound probe encased in a sterile sleeve, the greater saphenous vein is identified at or below the level of the knee (FIGURE 2). If not using general anesthesia, the skin is anesthetized with 1% lidocaine, and a 21-gauge access needle is inserted into the vein. A 0.018-in micropuncture wire is inserted through the needle into the vein to secure access and the needle removed (FIGURE 3). A small nick is made in the skin where the wire exits and a 4F or 5F access sheath is inserted over the wire. The wire and sheath dilator are removed and a 0.035-in J-tipped wire is inserted through the access sheath and passed to the groin where its presence is confirmed by ultrasound. The access sheath

is removed and the long laser sheath with centimeter markings is placed on the thigh with the distal tip at the level of the femoral pulse to get an estimate of how much sheath will need to be inserted. The laser sheath is inserted over the wire (FIGURE 4) and the dilator removed. The laser fiber is inserted to the lock position (FIGURE 5) and the ultrasound is used to locate the fiber tip in the distal greater saphenous vein bulb. Care is used to make sure that the tip does not enter the femoral vein and is distal to the superficial epigastric vein.

The ultrasound now visualizes the catheter at the knee level and the area adjacent to the catheter is infiltrated with the tumescence solution for anesthesia. A 21-gauge needle attached foot–pedal-controlled pump is used to administer the tumescence fluid. Tumescence fluid is administered throughout the length of the laser sheath. Not only does the tumescence fluid provide anesthesia, but it also reduces the transfer of energy from the laser to the surrounding tissue. Laser safety goggles are now worn. The location of the distal laser tip is reconfirmed by ultrasound before the laser energy is applied. A diode laser is used with a wavelength of 980 nm at a power setting of 14 W. Any of a number of available lasers may be used. The laser is turned on and withdrawn at a rate of 50 J/cm until the signal markings at the end of the laser sheath are seen which indicate that adequate length of vein has been treated. The laser is turned off and the sheath and laser fiber removed. Hemostasis is obtained by direct pressure.

If there are no stab phlebectomies, the procedure is over and a Band-Aid placed over the puncture site. A thigh-length support stocking is then applied. However, if stab phlebectomies are to be performed, they are done now. A #11 blade or a narrow Beaver blade is used to make tiny incisions adjacent to the previously marked varicose veins (FIGURE 6A), and specially designed phlebectomy hooks are used to capture the vein below the skin surface (FIGURE 6B). The captured vein is pulled out through the skin incision and grasped with a hemostat. Tension is place on the vein by pulling on the hemostat and as much vein as possible is bluntly dissected by using a second hemostat to tease the surrounding tissue away from the vein. The vein is then removed by manual avulsion (FIGURE 6C) and pressure held on the wound for hemostasis. This process is repeated until as much varicose vein as possible is removed. When hemostasis is complete, the limb is wiped with saline and dried. Steri-strips are used to approximate the incision and dry sterile dressing are applied and held in place with clear plastic adhesive. The thigh-length support stocking is then applied, and the patient taken to the recovery area.

POSTOPERATIVE CARE The patient is ambulatory at the time of discharge and is encouraged to walk for a few minutes every hour while awake. Mild analgesics are all that is required for perioperative pain. The patient is usually able to return to normal function within several days. ■

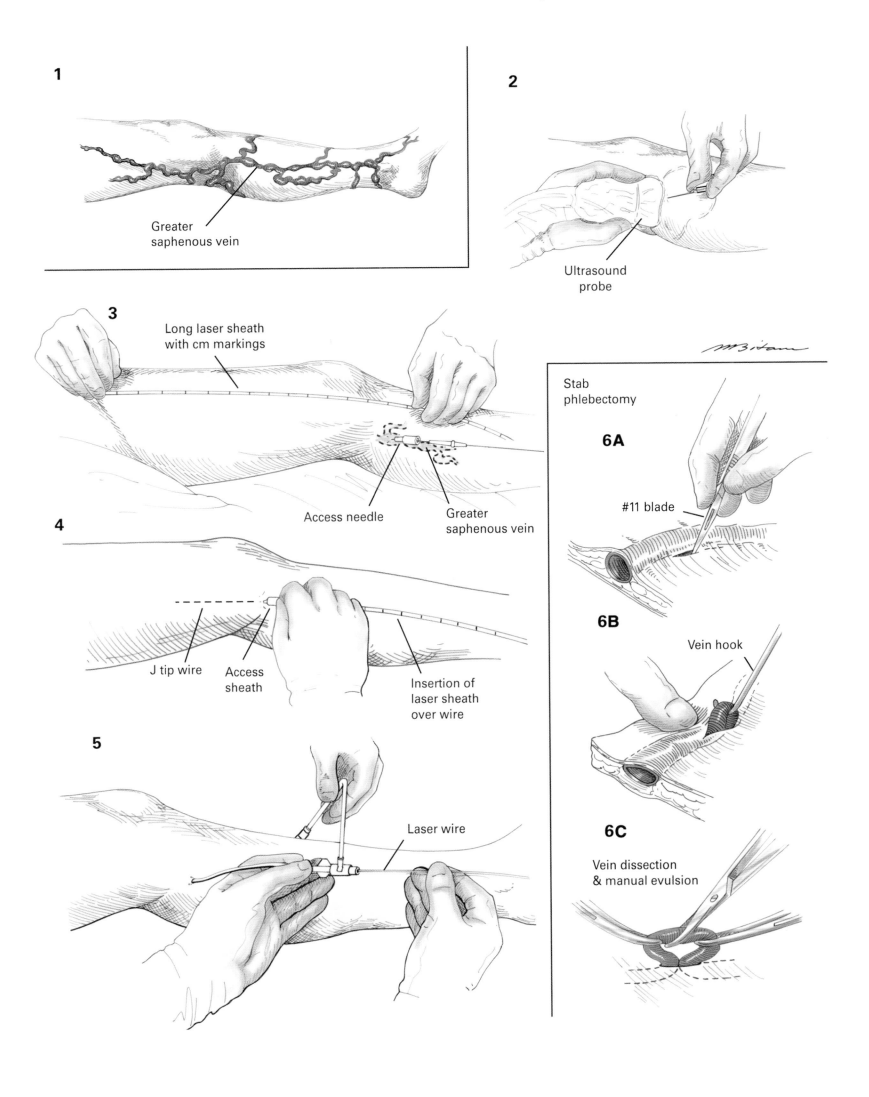

1

Greater saphenous vein

2

Ultrasound probe

3

Long laser sheath with cm markings

Access needle

Greater saphenous vein

4

J tip wire

Access sheath

Insertion of laser sheath over wire

5

Laser wire

Stab phlebectomy

6A

#11 blade

6B

Vein hook

6C

Vein dissection & manual evulsion

SHUNTING PROCEDURES FOR PORTAL HYPERTENSION

INDICATIONS Portal decompression is indicated in patients who have portal hypertension complicated by gastrointestinal hemorrhage from esophageal varices that are not effectively controlled with sclerotherapy injections. Some procedures completely interrupt portal venous flow to the liver (end-to-side portacaval shunt), while others selectively decompress the portal system via a collateral shunt (side-to-side portacaval, splenorenal, and mesocaval). The procedure selected will depend upon the patency of the portal and splenic veins, the results of liver function studies, the amount of portal venous blood being shunted, whether the patient is bleeding acutely, and whether the patient is a candidate for liver transplantation.

Selection of patients should be based on their clinical status, results of liver function studies, and interpretation of hepatic hemodynamics as determined by radiologic studies. Patients considered for shunting procedures generally should be under 60 years of age. Ideally, there should be no evidence of encephalopathy, jaundice, ascites, or muscle wasting. Serum albumin should be above 3 g/dL, prothrombin time greater than 1.5 times normal, or other evidence of intact hepatic synthetic function. Deviation from these criteria does not absolutely contraindicate surgery, but the surgical risk is directly proportional to the degree of hepatic decompensation.

Shunting procedures for portal hypertension can be divided into three types: portacaval, splenorenal, and mesocaval. FIGURES A to F show diagrammatically the basic surgical choices for diversion of the portal venous flow.

PORTACAVAL SHUNT The primary indication for portacaval shunt is the control of massive upper-gastrointestinal hemorrhage from varices which cannot be controlled with endoscopic ablation or by transjugular intrahepatic portosystemic shunts (TIPS). Portacaval shunts are sometimes preferred when there has been prior splenectomy, splenic vein thrombosis, reversal of flow in the portal vein, thrombosed splenorenal shunt, ascites, or hepatic vein thrombosis. The selection of a direct portacaval shunt, of course, depends upon the demonstration of a patent portal vein preoperatively or at laparotomy.

The side-to-side anastomosis (FIGURE A) has been preferred by some in the presence of portal hypertension with no evidence of a rise in pressure on the hepatic end of the temporarily occluded portal vein. This suggests that the arterial blood supply is going through the liver and that lowering of the portal pressure by the side-to-side anastomosis with the vena cava will not result in diversion of the arterial supply to the liver. Another advantage of this type of shunt is that it decompresses the hepatic sinusoids, and this may be beneficial in the treatment of patients with intractable ascites accompanied by variceal hemorrhage.

The usefulness of the portacaval shunt in the treatment of refractory ascites is not accepted universally, although several studies have suggested that this is an effective mode of therapy. If shunting is indicated to control ascites, a direct side-to-side shunt or a side-to-side H-shunt with an 8- or 10-mm ringed PTFE interposition graft is usually preferred. This is particularly true in unusual cases of hepatic vein thrombosis (Budd–Chiari). No decompressive procedure on the portal system has any beneficial effect on liver function. The end result of any such operation, therefore, will depend largely upon the progress of the basic liver disease.

In an end-to-side portacaval shunt (FIGURE B), the portal vein is ligated in the hilus of the liver, and the distal portion of the portal vein is anastomosed to the inferior vena cava. This shunt is particularly indicated when there is no evidence of ascites and when portal blood flow is reversed in the hepatoportal direction, as determined by a rising pressure in the hepatic end of the temporarily occluded portal vein. With the end-to-side anastomosis, all of the portal venous blood flow is shunted from the liver, while hepatic artery flow to the liver is preserved.

SPLENORENAL SHUNT In the presence of extrahepatic block of the portal vein, secondary hypersplenism, prior biliary surgery, and/or cavernomatous changes of the portal vein, a shunt between the splenic vein and left renal vein may be the procedure of choice, provided the splenic vein is patent and of adequate size (preferably 1 cm). If it is necessary or desirable to remove the spleen, a conventional splenorenal anastomosis (FIGURE C) may be performed. The distal splenorenal shunt (Warren shunt, FIGURE D) retains the spleen and, while selectively decompressing the esophageal varices, allows maintenance of portal pressure and perfusion of the liver, thus providing protection against hepatic encephalopathy. This shunt is particularly indicated in the presence of normal liver function, high volume of portal flow to the liver, minimal hepatocellular disease, marked splenomegaly, or idiopathic portal hypertension. The procedure consists of dividing the splenic vein at its junction with the superior mesenteric vein, ligating the proximal portion of the vein, and anastomosing the distal portion to the left renal vein. As an alternative to dividing the splenic vein, an interposition graft may be anastomosed between the splenic vein and the left renal vein, with ligation of the splenic vein proximal to the graft as well as ligation of the coronary and right gastroepiploic veins.

MESOCAVAL SHUNT In most instances portal decompression may be accomplished by portacaval or splenorenal shunt procedures. However, the Clatworthy mesocaval shunt (FIGURE E) is necessary in patients who have undergone splenectomy and have either thrombosis or cavernomatous changes of the portal vein. The mesocaval shunt is advisable in patients with excessive bleeding at surgery from periportal or perisplenic vessels. Finally, it should be the procedure of choice in small children in whom the splenic and/or portal veins may be too small for a successful procedure (minimal size approximately 1 cm in diameter). Elective shunts in children should be postponed, if possible, until the age of 4 years. The procedure consists of division of the superior vena cava and anastomosis side to end with the superior mesenteric vein.

In cases of emergency, a lesser technical procedure without division of the inferior vena cava can be accomplished by the interposition of a large knitted Dacron graft between the vena cava and superior mesenteric vein at the level of its first branches (FIGURE F). This modification of the mesocaval shunt (interposition mesocaval shunt or Drapanas shunt) offers the advantages of a simplified technical approach with minimal blood loss.

The details of these procedures are available online in the Historical Supplement at www.ZollingersAtlas.com. ■

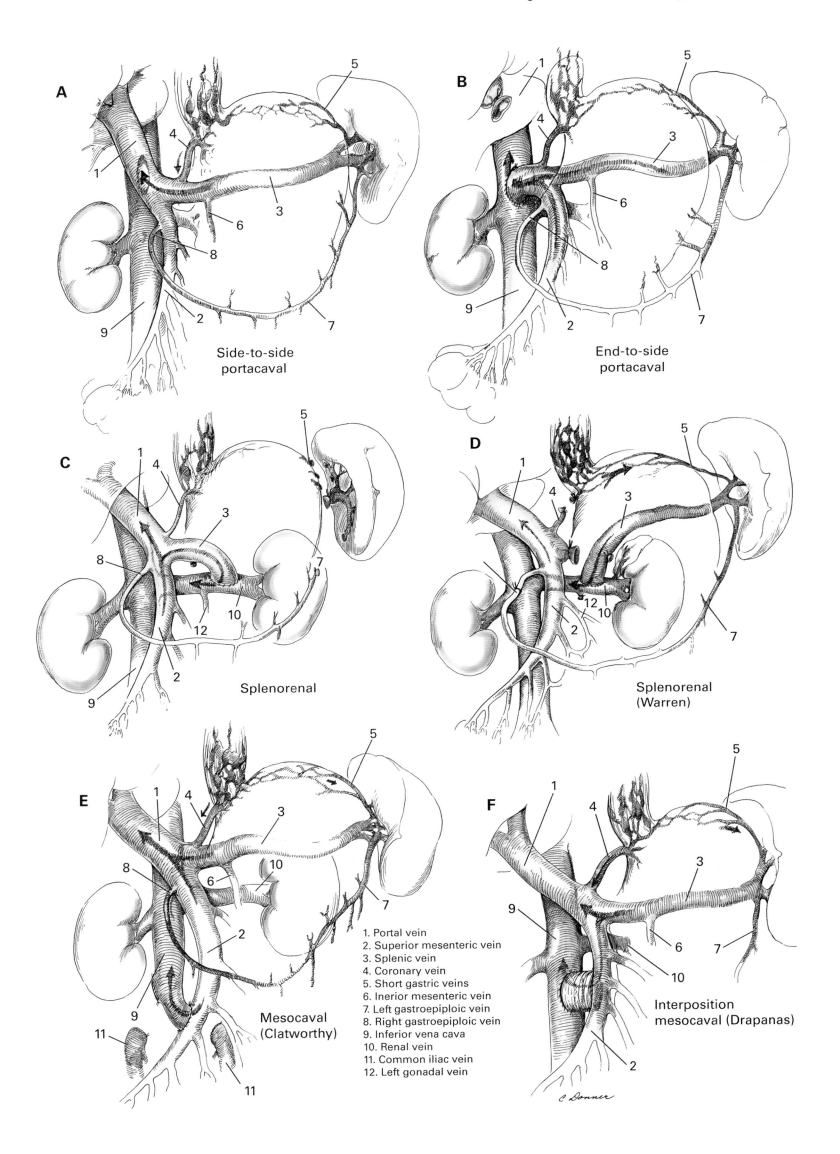

A Side-to-side portacaval

B End-to-side portacaval

C Splenorenal

D Splenorenal (Warren)

E Mesocaval (Clatworthy)

F Interposition mesocaval (Drapanas)

1. Portal vein
2. Superior mesenteric vein
3. Splenic vein
4. Coronary vein
5. Short gastric veins
6. Inerior mesenteric vein
7. Left gastroepiploic vein
8. Right gastroepiploic vein
9. Inferior vena cava
10. Renal vein
11. Common iliac vein
12. Left gonadal vein

C Donner

SECTION XIV
EXTREMITIES

INDICATIONS Compartment syndrome develops as the result of increased pressure within the confines of a fixed space. This may occur in the extremities as the result of ischemia, trauma, or burn injuries. Management involves not only the treatment of the underlying pathology, but also the physical release of the compartment to prevent further damage due to impaired capillary perfusion and increased venous resistance.

Diagnosis of compartment syndrome can be made by obtaining formal intracompartmental pressures (tissue perfusion becomes impaired around 20 mm Hg) (FIGURE 1) or based on physical signs and symptoms. These may include tense and tender muscle groups, pain on passive motion, and numbness or impaired motor function in the distribution of the nerve within the compartment. The most common site for compartment syndrome is the lower leg, often due to ischemia or the restoration of flow after a period of ischemia. To be complete, all four compartments, anterior, lateral, superficial posterior, and deep posterior, should undergo fasciotomy (FIGURES 2A and 2B).

PREOPERATIVE PREPARATION Attention should be given to hemodynamic stability of the patient, as well as close fluid and electrolyte management. Preoperative antibiotics are essential to prevent infection.

ANESTHESIA In the case of fasciotomy, general anesthesia and close hemodynamic monitoring will usually be required due to the complex nature of these patients. As is routine before making any type of skin incision, the skin should be prepared with topical cleansers.

PROCEDURAL DETAILS For lower-leg fasciotomy the entire leg should be prepared and draped in the usual fashion. This may have been preceded by a procedure to restore flow to the leg (i.e., thrombectomy/embolectomy, bypass, or thrombolytic therapy). The most common approach to a four compartment fasciotomy can be accomplished through two lower-leg incisions (FIGURE 3).

The posterior compartments are approached through a skin incision made over the medial calf, 1 cm posterior to the posterior edge of the tibia, for a similar length and the superficial posterior compartment fascia is incised in a similar fashion (FIGURE 4). To access the deep posterior compartment, the gastrocnemius–soleal muscle complex is taken down from its attachments to the tibia (FIGURE 2B).

For the anterior and lateral compartments an incision is made several centimeters lateral to the anterior tibia for a length of approximately 10 cm. The anterior compartment fascia is encountered and incised for the length of the skin incision, taking care not to invade into the underlying muscle to avoid bleeding, especially if the patient is anticoagulated postoperatively. The tip of Metzenbaum scissors are inserted into the edges of the fascial incision proximally and distally and advanced under the skin, completing the fasciotomy (FIGURE 5). The lateral compartment is incised similarly within the same site. Care is taken not to injure the superficial branch of the peroneal nerve which lies adjacent to the intermuscular septum between the anterior and lateral compartments (FIGURE 2A,B).

POSTOPERATIVE CARE The leg wounds are dressed with saline wet-to-dry dressings. Often the leg may need elevated to minimize edema and sometimes an elastic wrap is appropriate, taking care not to impair perfusion further. Wounds are inspected at least daily and assessed as to the ability to close them primarily or if an alternate management would be more appropriate (i.e., vacuum-assisted closure, healing by secondary intention, or skin grafting). Infection, bleeding, and nerve injury are the most common complications. ∎

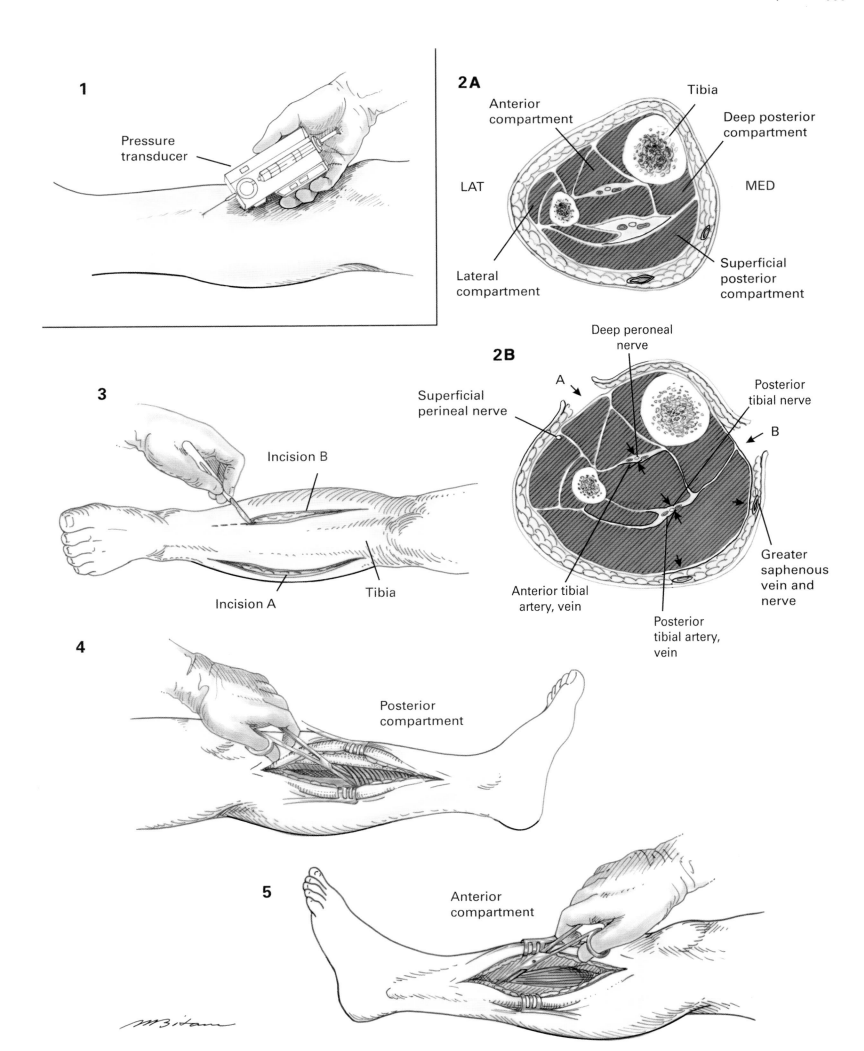

1

Pressure transducer

2A

Anterior compartment

Tibia

Deep posterior compartment

LAT

MED

Lateral compartment

Superficial posterior compartment

3

Incision B

Incision A

Tibia

2B

Deep peroneal nerve

Superficial perineal nerve

A

Posterior tibial nerve

B

Anterior tibial artery, vein

Greater saphenous vein and nerve

Posterior tibial artery, vein

4

Posterior compartment

5

Anterior compartment

ESCHAROTOMY

INDICATIONS When the skin suffers a full-thickness burn (eschar) it loses its elasticity. At the same time, there is a shifting of fluid in the underlying subcutaneous tissues into the adjacent interstitial space. With this fluid shift comes an increase in tissue pressure. The inelasticity of the overlying burned skin, when it is circumferential on an extremity, can cause these tissue pressures to exceed the pulse pressure, thereby compromising blood flow to the extremity. On the anterior trunk, a full-thickness burn eschar can compromise respiratory mechanics, which is seen clinically as the inability of the patient to ventilate followed by the inability to oxygenate. To relieve these pressures and restore perfusion and/or correct respiratory mechanics, escharotomies are performed.

PREOPERATIVE PREPARATION Attention should be given to hemodynamic stability of the patient, as well as close fluid and electrolyte management in the case of burn patients. Preoperative antibiotics are essential to prevent infection.

ANESTHESIA Because all cutaneous nerves have been destroyed in the area of full-thickness burn, no anesthetic is required prior to performing an escharotomy.

DETAILS OF PROCEDURE For escharotomy, using either a scalpel or electrocautery set to "CUT," incisions are made through the entire thickness of the circumferential eschar until subcutaneous fat is observed. The escharotomy incision should be placed on the medial and lateral aspect of the circumferential full-thickness extremity burn and should extend the entire length of the eschar (FIGURES 1 and 2). On the anterior chest, the escharotomies should be made along the lateral aspects of the trunk, with additional incisions placed across the upper trunk and lower trunk so that they form a rectangle (FIGURE 3). When performing escharotomies on the hand, the incisions should be placed on the dorsum between the metacarpals. If necessary, they can be extended onto the ulnar aspect of each digit (FIGURE 4).

When correctly made, the eschar will expand open and the subcutaneous fat will be seen (FIGURE 1). If subcutaneous fat is not observed, the escharotomy should be made deeper. Any bleeding encountered after the escharotomy has been performed is venous and will stop with application of thrombin-soaked pads.

POSTOPERATIVE CARE Escharotomies are covered with the same burn dressings being used to cover the associated full-thickness burn. Escharotomies are not closed. Because they exist in full-thickness burn, eventually they will be included in the debridement of the burn wound. Management of the patient's concomitant medical problems is of utmost priority. ■

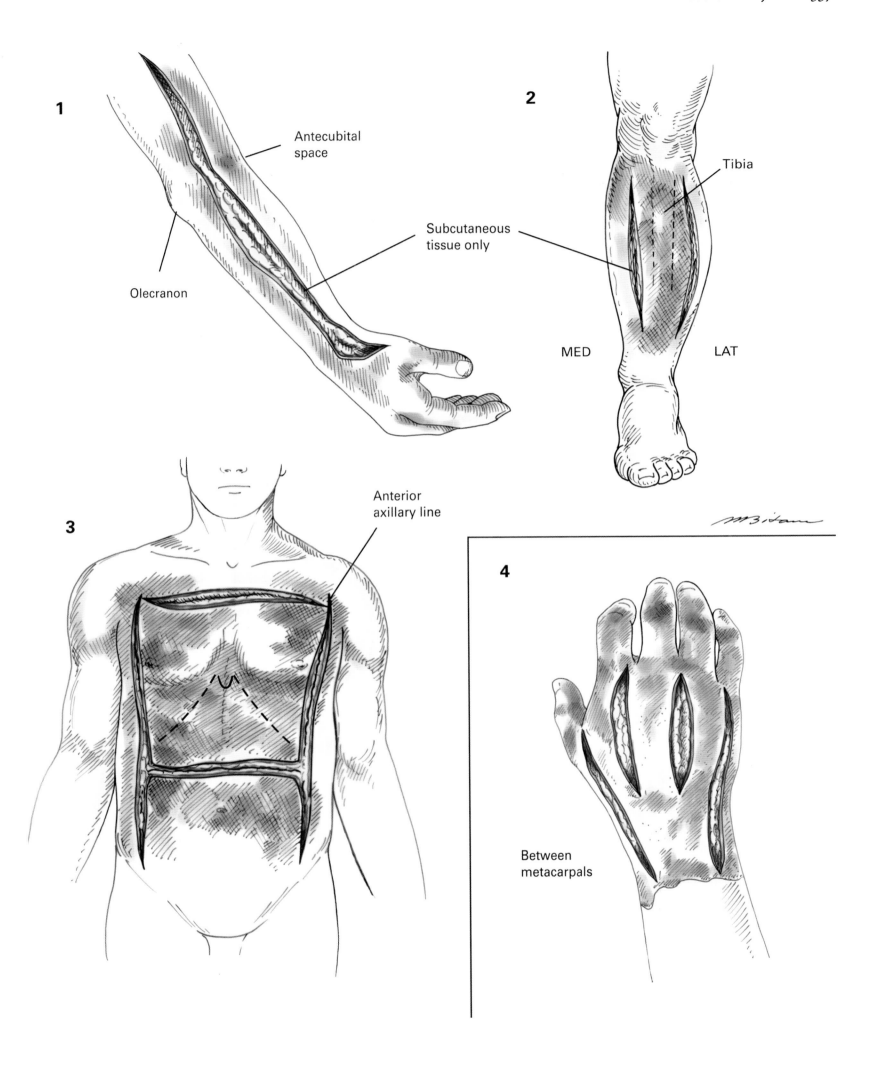

1

Antecubital space

Olecranon

Subcutaneous tissue only

2

Tibia

MED   LAT

3

Anterior axillary line

4

Between metacarpals

PRINCIPLES OF AMPUTATION

INDICATIONS The common factors indicating amputation of a part of the body are trauma, interference with the vascular supply, malignant neoplasm, chronic osteomyelitis, life-threatening infections, inoperable congenital limb deformity in children, the need to increase function, and, occasionally, the cosmetic effect.

PREOPERATIVE PREPARATION In the presence of trauma, it is first necessary to evaluate carefully the overall health and status of the patient to evaluate if limb salvage is possible. Next, the extent of tissue and vascular damage in the extremity must be evaluated. With the recent advances in peripheral vascular repair and grafting, reestablishment of distal blood is often possible. With diabetes or advanced vascular disease, the usual strict medical measures are taken to regulate these associated diseases. If there is localized skin infection at the proposed level for amputation, the procedure is delayed whenever possible. In the presence of wet gangrene, packing the leg in ice or dry ice combined with the application of a tourniquet just below the site of proposed amputation not only may lessen toxicity but also may decrease the incidence of wound infection, since the lymphatics may be cleared before amputation. The threat of gas gangrene may be a real one when the arterial supply to the extremity has been severely compromised, either by intra-arterial occlusion or trauma with inadequate debridement and a closed-space infection. A staged amputation with the first surgery providing a "drainage amputation" may help prevent wound problems at the final level of amputation.

ANESTHESIA Spinal anesthesia is commonly used for major amputation of the lower extremities, inhalation anesthesia for major amputations of the upper extremities, and plexus block or local infiltration anesthesia for amputation of the fingers and toes.

POSITION (See Chapter 148, page 561, FIGURE 1) In amputations of the upper extremity, the patient is placed near the edge of the table with the arm extended and abducted to the desired position. For amputations of the lower extremity, the leg may be elevated with several sterile towels under the calf.

OPERATIVE PREPARATION In the absence of infection, the extremity is elevated to encourage venous drainage before a tourniquet is applied. The tourniquet is placed above the knee for amputations of the lower leg and foot, high in the thigh for amputations of the knee and lower thigh, and above the elbow to control the brachial artery for major amputations of the forearm. In cases of arteriosclerosis, the tourniquet should not be used because of the possibility of damaging the blood supply to the stump. Sterile elastic bands may be applied to the base of the digit for minor amputations. The skin is prepared with the usual antiseptic solutions well above and below the proposed site of amputation. In major amputations, the entire extremity may be wrapped in and impervious stockinette to enable the assistant to hold it and change its position as desired.

SITES FOR AMPUTATION The efficiency of modern prosthesis has eliminated the time-honored "sites of election." Generally, the pathology dictates the site of amputation, with the goal of preserving all possible length. This is particularly true of the upper extremity, although in the lower extremity, whenever possible, the knee should be saved, since it provides major functional advantages. Although the blood supply to the upper extremity is usually adequate, the reverse is often true for the lower extremity. Since an inadequate blood supply, often after failure of a vascular bypass graft, is the most common indication for amputating the lower extremity.

Since the profunda femoral artery tends to be the main channel after occlusion of the superficial femoral vessels or thrombosed femoral-popliteal bypass graft, the site of amputation must be selected well within the zone adequately supplied by the vessel. Accordingly, the amputation is frequently above the knee (See FIGURE 1C). Knee disarticulation (C) and transcondylar

amputation (B) yield an enlarged, rounded end that is cumbersome and difficult to fit with a prosthesis.

The rule of saving all possible length does not necessarily apply to below-knee amputation. Since the anterior margin of the tibia is usually beveled to prevent a pressure point at the stump, there must be enough solid tissue with good blood supply to cover it, as provided by a long posterior flap which is transposed anteriorly over the stump. A short below-knee stump is preferable to knee disarticulation. Ideally, for a below the knee amputation, at least 8 cm of tibia (as measured from the tibial tuberosity) should be preserved to fit into a prosthetic. A below-knee amputation longer than 20 cm is probably not any more functionally effective. A very short fibula tends to migrate laterally and may be removed in a short below-knee stump.

Although ankle and midfoot amputations have few indications, chiefly trauma, the Syme amputation lends itself to a very serviceable end–weight-bearing prosthesis, but it has cosmetic disadvantages in females (FIGURE 1 D). There is general agreement that a most satisfactory foot amputation is the transmetatarsal (see FIGURE 5, A-A and Long Plantar Flap). In the presence of vascular insufficiency to the lower extremity, amputations about the ankle or foot should be rarely performed only for secure indications, because they frequently heal poorly, necessitating higher level amputations.

Formerly, the junction of the lower and middle thirds of the forearm was considered the optimum site for amputations; however, newer artificial limbs that include pronation and supination movements make it desirable to save all possible length (FIGURE 2). Length is again important in the hand, where a partial amputation of the fingers or of all fingers, leaving an opposing surface at the thumb for gripping, allows better function than can be provided by any prosthesis. A stump of any length in the forearm will give better function than an amputation above the elbow, and it eliminates an elbow hinge in a prosthesis.

TYPES OF FLAPS As a general rule it is desirable to have the scar in the posterior of the stump in the upper extremity, since the prosthesis bears largely on the distal surfaces of the stump. The scar for end-bearing stumps of the lower extremity should preferably be placed away from areas of direct pressure. In minor amputations of the fingers and toes, long palmar and plantar flaps are made to cover the stump with a thick, protective pad of tissue (FIGURES 3, 4, and 6A). Racket incisions are advisable for amputations of the toes, since they may be extended upward to permit exposure of the metatarsals (FIGURE 5), or they may be used for amputations of digits where all possible length must be preserved. This is especially true for injuries of the thumb (Incisions B, C, and D, FIGURE 6). Racket incisions with removal of the head of the metacarpal or metatarsal give a good appearance to the extremity but considerably diminish the breadth of the foot or palm.

DETAILS OF PROCEDURE Sufficient soft tissue must be present to approximate easily over the end of the bone, but excessive amounts are avoided, since bulky soft tissue hinders the fitting of a prosthesis. Arteries and veins should be tied individually. Nerves are divided with nonabsorbable sutures at as high a level as possible and buried within muscle bellies to prevent neuroma formation. It should be remote from scar and away from areas of pressure, since a neuroma becomes symptomatic when pressure is applied. The bone should be divided at a sufficiently high level to permit the soft parts to approximate, producing a thick covering for its end. The sharp margins of bone are beveled either with a rongeur or rasp.

CLOSURE Hemostasis is achieved and a closed-suction drain may be placed in the deep space in larger amputations. The investing fascia is loosely approximated with interrupted absorbable sutures. If a guillotine "drainage" type of amputation was carried out in the presence of a progressing infection, the wound is left open to be closed secondarily later, or the extremity is reamputated later at a higher lever to permit primary closure.

POSTOPERATIVE CARE (See Chapter 148, page 562). ∎

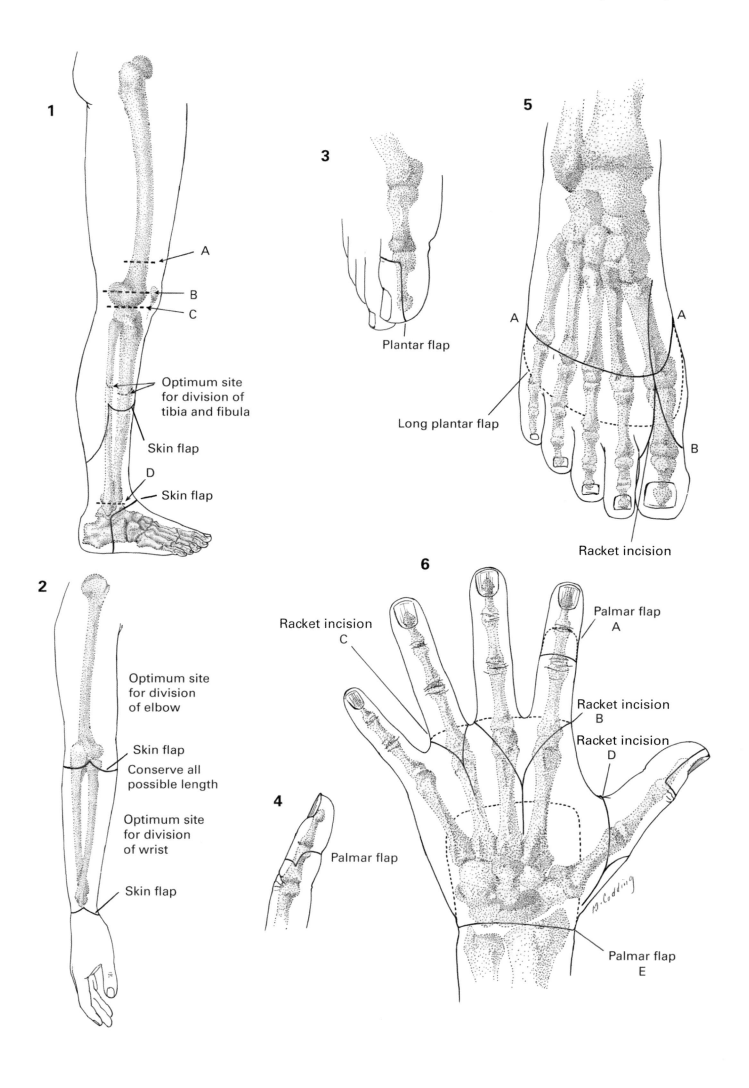

1

A
B
C

Optimum site
for division of
tibia and fibula

Skin flap

D

Skin flap

2

Optimum site
for division
of elbow

Skin flap
Conserve all
possible length

Optimum site
for division
of wrist

Skin flap

3

Plantar flap

4

Palmar flap

5

A   A

B

Long plantar flap

Racket incision

6

Racket incision
C

Palmar flap
A

Racket incision
B

Racket incision
D

Palmar flap
E

INDICATIONS Common indications for supracondylar amputation include trauma, poor blood supply, tumor, and progressive untreatable. Amputation should not be performed unless all conservative measures have failed.

The amputation at the level of the thigh is described in detail here. This is a frequent site following failure of reconstructive or bypass arterial procedures or in the presence of unreconstructable circumstances as documented with proximal and distal arteriography.

PREOPERATIVE PREPARATION The preoperative preparation must of necessity vary with the indications for amputation as outlined in the preceding section. Careful evaluation must be made to determine whether there is a localized arterial obstruction, and arteriography is essential. If localized obstruction is present, a proximal (e.g., an iliac stent or aortofemoral) reconstructive procedure may restore an adequate blood inflow, or a distal (e.g., femoropopliteal) bypass arterial graft may eliminate the need for amputation.

When infection is present, aggressive surgical debridement is the most critical step for success. Appropriate antibiotic regimens should be tailored based on documented sensitivities. Should there be a localized skin infection at the proposed level of amputation, the procedure is delayed if improvement is possible. In the presence of an advancing infection a guillotine or open amputation is done above the level of infection, with a subsequent definitive amputation at a higher point a few days later or when sepsis has cleared.

For elective amputations, preoperative consultation with physical therapy and a prosthetist can help the patient be emotionally and physically ready for the rehabilitation required after amputation surgery.

ANESTHESIA Low spinal anesthesia is used most frequently, although inhalation anesthesia may be administered unless the patient's condition contraindicates it.

POSITION The patient is placed with the hip on the affected side out to the margin of the table to allow full abduction of the thigh by an assistant, and the calf or ankle may be elevated with several sterile towels. The hair is clipped at the operative level.

OPERATIVE PREPARATION The skin from the lower abdomen to well below the knee is prepped. A sterile sheet is placed beneath the thigh. The foot and lower leg up to the knee are covered with an impervious stockinette (FIGURE 1). Unless there is evidence of progressive infection, the extremity is elevated by the assistant to encourage venous drainage. If a low amputation is planned, a sterile tourniquet can be applied high on the thigh.

INCISION AND EXPOSURE The type of flap that is used varies. With progressive infection of the lower leg, a circular incision is made for a guillotine amputation. However, when possible, anterior and posterior flaps are outlined with a sterile marking pen, ensuring an appropriate stump length (FIGURE 1). Either equal anterior and posterior flaps are used or, more commonly, a larger anterior flap is utilized to place the final closure line away from the pressure points of the prosthesis.

The surgeon stands on the inner side of the thigh so as to visualize better the main arterial and nerve supply, and outlines the selected incision. Since the skin and soft tissues retract considerably and to allow for rotation of the skin edges, the skin incision should extend 10 to 15 cm below the point where the bone is to be divided. The incision is carried through the skin and subcutaneous tissue down to the fascia over the underlying muscles.

DETAILS OF PROCEDURE The surgeon must be familiar with the location of the major nerves and vessels (FIGURE 2). The most superficial vessels to be ligated is the great saphenous vein, located on the medial or posteromedial aspect of the thigh, depending on the level of amputation (FIGURES 2 and 3). The muscles should be divided at a slightly higher level than the skin and fascia and allowed to retract upward so that the final flaps for closure will consist chiefly of skin and fascia (FIGURE 4). The median incision into the muscle layer is made carefully and the femoral vessels are identified deep to the vastus medialis muscle (FIGURE 5). If a tourniquet has not been applied, the surgeon should locate the major vessel by palpation or by its visible pulsation. If a tourniquet has been used, the dissection is carried out directly until the femoral vein is exposed. This is divided between half-length clamps. Both artery and vein are tied separately (FIGURE 5), and, if desired, a transfixing tie may be added distal to the original ligature on the femoral artery.

The sciatic nerve is located posterior to the femoral vessels and is isolated from the surrounding tissues. In the event of a high amputation with bifurcation of the sciatic nerve, the tibial and peroneal nerves are individually ligated. In an effort to minimize the formation of an amputation neuroma, the nerve is pulled down as far as possible, and a strong straight Ochsner clamp is applied. A second similar crushing clamp is applied about 5 mm distal to the first clamp and the nerve divided immediately below the second clamp. The proximal clamp is removed, and the crushed area is ligated with a heavy 0 ligature of nonabsorbable suture (FIGURE 6). Fine ligatures are avoided, lest the epineural sheath be cut through, permitting the formation of a neuroma. Absorbable ligatures are avoided since they may be absorbed before the epineural sheath has united, causing the sheath to reopen with the formation of a neuroma. The distal clamp is then removed, leaving a crushed and flattened short segment of nerve that tends to prevent the ligature from slipping off. The nerve is allowed to retract well upward into the muscle layers. It should never be anchored to adjacent structures. When the sciatic nerve has retracted upward, the tissues are further freed from the posterior surface of the femur. The profunda femoris artery and vein must be secured and ligated in the posterior group of muscles (FIGURE 2). **CONTINUES ▶**

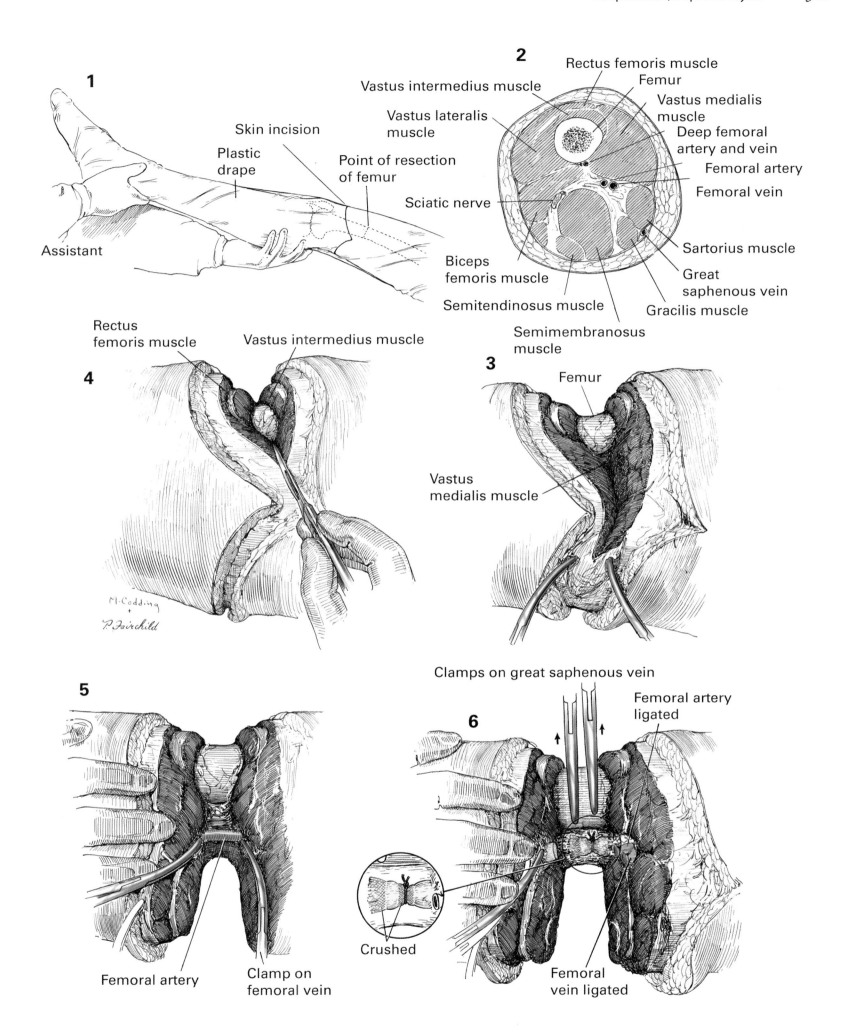

1

Assistant

Skin incision

Plastic drape

Point of resection of femur

2

Rectus femoris muscle

Femur

Vastus intermedius muscle

Vastus medialis muscle

Vastus lateralis muscle

Deep femoral artery and vein

Femoral artery

Femoral vein

Sciatic nerve

Biceps femoris muscle

Sartorius muscle

Great saphenous vein

Gracilis muscle

Semitendinosus muscle

Semimembranosus muscle

4

Rectus femoris muscle

Vastus intermedius muscle

M. Codding
+
P. Fairchild

3

Femur

Vastus medialis muscle

5

Femoral artery

Clamp on femoral vein

6

Clamps on great saphenous vein

Femoral artery ligated

Crushed

Femoral vein ligated

DETAILS OF PROCEDURE ◀CONTINUED▶ The femur is then circumferentially freed from all soft tissue and the level of bone amputation is identified with preservation of good anterior and posterior skin flaps. A circular incision is made through the periosteum of the femur at the level of the amputation (FIGURE 7), and the inferior periosteum is elevated to allow for clean bone to be cut (FIGURE 8). Retraction and protection of the muscle are maintained while the femur is divided with a power saw at the desired level (FIGURE 9). The amputated part is removed from the surgical field.

The sharp margins of the bone at the site of amputation are beveled off with a rongeur or rasp (FIGURE 10). If a tourniquet has been used, it is now removed, and any additional bleeding points are clamped and tied. The muscle surface is washed with warm isotonic saline until the surgeon is assured that there is good hemostasis and all bone fragments are washed away. A deep drain may be placed and is left to the discretion of the surgeon and the condition of the wound.

CLOSURE The anterior and posterior flaps are inspected for appropriate length and they can be trimmed as needed to allow for a snug (but not tight) closure. The deep investing muscle fascia anteriorly and posteriorly are approximated with interrupted sutures over the end of the femur (FIGURE 11). Scarpa's fascia is next approximated with interrupted absorbable sutures (FIGURE 11) to take tension off of the skin closure. If a guillotine type of amputation was carried out, the wound is left open to be closed later in a delayed manner, or the limb may be reamputated at a higher level to permit primary closure.

The skin flaps are tailored to an appropriate shape and skin closure is performed by the surgeon's preference (FIGURES 11 and 12). In general, interrupted nonabsorbable monofilament sutures provide good closure without undue tissue ischemia, and forceps trauma to the skin edges should be avoided.

POSTOPERATIVE CARE The stump is covered with a nonadherent dressing and fluffs of sterile gauze and is encased in a dressing that is snug but not too tight. This dressing may have to be changed in 24 hours, since the stump may swell, resulting in pain as well as interference with the blood supply. If edema of the tissues is a concern, an incisional vacuum sponge dressing along the incision lines can be placed over nonadherent gauze. The immediate postoperative care includes continued insulin regulation in the diabetic. To combat swelling, the foot of the bed but not the stump may be elevated. Splints may be applied at the time of surgery to maintain exten-

sion and prevent flexion contractures, but these must be removed early so that exercises can be started in a few days.

Guillotine amputations require special care if no further surgical intervention is planned. If eventual higher level amputation is planned, regular dressing changes are performed until surgery. For guillotine amputations which will be required to heal (usually due to patient factors that prevent them from having further surgery), progressive skin traction devices can be applied to the skin to facilitate skin edge migration. In some cases this will be sufficient to cover the bone ends, and healing will take place; however, when the skin cannot be brought together in this way, dressing changes can be performed until there is secondary closure.

After initial healing of the wound, efforts to contour the amputation stump to fit a prosthesis are performed. With the assistance of occupational therapy, cotton-elastic bandages can be wrapped around the stump and worn continuously to aid shrinkage of the stump. The bandages are removed and reapplied every 4 hours and at bedtime, and a clean bandage is used every day. The amputee or members of the family are taught to apply the bandage. Another option is a heavy elastic sock called a "stump shrinker" that fits over the stump and applies circumferential pressure.

Crutch walking requires more energy than walking with a prosthesis. The best single indicator of whether the patient will be able to use a prosthesis is whether he was ambulatory prior to the amputation. Important also is the presence of other serious illnesses, poor vision, condition of the other leg, degree of cooperation and alertness, as well as balance and degree of coordination. Patients who can walk with crutches likely can walk with a prosthesis.

Most patients after amputation describe phantom sensations and should be considered a normal part of the recovery. Phantom sensations in the lower extremity always remain in a normal relation to other parts of the body and disappear in most instances when a prosthesis is applied. The degree of phantom pain is largely dependent upon the degree of pain before amputation, but it may occur because of radiculopathy, position during operation, or when a neuroma is caught in the scar or in an area vulnerable to pressure. Exercising the phantom can be helpful and referral to physical and occupational therapy can help alleviate symptoms. A planned program of rehabilitation is very important regardless of the type and extent of the amputation, and a coordinated follow-up involving the surgeon, physical therapist, and prosthetist is necessary. When elective amputation is planned, the physical therapist can teach crutch walking and instruct the patient in proper exercise before operation. ■

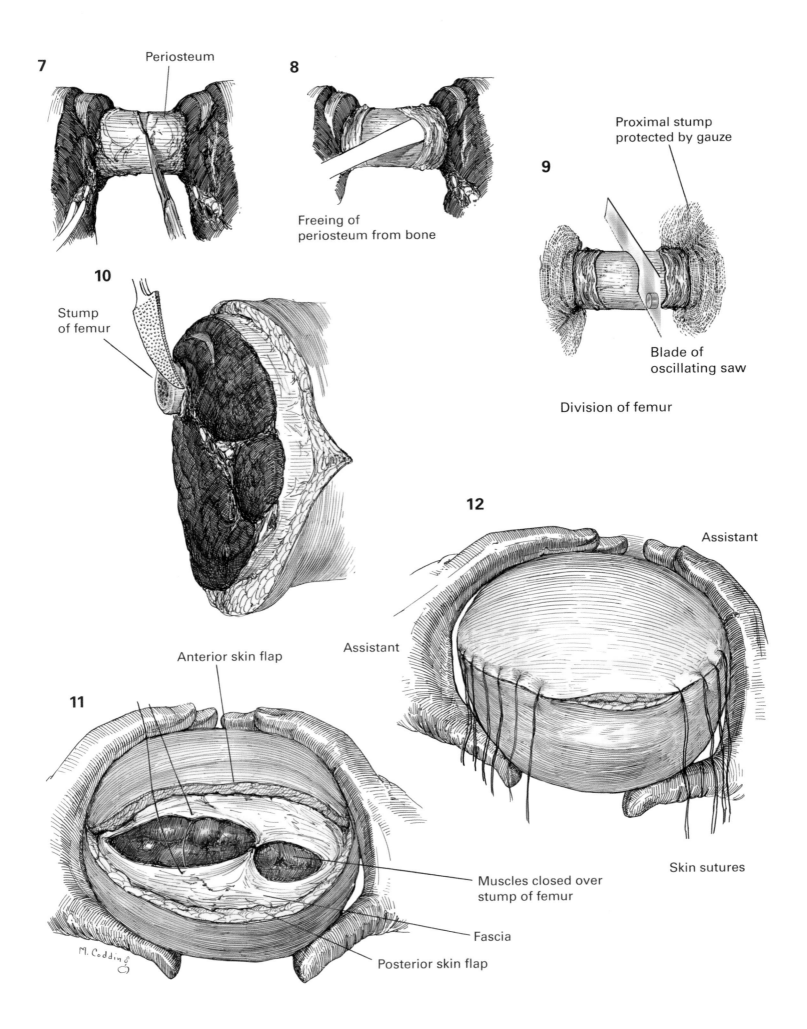

7

Periosteum

8

Freeing of
periosteum from bone

9

Proximal stump
protected by gauze

Blade of
oscillating saw

Division of femur

10

Stump
of femur

12

Assistant

Assistant

Skin sutures

11

Anterior skin flap

Muscles closed over
stump of femur

Fascia

Posterior skin flap

M. Codding

INCISION AND DRAINAGE OF INFECTIONS OF THE HAND

INDICATIONS Although definitive indications for incision and drainage of infections of the hand vary with the location, duration, extent, and severity of the infection, most localized infections warrant incision and drainage or operative debridement. Particular attention must be paid to patients with immunocompromised conditions that might mask an adequate inflammatory response and delay diagnosis and treatment. Most infections arising on the volar surface of the hand produce maximal swelling on the dorsum; however, dorsal drainage is used only when suppuration presents on the dorsum. If necrotizing fasciitis is suspected, either streptococcal or polymicrobial, emergent and aggressive operative debridement is warranted.

PREOPERATIVE PREPARATION If surgery cannot be performed immediately or the diagnosis of deep infection is uncertain, immobilization, rest, and elevation of the extremity in combination with aggressive broad-spectrum antibiotic therapy are initial treatments. Once the diagnosis of abscess is made, incision and drainage are performed. Patients with comorbidities must be evaluated and treated appropriately, particularly glucose control in diabetic patients. Patients with a history of tobacco abuse should be counseled to stop all nicotine products to facilitate wound healing.

ANESTHESIA Various anesthetic blocks can be used depending on the level and extent of anesthesia required. Axillary, brachial plexus, and Bier blocks may be used for complete anesthesia of the forearm and hand. Regional blocks of the median, ulnar, or radial nerve at the wrist can be performed with a high level of reliability. Digital blocks can be performed either through a volar or dorsal approach, taking care to prevent excessive infiltration around the base of the digit, which can cause digital compartment syndrome and threaten circulation. Epinephrine in the can be used in a dilute solution, but care should be taken, especially in patients with poor circulation. General anesthesia is used for more extensive infections or in cases where regional anesthesia cannot be performed safely.

POSITION The patient is placed in a supine position with the involved hand on an arm table.

OPERATIVE PREPARATION Routine skin preparation of the hand is performed. Except for minor procedures, a tourniquet set to 250 mm Hg is placed on the upper arm. In infectious cases, gravity exsanguination is preferred over active (elastic bandage) exsanguination to prevent the hematologic spread of infection.

A. FELON

DETAILS OF PROCEDURE Immediate drainage is imperative to relieve increased tension and prevent development of osteomyelitis of the distal phalanx. For a deeply situated abscess, the incision can be made longitudinally along the ulnar side of the digit 3-mm volar to the nail edge. Incisions along the radial side of the digit should be avoided to prevent painful scar with pinch maneuvers. Alternatively, a longitudinal incision centered on the volar pad can be performed. Regardless of the approach, blunt dissection volar to the distal phalanx through the septae of the pulp should be thorough, releasing all compartments where infection could reside (FIGURES 1 to 3). Care must be taken not to enter the tendon sheath. The wound should be copiously irrigated and packed with light gauze and the wound left to heal secondarily.

B. PARONYCHIA

DETAILS OF PROCEDURE Acute paronychia is the most common infection of the hand. Acute unilateral paronychia requires elevation of the cuticle from the nail at the site of infection (FIGURE 4). If the infection is advanced or proximal abscess is present, removal of the proximal portion of the nail plate is performed (FIGURES 4 and 5). Minor infections may be treated by incising both cuticles longitudinally and then placing a piece of foil from the suture package or a medicated gauze as a stent beneath to prevent closure of the eponychial fold (FIGURES 6A, B and C). The entire nail plate may need to be removed in more extensive infection. Recurrent or chronic paronychia should be evaluated for fungal infection and may need marsupialization of the nail plate (FIGURES 7A, B and C).

C. INFECTIONS OF TENDON SHEATHS

DETAILS OF PROCEDURE The flexor sheaths originate just distal to the distal interphalangeal joint and extend to the palmar flexion crease. The sheath of the flexor pollicis longus continues to the radial bursa and the flexor sheath of the little finger is confluent with the ulnar bursa (FIGURE 8). For early infections (less than 24 hours) without evidence of abscess, conservative treatment with broad-spectrum intravenous antibiotics, splinting, elevation, and frequent physical examination can be performed. If moderate infection is present, drainage can be performed with a limited incision approach proximally and distally in the sheath to allow for an indwelling irrigation catheter (FIGURE 9). The proximal incision is transversely oriented at the distal palmar flexion crease and the distal incision is obliquely oriented over the middle phalanx or along with midlateral line to expose the flexor tendon sheaths. Care is taken to prevent injury to the neurovascular bundles by staying central over the volar aspect of the digit. Longitudinal spreading of tissues can help expose the tendon sheath while protecting the neurovascular structures from injury. Extensive infection should be approached through ulnar midaxial incisions on digits 2, 3, and 4 and radial on the thumb and small finger (FIGURE 10). Care must be taken to avoid the digital neurovascular structures. After drainage, loose approximation of the skin is performed with interrupted permanent sutures to allow for any postoperative drainage. A postoperative splint should be applied for comfort. For all infections, cultures and sensitivities should be performed with directed antibiotic coverage.

D. INFECTIONS OF THE DEEP PALMAR SPACES

DETAILS OF PROCEDURE Most abscesses of the interdigital spaces may be drained through incisions placed longitudinally over the dorsal web-space, preventing a painful scar on the volar surface (FIGURE 11). If the infection is near the volar surface, a second volar incision may be indicated. Midpalmar space infections should be approached volarly in a curved longitudinal incision (FIGURE 10). Isolated deep infections of the thenar and hypothenar spaces are rare and can be approached through a longitudinal dorsal approach (FIGURE 11). Parona's space connects the thenar and midpalmar spaces in the distal forearm, just superficial to the pronator quadratus. It can be approached through a longitudinal incision just ulnar to the palmaris tendon (FIGURE 11). Care should be taken to prevent injury to the median nerve. As in the case for most infections, cultures should be obtained and broad-spectrum antibiotics administered until culture-directed treatment can be implemented.

POSTOPERATIVE CARE For felons and paronychia, dressing changes and early return of motion are indicated, usually on the following day with gradual increase in range of motion. For tendon sheath and deep space infections, antibiotics are continued in a culture-directed manner. Dressing changes are performed several times a day. Irrigation catheters can usually be removed 2 to 3 days after placement. Once overt infection has improved, gentle movements are encouraged and increased as tolerated. Elevation of the extremity to heart level will lessen discomfort during the period of immobilization until swelling has cleared. Frequently, these patients need to be evaluated and treated by dedicated hand therapy specialists to maximize recovery. ■

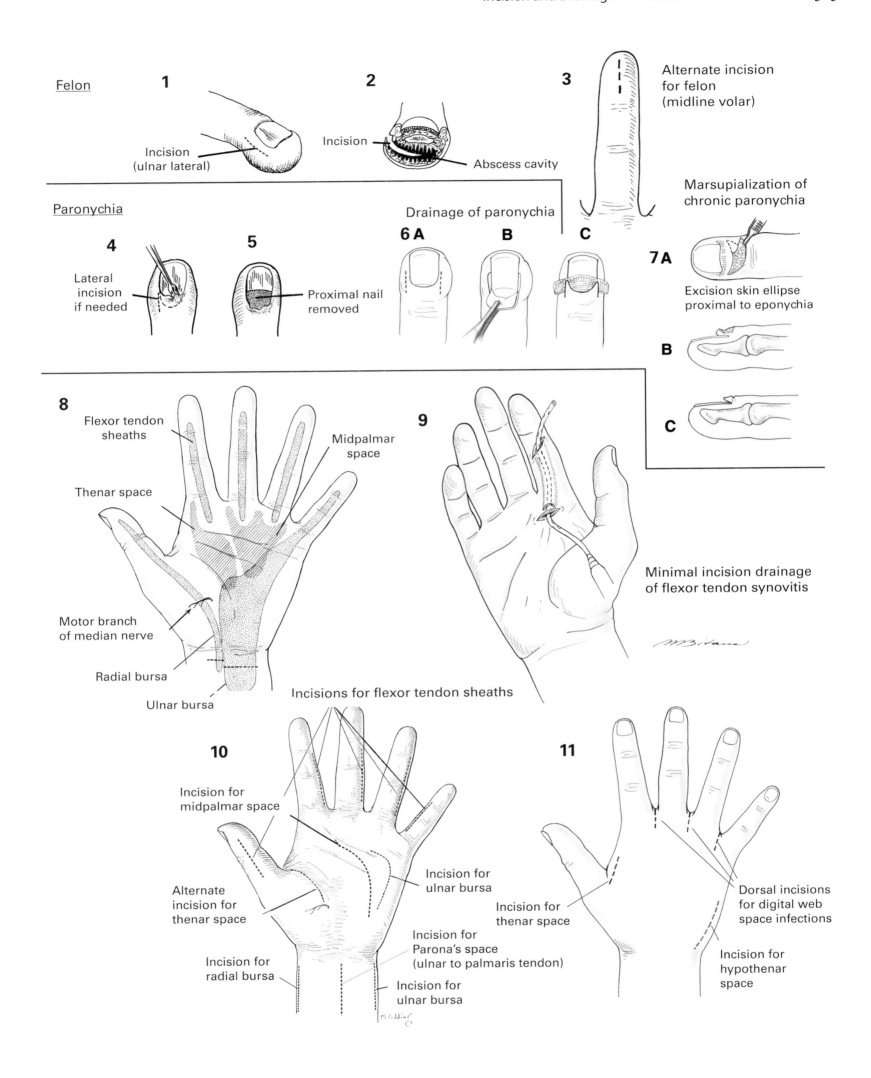

Felon

1

Incision
(ulnar lateral)

2

Incision

Abscess cavity

3

Alternate incision
for felon
(midline volar)

Paronychia

4

Lateral
incision
if needed

5

Proximal nail
removed

Drainage of paronychia

6 A   **B**   **C**

Marsupialization of
chronic paronychia

7A

Excision skin ellipse
proximal to eponychia

B

C

8

Flexor tendon
sheaths

Midpalmar
space

Thenar space

Motor branch
of median nerve

Radial bursa

Ulnar bursa

9

Minimal incision drainage
of flexor tendon synovitis

Incisions for flexor tendon sheaths

10

Incision for
midpalmar space

Alternate
incision for
thenar space

Incision for
radial bursa

Incision for
ulnar bursa

Incision for
Parona's space
(ulnar to palmaris tendon)

Incision for
ulnar bursa

11

Incision for
thenar space

Dorsal incisions
for digital web
space infections

Incision for
hypothenar
space

SUTURE OF TENDON

INDICATIONS Repair of the lacerated flexor tendon should only be performed under ideal conditions, because the best (and sometimes only) opportunity for a good functional result is the first attempt at repair. Presence of severe contamination, infection, or massive tissue destruction should be a contraindication for immediate repair. Debridement and wound preparation should be performed first with delayed repair performed at a later time.

There are five zones of injury for flexor tendons (FIGURE 1). Each zone has its own method of repair. Traditionally, zone II injuries (within the flexor tendon sheath) were known as "no man's land" because of the poor results of repairs in this zone. Today, with proper surgical repair and aggressive and comprehensive rehabilitation by a specialized hand therapy service, even these patients can have satisfactory return of function.

ANESTHESIA General or axillary block anesthesia may be used. Regional blocks of the wrist or elbow of the median, ulnar, and radial nerves can also be performed. These blocks can be of benefit in the emergency room while the patient is awaiting surgery. Digital blocks are generally of little use in this setting.

OPERATIVE PREPARATION Prior to surgery, the wound should be cleansed thoroughly (as tolerated) in the emergency room and a sterile dressing applied. Once adequate anesthesia is obtained, exsanguination of the arm is performed with gravity or an elastic bandage and a tourniquet should be placed on the upper arm. In the normal adult, a blood pressure cuff is inflated to 250 mm Hg, or at least 80 mm Hg above systolic blood pressure. This tourniquet may be left inflated for 2 hours. It may be reinflated again after a 20-minute period of normal circulation. The wound is then uncovered and thoroughly irrigated with several liters of warm saline.

INCISION AND EXPOSURE Exposure must be adequate. It is usually necessary to extend the original limits of the wound (FIGURE 2). However, care must be taken that the extending incisions do not injure neurovascular structures and will not cause scar contracture across the joints. Incisions in the digits should be based on the laceration pattern. For oblique lacerations on the digit, Brunner-style diagonal extensions between interphalangeal joints should be utilized, creating a zig-zag pattern along the volar surface. For transverse lacerations, midaxial incisions should be performed to prevent narrow skin flaps. It is imperative to keep the digital skin flaps widely based to prevent ischemia. The neurovascular bundles of the digits lie along the lateral volar surface of the digit and should be protected at all costs. Poorly made incisions may result in skin compromise and deformity.

DETAILS OF PROCEDURE Debridement and exploration of the involved area are carried out. Adjacent nerves and vessels are identified and retracted. Frequently nerve and vascular injury can be identified and should be repaired. If possible, the tendon ends are located in the wound and gently grasped with forceps (FIGURE 3). Gentle tissue handling is of utmost importance, as crush injury to the tendon can lead to poor healing, gapping of the repair, and eventual failure. In general, lacerations that involve less than half of the cross section of the tendon do not need to be repaired. The loose fibers should only be trimmed to prevent catching of the tendon on the flexor pulleys. Larger cross-sectional injuries require repair. Depending on the location of the laceration, the proximal tendon stump may retract and require maneuvers to retrieve it. Retrieval should be atraumatic and under direct visualization if possible. Flexing the wrist and elbow and squeezing the volar muscles of the forearm can help deliver the proximal stump to

the incision. Sometimes counter incisions proximal in the palm or forearm need to be performed to identify the tendon. Generally, the distal segment is identified easily with finger flexion. In multiple tendon injury cases, care must be taken to confirm the anatomy and orientation of the proximal and distal tendons. General principles of tendon suturing have evolved over time, with both multistrand core sutures and epitendinous sutures maximizing outcomes. A running, epitendinous suture line of 6-0 permanent monofilament suture provides both strength and a smooth gliding surface. Frequently the "back wall" epitendinous repair will be performed first, followed by a multistrand core suture repair with 3-0 or 4-0 permanent suture, finished by epitendinous repair of the "front wall" to complete the repair. For both epitendinous and core suturing, there are several methods described (FIGURES 4 and 5). The most reliable core sutures are performed with locking four-strand repair techniques and most epitendinous repairs are performed in a running fashion (simple, locking, or horizontal mattress techniques).

Zone I injuries (distal to the insertion of the flexor digitorum superficialis tendon on the middle phalanx) usually require percutaneous button suturing of the proximal tendon to the distal phalanx due to the frequent shortage of distal tendon available (FIGURE 6). If a bone fragment is attached to the tendon, K-wire fixation can be performed. Zone II injuries (within the flexor sheath) are the most difficult cases and should only be attempted by a surgeon experienced with these injuries. Both the flexor digitorum superficialis and profundus tendons (FDS and FDP, respectively) should be repaired. Zone III injuries (in the palm) are generally more straightforward and heal well. Zone IV injuries (within the carpal tunnel under the transverse carpal ligament) are rare and are frequently associated with injuries to the median nerve. Zone V injuries (in the forearm) can be complicated if the injury occurs at the musculotendinous junction, as muscle does not hold sutures securely. Potential injury to the arteries and nerves of the forearm needs to be evaluated.

Once all repairs have been completed, the tourniquet is released and meticulous hemostasis is achieved. The field must be dry before closure is attempted.

CLOSURE Deep soft tissues are approximated to eliminate dead space; subcutaneous tissue and skin are closed in the usual manner with fine sutures.

Nonadherent gauze is placed over the wound and a dorsal block splint is fashioned to prevent extension of the wrist and fingers. It is important to make sure the splint extends beyond the ends of the fingers. The splint is fashioned to keep the fingers and wrist in slight flexion to keep tension off the flexor tendon repair (FIGURE 7). Postoperatively, the hand is kept elevated to reduce edema.

POSTOPERATIVE CARE The initial dressing and splint are kept in place for a couple of days. The patient then is enrolled in a comprehensive hand therapy program monitored by the surgeon and a certified hand therapist. Most programs start with passive exercises in the first week. Depending on the patient's compliance and motivation and the quality of the tendon repair, some patients may start an early active motion protocol. Early motion of tendon repairs has been shown to reduce the amount of scarring and subsequent stiffness in repaired tendons, but is balanced by the increased risk of tendon repair rupture if therapy is more aggressive than the repair can support. Patient compliance with the postoperative therapy is the largest determinant of outcome for tendon laceration repairs. ■

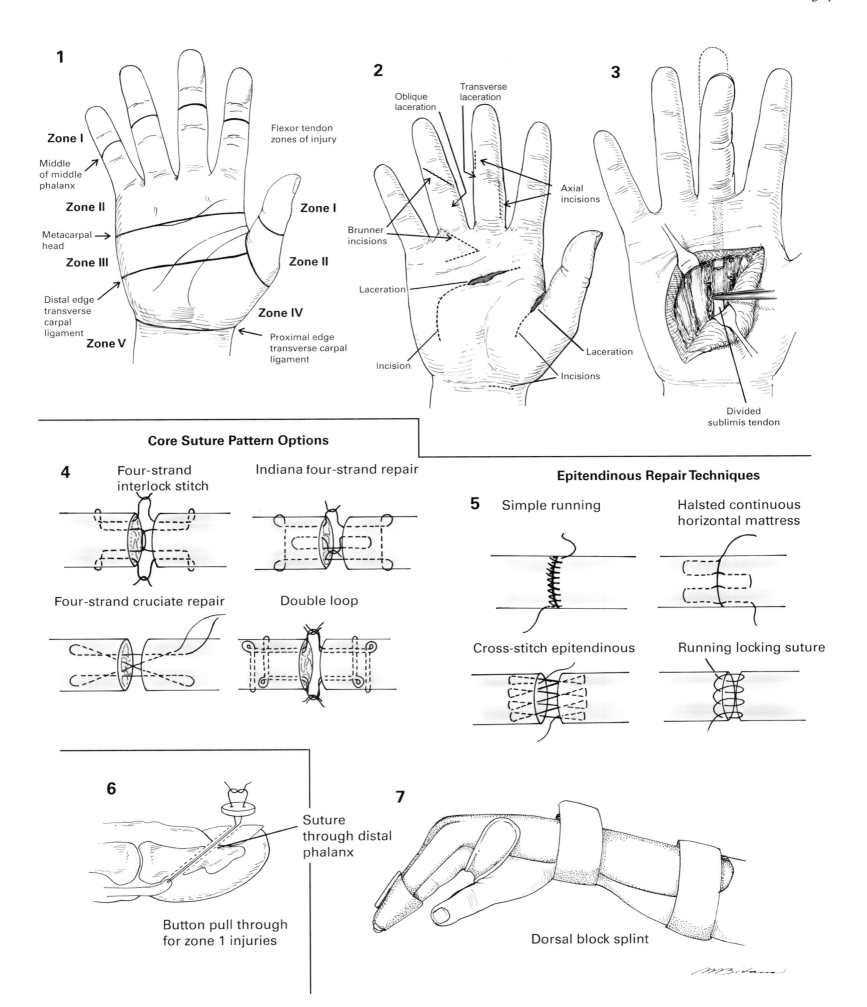

1

Zone I

Middle of middle phalanx

Zone II

Metacarpal head

Zone III

Distal edge transverse carpal ligament

Zone V

Flexor tendon zones of injury

Zone I

Zone II

Zone IV

Proximal edge transverse carpal ligament

2

Oblique laceration

Transverse laceration

Brunner incisions

Axial incisions

Laceration

Incision

Laceration

Incisions

3

Divided sublimis tendon

Core Suture Pattern Options

4

Four-strand interlock stitch

Indiana four-strand repair

Four-strand cruciate repair

Double loop

Epitendinous Repair Techniques

5

Simple running

Halsted continuous horizontal mattress

Cross-stitch epitendinous

Running locking suture

6

Suture through distal phalanx

Button pull through for zone 1 injuries

7

Dorsal block splint

INDEX

Note: Page number followed by f indicates figure only.